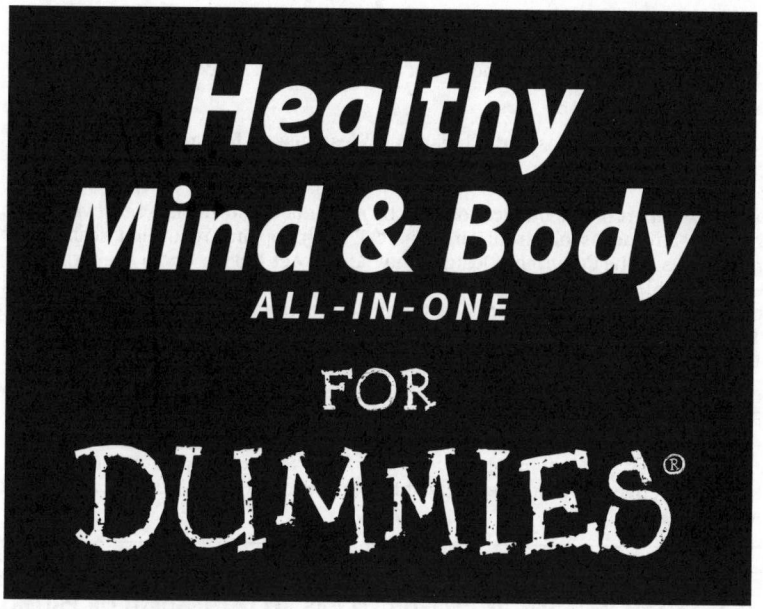

Healthy Mind & Body
ALL-IN-ONE
FOR DUMMIES®

By Sue Baic, Nigel Denby, Allen Elkin,
Charles Elliott, Georg Feuerstein, Ellie Herman,
Elaine Iljon Foreman, Liz Neporent, Larry Payne,
Carol Ann Rinzler, Suzanne Schlosberg
and Laura Smith

Edited by Gillian

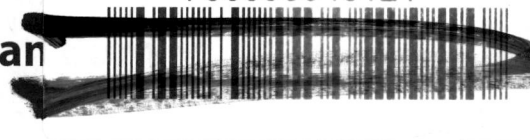

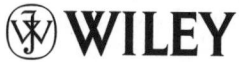

WILEY

A John Wiley and Sons, Ltd, Publication

Healthy Mind & Body All-in-One For Dummies®

Published by
John Wiley & Sons, Ltd
The Atrium
Southern Gate
Chichester
West Sussex
PO19 8SQ
England

Email (for orders and customer service enquires): cs-books@wiley.co.uk

Visit our Home Page on www.wiley.com

For general information on our other products and services, please contact our Customer Care Department within the US at 800-762-2974, outside the US at 317-572-3993, or fax 317-572-4002.

For technical support, please visit www.wiley.com/techsupport.

Wiley also publishes its books in a variety of electronic formats. Some content that appears in print may not be available in electronic books.

British Library Cataloguing in Publication Data: A catalogue record for this book is available from the British Library

ISBN: 978-0-470-74830-5

Printed and bound in Great Britain by TJ International Ltd, Padstow, Cornwall

10 9 8 7 6 5 4 3 2 1

WILEY

About the Authors

Sue Baic is a Lecturer in Nutrition and Public Health in the Department of Exercise and Health Sciences at Bristol University. She has a first degree from Bristol University followed by a Master of Science in Human Nutrition from London University. Sue is a Registered Dietitian (RD) with over 15 years' experience in the field of nutrition and health in the NHS and as a freelance consultant. She feels strongly about providing nutrition information to the public that is evidence-based, up to date, unbiased and reliable.

As a member of the public relations committee of the British Dietetic Association she has written for the media on a variety of nutrition-related health issues. Sue lives in Bristol and spends her spare time running up and down hills in the Cotswolds in an attempt to get fit.

Sue is the co-author of *Nutrition For Dummies* and *The GL Diet For Dummies*.

Gillian Burn has been working in the field of mind and body health for over 25 years. Her background covers nursing, midwifery and health visiting, including experience with the Flying Doctor Service in the Australian outback.

Gillian has an MSc in Exercise and Health and is a qualified master practitioner in Neuro-Linguistic Programming, time line therapy and in creating healthy environments. She is a licensed instructor for Mind Mapping techniques and speed reading with Tony Buzan, and a licensed instructor in Body Control Pilates with the Body Control Pilates Academy.

Gillian is the Director of Health Circles Ltd (www.healthcircles.co.uk), providing training programmes and consultancy services focusing on improving health and quality of life for individuals and companies. Her workshops focus on training people to use their minds and bodies to increase energy and performance. This includes nutrition and exercise advice, understanding the mind and body connection, creating balance and techniques to increase creativity and effectiveness.

Gillian also provides life coaching to help clients create a compelling future to reach their full potential and peak performance. She teaches Pilates classes each week. Gillian aims to practice what she preaches! She rows on the river and enjoys walking, cooking and Pilates while bringing up her young daughter with her partner, John.

Gillian is the Editor of *Personal Development All-in-One For Dummies* published in 2007, and the author of *Motivation For Dummies* published in 2008, both by Wiley. She writes regularly on health related topics.

Nigel Denby trained as a dietitian at Glasgow Caledonian University, following an established career in the catering industry. He is also a qualified chef and previously owned his own restaurant.

His dietetic career began as a Research Dietitian at the Human Nutrition Research Centre in Newcastle upon Tyne. After a period working as a Community Dietitian, Nigel left the NHS to join Boots Health and Beauty Experience where he led the delivery and training of Nutrition and Weight Management services.

In 2003 Nigel set up his own Nutrition Consultancy, delivering a clinical service to Hammersmith and Queen Charlotte's Hospital Women's Health Clinic and the International Eating Disorders Centre in Buckinghamshire as well as acting as Nutrition Consultant for the Childbase Children's Nursery Group.

Nigel also runs his own private practice in Harley Street, specialising in weight management, PMS, menopause and irritable bowel syndrome.

Nigel works extensively with the media, writing for the *Sunday Telegraph Magazine*, *Zest*, *Essentials* and various other consumer magazines. His work in radio and television includes BBC and ITN news programmes, Channel 4's *Fit Farm*, BBC *Breakfast* and BBC *Real Story*.

He is the co-author of *Nutrition For Dummies* and *The GL Diet For Dummies*.

Allen Elkin, PhD, is a clinical psychologist, a certified sex therapist, and the director of The Stress Management & Counseling Center in New York City and is known for his expertise in the field of stress and emotional disorders. Dr Elkin holds workshops and presentations for professional organisations and corporations, including the American Society of Contemporary Medicine and Surgery, the Drug Enforcement Agency, Morgan Stanley, IBM, PepsiCo and the New York Stock Exchange.

His first book, *Urban Ease: Stress-Free Living in the Big City*, was published by Penguin Putnam (Plume, 1999). He is also the author of *Stress Management For Dummies*.

Charles H. Elliott, PhD, is a clinical psychologist and a member of the faculty at the Fielding Graduate Institute. He has a part-time private practice in Albuquerque, New Mexico, that specialises in the treatment of anxiety and depression. He is a Founding Fellow in the Academy of Cognitive Therapy, an internationally recognised organisation that certifies cognitive therapists for treating depression, anxiety, panic attacks and other emotional disorders. He has made numerous presentations nationally and internationally on new developments in assessment and therapy of emotional disorders. He is co-author of *Overcoming Depression For Dummies* (Wiley), *Overcoming Anxiety*

For Dummies (Wiley), *Anxiety & Depression Workbook For Dummies* (Wiley), *Why Can't I Get What I Want?* (Davies-Black, 1998; A Behavioral Science Book Club Selection), *Why Can't I Be the Parent I Want to Be?* (New Harbinger Publications, 1999), and *Hollow Kids: Recapturing the Soul of a Generation Lost to the Self-Esteem Myth* (Prima, 2001).

Georg Feuerstein, PhD, has been studying and practicing Yoga since his early teens. He is internationally respected for his contribution to Yoga research and the history of consciousness and has been featured in many national magazines both in the United States and abroad. He has authored over 30 books, including *The Yoga Tradition, The Shambhala Encyclopedia of Yoga, Tantra: The Path of Ecstasy,* and *Lucid Waking.* In the early '70s, he taught Hatha Yoga (physical exercises) to the British women's Olympic ski team for one season, but his main focus is on Jnana Yoga (the path of wisdom) and Raja Yoga (the royal path of meditation).

Georg is founder-director of the Yoga Research Center in Northern California, a coeditor of *Yoga World,* a patron of the British Wheel of Yoga, a fellow of the Indian Academy of Yoga, a contributing editor of *Yoga Journal* and *Intuition* magazine, and he also serves on the advisory board of the Integral Health Network. He's the co-author of *Yoga For Dummies.*

Ellie Herman, MS, Lac, runs two thriving Pilates studios, one in San Francisco and one in Oakland. The Ellie Herman Studios offer annual teacher training intensives in Northern California. Ellie has certified instructors locally, nationally and internationally. She has taught Pilates for over ten years and has developed a unique language to communicate the essence of the Pilates method. She was first introduced to Pilates in 1988 as a rehabilitation patient at Saint Francis Hospital Dance Medicine in San Francisco. She received her formal Pilates training in 1991 in New York City, where she studied with two of the original Pilates protégés, Romana Kryzanowska and Kathy Grant.

Formerly a professional dancer and choreographer with her own dance company, Ellie has a background that includes contemporary dance techniques, yoga, gymnastics, kinesiology and anatomy. She is a licensed acupuncturist with a Master of Science degree in acupuncture and Chinese herbal medicine. In her studios, Ellie combines Pilates with acupuncture and body work to offer a complete rehabilitation and wellness environment. Ellie strives to integrate her studies and continually expand her approach to bring balance back to the body.

She is the author of *Pilates For Dummies.*

Elaine Iljon Foreman MSc, AFPBSs is a Chartered Clinical Psychologist and Associate Fellow of the British Psychological Society. She specialises in the treatment of fear of flying plus other anxiety and depression related problems. Elaine is a Consultant Specialist in Cognitive Behavioural Therapy, accredited with the British Association for Behavioural and Cognitive Psychotherapy, a Fellow of the Institute of Travel and Tourism, and chairs the UKCP Ethics Committee. Her highly specialised Freedom to Fly Treatment Programme for the fear of flying (www.freedomtofly.biz), and the Freedom from Fear approach for other depression and anxiety-based problems have been developed from over thirty years of clinical experience. Elaine co-ordinates international research into the field of treatment for fear of flying. Her presentations and workshops are given both nationally and internationally to professional and self-help audiences.

Elaine's most recent publications are *Overcoming Anxiety For Dummies*, *Overcoming Depression For Dummies*, *Anxiety & Depression Workbook For Dummies*, and *Fly Away Fear, A Self-Help Guide to Overcoming Fear of Flying* co-authored with Lucas Van Gerwen, and published by Karnac in May 2008.

Liz Neporent is a certified trainer and president of Plus One Health Management, a fitness consulting company in New York City. Her job is to make sure the members of more than a dozen fitness centres in hotels and corporations throughout New York are happy, motivated and exercising on a regular basis.

Liz holds a Master's degree in exercise physiology and is certified by the American Council on Exercise, the American College of Sports Medicine, the National Strength and Conditioning Association and the National Academy of Sports Medicine. She is co-author of *Abs of Steel, Buns of Steel: Total Body Workout, Weight Training For Dummies, Fitness Walking For Dummies* and *Fitness For Dummies*. Additionally, she is the Gear Editor for *Shape* magazine and a regular contributor to *The New York Times*. She appears regularly on TV and radio as an authority on fitness and exercise.

Liz is an avid runner and has competed in more than two dozen marathons and ultra-marathons. She's also a devoted sports climber, walker, hiker, and weight trainer. She lives in New York City with her husband, Jay Shafran, and her greyhound, Zoomer.

Larry Payne, PhD, is an internationally prominent Yoga teacher and workshop leader. He used Yoga to overcome his own serious back problems which he developed during his previous career as an advertising sales executive. Larry regards his own early injuries from numerous competitive sports, his experience in a high-stress profession, and a previously inflexible body as invaluable preparation for helping others.

In Los Angeles, Larry is the founder of the corporate Yoga programme at the J. Paul Getty Museum, cofounder of the Yoga program at the UCLA

School of Medicine, and also founded similar programs for Rancho La Puerta Fitness Spa, The Ritz Carlton and Lowes Hotels, and numerous corporations. Larry is chairman of the International Association of Yoga Therapists and has received Outstanding Achievement Awards for Yoga in Europe, South America and the United States. Larry has appeared on national television, syndicated radio and has been featured in numerous international magazines, as well as *The New York Times* and the *Los Angeles Times*. He's the co-author of *Yoga For Dummies*. His website is www.samata.com.

Carol Ann Rinzler is a noted authority on health and nutrition and holds an MA from Columbia University. She writes a weekly nutrition column for *The New York Daily News* and is the author of more than 20 health-related books, including *Nutrition For Dummies, Controlling Cholesterol For Dummies, Weight Loss Kit For Dummies* and the highly acclaimed *Estrogen and Breast Cancer: A Warning for Women*. Carol Ann lives in New York with her husband, wine writer Perry Luntz, and their amiable cat, Kat.

Suzanne Schlosberg is a magazine writer known for her humorous approach to health and fitness. She is a contributing editor to *Shape* and *Health* magazines and co-author of *Weight Training For Dummies, Fitness For Dummies* and *Kathy Smith's Fitness Makeover*. She is also the author of *The Ultimate Workout Log*, Second Edition, and an instructor in UCLA Extension's Certificate in Journalism Program.

Suzanne writes frequently about her fitness adventures – from her failed tryout for The American Gladiators to her record-setting victory in Nevada's Great American Sack Race, a quadrennial event in which competitors run 5 miles while carrying a 50-pound sack of chicken feed on their shoulders. Suzanne chronicled her two bicycle treks across the United States. She never travels without her weight-lifting gloves and has put them to good use at gyms in Zimbabwe, Morocco, Guam and the Micronesian island of Yap.

Laura L. Smith, PhD, is a clinical psychologist at Presbyterian Behavioral Medicine, Albuquerque, New Mexico. At Presbyterian, she specialises in the assessment and treatment of both adults and children with anxiety and other mood disorders. She is an adjunct faculty member at the Fielding Graduate Institute. Formerly, she was the clinical supervisor for a regional educational cooperative. In addition, she has presented on new developments in cognitive therapy to both national and international audiences. Dr Smith is co-author of *Hollow Kids* (Prima, 2001) and *Why Can't I Be the Parent I Want to Be?* (New Harbinger Publications, 1999). She is the co-author of *Overcoming Anxiety For Dummies, Overcoming Depression For Dummies* and *Anxiety & Depression Workbook For Dummies*.

Publisher's Acknowledgments

We're proud of this book; please send us your comments through our Dummies online registration form located at www.dummies.com/register/.

Some of the people who helped bring this book to market include the following:

Acquisitions, Editorial, and Media Development

Project Editor: Rachael Chilvers

Content Editor: Jo Theedom

Commissioning Editor: Wejdan Ismail

Assistant Editor: Jennifer Prytherch

Production Manager: Daniel Mersey

Cover Photos: Front cover: © JLP/Corbis. Back cover (vegetables): © The Daniel Heighton Food Collection / Alamy; back cover (yoga): © Radius Images/Corbis

Cartoons: Ed McLachlan

Composition Services

Project Coordinator: Lynsey Stanford

Layout and Graphics: Tim Detrick, Andrea Hornberger

Proofreader: Jessica Kramer

Indexer: Ty Koontz

Contents at a Glance

Table of Contents

Introduction

*W*elcome to *Healthy Mind & Body All-in-One For Dummies*, your guide to understanding the impact of food, exercise and your state of mind on how healthy you feel and how much you enjoy life. Having a healthy mind and body are what many people strive for. You're probably aware of the importance of eating healthy food, taking regular physical exercise and feeling positive about life, but often struggle to bring all the elements together, especially when the pressure or challenges of everyday life take over.

This book is designed to provide ideas that you can use every day to have a positive impact on your health. You can explore healthier food choices, try a range of exercises to tone and strengthen your body, and discover a variety of techniques to deal with stress and pressure to enhance your sense of well-being.

About This Book

Healthy Mind & Body All-in-One For Dummies provides you with tips and ideas to make healthy choices about nutrition, exercise and enhance your mental well-being.

This book aims to boost your health by focusing on:

- ✔ Specific ideas to improve your nutrition and maintain a healthy diet
- ✔ Practical ways to incorporate a range of exercises into your daily life
- ✔ Solutions to deal with stress, anxiety and depression

The range of information described in this book is applicable throughout your life and covers different life circumstances, whether you want to shed a few pounds, are busy with family life or dealing with a stressful work situation.

Healthy Mind & Body All-in-One For Dummies draws on advice from several other *For Dummies* books, which you may want to check out for more in-depth coverage of certain topics (all published by Wiley):

- ✔ *Fitness For Dummies* (Suzanne Schlosberg, Liz Neporent)
- ✔ *The GL Diet For Dummies* (Nigel Denby, Sue Baic)
- ✔ *Nutrition For Dummies* (Nigel Denby, Sue Baic, Carol Ann Rinzler)

- *Overcoming Anxiety For Dummies* (Elaine Iljon Foreman, Charles Elliott, Laura Smith)

- *Overcoming Depression For Dummies* (Elaine Iljon Foreman, Charles Elliott, Laura Smith)

- *Pilates For Dummies* (Ellie Herman)

- *Stress Management For Dummies* (Allen Elkin)

- *Yoga For Dummies* (Georg Feuerstein and Larry Payne)

Conventions Used in This Book

The following conventions are used throughout the text to make things consistent and easy to understand:

- All web addresses appear in `monofont`.

- New terms appear in *italic* and are closely followed by an easy-to-understand definition.

- **Bold** is used to highlight the action parts of numbered steps.

- In the Food and Nutrition chapters we use metric terms such as gram (g), milligram (mg), and microgram (mcg) to describe quantities of protein, fat, carbohydrates, vitamins, minerals and other nutrients in the recipes.

- Nutritionists measure food in 100-gram portions. So 'a portion' in this book means a 100-gram dollop unless we state otherwise.

- In the recipes both the imperial and metric measurements are included. Follow either one – just don't switch halfway through a recipe!

- In the exercise chapters we provide helpful photos or illustrations to help you along. Because breathing is such an important part of many of the exercises, we include the words *Inhale* or *Exhale* to help you breathe properly.

- For your safety, when practising the exercises, be sure to read all the instructions. Although the illustrations are very helpful tools, they don't give you the whole story needed to practice safe and effective exercise.

Foolish Assumptions

In writing this book we've made several assumptions about you:

- ✔ You're generally interested in your health and are aware of the importance of exercise and nutrition to boost your sense of well-being.

- ✔ You're keen to make some positive changes and need some guidance on what exercises to do to tone and strengthen your body.

- ✔ You want some advice to solve the confusion about healthy food and to know how to maintain a balanced and nutritious diet every day.

- ✔ You want to understand the effects of stress and anxiety, and learn some techniques to help make a positive difference.

How This Book Is Organised

The following is a brief summary of each part in *Healthy Mind & Body All-in-One For Dummies*. You can use this as a fast guide to check out what you want to read first.

Book I: The Importance of Your Health

Chapter 1 helps clarify the basic elements of healthy nutrition so you know how food is digested and the effect of hunger and taste on what you eat. You explore how to make wise food choices so you have no excuses for considering some healthy options. Chapter 2 gives you some ideas to kick-start an active lifestyle to boost your health. You'll also find an overview of how to stay safe with exercise and the benefits of Pilates. In Chapter 3 we start assessing your state of mind to find out how you're feeling and identify things that can cause you stress or anxiety.

Book II: Food and Nutrition

Chapter 1 gives you the facts about a healthy diet, tips on avoiding unhealthy foods and emphasises the value of water. Chapter 2 takes you on a tour of proteins, vitamins, minerals and carbohydrates, and gives you the lowdown on cholesterol. In Chapter 3 we explore the effect of food on health and how to balance the calories to control your weight. Chapter 4 delves into the GL (Glycaemic Load) Diet so you can understand the science behind it and gives you some sample recipes to start putting the eating plan into practice. In Chapter 5 we highlight the key elements of the GL Diet so you can shop with confidence and incorporate the principles into a healthy eating plan.

Book III: Physical Health: Achieving Fitness

Chapter 1 highlights the benefits of being physically active and introduces some simple stretches to get you started. Chapter 2 helps you set some fitness goals and personal rewards for making new exercise habits. Chapter 3 takes a more active approach to fitness, showing you the elements of a cardio workout followed by a few moments to relax! Chapter 4 explores a variety of exercises to suit your lifestyle from walking, running, cycling and swimming to circuit training and using weights to help build up your strength.

Book IV: Exploring Yoga and Pilates

This part considers Yoga and Pilates in more detail. As you turn to Chapter 1 you're introduced to the basics of Yoga and Pilates so you can understand the key principles. Chapter 2 brings breathing into your Yoga practice and includes ideas on meditation. Chapter 3 illustrates a variety of Yoga exercises you can try out, starting with some warm-up exercises. Chapter 4 delves further into Yoga, providing a variety of postures incorporating standing, sitting and balancing – including exercising your abdominals! In Chapter 5 we turn you upside down to improve your health with some inversion postures, bending and twisting. If you still have some energy left, in Chapter 6, you have the opportunity to take your whole body through the classic Yoga formula.

Chapter 7 focuses on the key principles of Pilates and introduces some basic mat exercises as a taster. Chapter 8 takes you through a variety of exercises to work your whole body to help you feel stronger. Chapter 9 brings in some advanced Pilates exercises for you to try after mastering the basics if you want to challenge yourself further to tone your bottom, legs and thighs. The exercises are illustrated with step-by-step instructions to make the routines easier to follow.

Book V: Mental Health

As you move into Part V the focus changes to your mind and thoughts. Chapter 1 helps you to acknowledge the importance of your personal well-being and how stress can affect you. You explore the value of sleep to boost your mental well-being with some tips for getting a good night's rest. Chapter 2 helps get to the root of depression by identifying some of the causes and examines the main types of depression. In Chapter 3 we describe a selection of techniques to help overcome depression by addressing your thinking process, and ways to tackle previous difficult memories. We explain the concept of mindfulness and give you suggestions to minimise the risk of relapse.

In Chapter 4 we examine the seven main types of anxiety and unearth some of the root causes. Chapter 5 gives you ideas on conquering anxiety by watching out for worry words and taking one step at a time to restore calm and relaxation.

Chapter 6 turns to stress management. We look at common signs and symptoms to help you understand stress in your life. Chapter 7 helps you manage stress proactively by letting go of tension, calming your mind and overcoming anger to help you worry less. You also consider how to build a stress-resilient lifestyle and bring some fun back into your life.

Icons Used in This Book

For Dummies icons are a handy way to draw your attention to particular segments as you slide your eyes down the page. Each icon has its own special meaning:

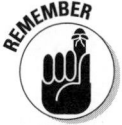

Check out these snippets of useful information to bear in mind.

This icon alerts you to explanations of technical terms and processes – details that are interesting but not necessarily critical to your understanding of a topic. In other words, skip them if you want, but try a few first.

Bull's-eye! This is time and stress saving information that you can use to improve your exercise, diet and health.

This warning icon alerts you to pitfalls to be aware of that may do more damage than good to your health.

Where to Go from Here

Ah, here's the best part. *For Dummies* books aren't linear (a fancy way of saying that they don't proceed from A to B to C . . . and so on). In fact, you can dive right in anywhere, say at L, M or N, and still make sense of what you're reading because we've made sure each chapter delivers a complete message.

For example, if you think Pilates is your passion, go right to Chapter 7 in Book IV. If you want to cook some new GL recipes head to Chapter 5 in Book II. You can use the Table of Contents to find broad categories of information or the Index to look up more specific things.

If you're not sure where you want to go, you may want to start with Part I. It gives you all the basic info you need to understand mind and body health.

You can dive in absolutely anywhere and still come up with tons of ideas to improve how you're feeling and understand how aspects of your diet and exercise can impact your health and well-being.

Book I
The Importance of Your Health

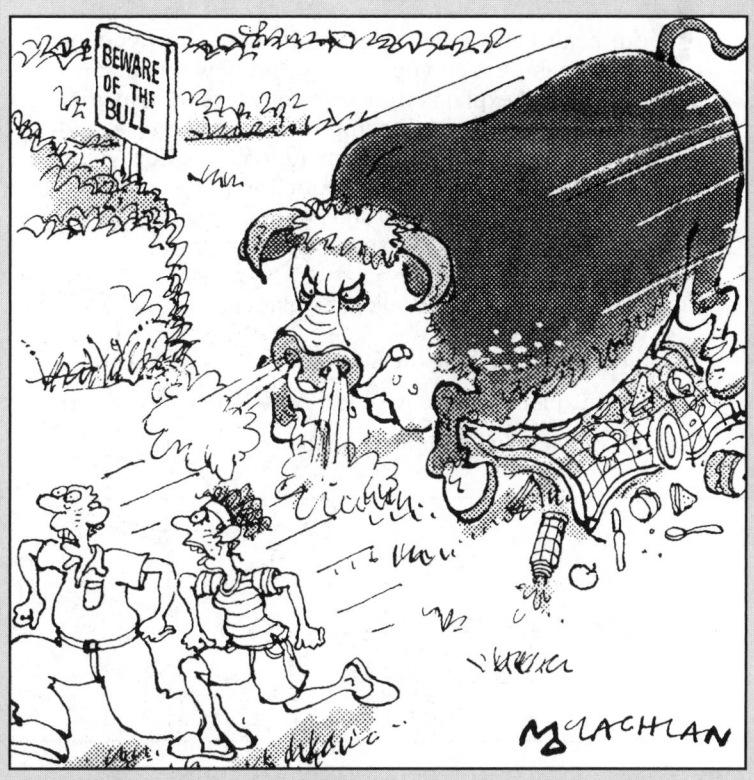

'You and your healthy picnic in the countryside
with plenty of exercise.'

In this book . . .

Your health is vitally important; it affects how you feel and can impact on your energy and how much you enjoy life. Book I explains the basic concepts to help you understand healthy food, the importance of exercise, and helps you start tuning into your mind to check how you're feeling. In short, it's a handy introduction to the rest of the book and a good place to start to help you decide which section you want to explore next.

Here are the contents of Book I at a glance:

Chapter 1: Understanding the Elements of Healthy Nutrition

Chapter 2: Exploring an Active Lifestyle to Boost Your Health

Chapter 3: Examining Your State of Mind

Chapter 1

Understanding the Elements of Healthy Nutrition

*T*o understand why nutrition matters you need a firm grasp of the basics. In this chapter not only do we explore what happens to food as it passes through your body (yuk!), but we also explain which foods are particularly important to your health. You'll also discover how to manage your diet so that you can get the biggest return (nutrients) from your investment (food).

Why Nutrition Matters

Technically speaking, *nutrition* is the science of how the body takes in and uses food. All living things need food and water just to stay alive. If you want to live *well*, then you need not only food but *good* food, meaning food with the essential nutrients. Without these nutrients:

✔ Your bones can become brittle (not enough calcium or vitamin D).

✔ Your gums may bleed (not enough vitamin C).

✔ You may feel tired and short of breath (not enough iron).

But optimal nutrition isn't just about avoiding deficiency diseases. We now know that a good diet can help to:

✔ Protect against common health problems such as heart disease, stroke, cancer and high blood pressure.

✔ Provide enough of the right fuel and fluid for regular physical activity.

✔ Improve your mood and your concentration levels.

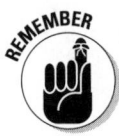

Nutrition is about why you eat what you eat and how it affects your health and well-being.

You are what you eat

I bet you've heard that before! However, it's worth repeating because the human body really is built from the things it gets from food: water, protein, fat, carbohydrates, vitamins and minerals. Your diet provides the energy and building blocks you need to construct and maintain every cell and organ in your body. To do this you need a range of nutrients from two different and distinct groups:

✔ **Macronutrients (macro = big):** Energy, protein, fat, carbohydrates and fibre

✔ **Micronutrients (micro = small):** Vitamins and minerals

Daily requirements for *macronutrients* are always in the order of several grams. For example, an average man needs about 55 grams of protein a day and 18 grams of fibre.

Your daily requirements for *micronutrients* are much smaller. For example, the *reference nutrient intake* (RNI) for vitamin C is measured in milligrams (⅟1,000 of a gram), while the RNIs for vitamin D, vitamin B12 and folate are even smaller and are measured in micrograms (⅟1,000,000 of a gram).

Energy from food

Energy is your power supply. Virtually every mouthful of food you eat is burnt or metabolised by your body cells to give you energy, even when it doesn't give you many other nutrients. The amount of energy released from food in this way is measured in *kilocalories* (kcal) or in *kilojoules* (kJ). Kilojoules is the standard international (SI) unit for energy and as such is the more scientifically accurate way to express energy. However, most of us are more familiar with food energy expressed as kcals or even more usually as calories. One kilocalorie is equal to one calorie, which is equal to 4.18 kJ.

The main thing to remember for now is that food is the fuel on which your body runs. If you don't eat enough food, you won't get enough energy.

What's a body made of?

On average approximately 60 per cent of your weight is water, 20 per cent is body fat (slightly less for a man), and 20 per cent is a combination of mostly protein, plus carbohydrates, minerals, vitamins and other naturally occurring biochemicals.

An easy way to remember this formula is to think of it as the *60-20-20 rule*.

Based on these percentages, you can reasonably expect that an average 70 kg person's body weight consists of about:

✔ 40 kg of water

✔ 15 kg of body fat

✔ 15 kg of a combination of protein (up to about 80–90 per cent), minerals (up to 20–30 per cent), carbohydrates (up to 5 per cent) and vitamins (a trace). The exact proportions vary from person to person.

For example, a young person's body has proportionately more muscle and less fat than an older person's, while a woman's body has proportionately less muscle and more fat than a man's. As a result, more of a man's weight comes from protein and calcium, while more of a woman's weight comes from fat. Protein-packed muscles and mineral-packed bones are denser tissue than fat, so if you weigh a man and a woman of roughly the same height and size, the man is likely to be the heavier every time.

Other nutrients in food

Your body needs other nutrients to build, maintain and repair tissues. Nutrients also empower cells to send messages back and forth and conduct essential chemical reactions, such as the ones that make it possible for you to move, see, hear, eliminate waste, and do everything else natural to a living body.

Understanding essential nutrients

In nutritionspeak, an *essential nutrient* is a very precious thing:

✔ **An essential nutrient cannot be manufactured in the body.** You have to get essential nutrients from your diet or from a nutritional supplement.

✔ **The lack of an essential nutrient in your diet is often linked to a specific deficiency disease.** For example, people who go without protein for extended periods of time develop the protein-deficiency disease *kwashiorkor*. Those who do not get enough vitamin C develop the vitamin C-deficiency disease *scurvy*. A diet or supplement rich in the essential nutrient cures the deficiency disease, but you need the proper nutrient. In other words, you can't cure a protein deficiency with extra amounts of vitamin C.

✔ **Not all nutrients are essential for all species of animals.** For example, vitamin C is only essential for human beings, apes and guinea pigs. All other animals, including cats, dogs and horses, can make all the vitamin C they need in the liver just from a type of sugar called glucose.

Essential nutrients for human beings include many well-known vitamins and minerals, along with several *amino acids* (the building blocks of proteins) and some fatty acids.

Introducing the Digestive System

Your digestive system may never win an Oscar, but it certainly deserves an award for its ability to translate complex food into basic nutrients. Digestion is a major performance requiring not a cast of thousands, but a group of digestive organs, each designed specifically to perform a cameo role in the digestion process.

The digestive organs

While exceedingly well organised, your digestive system is basically one long tube that starts at your mouth, continues down through your throat to your stomach, then on to your small and large intestines, and past the rectum to end at your anus.

In between, with the help of the liver, pancreas and gall bladder, the digestible parts of everything you eat are converted to simple chemicals that your body can easily absorb to burn for energy or build new tissue. The indigestible residue is bundled off and eliminated at the other end as waste.

Figure 1-1 shows the body parts and organs that comprise your digestive system.

Digestion: A performance in two acts

Digestion is really a two-part process – half mechanical, half chemical:

- *Mechanical digestion* takes place in your mouth and your stomach. Your teeth break food into small pieces that you can swallow without choking. In your stomach, a churning action continues to break food into even smaller particles.

- *Chemical digestion* occurs at every point in the digestive tract where enzymes and other substances such as *hydrochloric acid* (from cells in the stomach lining) and *bile* (from the gall bladder) dissolve food, releasing the nutrients inside.

Each organ in the digestive system plays a specific role in the digestive drama. But the first act occurs in two places that are never listed as part of the digestive tract: Your eyes and your nose.

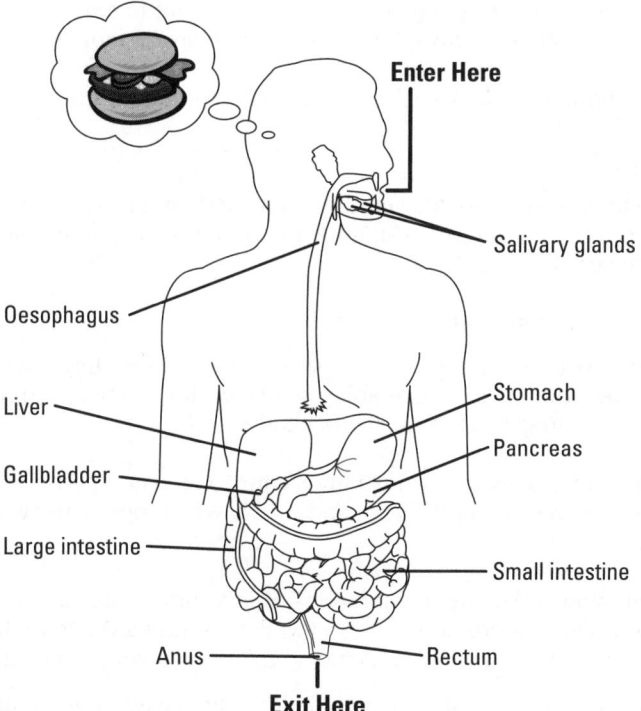

Enter Here

Salivary glands

Oesophagus

Liver

Gallbladder

Large intestine

Stomach

Pancreas

Small intestine

Anus

Rectum

Exit Here

Figure 1-1:
Your
digestive
system in all
its glory.

The eyes and nose

When you see appetising food, you experience a conditioned response. In other words, your thoughts – mmm, that looks good! – stimulate your brain to tell your digestive organs to get ready for action.

What happens in your nose is purely physical. The aroma of good food is transmitted by molecules that fly from the surface of the food to settle on the membrane lining of your nostrils, stimulating receptor cells on olfactory nerves that stretch from your nose to your brain. When the receptor cells communicate with your brain – something smells delicious! – your brain sends encouraging messages off to your mouth and digestive tract.

The messages say: 'Start the saliva flowing. Warm up the stomach. Alert the small intestine.' In other words, the sight and scent of food make your mouth water and your stomach rumble in anticipatory hunger pangs.

But wait! Suppose you hate what you see or smell? For some people, even the thought of liver is enough to make them nauseous. At that point, your body takes up arms to protect you: You experience a *rejection reaction* – a reaction similar to that exhibited by babies given something that tastes bitter or sour. Your mouth purses and your nose wrinkles as if to keep the food (and its odour) as far away as possible. Your throat tightens and your stomach heaves – muscles contracting not in anticipation but in movements preparatory to vomiting up the unwanted food. Not a pleasant moment.

But let's assume you like what's on your plate and take a bite.

The mouth

Once you lift your fork to your mouth, your teeth and salivary glands swing into action. Your teeth chew, grinding the food, breaking it into small, manageable pieces. As a result:

- ✔ You can swallow without choking.
- ✔ You break up the indigestible layer of fibre surrounding the edible parts of some foods (fruits, vegetables, whole grains) so that your digestive enzymes can get to the nutrients inside.

At the same time, salivary glands under your tongue and in the back of your mouth secrete the watery liquid called *saliva,* which performs two important functions:

- ✔ Moistening and compacting food so that your tongue can push it to the back of your mouth and you can swallow, sending the food down the slide of your throat (oesophagus or gullet) into your stomach.
- ✔ Providing *amylases*, enzymes that start the digestion of complex carbohydrates (starches), breaking the starch molecules into simple sugars. (No protein or fat digestion occurs in your mouth.)

Chewing your food well also helps stimulate the release of digestive juices further down your gut. It also makes you eat more slowly, giving your brain a chance to recognise when your body has had enough food so helping to stop you overeating.

The stomach

If you were to lay your digestive tract out on a table, most of it would look like a rather narrow tube. The exception is your stomach, a pouchy part just below your throat (oesophagus).

Like most of the digestive tube, your stomach is circled with strong muscles whose rhythmic contractions – called *peristalsis* – move food briskly along and turn your stomach into a sort of food processor that mechanically breaks pieces of food into ever smaller particles. While this is going on, cells in the stomach wall are secreting *stomach juices* – a potent blend of enzymes, hydrochloric acid and mucus (the mucus protects the stomach from the acid and enzymes). Ugh, it's enough to turn your stomach.

One stomach enzyme – *gastric alcohol dehydrogenase* – digests small amounts of alcohol, an unusual nutrient that can be absorbed directly into your bloodstream even before it has been digested.

Other enzymes, plus stomach juices, begin the digestion of proteins and fats, separating them into their basic components – amino acids (from protein) and fatty acids.

For the most part, digestion of carbohydrates comes to a screeching – though temporary – halt in the stomach, because the stomach juices are so acidic that they inactivate amylases, the enzymes in your saliva that break complex carbohydrates apart into simple sugars. Stomach acid can break some carbohydrate bonds, so a bit of carbohydrate digestion does take place.

Eventually, your churning stomach blends its contents into a thick soupy mass called *chyme* (from *cheymos*, the Greek word for juice). When a small amount of chyme spills past the stomach into the small intestine, the digestion of carbohydrates resumes in earnest, and your body begins to extract nutrients from food.

The small intestine

Open your hand and put it flat against your belly button, with your thumb pointing up to your waist and your little finger pointing down. Your hand is now covering most of the relatively small space into which your 3 metre (10 foot) long so-called small intestine is neatly coiled. When chyme spills from your stomach into this part of the digestive tube, a whole new load of digestive juices is released. These juices include:

- ✔ *Pancreatic and intestinal enzymes* that finish the digestion of proteins into amino acids (the building blocks for the body) and help digest fat and polysaccharides (type of carbohydrate).
- ✔ *Bile*, a greenish liquid (made in the liver and stored in the gall bladder) that enables fats to mix with water.
- ✔ *Alkaline pancreatic juices* that make the chyme less acidic so that amylases (the enzymes that break down carbohydrates) can go back to work transforming complex carbohydrates into simple sugars.
- ✔ *Intestinal alcohol dehydrogenase* that digests alcohol not previously absorbed into your bloodstream.

While these chemicals are working, peristaltic contractions of the small intestine continue to move the food mass down through the tube so that your body can absorb sugars, amino acids, fatty acids, vitamins and minerals into cells in the intestinal wall.

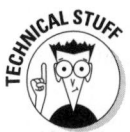

The lining of the small intestine is a series of folds covered with projections like little fingers. The technical name for these small fingers is *villi* (single: villus). Each villus is covered with smaller projections called *microvilli*, and every villus and microvillus is programmed to accept a specific nutrient – and no other. Pretty impressive, eh?

Nutrients are absorbed according to how fast they're broken down into their basic parts:

✔ Carbohydrates, which separate quickly into single sugar units, are absorbed first.

✔ Proteins (as amino acids) go next.

✔ Fats, which take longest to break apart into their constituent fatty acids, are last.

✔ Water-soluble vitamins such as B and C, and minerals are absorbed earlier than those that dissolve in fat.

After you've digested your food and absorbed its nutrients through your small intestine, a number of processes happen:

✔ Amino acids, sugars, vitamin C, the B vitamins, minerals including iron, calcium and magnesium, and trace elements are carried through the bloodstream to your liver, where they are processed and sent out to the rest of the body.

✔ Fatty acids, cholesterol and fat soluble vitamins including A, D, E and K go into the lymph system (another fluid transport system which, like blood, runs throughout the body bathing all the cells). From there they are passed into the blood itself. They, too, end up in the liver, are processed, and are sent out to other body cells.

Inside the cells, nutrients are *metabolised*: burned for heat and energy or used to build new tissues.

The large intestine

After every useful, digestible ingredient other than water has been wrung out of your food, the rest – indigestible waste – moves into the top of your large intestine, the area known as your *colon*. The colon's primary job is to absorb water from this mixture and then to squeeze the remaining matter into the smelly compact bundle known as faeces.

Faeces (whose brown colour comes from leftover bile pigments) are made of indigestible material from food, plus cells that have sloughed off the intestinal lining, and bacteria – quite a lot of bacteria. In fact, about 30 per cent of the entire weight of the faeces is bacteria. No, these bacteria aren't a sign you're ill. On the contrary, they prove that you're healthy and well. Some of these bacteria are good for you, microorganisms that live in permanent colonies in your colon where they:

✔ Break down previously undigested nitrogen containing compounds, releasing nitrogen gas.

✔ Feast on previously indigestible carbohydrates (fibre), producing the gases such as methane, carbon dioxide and hydrogen that sometimes makes you physically uncomfortable (or a social outcast) as well as hydrogen sulphide (a mix of hydrogen with sulphur which makes faeces smell so horrible).

✔ Ferment fibre to produce short chain fatty acids (SCFA) that help protect the cells in the colon against damage from cancer causing chemicals.

When the bacteria have finished, the faeces – the small remains of yesterday's food – pass down through your rectum and out through your anus.

Digestion's complete!

Combating digestive problems

Eating regular meals based on the principles of healthy eating can help many common digestive complaints. However, specific strategies can also help with digestive problems:

✔ **Indigestion** or feeling full and uncomfortable after eating is usually caused by eating too fast or too infrequently, especially eating just one heavy meal late at night. Try to eat smaller meals more often and make time to relax and digest – and enjoy your food!

✔ **Heartburn** (or *gastro-oesophageal reflux*) is caused by stomach acid coming backwards into the oesophagus and causing pain, usually after a meal. Drugs such as antacids are very effective treatment but sitting calmly after meals and avoiding bending or lying down can also help. Losing weight from around your waist helps because it reduces abdominal pressure, which makes heartburn worse. Some people also report a benefit from avoiding very spicy or very fatty foods, excessive tea, coffee, tobacco and alcohol.

✔ **Constipation** is helped by choosing high-fibre foods to stimulate movement of the gut. Try wholegrain bread and breakfast cereals, as well as fruit and vegetables, pulses and beans. Don't forget to drink plenty of fluids to allow the fibre to expand and soften. Try regular physical activity that improves muscle function, including movement of the gut muscle.

✔ **Irritable Bowel Syndrome (IBS)** can be characterised by diarrhoea or constipation, or sometimes both together with pain and bloating. Experts still don't really know what causes it or how to treat it, or even if what you eat really makes any difference at all. If constipation is the main symptom, extra fibre may help but if you suffer from diarrhoea you may benefit from actually reducing cereal fibre, fruit and vegetable skins, seeds and spicy foods. If you feel bloated, avoid pulses, onions and brassicas like cabbage.

If none of this helps, you could try a trial exclusion diet. Sometimes cutting out milk or wheat can help, but make sure you replace the valuable nutrients found in these foods (such as calcium) with an alternative source. Increasing your friendly gut bacteria from the 'probiotics' found in yoghurts and drinks may also help. For more information on IBS visit www.ibsnetwork.org.uk.

Sometimes digestive problems can indicate an underlying medical problem so do visit your doctor if you have any concerns.

Understanding the Difference between Hunger and Appetite

People eat for two reasons. The first reason is hunger; the second is appetite. Hunger and appetite are *not* the same. In fact, hunger and appetite are entirely different processes.

Hunger is the *need* for food. Hunger is:

- A physical reaction that includes chemical changes in your body related to a naturally low level of glucose in your blood several hours after eating.
- An instinctive, protective mechanism that makes sure that your body gets the fuel it requires to function well.

Appetite is the *desire* for food. Appetite is:

- A sensory or psychological reaction (looks luscious! smells scrummy!) that stimulates an involuntary physiological response (salivation, stomach contractions).
- A conditioned response to food (see the sidebar on Pavlov's dogs).

The practical difference between hunger and appetite is this: When you're hungry, you eat one handful of peanuts. After that, your appetite may lead you to eat two more handfuls just because they look appealing or taste good.

In other words, appetite is the basis for the familiar saying: 'Your eyes are bigger than your stomach.' Not to mention the well-known advertising slogan: 'Once you pop, you can't stop' – the advertising gurus know exactly how your hunger and appetite work.

Refuelling: The cycle of hunger and satiety

Your body does its best to create cycles of activity that parallel a 24-hour day. Like sleep, hunger occurs at pretty regular intervals, although your lifestyle may make it difficult to follow this natural pattern – even when your stomach loudly announces that it's empty!

Recognising hunger

The clearest signals that your body wants food, right now, are the physical reactions from your stomach and your blood that let you know it is definitely time to eat.

Rumbly tummy

An empty stomach has no manners. If you don't fill it when it's empty, your stomach issues an audible – sometimes embarrassing – call for food. This rumbling signal is called a *hunger pang*.

Hunger pangs are actually plain old muscle contractions. When your stomach's full, these contractions and their continual waves down the entire length of the intestine – known as *peristalsis* – move food through your digestive tract. When your stomach's empty, the contractions squeeze only air, and that makes noise.

Feeling weak and wobbly

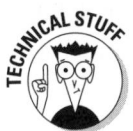

Every time you eat, your pancreas secretes *insulin*, a hormone enabling you to move blood sugar (glucose) out of the blood and into cells where it is needed for everyday chores like keeping you breathing, your heart pumping, and enabling you to carry out day-to-day physical work. *Glucose* is the basic fuel your body uses for energy. The level of glucose circulating in your blood rises and declines naturally, producing a vague feeling of emptiness, and perhaps weakness, that prompts you to eat. Most people experience the natural rise and fall of glucose as a relatively smooth pattern that lasts about four hours.

Knowing when you're full

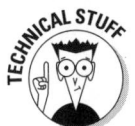

The satisfying feeling of fullness after eating is called *satiety*, the signal that says: I can't manage pudding, I've had plenty, and I need to leave the table.

Your *hypothalamus*, a small gland in the middle and towards the back of the brain on top of the *brain stem* (the part of the brain that connects to the top of the spinal cord), houses your appetite controls in an area of the brain where hormones and other chemicals that control hunger and appetite are made. The hypothalamus controls the release of neuropeptide Y (NPY) and peptide YY in the gut, two chemicals that tell us when we are full, or if we're empty it sends out a signal: More food!

Other body cells also play a role in knowing when you're full. In 1995, researchers at Rockefeller University in the United States discovered a gene in *fat cells* (the body cells where fat is stored) that directs the production of a hormone called *leptin* (from the Greek word for *thin*). Leptin appears to tell your body how much fat you have stored, thus regulating your hunger. Leptin also reduces the hypothalamus's secretion of NPY, the hormone that signals hunger. When the Rockefeller scientists injected leptin into specially bred fat mice, the mice ate less, burned food faster, and lost significant amounts of weight.

Eventually, researchers hope that this kind of information will lead to the creation of safe and effective drugs to combat obesity.

Beating those between-meal energy lows

Throughout the world, the cycle of hunger (namely, of glucose rising and falling) prompts a feeding schedule that generally provides four meals during the day: breakfast, lunch, tea (officially a mid-afternoon meal), and supper or dinner.

Our three-meal-a-day culture forces us to fight our natural rhythm by going without food from lunch at around 1 p.m. to dinner at around 7 p.m. or later. The result is that when glucose levels decline at around 4 p.m., you can get irritable and hungry, and then try to satisfy your natural hunger by grabbing the nearest food, often a high-fat, high-calorie snack.

Some people find that eating six small meals a day suits them much better than three large meals. Good evidence shows that avoiding those 'grab a chocolate bar', low-energy moments mid-morning or mid-afternoon is helpful for weight control.

Maintaining a healthy appetite

The best way to deal with hunger and appetite is to find out how to recognise and follow your body's natural cues.

If you're hungry, eat – in reasonable amounts that support a realistic weight. And remember: Nobody's perfect. Make one day's indulgence guilt free by reducing your calorie intake or increasing your calorie expenditure by exercising proportionately over the next few days. A little give here, a little take there, and you'll stay on target overall.

Responding to Your Environment on a Gut Level

Your physical and psychological environments definitely affect appetite and hunger, sometimes leading you to eat more or less than normal.

In the bleak midwinter

You're more likely to feel hungry in a cold environment than a warm place. And you're more likely to want high-calorie dishes in cold weather than in hot weather. Just think about the foods that tempt you in winter – stews, roasts, thick soups – versus those you find tempting on a simmering summer day – salads, chilled fruit, simple sandwiches.

This difference is no accident. Food gives you calories (energy). Calories keep you warm. Making sure that you get what you need, your body processes food faster when it's cold. Your stomach empties more quickly as food speeds along through the digestive tract, which means that those old hunger pangs show up sooner than expected, which, in turn, means that you eat more and stay warmer and . . . well, you get the picture.

Exercising more than your mouth

Everybody knows that exercising gives you a big appetite, yes? Well, actually, no. People who exercise regularly are likely to have a healthy (read: normal) appetite, but they're rarely hungry immediately after exercising because:

- ✔ Ordinary short bursts of exercise release stored energy (glucose and fat) from your body tissues, so your glucose levels stay steady and you don't feel hungry.

- ✔ Endurance exercise like marathon running or triathalon events eventually use up all stored energy in body tissues. If endurance athletes don't top up with glucose drinks they eventually 'hit the wall' – where the mind wants to keep going, but the body says 'No, I need more energy!'

- ✔ Exercise slows the passage of food through the digestive tract. Your stomach empties more slowly and you feel fuller for longer.

     Don't eat a heavy meal just before exercising or you may develop cramps or heartburn. Ouch.

- ✔ Exercise (including mental exertion) reduces anxiety. For some comfort-eaters, that means less desire to reach for a snack.

Tackling Taste: How Your Brain and Tongue Work Together

Your *taste buds* are sensory organs that enable you to perceive different flavours in food – in other words, to taste the food you eat.

Taste buds (also referred to as *taste papillae*) are tiny bumps on the surface of your tongue. Each taste bud contains groups of receptor cells that anchor an antenna-like structure called a *microvillus* that projects up through a pore in the centre of the taste bud. Imagine a thread sticking through the hole in a polo mint.

The microvilli in your taste buds transmit messages from flavour chemicals in the food along nerve fibres to your brain. Your brain translates the messages into perceptions: 'Oh, wow, that's delicious' or 'Ugh, that's revolting.'

The four (or five) basic flavours

Your taste buds definitely recognise four basic flavours: Sweet, sour, bitter and salt. Some people add a fifth basic flavour to this list. It's called *umami*, a Japanese word describing richness or a savoury flavour associated with certain amino acids such as glutamates – we talk more about monosodium glutamate (MSG) later in this section – and soya products such as tofu.

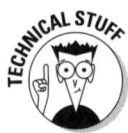

Early on, scientists thought that everyone had specific taste buds for specific flavours: Sweet taste buds for sweets, sour taste buds for sour, and so on. However, the prevailing theory today is that groups of taste buds work together so that flavour chemicals in food link up with chemical bonds in taste buds to create patterns that you recognise as sweet, sour, bitter and salt. The technical term for this process is *across-fibre pattern theory of gustatory coding*. Try saying that with a mouth full of tofu. Receptor patterns for the main four (sweet, sour, bitter, salt) have been tentatively identified, but the pattern for umami remains elusive.

Flavours are not frivolous. They are one of the factors that enable you to enjoy food. In fact, flavours are so important that MSG is used to make food taste better. MSG, most often found in food prepared in Chinese restaurants, stimulates brain cells. People who are sensitive to MSG may actually develop *Chinese restaurant syndrome*, characterised by tight facial muscles, headache, nausea, and sweating caused by overactive brain cells. The compound is banned from baby food. However, no real evidence indicates that a little MSG is a problem for people who aren't sensitive to it. That leaves only one question: How does MSG work? Does it enhance existing flavours or simply add that umami flavour on its own? Believe it or not, right now nobody knows. Sorry about that.

Your health and your taste buds

Some illnesses and medicines alter your ability to taste foods. The result may be partial or total *ageusia* (the medical term for loss of taste). Or you may experience *flavour confusion* – meaning that you mix up flavours, translating sour as bitter, or sweet as salt, or vice versa.

Table 1-1 lists some medical conditions that affect your sense of taste.

Table 1-1	These Things Make Tasting Food Difficult
This Condition	*May Lead to this Problem*
A bacterial or viral infection of the tongue	Secretions that block your taste buds
Injury to your mouth, nose, or throat	Damage to the nerves that transmit flavour signals
Radiation therapy to mouth and throat	Damage to the nerves that transmit flavour signals

Tricking your taste buds

Combining foods can short-circuit your taste buds' ability to identify flavours correctly. For example, when you sip wine (even an apparently smooth and silky one), your taste buds say, 'That alcohol's sharp.' Take a bite of cheese first, and the wine tastes smoother (less acidic) because the cheese's fat and protein molecules coat your receptor cells so that acidic wine molecules cannot connect.

A similar phenomenon occurs during wine tastings. Try two equally dry, acidic wines, and the second seems mellower because acid molecules from the first one fill up space on the chemical bonds that perceive acidity. Drink a sweet wine after a dry one, and the sweetness is often more pronounced.

Determining Deliciousness

When it comes to deciding what tastes good, all human beings and most animals have four things in common: They like sweets, crave salt, go for the fat, and avoid the bitter (at least at first).

These choices are rooted deep in biology and evolution. In fact, you can say that whenever you reach for something that you consider delicious to eat, the entire human race – especially your own ancestors – reaches with you. All right, cavemen didn't have ice cream, but that's what evolution's all about!

Listening to your body

Here's something to chew on: The foods that taste good – sweet foods, salty foods, fatty foods – are essential for a healthy body in the right doses:

✔ Sweet foods are a source of quick energy because their sugars can be converted quickly to glucose, the molecule that your body burns for energy.

Better yet, sweet foods make you feel good. Eating them tells your brain to release natural painkillers called *endorphins*. Sweet foods may also stimulate an increase in blood levels of *adrenaline*, a hormone secreted by the adrenal glands when circulating glucose is low. The glucose released from sweet foods doesn't stay in the bloodstream for long. It causes a sudden rise in blood glucose when we eat sweet foods but an equally rapid fall shortly after. Adrenaline is sometimes labelled the *fight-or-flight hormone* because it's secreted more heavily when you feel threatened and must decide whether to stand your ground – *fight* – or hurry away – *flight.*

✔ Salt is vital to life. It enables your body to maintain its fluid balance and to regulate chemicals called electrolytes that give your nerve cells the power needed to fire electrical charges that energise your muscles, power up your organs, and transmit messages from your brain.

✔ Fatty foods are even richer in calories (energy) than sugars. So the fact that you want them most when you're very hungry comes as no surprise. Which fatty food you want may depend on your sex. Several studies suggest that women like their fats with sugar – where's the chocolate? Men, on the other hand, seem to prefer their fat with salt – bring on the crisps!

Turning up your nose to tastes

Why some of us loathe broccoli but love olives (or vice versa) is still something of a mystery to the sensory experts. They suggest, but cannot prove, that your food preferences depend on your genes, your culture, and your personal experience.

If you're allergic to a food or have a metabolic problem that makes digesting it hard, you may eat the food less frequently but you may enjoy it as much as everyone else does. For example, people who cannot digest lactose, the sugar in milk, may end up gassy every time they eat ice cream, but they still like the way the ice cream tastes.

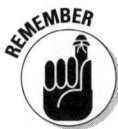

It's important to like your food. The simple act of putting food into your mouth stimulates the flow of saliva and the secretion of enzymes that you need to digest the food. Some studies suggest that if you really like your food, your pancreas releases as much as 30 times its normal amount of digestive enzymes.

However, if you truly loathe what you're eating, your body can refuse to take it in. No saliva flows; your mouth becomes so dry that you find it hard to swallow the food. If you do manage to choke it down, your stomach muscles and your digestive tract may convulse in an effort to be rid of the awful stuff.

No such ambivalence exists among people who've vomited after eating a specific food. When that happens to you, you naturally come to like its flavour less. Sometimes, your revulsion may be so strong that you'll never try the food again – even when you know that what actually made you sick was something else entirely, like riding a roller coaster just before eating, or having the flu, or being drunk!

Making Wise Food Choices

To help you make wise food choices you need some valuable nutrition tools – a food plate model (known as the Balance of Good Health) and some handy tips for choosing the best food whether you are planning , shopping, cooking or snacking.

Introducing the Balance of Good Health

The Balance of Good Health shown in Figure 1-2 is a pictorial representation of how to make up a healthy diet. It shows you know how much of each food group to consume.

The essential message of the Balance of Good Health is that you don't have to give up the foods you enjoy to be healthy – it's simply the balance you eat from the different food groups that counts.

Going deeper into the Balance of Good Health

To deliver this message, the Balance of Good Health is a plate divided into sections of differing sizes representing the five common food groups:

✔ **Bread, cereals and potatoes.** Includes breakfast cereals, pasta, rice, oats, corn, chapattis, yams and plantains.

✔ **Fruit and vegetables.** Includes fresh, frozen, tinned and dried varieties.

✔ **Milk and dairy foods.** Includes milk and calcium-fortified soya alternatives to milk, yogurt, cheese, and fromage frais, but not butter or cream.

✔ **Meat, fish and alternatives.** Includes red meat, poultry, offal, fish, eggs and vegetarian sources of protein such as nuts, beans, pulses, tofu and Quorn.

✔ **Fat and sugar.** Includes spreading fats, oils, cream, salad dressings and sauces, cakes, pies, biscuits, pastries, sweets, chocolate, savoury snacks such as crisps and soft drinks.

The Balance of Good Health

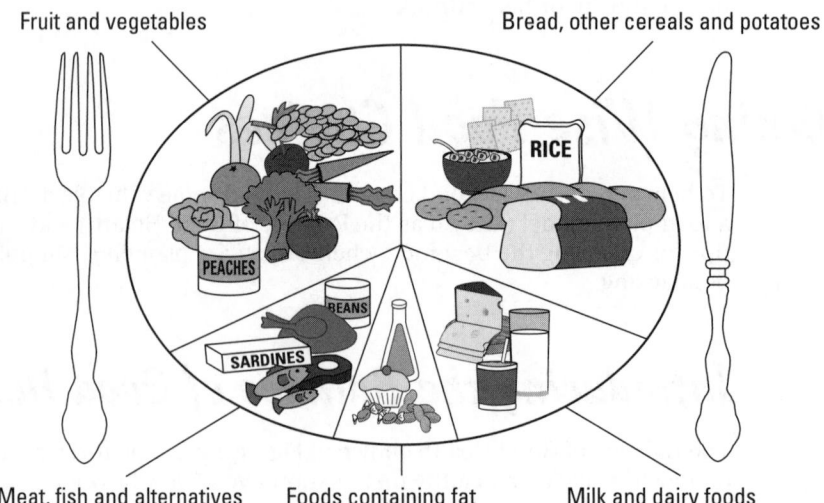

Figure 1-2: The Balance of Good Health shows the ideal quantities of different foods.

Adapted from model from the Food Standards Agency

Bearing the groups in mind, the Balance of Good Health delivers two important practical messages:

✔ **Proportion matters.** The different sections of the plate are not all the same size. They represent the proportions of the different food groups that should go up to make a healthy diet. Eat lots of the first two groups (bread and cereals, and fruit and veg) – each segment of the plate represents about one third of your diet. Eat the next two groups – meat and alternatives, and dairy foods – in moderate amounts, about one eighth of your daily food intake as meat (or alternative) and one sixth as dairy.

Fatty and sugary foods aren't essential to your diet but add choice and palatability. Consider them as occasional foods comprising a much smaller part of your food intake – moderation is the key here.

✔ **Variety counts.** You need a variety of the foods represented in the plate model to get all the nutrients you require. Choose different foods from within each group to increase your range of nutrients. The Balance of Good Health advises eating wholegrain varieties from the bread and cereal group where possible, and eating a wide variety of different types of fruit and vegetables. Choose low-fat versions of the foods from the meat and dairy groups whenever you can. These include semi-skimmed or skimmed milk, low-fat yogurts, and reduced-fat cheeses such as Edam, half-fat Cheddar, or Camembert. Choose lean meat and mince, poultry without skin, and fish without batter, and avoid frying where you can. Opt for lower-fat spreading fats, dressings, cakes, biscuits and ice cream where available.

Tailoring the Balance of Good Health to your needs

Different people have different energy (calorie) needs, which can be quite difficult to measure accurately. Healthy people with higher energy requirements need to eat larger portion sizes and more servings than those with lower energy expenditure. Nevertheless, the relative proportions of food from the different groups in the plate model should stay the same.

How much food you need is affected by your:

✔ **Gender:** Men generally need more food than women.

✔ **Age:** As you get older and are no longer growing you need less food.

✔ **Activity level:** The more active you are, the more energy you need.

A young, active person may eat more than someone who has retired, but the balance of the diet – the types of food and the proportions – should still stay the same.

The beauty of the Balance of Good Health is that using it enables you to eat practically everything you like – as long as you follow the guidelines on variety and proportion. The quantity is then determined by your own specific energy needs.

The principles of the Balance of Good Health apply to most adults of any ethnic origin, including vegetarians. It doesn't apply to children below the age of 2 (who need an energy-dense diet including full-fat dairy foods). However you can start to encourage children aged 2–5 years old to work towards the guidelines as they adopt a more adult diet.

Healthy shopping

The Balance of Good Health proves that you don't need to avoid certain foods forever; you don't need to avoid certain aisles in the supermarket either. Think of your local shops or supermarket like the plate in the Balance of Good Health. Make a shopping list based on the five sections and try to stick to it – and avoid shopping when you're hungry or you'll be tempted to buy all sorts of extras from the fatty and sugary group as a quick fix. Visit all the sections and make sure that your trolley looks like the picture when you've finished!

You could even try dividing your allocated shopping time in proportion to the food model too. Spend time checking out the range of exotic or seasonal fruit and vegetables and the huge variety of starchy foods from couscous to polenta. By contrast, just nip in to the cakes, biscuits and puddings section – don't browse there all day!

You can also read nutritional labels to check for ever-increasing portion sizes on ready meals and snacks such as sandwiches, crisps and chocolate bars. Just compare the fat content of a standard-size chocolate bar over a king-size bar and we think you'll pick the smaller bar every time!

Healthy meal planning

Back home in the kitchen, when you start deciding what to eat or preparing meals, the Balance of Good Health can help you plan anything from a nutritious packed lunch to a roast dinner. It's not always possible or practical to achieve the balance of all groups at every meal, but over the day it can help to get things in proportion.

What about dishes made up of more than one food group? Most of the food we eat is made up of a combination of different food groups, such as casserole, pies, pizza, lasagne, and even the humble sandwich. The trick here is to think about how the ingredients within the dish relate to the groups shown in the plate. Take the example of spaghetti bolognese. The pasta comes from the bread group; the beef from the meat and alternatives group; the Parmesan cheese from the dairy segment; the oil for frying from the fatty food group; and the tomatoes and onions in the sauce from the fruit and vegetables group. The healthy plate has a relatively larger serving of pasta with smaller servings of the vegetables, meat and cheese. You can see quite easily that the proportion of vegetables in the dish doesn't stand up to the balance of good health, but if you serve the meal with a side salad or add more vegetables to the sauce, it gets much nearer to the guidelines.

Healthy snacking

Our handy tools can even help you with health choices on the hoof. In the Balance of Good Health, snacks as well as meals count towards the proportions in your diet. Missed out on fruit and vegetables at breakfast? Well, what could be a handier mid-morning snack than unzipping a banana or cracking open a kiwi? Carrot sticks, celery, or mini cherry tomatoes are easy to eat. Dried fruit such as a mini box of raisins counts towards your intake of the fruit and veg group, as do individual tins of fruit – use the food label to find those with no added sugar.

Breadsticks, crumpets, muffins, crispbreads and oatcakes are alternatives to bread to fill that gap, and snacking on a bowl of cereal is another great way of increasing your starchy group. A bit low on your dairy group? Grab a smoothie made with fruit and milk, a pot of fruit yogurt, a fromage frais, or even a low-fat rice pudding.

With items such as cakes, biscuits and savoury snacks, use the nutritional information on the food label to compare them and choose the healthier varieties from each group. To get you started, Table 1-2 gives you some lower-fat alternatives to high-fat snacks. The lower-fat alternatives usually contain less than 10 grams of fat per 100 grams (less than 10 per cent fat).

Table 1-2	Snack Choices
High Fat Snack	*Lower Fat Choices*
Cakes	Scones, teacakes, malt loaf, currant buns, raisin bagel
Biscuits	Ginger nuts, Jaffa cakes, garibaldi, fig rolls
Savoury snacks	Plain popcorn, rice cakes, pretzels, rice crackers

Chapter 2

Exploring an Active Lifestyle to Boost Your Health

In This Chapter

▶ Understanding the benefits of staying active

▶ Getting started in an exercise programme

▶ Using Pilates and Yoga to tone your body

▶ Taking care while exercising

Maintaining an active lifestyle can help you throughout your life. Building up fitness early on is particularly beneficial to help you look and feel good, as well as giving you the strength and vigor to help reduce ailments and health problems. This chapter is a quick introduction to inspire you to get active.

Seeing Some of the Benefits from an Active Lifestyle

The secret to maintaining good health and ageing slowly is fitness. By staying active as you age, you reap substantial benefits from looking and feeling young and staving off life-threatening diseases. Your life can be enhanced by combining gentle cardio workouts (like walking or cycling) and strength training (lifting weights) several days a week:

✔ You have more energy.

✔ You experience less depression and anxiety.

✔ You have an easier time losing weight.

✔ You increase bone density, build muscle strength, and slow the muscle deterioration that comes with age.

- ✔ You improve your balance, which may prevent the falls that cause hip fractures.

- ✔ You reduce lower-back pain (this is especially true if you're lifting weights).

- ✔ You boost your immune system.

- ✔ You lower your blood pressure.

- ✔ You substantially cut your risk of heart disease, arthritis, diabetes, colon cancer and Alzheimer's and dementia.

- ✔ Your mind is more alert.

- ✔ You can be more independent in your daily activities.

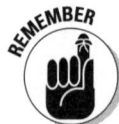

If you saw a pharmaceutical advertisement that listed even half of those benefits, you'd be lining up at your doctor's office for a prescription. So here's your exercise prescription: See your doctor for a check-up, and then, no matter what your age or experience with exercise, begin doing small amounts of cardio exercises, strength training, or a combination, three to five days per week. As your soreness wears off and your fitness improves, lengthen your workout times, improve your pace, and increase the amount of weight you're lifting.

Knowing where to begin

Do you find the idea of exercise daunting and just don't know where to start? Have you joined the gym but not attended yet, or are you one of those people that say you'll start exercising one day and still haven't started? If that sounds like you, you've come to the right place: this book. Just about all the information throughout this book applies to you, and you can visit the chapters that make the most sense to you. So, if you've never worked out before, flip to Book III to get some ideas on improving your fitness.

Getting fit does take time, but if you're doing a combination of cardio and weight training, you may notice small differences in just a week or two. After a month, your clothes may fit better, and within two or three months, your grandchildren will wonder how you're able to keep up with them. Exercise is its own fountain of youth, and while the magic potion does take a little time to make its way into your system, if you find an exercise you enjoy and stick with it, you'll be whistling a happy tune before you know it.

Cardio workouts for a healthy heart

Because cardio workouts (short for *cardiovascular*, the system that includes your heart and lungs) help lower your heart rate, improve your lung function, and make you feel more energised, be sure to include cardio as a part of your overall workout plan.

Resistance training for strength

Adding some resistance training to your exercise regime will make you stronger and tone and sculpt your muscles.

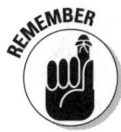

One of the major benefits of resistance training is that you improve your overall strength, which gives you more independence in your life. From carrying in groceries from the car to moving furniture around when it suits you, having greater strength allows you to do more without waiting for your son-in-law to show up.

Improving your balance

Both cardio workouts and weight training can improve your balance. Pilates also puts special emphasis on your body's *core* – your abdominal, back, hip, bottom and other nearby muscles – which, when strong, can greatly improve your overall balance.

Stretching and yoga for flexibility

Stretching can prevent your ligaments and muscles from shortening. Once you get into a routine of doing some simple yoga or stretching exercises every day, you will experience the wonderful relaxation you feel from a stretched body.

Seeing the Benefits from Pilates and Yoga

To help you get excited about starting your Yoga and Pilates programme, the following list shows some of the benefits you can achieve. You will feel some of the changes after only a few sessions, but it may take a little longer to see the difference in your body. Be patient and notice how different your body feels after each practice. But remember you do need to practice the exercise regularly, (at least twice a week) to start to feel and see the difference.

A firmer bottom

You should notice a definite change within a few weeks of doing Pilates regularly. Your bottom should be more toned and perhaps a little smaller.

Longer and leaner musculature

A ballet dancer was rejected from a ballet company because her body was too bulky and her 'line wasn't ideal'. This dancer did Pilates for a year and re-auditioned, and is now the principal dancer in this same company. Why? Because Pilates transformed this dancer's body to a more ideal shape. She started out with big hulking thighs that were strong but just too big to look perfect in a tutu. After doing Pilates for a year, her thighs got longer and leaner but still had the strength and flexibility required of a professional dancer.

If you are like this ballet dancer, and tend to bulk up when you work out, Pilates is an ideal strength-training programme for you. Pilates exercises accentuate the length of the limbs and change bulky muscles into longer and leaner ones. In general, Pilates exercise should lengthen your muscles and make you look taller.

Better posture

Better posture is something we can pretty much guarantee. And other people will surely notice this change in you after only a few Yoga and Pilates work-outs. If you take the lessons you learn from Yoga and Pilates to heart, you'll stand and sit taller and look more elegant. If you see no other changes, you'll see this one. If you don't see it, other people will.

Here are some important rules about posture to be aware of when standing:

- Pull your navel in toward your spine.
- Keep your head balanced on top of your hips (not forward or behind).
- Lengthen the back of your neck.
- Keep your shoulders back and down and keep your back wide.

Pilates exercises are almost always aimed at aligning the spine so that the head sits on top of the hips, not in front. If you think of one of our favourite images, 'imagine you have a golden string attached to the back of the top of your head, and it's pulling you up toward the heavens', you'll naturally correct your head posture.

Yoga and Pilates help address tight shoulder muscles by releasing tension in the neck and shoulder area, improving your posture and reducing stress and strain from desk and computer work.

The upper trapezius muscles work very hard. The trapezius muscles are at the top of your shoulders and at the back of your neck. The ones that could always use a nice massage. These muscles tend to hold tension. It's like they enjoy being tight and think they can just hold up the world. Actually, desk work and computer work are the man culprits that exacerbate neck and shoulder tension. Yoga and Pilates exercises help to address this problem (for example, shoulder shrugs in Book IV). Once you become aware of the tension that is constantly present in these muscles, you can begin to consciously release tension. Pilates teaches you how to relax the trapezius muscles and at the same time engage the opposing muscles to keep the trapezius muscles happy and tension-free.

A flatter tummy

The best way to get a flatter tummy is to lose a little weight. The second best way is to do Yoga and Pilates. If you're already thin but have a bulge in your middle, Yoga and Pilates can help you lose a notch in your belt. The most basic aspect of the Pilates method is pulling your navel in towards your spine or scooping your abdominals. If you apply this simple technique to your everyday life – when standing, walking, and so on – your tummy will be flatter and more attractive.

Less back pain

Most back pain results from faulty posture and a sedentary lifestyle. Yoga and Pilates address all the muscles that most typically contribute to back pain, namely the abdominals and the bottom muscles. They also stretch out the back muscles.

Using your body properly is another element of diminishing back pain. If you do Yoga and Pilates carefully, you'll understand how to use your body in ways that protect your back from injury. Yoga and Pilates are two of the best methods to use to keep your back healthy, no matter what your age or vocation, or what other exercise regimens you may do.

More flexibility

Yoga and Pilates exercises stretch the muscles and the joints while they strengthen the body. If you find that your spine has lost some of its range of motion and flexibility, Yoga and Pilates very quickly improve this problem. Everyone has physical limitations that depend on age, genetics and lifestyle. If you do a regular exercise programme, your body can reach its potential in flexibility and strength.

Better sex

Yoga and Pilates bring about a newfound body control that affects all aspects of life, including sex. You may find that, because of increased back and hip flexibility, you can get into positions that previously had been impossible. You may also discover increased control of your pelvic muscles, thereby enhancing sexual pleasure. If having sex hurts your back, you may find that you're going to love what Yoga and Pilates can do for you! And so will your partner.

More awareness

If nothing else, doing Yoga and Pilates should give you a new awareness of your body. You may never have thought about pulling in your tummy, sitting up tall, or keeping your shoulder blades down away from your ears. And you may never have thought a lot about how you breathe. All these images will start to filter into your consciousness, and you may find that you correct your own posture and habits naturally.

Better balance

Any gymnast knows that to avoid falling off the balance beam, you need to pull in your stomach and squeeze your bottom. In order to have good balance, you need to have a strong centre, and you need to know how to find it without a lot of thought. Yoga and Pilates exercises strengthen the core. After doing Yoga and Pilates regularly, you may not be able to do a back flip on the balance beam, but you'll definitely find increased co-ordination and balance.

Greater strength

Any exercise regimen should increase your body's overall strength, or else what's the point? But Yoga and Pilates strengthen the muscles in your body that you may actually notice on a day-to-day basis. Yoga and Pilates are meant to improve your daily life: They can help you get up from bed, if that's hard for you, or they can help you do a triple back flip off the diving board, if that's your goal. Whatever activity you do, you'll find that Yoga and Pilates exercises improve strength in meaningful ways and can help with the overall health of your spine. Doing Yoga and Pilates can prevent injuries, too!

Staying Safe

Before beginning an exercise programme, make an appointment with your doctor, just to make sure you're safe to do so. As you get yourself into a workout routine, keep the following safety tips in mind:

- ✔ Always warm up and cool down; stretch as often as possible.

- ✔ Check that you can carry on a conversation while exercising. If speaking is difficult, reduce your intensity or stop exercising.

- ✔ Never hold your breath while exercising, especially while lifting weights.

- ✔ Keep yourself hydrated. Remember that by the time you feel thirsty, you've started to become dehydrated.

- ✔ In hot weather, wear high-tech fabrics that let heat escape, and always wear sunscreen and a cap.

- ✔ During winter, layer your clothing so you can remove layers as your body heats up.

- ✔ When you have a cold or – worse yet – the flu, take a few days off of your exercise routine.

- ✔ Stop exercising if you feel any of the following:

    - Nausea, faintness, lightheadedness

    - Racing pulse or any abnormal heart rate

    - Cold sweat

    - Chest or neck pain or tightness

    - Muscular pain

    - Excessive fatigue or weakness

Using exercise as a social event

Exercise is a great way to meet and spend time with people of all ages, especially if you join a gym or a fitness group. If you don't have a gym in your town, check with your local community centre to see what classes or workout groups meet in the area – or start your own running or cycling club with friends and family. From meeting new friends at the gym to walking with your grandchildren a few days per week, you can use exercise as an opportunity for social interaction.

Chapter 3

Examining Your State of Mind

In This Chapter

▶ Looking at the symptoms of depression

▶ Discovering what makes you anxious

▶ Measuring stress

*T*aking time to tune into your feelings is an important first step in examining your state of mind and helping you overcome negative thoughts.

It's okay to experience good and bad days. It's knowing how to deal with life's challenges that makes the difference in how you are feeling and coping. When the pressure or challenges become too much you may find yourself experiencing some of the aspects of depression, anxiety and stress which this chapter will focus on.

Tuning Into Your Mind

To help tune into your mind, consider the following ways to analyse your thoughts and feelings to help detect depression and anxiety and assess your stressors.

Detecting depression

Depression takes many forms, and develops in different ways. Sometimes it deepens slowly but surely, gradually taking over your whole life. At other times depression overwhelms you, giving little, if any, warning. Some people don't realise that they have depression, but others fully recognise the signs. And sometimes depression has no obvious cause, often masquerading as a set of physical complaints including fatigue, sleeplessness, changes in appetite, and even indigestion.

Depression is a disorder of extremes. It can destroy your appetite – or make you insatiably hungry. It can deprive you of sleep – or make you overwhelmingly fatigued, confining you to bed for days at a time. When you are depressed you find yourself pacing to and fro frantically – or frozen with fear. Depression may last for months or years, but it can also lift within a very brief time.

Recognising the damage of depression

Everyone feels low at times. Financial setbacks, health problems, loss of loved ones, divorce, or failure to meet work targets – events like these can make anyone feel upset or sad for a while. But depression is more than a normal reaction to unpleasant events and losses. Depression is more intense and goes well beyond sadness, affecting both mind and body in disturbing ways.

Depression can affect all areas of your life. There are a several types of depression and they can all affect four main areas of your life. But although depression appears in different forms, they all can disrupt:

- ✔ Thoughts
- ✔ Behaviours
- ✔ Relationships
- ✔ Your body

In the following sections, we consider how depression affects each of these areas of your life.

Dwelling on dark thoughts

When you get depressed, your view of the world changes. The sun shines less brightly, and the sky's covered by dark cloud. Those around you seem cold and distant, and the future looks black. Your mind may focus on recurrent thoughts of worthlessness, self-loathing and even death. Typically, depressed people experience difficulty in concentrating, remembering, and in making decisions.

Does your mind dwell on negative thoughts? If so, you may be suffering from depression. The following 'Depressive Thoughts Quiz' gives you a sample of typical thoughts that go with depression. Tick each thought that you often have:

❑ Things are getting worse and worse for me.

❑ I think I'm worthless.

❑ No one would miss me if I were dead.

❑ My memory has gone to pieces.

❑ I make too many mistakes.

❑ Overall, I think I'm a failure.

❑ Lately, I find it impossible to make decisions.

❑ I don't look forward much to anything.

❑ I've been feeling down and pretty hopeless over the past month.

❑ The world would be a better place without me.

❑ Basically, I'm extremely pessimistic about things.

❑ I can't think of anything that sounds interesting or enjoyable.

❑ I've found little interest or pleasure in the things I used to do and enjoy.

❑ My life is full of regrets.

❑ Lately, I can't concentrate, and I forget what I've just read.

❑ I don't see my life getting better in the future.

❑ I'm deeply ashamed of myself.

Unlike many of the questionnaires you see in magazines or newspapers, there is no specific score in this one to identify your level of depression. Merely ticking a few items doesn't necessarily mean you're depressed. But the more items you tick, the greater possibility of depression. And if you tick any of the items related to death or suicide, it may well be cause for concern, and a signal to take action.

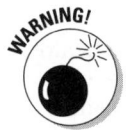

If you're having suicidal thoughts, you need immediate assessment and treatment. If the thoughts include a plan that you believe you may actually carry out either now, or in the very near future, go to your GP, the local Community Mental Heath Resource Centre, or a hospital Accident and Emergency Department. They have trained staff who can help. If you're not able to get yourself to any of these places, phone 999 for an ambulance.

Dragging your feet: Depressed behaviour

Not everyone who's depressed behaves in the same way. Some people find themselves speeding up and others find themselves slowing down. While some people can't stay awake, others suffer horribly from lack of sleep.

Douglas drags himself out of bed in the morning. Even after ten hours' sleep, he still feels exhausted, with no energy for anything. He starts being late for work, and frequently takes sick leave. He stops going to the gym, an activity he used to enjoy. He tells himself he'll go back when he finds the energy. His friends ask him what's going on, because lately they hardly see him. He says that he doesn't really know. He's always just so very tired.

Cheryl, on the other hand, has about three and a half hours of sleep a night. She wakes around 3 a.m. with thoughts racing through her mind. When she gets up, she feels a frantic pressure and can't seem to settle to anything. Irritable and bad-tempered, she snaps at her friends and colleagues. Unable to sleep at night, she starts drinking too much. Sometimes she cries for no apparent reason.

Although everyone is different, certain behaviours are typical of depression. Depressed people can feel like they're wading through treacle, or running full speed on a treadmill. Do you feel concerned about your behaviour? The following 'Depressed Behaviour Quiz' can tell you if your behaviour points to a problem. Tick each item that applies to you:

❑ I've been having unexplained crying spells.

❑ The few times I force myself to go out, I don't have much fun.

❑ I can't make myself exercise like I used to.

❑ I haven't been going out nearly as much as usual.

❑ I've been skipping work quite a bit lately.

❑ I can't get myself to do much of anything, even important projects.

❑ Lately I've been fidgety and can't sit still.

❑ I'm moving at a slower pace than I usually do, for no good reason.

❑ I haven't been doing things for fun as I usually do.

All these items are typical of depressed behaviour or, in some cases, a health problem. On a bad day, anyone is likely to tick one or two items. However, the more items you tick, the more likely it is that something's wrong, especially if the problem has been around for more than two weeks.

Struggling with relationships

Depression affects the way you relate to others. Withdrawal and avoidance are the most common responses to depression. Sometimes depressed people get irritable and critical with the very people they care most about.

Tony trips over a toy left on the living room floor and snaps at his wife Sylvia, 'Can't you get the kids to pick up their damn toys for once?' Hurt and surprised by the attack, Sylvia apologises. Tony fails to acknowledge her apology and turns away. Sylvia quickly picks up the toy and wonders what's happening to her marriage. Tony hardly talks to her any more, other than to complain or tell her off about something trivial. She can't remember the last time they had sex. She worries that he may be having an affair.

Have you or perhaps someone you care about been behaving differently within one or more of your relationships? The following 'Depression and Relationships Quiz' explores some of the ways in which depression affects relationships. Tick the items that describe your situation:

- ❑ I've been avoiding people more than usual, including friends and family.
- ❑ I've been having more difficulty than usual talking about my concerns.
- ❑ I've been unusually irritable with others.
- ❑ I don't feel like being with anyone.
- ❑ I feel isolated and alone.
- ❑ I'm sure that no one cares about or understands me.
- ❑ I haven't felt like being physically intimate with anyone lately.
- ❑ I feel like I've been letting down those who are close to me.
- ❑ I believe that others don't want to be around me.
- ❑ Lately, I don't seem to care about anyone the way I should.

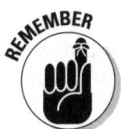

When you're depressed, you tend to turn away from the very people that may have the most support to offer you. You feel that they don't care about you, or perhaps you can't find any positive feelings for them. You may avoid others or find yourself irritated and snappy.

The more items you ticked in the 'Depression and Relationships Quiz', the more likely it is that depression is affecting your relationships.

Feeling foul: The physical signs of depression

Depression usually shows some physical symptoms. They include changes in appetite, sleep and energy. However, for some people, the experience of depression *primarily* consists of these physical symptoms and doesn't noticeably affect mood and relationships.

 Are you experiencing certain changes in your body you can't explain? The following 'Depression in the Body Quiz' highlights some of the ways that depression can show itself within your body. You know what to do – tick each item that applies to you:

❑ My blood pressure has risen lately for no obvious reason.

❑ I have no appetite these days.

❑ I haven't been sleeping nearly as well as usual.

❑ My diet is the same, but I'm having frequent constipation for no reason.

❑ I often feel nauseous.

❑ I suffer from loads of aches and pains.

❑ I'm sleeping much more than usual.

❑ I'm always hungry, and for no reason.

❑ My energy has been very low lately.

❑ I've gained (or lost) more than 2 kilograms (about 4.5 pounds), and I can't work out why.

Like the other three quizzes in this chapter, it really doesn't matter exactly how many of the items apply to you. However, be aware that the more items you tick, the greater the chance that you are suffering from depression.

If your depression shows itself in physical symptoms, medication or some other physical remedy is likely to be the best choice for you.

 The experiences listed in the quizzes may be caused by other health-related problems, not just depression. Therefore, if you're having any worrying physical problems, see your doctor, especially if the symptoms last for more than a week or two.

Analysing Anxiety

Anxiety, stress and worries. Everyone has these experiences. They are part of normal life – no way can we expect to go through life without experiencing them. But sometimes they get out of hand. Then anxiety causes pain, for a surprising number of people. Anxiety can create havoc in the home, destroy relationships, make employees lose time from work, and prevent people from living full, productive lives.

When people talk about their anxiety, you may hear any one or all of the following descriptions:

Book I

The Importance of Your Health

- ✔ I just can't find the right words to describe my feelings. It's like dread and doom, but a thousand times worse. I want to scream, cry for help, but I'm paralysed. It's the worst feeling in the world.

- ✔ When my panic attacks begin, I feel tightness in my chest. It's as though I'm drowning or suffocating, and I begin to sweat; the fear is overwhelming. I feel like I'm going to die, and I have to sit down because I'm convinced I'm going to faint.

- ✔ I'm lonely. I've always been painfully shy. I want friends, but I'm too embarrassed to contact anyone. I guess I feel anyone I call will think that I'm not worth talking to.

- ✔ I wake up worried every day, even at the weekends. I never feel I've caught up – there's always a list and always responsibility. I worry all the time. Sometimes, when it's really bad, I think about going to sleep and never waking up.

Anxiety: You can't escape it

Anxiety is the most common of all the so-called mental disorders. Estimates suggest that around 6.5 million people in the UK suffer from an anxiety disorder in any given year, and some calculate that as many as 25 per cent may suffer from an anxiety disorder at one point or another over a lifetime. Statistics around the world vary somewhat from country to country, but anxiety is the most common mental disorder worldwide. And even if you don't have an actual anxiety disorder, you may experience more anxiety than you want. In other words, you definitely aren't alone if you have unwanted anxiety.

Anxiety costs. It costs the sufferer in emotional, physical and financial terms. But anxiety doesn't stop there. Anxiety also incurs a financial burden for everyone. Stress, worry and anxiety disrupt relationships, work, leisure and family.

Sorting out what's normal from what's not

Anxiety is good for you! It prepares you to take action. It mobilises your body for emergencies. It warns you about potential problems. Be glad you have some anxiety. Your anxiety helps you stay out of trouble.

Anxiety only poses a problem for you when:

✔ Anxiety lasts uncomfortably long or occurs too often.

✔ It interferes with doing what you want to do.

✔ Anxiety greatly exceeds the level of actual danger or risk. For example, when your body and mind feel like an avalanche is about to bury you, but all you have to do is take a test at school, your anxiety has gone too far.

✔ You struggle to control your worries, but they keep disturbing you and never let up.

Recognising the symptoms of anxiety

You may be unaware that you suffer from anxiety or an anxiety disorder. That's because anxiety involves a rather wide range of symptoms. Each person experiences slightly different symptoms. And your own specific symptoms determine what kind of anxiety disorder you may have.

For now, you should know that some signs of anxiety appear in the form of *thoughts* or *beliefs*. Other indications of anxiety manifest themselves in *bodily sensations*. Still other symptoms show up in various kinds of anxious *behaviours*. Some people experience anxiety signs in all three ways, while others only notice their anxiety in one or two areas.

Thinking anxiously

In Book V Chapter 5, we discuss anxious thinking in great detail. For starters, people with anxiety generally think differently from other people. Look out for the following: You're probably thinking anxiously if you experience:

✔ **Approval addiction:** If you're an approval addict, you worry a great deal about what other people think about you.

✔ **Living in the future and predicting the worst:** When you do this, you think about everything that lies ahead and assume the worst possible outcome, a type of thinking known as *catastrophising*.

✔ **Magnification:** People who magnify the importance of negative events usually feel more anxious than other people do.

✔ **Perfectionism:** If you're a perfectionist, you assume that any mistake means total failure.

✔ **Poor concentration:** Anxious people routinely report that they struggle to focus their thoughts. Short-term memory sometimes suffers as well.

> ✔ **Racing thoughts:** When thoughts race, they run through your mind in a stream of almost uncontrollable worry and concern.

Finding anxiety in your body

Almost all people with severe anxiety experience a range of physical effects. These sensations don't simply occur in your head; they're as real as this book you're holding. The responses to anxiety vary considerably from person to person and include:

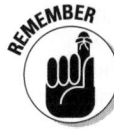

- ✔ Accelerated heart beat
- ✔ A spike in blood pressure
- ✔ Blurred vision
- ✔ Dizziness
- ✔ Fatigue
- ✔ Feelings of unreality
- ✔ Gastro-intestinal upset
- ✔ General aches and pains
- ✔ Muscle tension or spasms
- ✔ Sweating

These are simply the temporary effects that anxiety exerts on your body. Chronic anxiety left untreated can pose serious risks to your health.

Behaving anxiously

We have three words to describe anxious behaviour: avoidance, avoidance and avoidance. Anxious people inevitably attempt to get away, and stay away, from the things that make them anxious. Whether it's snakes, heights, crowds, motorways, parties, paying bills, reminders of bad times, or public speaking, anxious people search for escape routes.

One of the most common and obvious examples of anxiety-induced avoidance is how people react to their phobias. Have you ever seen the response of a spider-phobic when confronting one of the beasties? Usually, the phobic beats a hasty retreat.

In the short run, avoidance decreases anxiety. It can make you feel a little better. However, in the long run, avoidance actually maintains and heightens anxiety.

Assessing Your Stressors

Some people thrive on stress and they need a certain amount of pressure to keep them motivated. Carrying out an assessment of your own stressors can help you decide if stress is becoming a problem for you, or whether you're relishing the challenges around you.

Just how stressed are you?

Certainly, one of the very first steps in mastering your stress is knowing just how stressed you are. You may think that measuring stress is a relatively simple matter. The fact is, measuring your stress level is a tricky business. Part of the difficulty stems from the multifaceted nature of stress. It's both a stimulus and a response. It's what's on your plate, and it's how you react to what's on your plate. Stress also appears in the form of various biochemical and physiological changes in your body. It would be nice if you could be hooked up to a machine and measure your stress level as easily as your doctor measures your blood pressure or heart rate. Alas, this is not the case. However, measuring your stress is still possible. Below are some relatively easy ways of finding the number that tells you just how stressed you are.

The simplest way to measure your stress

Oddly enough, one of the better ways of measuring your stress is asking yourself this simple question:

> 'How much stress am I currently feeling?'

In an age of high-tech, computer-driven, digitally monitored gadgets and gear, this lowest-of-low tech ways of measuring your stress may seem like a joke. Yet it really is an incredibly useful way of assessing your stress level. This subjective measure of your stress has some advantages. It measures those aspects of your stress that you feel truly reflect your stress. This may take the form of anxiety, anger, muscle tension, or some other manifestation of your stress. This measure is also sensitive to the ways in which your stress level can change from day to day and even from moment to moment. All in all, it's not a bad measure to start with.

Use a stress gauge

To help you put a number on your stress level (and to give this approach the appearance of technological sophistication), we suggest that you use a simple 10-point scale that permits you to calibrate your level of stress in a more quantitative way.

10	
9	I feel extremely stressed.
8	
7	
6	I feel a moderate amount of stress.
5	
4	
3	
2	I feel only a little stress.
1	
0	I don't feel any stress.

So, right now, you may say to yourself, 'I'm feeling a little 5-ish.' This morning when you were stuck in major traffic you probably described your stress level as a 7.

Knowing where your stress is coming from

This scale helps you assess not only the amount of stress you are experiencing now, but also helps you identify where that stress is coming from. Items in the scale include major life changes, important issues, and worries and concerns that you may be now be experiencing. Use this simple scale to help you:

- ✔ N = No stress
- ✔ S = Some stress
- ✔ M = Moderate stress
- ✔ G = Great stress

Conflicts or concerns about your marriage or relationship	_____
Concerns or worries about your children	_____
Concerns or worries about your parents	_____
Pressures from other family members/in-laws	_____
Death of a loved one	_____
Health problems or worries	_____
Financial worries	_____

(continued)

(continued)

Concerns related to work/career	_____
Long or difficult commute to work	_____
Change in where you are living or will live	_____
Concerns with current residence or neighbourhood	_____
Household responsibilities	_____
Home improvements or repairs	_____
Balancing demands of work and family	_____
Relationships with friends	_____
Limited personal time	_____
Concerns with social life	_____
Concerns with your appearance	_____
Issues with your personal traits or habits	_____
Boredom	_____
Feelings of loneliness	_____
Feelings about growing old	_____

Note that this scale was not designed to provide you with a quantitative measure of your overall stress level. Rather, it is a tool that helps you pinpoint specific stresses in your life and assess the impact each might be having on your life at the present time. It is an index of what is 'on your plate'.

Keep a simple stress diary

To effectively manage your stress, you need to become aware of when you are feeling stressed and be able to identify the sources of that stress. A stress diary can help you do just that. Your diary shows you, very specifically, when you experienced stress and pinpoints the situations or circumstances that triggered those stresses. Your diary acts as a cue or prompt, reminding you that you should take some action and make use of one or more of the stress-management tools you have mastered. By keeping a longer-term record of your daily stress, you are in the best position to formulate a comprehensive programme of stress management that can integrate the various stress-reducing strategies and tactics.

Finding Your Stress Balance

Determining your stress balance is one of the best ways of finding out whether you are overreacting to the stress in your life. Knowing your stress balance also helps you regain any lost perspective. This technique is invaluable, and you can use it anywhere, at anytime. It may quickly prove to be your favourite tool in helping to manage and reduce your stress. And it's simple to use. Just follow the steps in the next three sections.

Step 1: Rate your stress level

First rate the amount of stress you are feeling about a particular stressful episode using this 10-point scale:

10	
9	I was extremely distressed.
8	
7	
6	I was moderately distressed.
5	
4	
3	
2	I was only a little distressed.
1	
0	I wasn't distressed at all.

The term *distress* here refers to any one of the many forms of stress – frustration, aggravation, upset, annoyance, worry, anger, sadness, disappointment and so on.

Step 2: Rate the relative importance of the stress

Whenever you experience some stress, attempt to identify what is the source of your stress and rate its *relative importance* on a similar 10-point scale.

10	
9	Major importance
8	
7	
6	Moderate importance
5	
4	
3	
2	Minor importance
1	
0	Not important at all

To help you get the feel of the scale, think of three major life stresses that could happen or have happened to you. These are your 9s and 10s, the major life-altering events that everyone fears, and some people dread.

If you're having trouble coming up with anything, you may consider these possibilities: the death of a loved one, a major financial loss, a life-threatening illness, the loss of your job, chronic pain and so on. Again, these are given an importance rating of a 9 or a 10.

Step 3: Evaluate your stress balance

Now simply ask yourself, 'Does the stress I'm feeling match the importance of the situation?'

If it doesn't, you are off balance. Your stress level is out of line. Edith was off balance when she had a level-3 stress response because she had to wait for a while in a stalled underground train (a level 1 in importance). Her son's emotional outburst (a 7) when he was told that his favourite pair of trousers were in the wash (a 1 or 2), and her neighbour's great upset when he discovered that his newspaper was missing are examples of being off balance. In each case, the people were experiencing too much stress relative to the importance of the situations. These problems, situations and circumstances do not deserve this kind of emotional investment. Knowing you are off balance tells you that you are overreacting to a situation. Your stress button is bigger than it has to be, and you are causing yourself more stress than is necessary.

Take the triple-A approach

To effectively manage your stress, you may need a systematic way of looking at your stress and then determining how to go about reducing it. I have found that a three-step approach, or what I call the triple-A approach to stress management, is a useful and easy way to help you plan a programme of stress reduction. It tells you where to begin and what to do after you've started.

Here's what each of the three As refers to:

- ✔ **Awareness:** Know what your stress looks like and where it comes from. Your stress can be an unpleasant work environment, a major deadline, being caught in traffic, or any one of an endless number of other potential stresses.

- ✔ **Analysis:** The process of determining the best way or ways of managing this stress. Your options may include changing the situation or circumstances, changing yourself – the ways in which you react to a particular stress trigger – or possibly changing both.

- ✔ **Action:** What you do about your stress. Your action could be to do one of the many relaxation exercises, delegate more effectively, meditate, get some sleep – or use another of the methods and techniques described in this book.

This book can help you reduce and manage your stress at all three levels. You build a repertoire of skills, strategies and tactics. The goal is to maximise your ability to manage and control the stress in your life.

Book II
Food and Nutrition

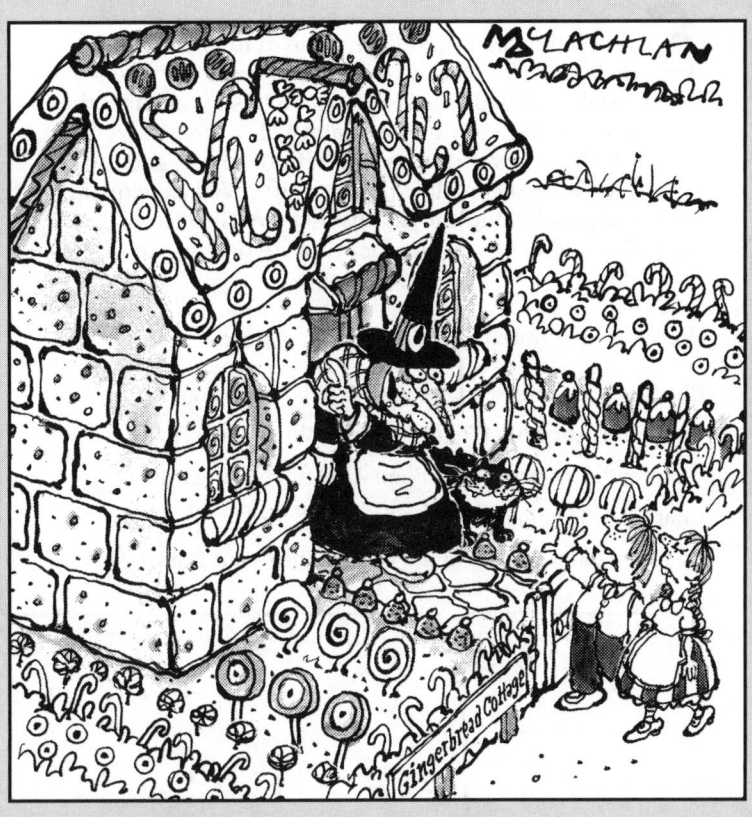

'No thanks — we're detoxing.'

In this book . . .

So much information on the value of food and nutrition is available that it's easy to become very confused. Book II goes through the key facts so you know the steps you can take towards a healthy diet. We give you information on what to eat and what not to eat, and explore how food can affect your health. We also explain the principles behind the highly-effective Glycaemic Load (GL) Diet, and how you can incorporate healthy ideas every day to boost your well-being.

Here are the contents of Book II at a glance:

Chapter 1

The Key Facts about Healthy Nutrition

In This Chapter

▶ Introducing dietary guidelines

▶ Striving for fitness

▶ Eating healthily

▶ Understanding why you need water

▶ Discovering ten superfoods

*O*ver the years many organisations have provided advice on healthy eating including The British Heart Foundation, The World Cancer Research Fund, The Food Standards Agency and Diabetes UK. The 1997 Guidelines for a Healthy Diet brought all the key messages together. This chapter helps you understand the key facts and shows you how to incorporate them in your own healthy eating regime.

Introducing the Guidelines for a Healthy Diet

The *Guidelines for a Healthy Diet* are a collection of sensible suggestions first published by the Ministry of Agriculture, Fisheries and Food and the Health Education Authority in 1991, and revised in 1997. The guidelines describe food and lifestyle choices that promote good health, provide the energy for an active life, and may reduce the risk or severity of chronic illnesses, such as diabetes and heart disease.

The best thing about these guidelines is that they seem to have been written by real people who actually like food. You can see this good attitude to food from the word go in the very first paragraph, which begins: 'Eating should be a pleasant aspect of life.' Hallelujah!

The guidelines work best in conjunction with the *Balance of Good Health*, which groups foods into categories and suggests the proportions of each you need to consume every day. You can read more about the Balance of Good Health in Book I Chapter 1. Right now, however, the job is spelling out the guidelines themselves.

The Guidelines for a Healthy Diet deliver eight basic health messages:

- ✔ Enjoy your food.
- ✔ Eat a variety of different foods.
- ✔ Eat the right amount to be a healthy weight.
- ✔ Eat plenty of foods rich in starch and fibre.
- ✔ Eat plenty of fruit and vegetables.
- ✔ Don't eat too many foods that contain a lot of fat.
- ✔ Don't have sugary foods and drinks too often.
- ✔ If you drink alcohol, drink sensibly.

The Scientific Advisory Committee on Nutrition (SACN) (2003) report suggests we add another guideline:

- ✔ Choose and prepare foods with less salt.

Throughout this chapter, we expand on what each of these suggestions means.

Stepping Out towards a Healthier Lifestyle

Healthy eating doesn't mean that any foods are completely banned or that others are obligatory. In order to maximise health and minimise the risk of disease you need to achieve nutritional balance. That means you don't need to restrict foods, you don't need to live in 'nutritional purgatory', and that sometimes a little of what you fancy does you good!

Eat a variety of foods

The greater the variety of foods you eat, the more likely that your diet will contain all the essential nutrients (including vitamins and minerals) that you need to be healthy. Mother Nature is pretty good at giving us everything we need in the foods we eat. The Balance of Good Health (Book I Chapter 1) shows the perfect model for what a healthy balanced diet should look like.

Eat the right amount for a healthy weight

Being overweight leads to many health problems. It places greater stress on the bones and joints, and raises blood pressure and cholesterol. It worsens breathing difficulties and increases the risk of developing diabetes, heart disease, stroke, and some forms of cancer. Eating the right diet and being physically active are essential to maintain a healthy weight.

So how do you go about managing your weight?

Book II

Food and Nutrition

- ✔ **Evaluate your body weight.** The best test of whether or not you're overweight is the Body Mass Index (BMI), a measure of body fat versus lean tissue or muscle that predicts the risk your weight poses to your health.

- ✔ **Manage your weight.** Weight management is about a lifelong lifestyle approach to food and activity. Quick fixes that sound too good to be true usually are!

- ✔ **If you need to lose weight do it gradually.** Forget the 'lose 2 stone in a month' headlines. Depending on how much weight you have to lose, anything between ½ and 2 pounds a week is a safe, maintainable weight loss. If you're overweight, losing just 10 per cent of your body weight brings significant health benefits, so it's not all about getting down to the weight you were at 16!

- ✔ **Encourage healthy weight in children.** It's sad but true that overweight kids usually become overweight adults. Helping children keep to a healthy weight from the start reduces the likelihood of them having weight problems later.

A few words about activity

When you take in more calories from food than you use up running your body systems (heart, lungs, brain, and so forth) and doing a day's normal activity, you end up storing the extra calories as body fat. In other words, you gain weight. The reverse is also true. When you use more energy in a day than you take in as food, you release the extra energy you need out of stored fat and you lose weight.

Even being mildly active increases the number of calories you can wolf down without gaining weight. The more strenuous the activity, the more plentiful the calorie allowance. If you're a 25-year-old man who weighs 10 stone, you require 1,652 calories a day to run your body systems. Clearly, you need more calories for doing your daily physical work, simply moving around, or exercising. Research shows that different levels of physical activity require different levels of energy or calorie intake. For example:

- Mild activity, such as gardening or housework, increases the number of calories you can consume each day without gaining weight to 2,645.

- Moderate activity, such as walking briskly at up to 4 miles per hour, raises the total number of calories you can consume each day without gaining weight to 2810.

- Working full out at a heavy activity, such as playing football or digging, pushes the number of calories you can consume each day without gaining weight up to 3,471.

In other words, a 10-stone man who steps up his physical activity from *mild* to *heavy* can consume 826 extra calories without gaining weight. That happens to be just about the amount of calories in a normal serving of spaghetti bolognaise. Now we're talking!

The following list describes some forms of moderate activity for healthy adults as recommended by the Chief Medical Officer's Report (2004) on Physical Activity and Health:

- Brisk walking (at the rate of 3 to 4 miles per hour)
- Playing active games with your children
- Table tennis
- Mowing the lawn
- Golf
- DIY, such as painting the walls
- Jogging
- Swimming
- Cycling (at the rate of less than 10 miles per hour)
- Gardening
- Dancing

Eat plenty of food rich in starch and fibre

Contrary to popular belief, foods like bread and potatoes are not necessarily fattening and provide essential nutrients such as vitamins and fibre. Other starchy, fibre-rich foods like cereals, pasta, and rice are filling and relatively cheap. These types of foods should be a major part of each meal and your diet as a whole.

Working out why you need to work out

Weight control is a good reason to step up your exercise level, but it isn't the only one. Here are four more:

✔ **Exercise increases muscles.** You can increase your muscle mass just by taking more regular exercise than you do at the moment. Because muscle tissue weighs more than fat tissue, some people may end up weighing more than they did before they started exercising to lose weight. But what your body weight is made up from is more important than the weight itself.

✔ **Exercise reduces the amount of fat stored in your body.** People who are fat around the middle as opposed to the hips (in other words an apple shape versus a pear shape) are at higher risk of weight-related illness. Exercise helps reduce abdominal fat and thus lowers your risk of weight-related diseases. Use a tape measure to identify your own body type by comparing your waistline to your hips (around the buttocks). If your waist (abdomen) is bigger, you're an apple. If your hips are bigger, you're a pear.

✔ **Exercise strengthens your bones.** *Osteoporosis* (a thinning of the bones that leads to repeated fractures) doesn't happen only to little old ladies. True, on average, a woman's bones thin faster and more dramatically than a man's, but after the mid-30s, everybody – male and female – begins losing bone density. Exercise can slow, halt, or in some cases even reverse the process. In addition, being physically active develops muscles that help support bones. Stronger bones equal less risk of fracture, which, in turn, equals less risk of potentially fatal complications.

✔ **Exercise increases brainpower.** You know that aerobic exercise increases the flow of oxygen to the heart, but did you also know that it increases the flow of oxygen to the brain? When a heavy workload keeps you up working into the night, a gentle exercise break can keep you going. Dr Judith J. Wurtman is a nutrition research scientist at Massachusetts Institute of Technology and author of *Managing Your Mind and Mood Through Food*. She discovered that when you're awake and working during hours that you'd normally be asleep, your internal body rhythms tell your body to cool down, even though your brain is racing along. Simply standing up and stretching, walking around the room, or doing a couple of sit-ups every hour or so speeds up your metabolism, warms up your muscles, increases your ability to stay awake, and, in Dr Wurtman's words, 'prolongs your ability to work smart into the night'.

Book II

Food and Nutrition

Let the Balance of Good Health guide your food choices

The Balance of Good Health is a guide that shows you exactly how to fill your plate. You can use it to help you plan a daily or weekly menu. See Book I Chapter 1 for more about the Balance of Good Health.

Eat plenty of fruit and vegetables

Fruits and vegetables are special because they:

- Add plenty of bulk but few calories to your diet, so you feel full without adding weight.

- Are usually low in fat and have no cholesterol, which means that they reduce your risk of heart disease.

- Are high in fibre, which reduces the risk of heart disease; prevents constipation; reduces the risk of developing haemorrhoids (or at least makes existing ones less painful); moves food quickly through your digestive tract, thus reducing the risk of diverticular disease (inflammation caused by food getting caught in the folds of your intestines and causing tiny pouches of the weakened gut wall); and lowers your risk of cancer of the mouth, throat (oesophagus and larynx), and stomach.

- Are rich in beneficial substances called phytochemicals and antioxidants, also believed to reduce your risk of heart disease and cancer.

For all these reasons, the British Dietetic Association, the British Heart Foundation, and just about every other agency with an interest in health recommends that we eat at least 5 portions of different-coloured fruit and vegetables every day.

People are often confused about what constitutes a portion, so here's a guide to help:

- 2 small pieces of fruit such as 2 plums or 2 apricots.

- 1 medium fruit such as 1 banana or 1 apple.

- 1 big slice of large fruit such as 1 large slice of melon or pineapple.

- 1 handful of berries such as strawberries or grapes.

- 2 tablespoons of dried, cooked, or tinned fruit in natural juice.

- 150 millilitres (5 fluid ounces or a small glass) of unsweetened fruit or vegetable juice – sorry, you can only count fruit juice once a day!

- 3 heaped tablespoons of beans (pulses also only count once a day).

- 2 tablespoons of raw or cooked vegetables.

- 1 cereal bowl full of mixed, undressed salad.

- ½ an avocado.

Walking Away from Unhealthy Food

Nutritionists don't like talking about 'good' or 'bad' foods, but you can benefit from eating less of certain foods. While a little of what you fancy really can do you good, too much of a good thing upsets the balance.

Don't eat too many fatty foods

Eating too much fat tends to raise blood cholesterol levels and increases the risk of obesity and heart disease. Most of us would benefit from eating less fat in general and in particular less saturated fat. With fats like butter, margarine, and cooking oils, and fried food, full-fat dairy products, and fatty meat, you can usually see the fat so it's easy to cut down. A lot of foods such as pastry, pies, biscuits, cakes, and savoury snacks contain a lot of hidden fat that you can't see so easily).

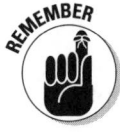

No foods are inherently good or bad, and fats are a good example. Fat is an essential nutrient but certain fats, especially the saturated fats mainly found in animal foods, increase our blood cholesterol levels. Other types such as monounsaturated fat, polyunsaturated fat, and omega 3 and 6 fatty acids are positively healthy. You've guessed it: It's all a question of balance.

Book II

Food and Nutrition

Counting the fat calories

To calculate the percentage of fat in any food, you need to know two numbers: The total calories in the serving and the number of grams of fat. Take, for example, one wedge of Camembert cheese. The label says that the cheese wedge has 115 calories and 9 grams of fat. One gram of fat has nine calories. Use the following equation to find out the percentage of calories that come from fat:

1. Multiply the number of grams of fat by 9 (the number of calories in one gram of fat).

   For the Camembert cheese example, 9 grams multiplied by 9 calories per gram gives you the number of calories from fat, or 81.

2. Divide the result from Step 1 by the total number of calories. The result is the percentage of calories from fat.

   Continuing the cheese example, divide 81 (the number of calories from fat) by 115 (the total number of calories in the wedge) and multiply by 100. The result: 70 per cent of the calories come from fat in one wedge of Camembert cheese.

The good news is that most packaged food sold in the UK carries nutritional information, including the fat content. Milk, peas, soup, chocolate cake – you name it, and you can find the total and saturated fat content per serving right there on the food label, which means you can also figure out the percentage of calories from fat.

Overall, the Guidelines for a Healthy Diet suggest that adults should derive no more than 30 to 35 per cent of calories from fat, with no more than 10 per cent of calories from saturated fat.

Don't have sugary foods and drinks too often

Sweet foods and drinks are fine as occasional treats, but too many, too often are likely to put your diet in an energy or calorie excess, which means you're likely to put on weight. If you're substituting fruits, vegetables, and starchy high-fibre foods with lots of sweet foods and drinks you're missing out on essential vitamins and minerals – too much sugar, too often is a double whammy for unbalancing your diet.

Frequent intakes of sugar-rich foods and drinks can also cause tooth decay. Brush teeth twice a day with a fluoride toothpaste and floss regularly. Chewing sugar-free gum can also stimulate the saliva flow to protect the teeth.

Question: Which is worse for your teeth, a piece of chocolate or a couple of raisins? Yes, this is a trick question. Yes, the answer is raisins.

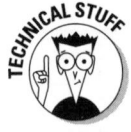

The explanation's simple. Both foods have lots of sugar, but the chocolate is less detrimental to your teeth because it dissolves quickly and is washed out of your mouth (and off your teeth) by your saliva. Raisins, on the other hand, are sticky. Unless you brush and floss thoroughly they cling to your teeth, providing a longer-lasting banquet for those pesky tooth-decay bacteria.

You can assume the food is high in sugar whenever the word sugar is one of the first ingredients listed on the food product's ingredient list. Although sugars occur naturally in fruits and vegetables, the safe bet is that most of the sugar in your diet comes as 'added sugar' in processed foods. These added sugars may be listed on food labels in any of the forms in the list that follows:

- Brown sugar
- Corn sweetener
- Corn syrup
- Fructose
- Fruit juice concentrate
- Glucose (dextrose)
- High-fructose corn syrup
- Honey

✔ Invert sugar (50:50 fructose–glucose)

✔ Lactose

✔ Maltose

✔ Molasses

✔ Raw sugar

✔ Sugar (sucrose)

✔ Syrup

If you drink alcohol, drink sensibly

Modest amounts of alcohol aren't harmful to most people and may even have health advantages in some circumstances. Men and postmenopausal women seem to get some reduced risk of heart disease from drinking in moderation. But what's *moderation*, anyway? Nutritionists define *moderate* as the amount of alcohol your body can metabolise without increasing your risk of serious illness such as cancer or liver damage.

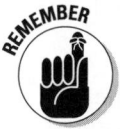

The Government defines sensible drinking limits as 3–4 units per day for men or 2–3 units per day for women. However, the Government also says that consistently drinking 4 units a day (3 for women) is not recommended because of the progressive health risk it carries.

One unit is:

✔ ½ pint of ordinary strength beer lager or cider.

✔ 1 small glass of wine (100ml).

✔ 1 single measure of spirits (25ml).

✔ 1 small glass of sherry (50ml).

The safe levels for women are lower than for men because women are on average smaller than men and their bodies contain proportionately less water and more fat. They can tolerate less alcohol before damage occurs to their organs and can feel its effects faster and more intensely. The old wives' tale that *he can drink her under the table* is no myth. It's physiology.

Some people shouldn't drink at all, not even in moderation, including people who suffer from alcoholism, people who plan to drive a car or take part in other activities that require attention to detail or physical skill, and people using certain types of medication (prescription drugs or over-the-counter products).

Choose and prepare foods with less salt

Sodium is a mineral that helps regulate your body's *fluid balance*, the flow of water into and out of every cell. This balance keeps just enough water inside the cell so that it can perform its daily jobs, but not so much that the cell explodes.

Most of us get far more sodium than we need, mainly from salt or sodium chloride in our diet. As a result high blood pressure is very common, and this in turn can increase the risk of heart disease and stroke. Salt or sodium makes your blood hold onto more water, which creates more pressure. If you already have high blood pressure, you can help reduce it by lowering the amount of salt you eat. If your blood pressure is normal you can help keep it that way by watching your salt intake.

For a few people reducing salt intake has another, unadvertised benefit. It may lower weight a bit. Why? Because sodium is *hydrophilic* (*hydro* = water; *philic* = loving). Sodium attracts and holds water. Eating less salt means that some people retain less water and feel less bloated.

Don't reduce salt intake drastically without first checking with your doctor. Remember, some sodium is essential, and the guidelines advocate moderate use, not no use at all.

The obvious question: What's moderate use? Current intakes are in the region of 9 grams of salt (3,600 milligrams of sodium) per day – that's about one and a half teaspoons. The Guidelines for a Healthy Diet recommend you aim for no more than 6 grams of salt (2,400 milligrams of sodium) or 1 teaspoon per day. (One gram of salt = 400 milligrams of sodium. To convert sodium to salt, multiply the sodium content by 2.5.)

Like sugar, sodium occurs naturally in foods. However, only about 15 per cent of sodium intake comes via this route. Another 15 per cent is added at the table or in cooking. A whopping 70 per cent comes from manufactured or processed foods. For example, a portion of frozen peas cooked in unsalted water has only a trace of sodium, but a portion of tinned peas has over 200 milligrams of sodium.

Look out for tinned and processed vegetables in lower-salt versions. The difference is notable: A tin of reduced-salt baked beans has approximately half the salt content of regular baked beans.

You also get salt from fast foods, sauces, and pickles. Not all the sodium you eat is sodium chloride. Sodium compounds are also used as preservatives, thickeners, and flavour enhancers, and these all add to the load.

To find out more about salt check out www.salt.gov.uk.

Table 1-1 lists several different kinds of sodium compounds in food.

Table 1-1	The Sodium Compounds Found in Food
Compound	*What It Is or Does*
Monosodium glutamate (MSG)	Flavour enhancer
Sodium benzoate	Food preservative
Sodium caseinate	Thickens foods
Sodium chloride	Table salt (flavouring agent)
Sodium citrate	Keeps drinks fizzy
Sodium hydroxide	Makes it easy to peel the skin off tomatoes and fruits before they're tinned
Sodium nitrate/nitrite	Keeps food preserved and gives them their distinctive red colour (e.g. cured meats)
Sodium saccharine	Artificial sweetener

Relaxing Once in a While

Life is not a test. You won't fail if you don't manage to follow the Guidelines for a Healthy Diet every single day of your life. Nobody's perfect, and the guidelines are meant to be broken once in a while. For example, ideally you should keep your daily fat intake to around 35 per cent of your total calories. But you can bet that you'll exceed that amount this Saturday as you stroll up to the buffet table at your best friend's wedding and see:

- ✔ Camembert cheese (70 per cent of the calories from fat).
- ✔ Sirloin steak (56 per cent of the calories from fat) and salad with Thousand Island dressing (90 per cent of the calories from fat).
- ✔ Hot chocolate fudge cake and cream (we can't count that high).

Is this a crisis? Should you stay at home? Must you keep your mouth shut tight all night? Are you joking? Here's the solution: Let your hair down every once in a while. After the party's over, compensate. For the rest of the week, eat lots of the nutritious, delicious, low-fat foods that should make up most of your regular diet:

- ✔ Fresh fruit (virtually no calories from fat).
- ✔ Salads (ditto – but watch that dressing!).
- ✔ Roast white meat (such as turkey), with no skin (20 per cent of its calories from fat).
- ✔ Pasta (5 per cent) with tomato-based sauces (2–3 per cent).

By the end of the week, you're likely to have averaged out to a desirable amount with no problem and be right in line with that headline from the first page of the guidelines that we mention in the beginning of this chapter: 'Enjoy your food.' Amen to that.

Investigating the Many Ways Your Body Uses Water

Water is a solvent. It dissolves other substances and carries nutrients and other material (such as blood cells) around the body, making it possible for every organ to do its job. You need water to:

✔ Digest food, dissolving nutrients so that they can pass through the intestinal cell walls into your bloodstream, and move food along through your intestinal tract.

✔ Carry toxins and waste products out of your body via urine from the kidneys.

✔ Provide a medium in which chemical reactions such as metabolism occur.

✔ Send electrical messages between cells so that your muscles can move, your eyes can see, your brain can think, and so on.

✔ Act as a lubricant for mucous membranes.

✔ Prevent overheating just like the water in a car radiator – cooling your body with moisture (sweat) that evaporates from your skin.

Maintaining the right amount of water in your body

Of the 45 litres of water in an average adult body, about 30 litres or 2/3 is in the *intracellular fluid*, the liquid inside body cells. The remaining 15 litres is in the *extracellular fluid*, which is all the other body liquids, such as:

✔ Interstitial fluid (the fluid surrounding the cells).

✔ Blood plasma (the clear liquid in blood).

✔ Lymph (a clear, slightly yellow fluid collected from body tissues that flows through your lymph nodes and eventually into your blood vessels).

A healthy body has just the right amount of fluid inside and outside each cell, a situation that health professionals call *fluid balance*. Maintaining your fluid balance is essential to life. If too little water is inside a cell, the cell shrivels and dies. Too much water, and the cell bursts.

A balancing act: The role of electrolytes

Your body regulates its fluid balance through the action of substances called *electrolytes*, essential minerals which dissolve in water into electrically charged particles called ions and which are found in every body fluid.

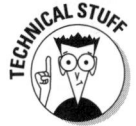

Many minerals, including calcium, phosphorus, and magnesium, form compounds that dissolve into charged particles. But nutritionists generally use the term electrolyte to describe sodium, potassium, and chlorine (as chloride). The most familiar source of electrolytes is the one found on every dinner table – sodium chloride, plain old table salt. (In water, its molecules dissolve into two ions: One sodium ion and one chloride ion.)

Under normal circumstances, the fluid inside your cells has more potassium than sodium and chloride. The fluid outside is just the opposite: More sodium and chloride than potassium rather like seawater. The cell wall is a *semipermeable membrane*; some things pass through, but others do not. Water molecules and electrolytes flow through freely, but larger molecules such as proteins do not. Changes in fluid balance alter the concentration of these electrolytes either diluting them or concentrating them, which in turn controls the body's response to loss of water.

The body uses this changing concentration of electrolytes to draw water between the cells and maintain a balance between the extra and intra cellular areas. When your body loses too much fluid, your thirst centre in the brain is stimulated by the increased concentration of electrolytes in the blood, especially sodium, causing you to drink more to replace the lost fluid.

Concentration of the plasma sodium also results in reduced urination, a protective mechanism triggered by *antidiuretic hormone (ADH)*, a hormone secreted by the hypothalamus, a gland at the base of your brain, which reduces the release of urine from the kidneys. If you drink too much the concentration of sodium goes down and the reverse occurs – you stop feeling thirsty and start producing more urine.

Dehydrating without enough water and electrolytes

Drink more water than you need, and the healthy body simply shrugs its shoulders, urinates more copiously, and readjusts the water levels. A healthy person on a normal diet would find it hard to drink himself or herself to death on water. However, some people with heart or kidney problems may be at risk of fluid overload and need to follow medically supervised fluid restrictions. Some marathon runners are also at risk of excessive consumption of water or sports drinks, leading to very low levels of sodium.

If you don't get enough water, your body lets you know pretty quickly. Rapid fluid depletion can occur in children with diarrhoea and can be fatal.

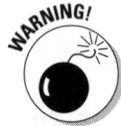

Chronic dehydration can be a problem for people if they have a low fluid intake. Children, nursing mothers, active adults, the elderly, and the unwell need to have lots of fluids. People on diuretic drugs (medication that increases the flow of urine) or those with swallowing difficulties also need to be careful. Recent studies show that as many as 1 in 4 people don't drink enough.

The thirst mechanism isn't really very sensitive in humans – by the time you feel thirsty, you've already lost about 1–2 per cent of your body weight as water and you may already be really quite dehydrated.

Signs of dehydration include:

- ✔ Constipation

- ✔ Headache

- ✔ Fatigue and irritability

- ✔ Lack of concentration or exacerbated existing mental confusion

- ✔ Loss of appetite

- ✔ Nausea or dizziness

- ✔ Concentrated dark urine

Severe dehydration can lead to urinary and kidney problems, circulatory collapse, and even death.

Getting the water you need

Unlike other nutrients, you don't store water, so you need to take in a new supply every day, enough to replace what you lose. Total daily water exchange for a reasonably sedentary individual in a temperate climate is about 2,800 millilitres a day from food and liquid. The average person in Britain uses 150 litres of water each day but only actually drinks 1 litre. You lose about 1400 millilitres or nearly 50 per cent of water in your urine. You lose another 150 millilitres in your faeces, and around 850 millilitres as sweat, and 400 millilitres in breath from your lungs.

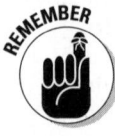

Not all of this lost water needs to be replaced by drinks. About 10 per cent of the water you need (around 300 millilitres) is created when you digest and metabolise food. The end products of digestion and metabolism are carbon dioxide (a waste product that you breathe out of your body) and water (composed of hydrogen from food and oxygen from the air that you breathe). Around a litre of water comes from your daily food intake. Fruit and vegetables are full of it. Lettuce, for example, is 90 per cent water. The rest of your fluid intake comes directly from drinks – around 1500 millilitres a day. This translates to about eight glasses a day. In a temperate climate, or if you're very active, you need more: You can lose 2–3 litres of sweat per hour. Yuk!

Any fluid, not just water, can contribute to your daily fluid intake. This includes milk, coffee, tea, soft drinks, and fruit juices. But here's an interesting fact: Not all liquids are equally rehydrating. Strong coffee, and the alcohol in beer, wine, and spirits, act as diuretics, or chemicals that make you urinate more copiously. But don't ditch your espresso machine: Recent studies show that standard servings of tea and coffee have very little diuretic effect and regular consumers are able to tolerate them.

Taking in extra water and electrolytes as needed

Most people regularly consume much more sodium than they need. It occurs naturally in many foods and is added in a variety of forms including sodium chloride and monosodium glutamate to foods during processing. In fact, high salt intakes may be responsible for high blood pressure especially the increase in blood pressure associated with getting older. Studies suggest that for many this can be which can be lowered if they reduce their sodium intake (For more about high blood pressure, check out *High Blood Pressure For Dummies* by Dr Alan Rubin).

Potassium and chloride are found in so many foods that dietary deficiency is virtually non-existent. However increasing dietary potassium has been shown to be a factor in helping to reduce high blood pressure. Particularly useful sources of potassium include fruit, vegetables and potatoes.

The daily reference nutrient intakes (RNIs) for adults for sodium, potassium, and chloride are:

- **Sodium:** 1600 milligrams
- **Potassium:** 3500 milligrams
- **Chloride:** 2500 milligrams

Most of us get much more as a matter of course, but sometimes you actually need extra water and electrolytes.

You've got an upset stomach

Repeated vomiting or diarrhoea drains your body of water and electrolytes. The normal faecal loss of water of 150 millilitres can increase to 1–2 litres with severe diarrhoea. Similarly, you also need extra water to replace the liquid lost in sweat when you have a temperature.

When you need it in a hurry, plain water won't replace that fluid as quickly as a rehydration solution with added electrolytes. Check with your pharmacist for a drink to hydrate your body without upsetting your stomach.

You're exercising or working hard in a hot environment

When you're warm, you sweat. The moisture evaporates and cools your skin so that blood circulating up from the centre of your body to the surface is cooled. The cooled blood returns to the centre of your body, lowering the temperature (your *core temperature*) there, too. If you don't replace the water lost in sweat things can get tricky. At first it's just your concentration and ability to keep going that's affected, but ultimately dehydration can lead to heat stroke and circulatory collapse.

Always make sure you start exercising well hydrated. For most recreational or competitive exercise, aim to drink up to 600–800 millilitres of water per hour at regular intervals to top up – don't wait until you feel thirsty. Rehydrate afterwards as soon as you can – and certainly before you head for the bar! Plain water is fine in most situations, but for exercise lasting more than an hour some sports drinks containing electrolytes may increase your fluid absorption and offer added carbohydrate for energy.

Ten Superfoods

All foods contain valuable nutrients – yes, even a deep-fried Mars Bar has some goodness. However, some superfoods have so many health-giving properties that eating them on a regular basis could be a real bonus. Here are our top ten superfoods based on the latest nutrition research.

Bananas

Did you know that bananas don't actually grow on trees but on giant herbs? It's also a myth that bananas are fattening. Bananas are slightly higher in energy than other fruits but the calories come mainly from carbohydrate; excellent for refuelling before, during or after exercise.

Bananas also make a very useful contribution to the recommended daily five portions of fruit and vegetables. All types of fruit and vegetables contain plant chemicals or phytochemicals known as *antioxidants*. These antioxidants protect cells in the body against damage from free radicals that can cause heart disease and cancer. Increasing your intake to five portions of fruit and veg a day reduces the risk of death from these chronic diseases by about 20 per cent. Bananas are also jam-packed with potassium, which helps lower blood pressure, and vitamin B6 for healthy skin and hair.

Water, water, everywhere

Water is the only substance on Earth that can exist as a liquid (water) and a solid (ice or snow) and a gas (steam). Water can be hard or soft depending on the mineral content.

✔ **Hard water** is water that rises to the Earth's surface from underground springs. It has lots of minerals that it picks up as it moves up through the ground. Much of the water in south-east England is hard.

Hard water may contain as many as 100 particles of calcium, magnesium, iron, and sodium for every 1 million parts of water (shorthand: 100 ppm) and can leave a deposit on the bath or a scale in your kettle and washing machine.

✔ **Soft water** is usually surface water collected from streams and hills, or rainwater that falls directly into reservoirs. Wales, Scotland, central and south-west England have soft water. Soft water has fewer minerals.

If you aren't sure about whether your drinking water is hard or soft, consider the source. In areas of the United Kingdom where the major part of the water supply comes from reservoirs, the water that flows from your tap is likely to be soft. In the other parts of the UK, the water is likely to be hard.

Tap water in the United Kingdom meets rigorous safety standards making it entirely suitable as your main source of fluid not to mention being more environmentally friendly than bottled water. However, some people either don't like the taste of their tap water, or they may wish to avoid added chemicals such as fluoride, chlorine used to kill microorganisms or traces of chemicals used in farming. As a result, the last decade has seen a massive explosion in the use of water filters and bottled water. In the United Kingdom people spend well over £2 million per year on bottled water, with the average purchaser spending £450. Who could have predicted that one day entire aisles of our supermarkets would be devoted just to bottled water? Here's what you can get:

✔ **Bottled water** is usually tap water that's purified to remove all chemicals by methods such as distillation, ionisation, or reverse osmosis. If carbon dioxide is added it's known as sparkling water.

✔ **Natural mineral water** must come from a natural underground source. It contains minerals leached from the rocks as it passes through. Generally the mineral level is quite low, but check the label if you are watching your salt intake, as some brand-name mineral water is high in sodium. For this reason don't use natural mineral water when making up infant formula.

✔ **Spring water** is water from a natural spring source. It can be fizzy or still and often has fewer mineral particles and a cleaner taste than mineral water. Some brands can still be major sources of sodium – always check the label.

Apples

An apple a day keeps the doctor away, or so we've always been told. Over 7,500 varieties of apple are grown throughout the world and any one counts as one of your five-a-day portions. Like bananas, apples are packed full of antioxidants, especially vitamin C for healthy skin and gums – one apple provides a quarter of your daily requirement of vitamin C. In addition apples contain a form of soluble fibre called pectin that can help to lower blood cholesterol levels and keep the digestive system healthy.

An apple is also a handy package of carbohydrate of the low glycaemic index (GI) type. Low GI foods are digested slowly; once they are finally broken down in the intestine they are gradually absorbed into the bloodstream as glucose, causing a gradual rise in blood sugar levels. This means that only a small amount of the hormone insulin needs to be released to keep blood sugar within the normal range. A regular inclusion of low GI foods such as apples may help to improve diabetics' long-term control of blood sugar levels. Low GI foods may also help with weight control and may be protective against heart disease.

Broccoli

The old advice to eat up your greens to stay healthy is also true. Although the intake of many vegetables has gone down in the UK, broccoli has increased in popularity in recent years. Just two florets – raw or lightly cooked – count as a portion.

Not only does broccoli contain antioxidants including vitamin C but it's a particularly good source of folate (naturally occurring folic acid). This B vitamin has been found to reduce levels of an amino acid known as homocysteine in the blood. High homocysteine is linked to an increased risk of heart disease and is now believed to be as important a risk factor as high cholesterol levels. Increasing your intake of folic acid is thought to be of major benefit in preventing heart disease, and studies are currently under way to investigate further. Recent research has linked high homocysteine to an increased risk of Alzheimer's disease and osteoporosis as well.

Broccoli also contains a particular antioxidant called lutein that can delay the progression of age-related macular degeneration (AMD). AMD affects 10 per cent of people over 60 (and 20 per cent over 80) and is a major cause of impaired vision and blindness. So it's not just carrots that are good for eyesight. As if all this good stuff isn't enough, broccoli contains another phytochemical called sulphoraphane that has specific anti-cancer properties.

Brazil nuts

All nuts are generally packed full of essential vitamins, minerals and fibre. Recent studies suggest that eating a small handful of nuts four to five times a week can help reduce heart disease, satisfy food cravings, and even control weight. Unsalted nuts are best, as most of us already get far too much salt from the rest of our food. Brazil nuts are one of the few good sources of selenium, which may help protect against cancer, depression and Alzheimer's disease. Just two brazil nuts a day meets your selenium requirement.

Olive oil

Olive oil is prized in many parts of the world for its taste and versatility and is the cornerstone of many great cuisines. In ancient medicine it was used to cure pretty much everything from mental illness to ulcers. Several large studies suggest that the monounsaturated fat in olive oil is good for the heart. Olive oil lowers bad cholesterol levels and increases the good levels (see Book II Chapter 2 for more on the goodies and baddies of the cholesterol world). Olive oil is also rich in antioxidants – in fact, it's probably one of the key protective aspects of the so-called Mediterranean diet. You can use olive oil for cooking or drizzled on salad. Olive oil-based spreads are an excellent alternative to butter.

Watch out for the calories – a little goes a long way: A tablespoon of oil contains 120 kilocalories, the same as a large slice of bread and butter. If you're not keen on the taste of olive oil, then rapeseed oil (often sold as blended vegetable oil) is nearly as good but just as high in calories.

Book II

Food and Nutrition

Salmon

All fish is a source of good-quality protein, vitamins and minerals, but oily fish such as salmon also contains omega 3 fats that reduce blood clotting (thrombosis) and inflammation. Studies show that eating oily fish dramatically reduces the risk of having a heart attack, even in older adults: It's never too late to start. Omega 3 fats have also been shown to have myriad other benefits. They help prevent depression, and protect against the onset of dementia. Yep, it's true, fish really is an all-round brain food.

Eat at least one serving of oily fish per week, increasing to two to three servings per week if you are at high risk of heart disease. Alternatives to salmon include pilchards, trout, herrings, mackerel and sardines. Tinned, fresh and smoked fish are all good.

Tea

Tea has a range of useful properties. The caffeine content is helpful for stimulating alertness, mood and motivation, especially when you're tired or run down. Tea drunk at typical UK levels contains insufficient caffeine to have any harmful diuretic effect. Tea counts towards the recommended eight cups or around 1,500 millilitres of fluid daily. Don't forget that this is a minimum needed to avoid dehydration, which can impair both physical performance and mental concentration. You need more if the weather's hot or you're very active.

Tea, whether black, green (more common in Asia) or red, is a rich source of a particular type of antioxidant called catechins. Studies suggest that catechins protect the artery walls against the damage that causes heart disease and prevent formation of sticky blood clots. Some population studies suggest that tea drinkers have less heart disease and as little as one cuppa a day seems to offer some protection. So pop that kettle on!

Whole-grain seeded bread

Breads containing a lot of seeds and whole grains (as well as rye bread, and barley and sunflower bread) have a low glycaemic index, which can protect against heart disease, reduce hunger pangs, and even help with weight control. Seeded and whole-grain breads are also packed with fibre, which keeps the gut working efficiently; and seeded breads contain essential fatty acids that offer a whole host of health-boosting properties.

Studies show that including four slices of soya and linseed bread a day can give a therapeutic dose of phyto-oestrogens, thought to relieve vasomotor symptoms or 'hot flushes' in menopausal women.

The downside is that bread contains a lot of salt. In 2000, more than a fifth of the average total intake of salt in the UK was from bread. However, the good news is that bread manufacturers have already started to use less salt – levels in pre-packed bread fell by about 13 per cent between 1998 and 2001. The Federation of Bakers, which represents most manufacturers of sliced wrapped bread, pledged to continue a gradual reduction in the salt added to bread by their members.

Yoghurt

To make yoghurt, a bacterial culture is added to warm milk. The bacteria feed on the milk sugar called lactose, and release lactic acid, which thickens the milk into the familiar creamy texture of yoghurt. Yoghurt is an easily absorbed source of calcium, one small carton providing 40 per cent of an adult's daily calcium needs. It's also a useful milk substitute for people who can't digest large amounts of the milk sugar, lactose.

When milk is made into yoghurt, the bacteria culture added to the milk produces lactase that breaks down lactose, the milk sugar.

Yoghurt has long been credited with a range of therapeutic benefits, many of which involve the health of the large intestine and the relief of gastro-intestinal upsets. At the beginning of the 1900s, the Russian researcher Metchinikov won the Nobel prize for his investigations into why people in some parts of eastern Europe live particularly active lives and stay in good health well into their nineties and beyond. He concluded that this phenomenon was attributable to the yoghurt in their diet.

The bacteria *Lactobacillus GG*, added to some yoghurt, are not digested, and reach the large intestine intact where they 'top up' the other friendly bacteria living there. The friendly bacteria fight harmful bacteria, including *Clostridium difficile*, which can cause diarrhoea after a course of antibiotics. Other strains of friendly bacteria like *Lactobacillus immunitas* have since been discovered; many now appear in yoghurts and other functional foods designed specifically to improve gut health. So as well as choosing between strawberry or raspberry yoghurt, you can also decide which type of friendly bacteria you want to snack on!

Book II

Food and Nutrition

Baked beans

The humble baked bean is a nutritional powerhouse of protein, fibre, iron and calcium. It contains carbohydrate that, like that in apples and seeded breads, is of the low GI variety.

The tomato sauce covering baked beans is also a good source of lycopene, another powerful antioxidant shown to help prevent heart disease and prostate cancer. Lycopene is found predominantly in tomatoes and appears to be more available to the body when tomatoes are processed or mixed with other foods. So the sauce with your beans is a lot more than a tasty accompaniment to make your toast soggy!

The insoluble fibre in baked beans is not digested but moves into the large intestine, or colon, where bacteria act on it and produce short-chain fatty acids. These fatty acids are thought to nourish the colon lining and protect it from carcinogenic (cancer-causing) invaders. Insoluble fibre adds to the physical bulk of the stools, helping them to move along more rapidly. This helps prevent the cancer-causing substances from attaching themselves to the colon wall.

Chapter 2

Knowing What and What Not to Eat

The human body needs all sorts of nutrients to function at its best. In this chapter we explain how powerful these nutrients are and see how much of each you need.

Powerful Protein

Protein is an essential nutrient, vital for the structure of your body and its functions.

How your body uses protein

Your body uses proteins to build new cells, maintain tissues and put together new proteins that make it possible for you to perform basic bodily functions.

Every day, you reuse more proteins than you get from the food you eat, so you need a continuous supply to maintain your protein levels. If your diet does not contain sufficient amounts of proteins, you start digesting the proteins in your body, including the proteins in your muscles and, in extreme cases of starvation, your heart muscle.

Complete proteins and incomplete proteins

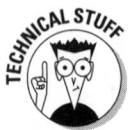

Another way to describe the quality of proteins is to say that they are either complete or incomplete, or have a high or low biological value. A *complete protein* with a *high biological value* is one that contains ample amounts of all essential amino acids; an *incomplete protein* or one with a *low biological value* does not. A protein low in one specific amino acid is called a *limiting protein* because it can build only as much tissue as the smallest amount of the necessary amino acid. You can improve the quality in a food containing incomplete or limited proteins by eating it with protein that contains sufficient amounts of amino acids. Matching foods to create complete proteins is called *complementarity*.

For example, grains are low in the essential amino acid lysine, and beans are low in the essential amino acid methionine. By combining the two by eating beans on toast, you improve (or complete) the proteins in both. Another example is combining grains with dairy products, such as eating pasta and cheese. Pasta is low in the essential amino acids lysine and isoleucine, but milk products (like cheese) have abundant amounts of these two amino acids. Shaking Parmesan cheese onto pasta creates a higher-quality protein dish. In each case, the foods have complementary amino acids.

Other examples of complementary protein dishes are peanut butter with bread, and milk with cereal. Many combinations of two or more types of plant proteins are a natural and customary part of the diet in parts of the world where animal proteins are scarce or very expensive. Table 2-1 shows how to combine foods to improve the quality of their proteins. Improving proteins is particularly important for people following a vegan or vegetarian diet.

Table 2-1	How to Combine Foods to Complement Proteins	
This food	*Complements this food*	*Examples*
Whole grains	Legumes (beans)	Rice and peas; beans on toast; dahl and rice; tofu and noodles; tortilla and refried beans; couscous and chick peas; falafel and pitta bread
Dairy products	Whole grains	Cheese sandwich with wholemeal bread; wholemeal pasta with cheese; pancakes (wheat and milk and egg batter); porridge and milk
Legumes (beans)	Nuts and seeds	Mixed bean salad with sesame seed dressing; hummus
Dairy products	Legumes (beans)	Baked beans with grated cheese
Dairy products	Nuts and seeds	Yogurt with chopped nuts; muesli with milk

Deciding how much protein you need

The Department of Health, which sets the requirements (known as *Dietary Reference Values*) for vitamins and minerals, also sets goals for daily protein consumption. As with other nutrients, the department has different recommendations for different groups of people; young or older, men or women.

Calculating the correct amount

As a general rule, the Department of Health says that healthy people need to get around 15 per cent of their daily calories from protein. As a secondary rule, an average healthy adult man or woman needs about 0.75 grams of high-quality protein for every kilogram (2.2 pounds) of body weight, slightly less than 0.35 grams for every pound.

Book II

Food and Nutrition

For example, a woman weighing 63 kilograms (9 stone 8 pounds) needs about 50 grams of protein a day, and a man weighing 79.5 kilograms (12 stone 7 pounds) needs about 63 grams. These amounts are easily obtained from two to three average servings of lean meat, fish, or poultry (21 grams each). If the woman is a vegetarian, she can get her 50 grams of protein from two eggs (32 grams) or two servings of soya products (28 grams), two slices of cheese (10 grams), four slices of bread (12 grams), and one serving of yogurt (10 grams). The number crunchers amongst you will quickly spot that these combinations add up to more than 50 grams; the point we are making is that it is very easy to get all the protein you need from a normal healthy diet so you can mix and match your protein sources without worrying if you'll be getting enough.

Boosting your protein intake: Special considerations

Anyone who is building new tissue quickly needs more than 0.75 grams of protein per kilogram (2.2 pounds) of body weight per day. For example:

- Infants need as much as 2.0 grams of protein for every kilogram of body weight per day.

- Adolescents need as much as 1.2 grams per kilogram per day.

- Pregnant women need an extra 10 grams a day, and breast-feeding women also need extra protein. This extra protein is used to build the foetal tissues and then to produce adequate amounts of nutritious breast milk.

Injuries also raise your protein requirements. An injured body releases above-normal amounts of protein-destroying hormones from the pituitary and adrenal glands. You need extra protein to protect existing tissues, and after severe blood loss, you need extra protein to make new haemoglobin. Cuts, burns, or surgical procedures mean that you need extra protein to make new skin and muscle cells. Fractures mean that extra protein is needed to make new bone. The need for protein is so important when you've been badly injured that if you cannot take protein by mouth, you'll be given an intravenous solution of amino acids with glucose (sugar) or emulsified fat.

The Lowdown on Fat and Cholesterol

The chemical family name for fats and related compounds such as cholesterol is *lipids* (from *lipos*, the Greek word for fat). Liquid fats are called *oils*; solid fats are called, well, *fat*. With the exception of *cholesterol* (a fatty substance that has no calories and provides no energy), fats are high-energy nutrients. Gram for gram, fats have more than twice as much energy potential (calories) as protein and carbohydrates (affectionately referred to as carbs): 9 calories per fat gram versus 3.75 calories per gram for proteins and 4 for carbs.

In this section, we cut the fat away from the subject of fats and home in on the essential facts you need to put together a diet with enough fat (yes, you do need fat) to provide the bounce that every diet requires. And then we'll deal with that ultimate baddie cholesterol. Surprise! You need some of that, too.

Finding the facts about fat

Fats are sources of energy that add flavour and texture to food – the sizzle on the steak, you could say. However, as most people know, fats can also be hazardous to your health. The trick is separating the good fats from the bad and getting the balance right.

Understanding why your body needs fat

A healthy body needs fat. Your body uses *dietary fat* (the fat that you get from food) to make tissue and manufacture biochemicals, such as hormones. Some of the body fat made from food fat is *visible*. Even though your skin covers it, you can *see* the fat in the *adipose* (fatty) *tissue* in female breasts, hips, thighs, buttocks and belly (all of which are part of the design to make women able to carry, bear and feed children), or male abdomen and shoulders.

This *visible* body fat:

- Provides a source of stored energy.
- Gives shape to your body.
- Cushions your skin (imagine sitting in a chair for a while to read this book without your buttocks to cushion your bones).
- Acts as an insulation blanket that reduces heat loss.

Other body fat is *invisible*. You can't see this body fat because it's tucked away in and around your internal organs. This hidden fat is:

✔ Part of every cell membrane (the outer skin that holds each cell together).

✔ A component of *myelin*, the fatty material that sheathes nerve cells and makes it possible for them to fire the electrical messages that enable you to think, see, speak, move and perform the multitude of tasks natural to a living body. Brain tissue is also rich in fat.

✔ A shock absorber that protects your organs as much as possible if you fall or injure yourself.

✔ A constituent of hormones and other biochemicals, such as vitamin D and bile.

Book II

Food and Nutrition

Releasing energy from fat

Although fat has more energy (calories) per gram than proteins and carbohydrates, your body has a more difficult time releasing the energy from fatty foods. When you drop a balloon into water, it floats. That's exactly what happens when you swallow fatty foods. The fat floats on top of the watery food and liquid mixture in your stomach, limiting the effect that *lipases* – fat-busting digestive enzymes in the mix below – can have on it. Because fat is digested more slowly than proteins and carbohydrates, you feel fuller (a condition called *satiety*) longer after eating high-fat food. In fact, very little digestion of fats takes place in the stomach at all – the fatty foods wait until they move through to the small intestine before the action starts.

Focusing on the fats in food

Food contains three kinds of fats: triglycerides, phospholipids and sterols.

✔ *Triglycerides* are the fats that you use to make adipose tissue and burn for energy.

✔ *Phospholipids* are hybrids – part lipid, part *phosphate* (a molecule made with the mineral phosphorus) – that act as transporters, ferrying hormones and fat-soluble vitamins A, D, E and K through your blood and backwards and forwards in the watery fluid that flows across cell membranes. By the way, the official name for fluid around cells is *extracellular fluid*. But for us, 'watery fluid' will do nicely!

✔ *Sterols* are fat and alcohol compounds with no calories. Vitamin D is a sterol. So is the sex hormone testosterone. And so is cholesterol, the base from which your body makes some hormones and vitamins. So you see, not all cholesterol is bad.

Getting the right amount of fat

Getting the right amount of fat in your diet is a delicate balancing act. Too much, and you increase your risk of obesity, diabetes, heart disease and some forms of cancer. (The risk of colon cancer seems to be linked to a diet high in fat.) Too little fat, and infants can't thrive, children don't grow, and everyone, regardless of age, is unable to absorb and use fat-soluble vitamins that smooth the skin, protect vision, bolster the immune system, and keep reproductive organs functioning.

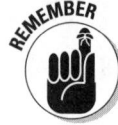

The Institute of Grocery Distributors in conjunction with The Department of Health and Ministry of Agriculture, Fisheries and Food developed guideline daily amounts (GDAs) of fat for average adults of normal weight. The guidelines suggest that men should consume up to 95 grams of total fat per day, of which no more than 30 grams should be saturated fat. Women should aim to consume up to 70 grams total fat with no more than 20 grams saturated fat per day. The GDA recommendations for fat assume that men and women consume the recommended number of calories per day, where as DRVs look at the amount of fat in the diet as a proportion of calories. Whether or not these meet recommendations can be confusing even to nutritionists! To make it simpler when you're shopping is that if a label says a food contains more than 20 grams of total fat and more than 5 grams of saturates per 100 grams, it contains a lot of fat. If the food contains less than 3 grams of total fat and 1 gram of saturated fat it contains 'a little' fat.

Finding fat in all kinds of foods

As a general rule:

- Fruits and vegetables have only traces of fat, primarily unsaturated fatty acids.

- Grains have small amounts of fat, up to 3 per cent of their total weight.

- Dairy products vary. Cream is a high-fat food. Normal milks and cheeses are moderately high in fat. Skimmed milk and skimmed milk products are low-fat foods. Most of the fat in any dairy product is saturated fatty acids.

- Red meat can be low to moderately high in fat depending on the cut, the breeding, and the species. A large part of fats in red meat are saturated fatty acids.

- Poultry without the skin is relatively low in fat.

- Fish can be high or low in fat. Fish with darker flesh (such as salmon, trout, or mackerel) is usually higher in fat. Its fats are composed primarily of unsaturated fatty acids.

- Vegetable oils, butter and lard are high-fat foods. Most of the fatty acids in vegetable oils are unsaturated; with the exception of coconut oil and cocoa butter most of the fatty acids in lard and butter are saturated.

- Processed foods, such as cakes, breads and tinned or frozen meat and vegetable dishes, are generally higher in fat (especially saturated and trans fats) than plain grains, meats, fruits and vegetables.

Defining fatty acids

Fatty acids are the building blocks of fats. Chemically speaking, a *fatty acid* is a chain of carbon atoms with hydrogen atoms attached and a *carbon–oxygen–oxygen–hydrogen group* (the unit that makes it an acid) at one end.

Comparing saturated and unsaturated fatty acids

Nutritionists characterise fatty acids as saturated, monounsaturated, or polyunsaturated, depending on how many hydrogen atoms are attached to the carbon atoms in the chain (we describe these categories in detail in the following section). The more hydrogen atoms, the more saturated the fatty acid, and the more likely the fat is to be solid at room temperature.

All the fats in food are combinations of fatty acids:

- A *saturated fat*, such as butter, has mostly saturated fatty acids. Saturated fats are solid at room temperature and get harder when chilled.

- A *monounsaturated fat*, such as olive oil, has mostly monounsaturated fatty acids. Monounsaturated fats are liquid at room temperature; they get thicker when chilled.

- A *polyunsaturated fat*, such as corn oil, has mostly polyunsaturated fatty acids. Polyunsaturated fats are liquid at room temperature; they stay liquid when chilled.

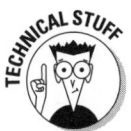

A fatty acid with extra hydrogen atoms is called a *hydrogenated fatty acid*. Some hydrogenated fatty acids are also trans fatty acids. *Trans fatty acids* are not healthy for your heart. Because of those added hydrogen atoms, they're more saturated, and they act like saturated fats, clogging arteries and raising the levels of cholesterol in your blood. To make it easier for you to control your trans fat intake, many food manufacturers now include how many grams of trans fats a product contains. The bottom line is: Keep them to a minimum. The best way to do that is avoid too much fast food and takeaways, and cook from scratch, using unprocessed ingredients when you can.

The good news is that you can buy trans fat-free margarines and spreads, including some that are made with plant sterols and stanols.

Cholesterol: The misunderstood nutrient

Every healthy body *needs* cholesterol. Honest. Cholesterol is in and around your cells, in your fatty tissue, in your organs, and in your glands. What's it doing there? Plenty of useful things. For example, cholesterol:

- Protects the integrity of cell membranes.
- Helps enable nerve cells to send messages backwards and forwards.
- Is a building block for vitamin D (a sterol), made when sunlight hits the fat just under your skin.
- Enables your gall bladder to make *bile acids*, digestive chemicals that, in turn, enable you to absorb fats and fat-soluble nutrients such as vitamin A, vitamin D, vitamin E and vitamin K.
- Is a base on which you build steroid hormones such as oestrogen and testosterone.

Cholesterol and heart disease

Cholesterol has its uses but it has a dark side. Cholesterol makes its way into blood vessels, sticks to the walls, and forms deposits that eventually block the flow of blood causing arteriosclerosis (clogging and hardening of the arteries), or can break away and cause a blood clot to form in an artery (thrombosis). The more cholesterol you have floating in your blood, the more cholesterol is likely to cross into your arteries, where it may increase your risk of heart attack or stroke.

As a general rule, an adult cholesterol level higher than 6.5 mmol/l is said to be a high risk factor for heart disease. A cholesterol level between 5.2 mmol/l and 6.5mmol/l is considered a moderate risk factor. A cholesterol level below 5.2 mmol/l is considered a low risk factor. These figures only apply to adults because we don't have cholesterol targets for children in the UK.

Diet and cholesterol

Most of the cholesterol you need is made right in your own liver, which churns out about 1 gram (1,000 milligrams) a day from the raw materials in the proteins, fats and carbohydrates that you consume. But you also get cholesterol from food of animal origin: meat, poultry, fish, eggs and dairy products. Although some plant foods, such as coconuts and cocoa beans, are high in saturated fats, no plants actually have cholesterol. Dietary cholesterol has a relatively small influence on blood cholesterol, so rather than bore you with long lists of the cholesterol content of masses of foods we've compiled Table 2-2, which shows groups of foods classified as being high, moderate, low, or cholesterol free. Eating a mixture of foods easily ensures that you get the 300mg of cholesterol each day you need from dietary sources.

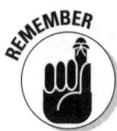

Plants don't have cholesterol, so no plant foods are on this list. No grains. No fruits. No veggies. No nuts and seeds.

Table 2-2	Sources of Dietary Cholesterol
Cholesterol Content	*Foods*
High	Liver, offal (and foods containing these such as pâté). Egg yolk, mayonnaise. Fish roes. Shellfish.
Moderate	Fat on meat, duck, goose and cold cuts such as salami. Full-fat milk, tinned milks, cream, ice cream, cheese, butter. Most manufactured pies, cakes, biscuits and pastries. Meat and fish products.
Low	Uncoated white and oily fish products, tinned fish in vegetable oil. Very lean meats, poultry (no skin). Skimmed milk, low-fat yoghurt, cottage cheese. Bread. Low-cholesterol margarine and spreads.
Cholesterol free	All vegetables and vegetable oils. Fruit including avocado and olives. Nuts. Cereals, pasta (without added egg), rice, popcorn (unbuttered). Egg white, meringue. Sugar.

Book II

Food and Nutrition

Carbohydrates: A Complex Story

Carbohydrates (the name means carbon plus water) are sugar compounds made by plants when the plants are exposed to light. This process of making sugar compounds is called *photosynthesis*, from the Latin words for 'light' and 'putting together'.

In this section, we shine the light on the different kinds of carbohydrates, illuminating all the nutritional nooks and crannies to explain how each contributes to your health, not to mention being a delicious daily staple.

Considering carbohydrates

Carbohydrates come in three varieties: simple carbohydrates, complex carbohydrates and dietary fibre. All are composed of units of sugar. What makes one carbohydrate different from another is the number of sugar units it contains and how the units are linked together.

- ✓ **Simple carbohydrates** are carbohydrates with only one or two units of sugar.
- ✓ **Complex carbohydrates,** also known as *polysaccharides* (poly = many), have more than two units of sugar linked together. Carbs with three to eight units of sugar are sometimes called *oligosaccharides* (oligo = many).

✔ **Dietary fibre** is a term used to distinguish the fibre in food from the natural and synthetic fibres (silk, cotton, wool, nylon) used in fabrics. Dietary fibre is a third kind of carbohydrate.

Dietary fibre is not like other carbohydrates. Human digestive enzymes cannot break the bonds that hold its sugar units together. Although the bacteria living naturally in your intestines convert very small amounts of dietary fibre to fatty acids, dietary fibre is not considered a source of energy.

How glucose becomes energy

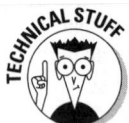

Inside your cells, the glucose from carbohydrates is burned to produce heat and *adenosine triphosphate* (ATP), a molecule that stores and releases energy as required by the cell. The transformation of glucose into energy occurs with oxygen or without it.

✔ Glucose is converted to energy with oxygen in the *mitochondria*, tiny bodies in the jelly-like substance inside every cell. This conversion yields energy (ATP and heat) plus water and carbon dioxide, a waste product.

✔ Red blood cells do not have mitochondria, so they change glucose into energy without oxygen. This yields energy (ATP and heat) and lactic acid.

✔ Glucose is also converted to energy in muscle cells.. Muscle cells have mitochondria, so they can process glucose with oxygen. But if the level of oxygen in the muscle cell falls very low, the cells can just go ahead and change glucose into energy without it. This is most likely to happen when you exercise so strenuously that you (and your muscles) are, literally, out of breath.

Being able to turn glucose into energy without oxygen is a handy trick, but here's the downside: One by-product is lactic acid. Why does that matter? Too much lactic acid makes your muscles ache.

Having too much of a good thing

Your cells use energy very carefully. Any glucose the cell does not need for its daily work is joined with other glucose cells and converted to *glycogen* (animal starch) and tucked away as stored energy in your liver and muscles. Glycogen is often called animal starch because it's the form of carbohydrate that only exists within animal cells; all other carbohydrates are produced within plant cells.

Your body can pack about 400 grams (14 ounces) of glycogen into liver and muscle cells. A gram of carbohydrates, including glucose, has 3.75 calories. If you add up all the glucose stored in glycogen to the small amount of glucose in your cells and blood, it equals about 1,800 calories of energy.

If your diet provides more carbohydrates (or any other energy source) than you need to produce this amount of stored calories in the form of glucose and glycogen in your cells, blood, muscles and liver, the excess will be converted to fat. If you really love your carbs, the way to combat expanding hips or any other area is to get more active and increase your need for energy – the bigger your need for energy, the bigger your plate!

Finding the carbohydrates you need

The most important sources of carbohydrates are plant foods – fruits, vegetables and grains. Milk and milk products contain the carbohydrate lactose (milk sugar), but meat, fish and poultry have no carbohydrates at all.

The dietary reference values (DRVs) for food energy and nutrients do not set specific recommendations for the amount of carbohydrate foods we should eat. However, most nutritionists recommend that 50 per cent of your daily calories need to come from carbohydrate foods. The Balance of Good Health makes it easy for you to build a nutritious carb-based diet with portion allowances based on how many calories you consume each day in:

Book II

Food and Nutrition

- ✔ 6 to 11 servings of complex carbohydrate foods (bread, cereals, pasta, rice and potatoes), plus
- ✔ At least 5 portions of fruit and vegetables

Dietary fibre

Dietary fibre is a group of complex carbohydrates that are not a source of energy for human beings. Because human digestive enzymes cannot break the bonds that hold fibre's sugar units together, fibre adds no calories to your diet and cannot be converted to glucose.

Just because you can't digest dietary fibre doesn't mean it isn't a valuable part of your diet. The opposite is true. Dietary fibre is valuable *because* you can't digest it!

Getting fibre from food

You find fibre in all plant foods – fruits, vegetables and grains. But you find absolutely no fibre in foods from animals – meat, fish, poultry, milk, milk products and eggs.

A balanced diet with lots of foods from plants gives you both insoluble and soluble fibre. In general terms soluble fibre helps to reduce glucose and cholesterol absorption, while insoluble fibre speeds up the time it takes food to pass through the gastrointestinal tract. Most foods that contain fibre have both kinds, although the balance usually tilts towards one or the other. For example, the predominant fibre in an apple is pectin (a soluble fibre), but apple peel also has some cellulose, hemicellulose and lignin.

How much fibre do you need?

The recommended dietary reference value (DRV) for adults is 18 grams of fibre a day. Children's intake should be proportionately lower than that of adults.

The amounts of dietary fibre recommended by DRVs are believed to give you the benefits you want without causing fibre-related unpleasantries.

If you eat more than enough fibre, your body tells you right away. All that roughage may irritate your intestinal tract, which will issue an unmistakable protest in the form of intestinal gas or diarrhoea. In extreme cases, if you don't drink enough fluid to carry the fibre you eat easily through your body, the dietary fibre may form a mass that can end up as an intestinal obstruction (for more about water, see Book II Chapter 1).

If you decide to increase the amount of fibre in your diet, follow our advice:

- ✔ Do it *very* gradually, a little bit more every day. That way you're less likely to experience the kind of intestinal distress we talked about earlier. In other words, if your current diet is heavy on no-fibre foods such as meat, fish, poultry, eggs, milk and cheese, and low-fibre foods such as white bread and white rice, don't load up on bran cereal (36.4 grams dietary fibre per 100 gram serving) or dried figs (6.9 grams per serving) all at once. Start by adding a serving of cornflakes (0.9 grams dietary fibre) at breakfast one day, then maybe an apple (1.8 grams) at lunch the following day, a pear (2.2 grams) at mid-afternoon later in the week, and a small tin of baked beans (6.9 grams) at dinner. Four simple additions, and already you're up to 18 grams of dietary fibre.

- ✔ Follow the recommendations of the Balance of Good Health (see Book I Chapter 1) and increase your consumption of grain products, vegetables and fruits – all good sources of dietary fibre.

- ✔ Always check the nutrition label whenever you shop. When choosing between similar products, just take the one with the higher fibre content per serving. For example, white pitta bread generally has about 2.2 grams of dietary fibre per serving. Wholemeal pitta bread has 5.8 grams. From a fibre standpoint, you know which works better for your body. Go for it!

By the way, dietary fibre is like a sponge. It soaks up liquid, so increasing your fibre intake may deprive your cells of the water they need to perform their daily work. Unless you're already drinking at least six large glasses of water every day, we and any other dieticians worth their salt suggest upping your fluid intake when you consume more fibre.

Vigorous Vitamins

Vitamins regulate a variety of bodily functions. They're essential for building body tissues such as bones, skin, glands, nerves and blood. They assist in metabolising (digesting) proteins, fats and carbohydrates, so that you can get energy from food. They prevent nutritional deficiency diseases, promote healing, and encourage good health.

This section is a guide to where you can find vitamins, how you add them to your diet, and how to tell if you're taking too many vitamins.

Book II

Food and Nutrition

Taking a look at the vitamins your body needs

Your body needs at least 11 specific vitamins: vitamin A, vitamin D, vitamin E, vitamin K, vitamin C, and the members of the B vitamin family: thiamin (vitamin B1), riboflavin (B2), niacin, vitamin B6, folate, and vitamin B12. Two more B vitamins, biotin and pantothenic acid, are also valuable to your well-being. You need only minuscule quantities of vitamins for good health. In some cases, the reference nutrient intake (RNI) determined by the Department of Health as the amount required by virtually every healthy person may be as small as just a few micrograms (µgs) or milligrams (mgs).

Nutritionists classify vitamins as either *fat soluble* or *water soluble*, meaning that they dissolve either in fat or in water. If you consume larger amounts of fat-soluble vitamins than your body needs, the excess is stored in body fat. Excess water-soluble vitamins are eliminated in urine.

Use this mnemonic to remember which vitamins are fat soluble and which dissolve in water: '**A**ll **D**ogs **E**at **K**idneys.' Vitamins A, D, E and K are fat soluble. All the rest dissolve in water.

Fat-soluble vitamins

Vitamin A, vitamin D, vitamin E and vitamin K are relatives that have two characteristics in common: All dissolve in fat, and all are stored in your fatty tissues. But like members of any family, they also have distinct personalities. One keeps your skin hydrated. Another protects your bones. A third keeps reproductive organs purring happily. And the fourth enables you to make special proteins. Because you can store fat-soluble vitamins, you could say that they work a bit more like a savings account where you can dip into your stash when you need it, whereas the water-soluble vitamins work more like your current account and need topping up regularly. For instance, the fat-soluble vitamin D is made in the skin from sunlight – we tend to build up stores in the summer but can still use those stores in the long, dark, damp winter months. Clever, eh?

Vitamin A

Vitamin A is the moisturising nutrient. This vitamin keeps your skin and *mucous membranes* (the smooth tissue that lines the eyes, nose, mouth, throat, vagina and rectum) smooth and supple. Vitamin A is also the vision vitamin, producing *rhodopsin* in the retina, making it possible to see when the lights are low. Vitamin A also promotes the growth of healthy bones and teeth, keeps your reproductive system healthy, and encourages your immune system to churn out the cells you need to fight off infection.

Vitamin D

If we say 'bones' or 'teeth', what nutrient springs most quickly to mind? If you answer calcium, you're only partly right. True, calcium is essential for hardening teeth and bones. But no matter how much calcium you consume, without vitamin D your body cannot absorb and use calcium. As well as it being vital for strong bones and teeth, some evidence points to the fact that failing to get enough vitamin D may increase the risks of diabetes and some forms of cancer.

Vitamin E

Every animal, including you, needs vitamin E to maintain a healthy reproductive system, nerves and muscles. Vitamin E is also an important antioxidant and because it's fat soluble, it's involved in protecting every body cell from the effects of *free radicals* (unstable compounds that damage healthy body cells).

Vitamin K

Vitamin K is a group of chemicals that your body uses to make specialised proteins found in blood *plasma* (the clear fluid in blood), such as prothrombin, the protein chiefly responsible for blood clotting and stopping you from bleeding to death when you cut yourself. You also need vitamin K to make bone and kidney tissues. Like vitamin D, vitamin K is essential for healthy bones. Vitamin D increases calcium absorption; vitamin K activates at least three different proteins that take part in forming new bone cells.

You get Vitamin K from dark green leafy vegetables (broccoli, cabbage, kale, lettuce, spinach and turnip greens), cheese, liver, cereals and fruits, but most of what you need comes from resident colonies of friendly bacteria in your intestines, an assembly line of busy bugs churning out the vitamin day and night.

Water-soluble vitamins

Vitamin C and the entire team of B vitamins (thiamin, riboflavin, niacin, vitamin B6, folate, biotin, pantothenic acid) are usually grouped together simply because they all dissolve in water.

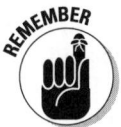

Because these vitamins dissolve in water, large amounts of these nutrients can't be stored in your body. If you take in more than you need to perform specific body tasks, you simply pee away virtually all the excess. The good news is that these vitamins rarely cause side effects. The bad news is that you have to take enough of these vitamins every day to protect yourself against deficiencies.

Vitamin C

Vitamin C, also called *ascorbic acid*, is essential for the development and maintenance of connective tissue (the fat, muscle and bone framework of the human body). Vitamin C speeds up the production of new cells in wound healing; helps with absorption of iron; and, like vitamin E, it's an antioxidant that keeps free radicals from joining up with other molecules to form damaging compounds that may otherwise attack your tissues. Vitamin C protects your immune system, helps you fight off infection, and may reduce the severity of allergic reactions. It plays a role in the synthesis of hormones and other body chemicals.

Book II

Food and Nutrition

The main sources of vitamin C are vegetables, fruit and fruit juices. The most concentrated sources are citrus fruit, but surprisingly you get around 16 per cent of your daily dose from the humble potato – not so much because potatoes are such a good source, but because us Brits typically eat so many of them. Vitamin C lies mainly beneath the potato's skin, so eating new potatoes with the skins on or using a peeler instead of a knife helps keep your vitamin C levels up.

Thiamin (vitamin B1)

This sulphur (*thia*) and nitrogen (*amin*) compound helps ensure a healthy appetite. It acts as a *coenzyme* (a substance that works along with other enzymes) essential to at least four different processes by which your body metabolises energy from carbohydrates, fats and alcohol. Thiamin also is a mild diuretic (something that makes you urinate more).

The richest dietary sources of thiamin are unrefined cereals and grains, lean pork, pulses, nuts and seeds. In the UK all flour (with the exception of wholemeal flour) is fortified with thiamin and most breakfast cereals are voluntarily fortified. Thiamin deficiency is rare and most likely to be seen in alcoholics (when the body is so busy dealing with alcohol it's less effective at absorbing nutrients) as Wernicke-Korsakoff syndrome (a form of dementia).

Riboflavin (vitamin B2)

Like thiamin, riboflavin is a coenzyme. Without it, your body can't digest and use proteins and carbohydrates. Like vitamin A, it protects the health of mucous membranes. You get riboflavin from foods of animal origin (meat, fish, poultry, eggs and milk), whole or enriched grain products, brewer's yeast, and dark green vegetables such as broccoli and spinach.

Niacin (Vitamin B3)

Niacin is one name for a pair of naturally occurring nutrients, nicotinic acid and nicotinamide. Niacin is essential for proper growth, and like other B vitamins, it's intimately involved in enzyme reactions. In fact, niacin is an integral part of an enzyme that enables oxygen to flow into body tissues. Like thiamin, it gives you a healthy appetite and participates in the metabolism of sugars and fats.

Niacin is available either as a preformed nutrient or via the conversion of the amino acid tryptophane. Preformed niacin comes from meat; tryptophane comes from milk and dairy foods. Some niacin is present in grains, but your body cannot absorb it efficiently unless the grain has been treated with lime (the mineral, not the fruit). This is a common practice in Central and South American countries where lime is added to cornmeal in making tortillas. In the United States and in the United Kingdom, breads and cereals are routinely fortified with niacin. Your body easily absorbs added niacin.

Vitamin B6 (Pyridoxine)

Vitamin B6 is another multiple compound, this one comprising three related chemicals: Pyridoxine, pyridoxal and pyridoxamine. Vitamin B6, a component of enzymes that metabolises proteins and fats, is essential for getting energy and nutrients from food. It plays an important role in removing excess amounts of homocysteine from your blood. A high level of *homocysteine*, an amino acid produced when you digest proteins, is an independent risk factor for heart disease, perhaps as important as your cholesterol levels.

The best food sources of vitamin B6 are liver, chicken, fish, pork, lamb, milk, eggs, brown rice, whole grains, beer, soya beans, potatoes, beans, nuts, seeds and dark green vegetables such as turnip greens. The RNIs for vitamin B6 are related to protein intake and although deficiencies are rare, people following a high-protein diet can be deficient. For the record the RNIs are 0.7–1.0 milligrams per day for children, adult men 1.4 milligrams per day, and adult women 1.2 milligrams per day.

Folate

Folate is an essential nutrient for human beings and other *vertebrates* (animals with backbones). Folate takes part in the synthesis of DNA, the metabolism of proteins, and the subsequent synthesis of amino acids used to produce new body cells and tissues. Folate is vital for normal growth and wound healing. An adequate supply of the vitamin is essential for pregnant women to enable them to create new maternal tissue as well as foetal tissue. In addition, an adequate supply of folate dramatically reduces the risk of neural tube defects (such as spina bifida).

Beans, dark green leafy vegetables, liver, yeast and various fruits are excellent food sources of folate, and all multivitamin supplements must now provide 400 micrograms of folate per dose. The RNIs for folate are 70–150 micrograms (µg) per day for children and 200 micrograms per day for adults.

During pregnancy this increases by 100 micrograms per day and by 60 micrograms per day while breast-feeding. Women who intend to become pregnant can consume an additional 400 micrograms per day. This level is difficult to achieve from diet alone, so folic acid is one of the few vitamins where supplements are strongly recommended before conception and during the first 12 weeks of pregnancy. High intakes of folate have no adverse effects.

Vitamin B12 (Cyanocobalamin)

Vitamin B12 makes healthy red blood cells. It protects *myelin*, the fatty material that covers your nerves and enables you to transmit electrical impulses (messages) between nerve cells. These messages make it possible for you to see, hear, think, move, and do all the things a healthy body does each day.

Vitamin B12 is unique. First, it is the only vitamin that contains a mineral, cobalt. (Cyanocobalamin, a cobalt compound, is commonly used as vitamin B12 in vitamin pills and nutritional supplements.) Second, it is a vitamin that cannot be made by plants. Like vitamin K, vitamin B12 is made by beneficial bacteria living in your small intestine. Meat, fish, poultry, milk products, and eggs are good sources of vitamin B12. Grains do not naturally contain vitamin B12, but like other B vitamins, it is added to many breakfast cereals in the UK. It is one of the few water-soluble vitamins that can be stored by the liver.

Book II

Food and Nutrition

Biotin

Biotin is a B vitamin, a component of enzymes that ferry carbon and oxygen atoms between cells. Biotin helps you metabolise fats and carbohydrates and is essential for synthesising fatty acids and amino acids needed for healthy growth. And it seems to prevent a build-up of fat deposits that may interfere with the proper functioning of liver and kidneys. (No, biotin won't keep fat from settling in more visible places, such as your hips.)

Your best food sources of biotin are liver, egg yolk, yeast, nuts and beans. If your diet doesn't give you all the biotin you need, bacteria in your gut synthesises enough to make up the difference. No RNIs for biotin exist, but intakes of between 10–200μg a day are thought to be adequate and safe.

Pantothenic acid

Pantothenic acid, another B vitamin, is vital to enzyme reactions that make it possible for you to use carbohydrates and create steroid biochemicals such as hormones. Pantothenic acid also helps stabilise blood sugar levels, defends against infection, and protects *haemoglobin* (the protein in red blood cells that carries oxygen through the body), as well as nerve, brain and muscle tissue. You get pantothenic acid from meat, fish and poultry, beans, wholegrain cereals, and fortified grain products. There are no RNIs for pantothenic acid, but the current average intake in the UK of 3–7milligrams a day is thought to be adequate. Large doses may cause diarrhoea and stomach upset.

Special circumstances: Taking extra vitamins as needed

The reference nutrient intakes set by the Department of Health are designed to protect healthy people from deficiencies, but sometimes the circumstances of your life (or your lifestyle) mean that you need something extra. You may need larger amounts of vitamins than the RDAs provide if you fit in with any of the following circumstances.

I'm taking medication

Many valuable medicines interact with vitamins. Some drugs increase or decrease the effectiveness of vitamins; some vitamins increase or decrease the effectiveness of drugs. For example, a woman who is using birth control pills may absorb less than the customary amount of the B vitamins.

I'm a smoker

You probably have low blood levels of vitamin C. More trouble: Chemicals from tobacco smoke create more free radicals in your body. International research organisations, which are often tough on vitamin overdosing, say that regular smokers need to take about 66 per cent more vitamin C – up to 100 milligrams a day – than non-smokers and should also increase their intake of beta-carotene from vegetable sources like carrots, red peppers, spinach, broccoli and tomatoes.

I'm vegan

If you follow a vegan diet (one that excludes all foods from animals, including milk, cheese, eggs and fish oils) you simply cannot get enough vitamin D without taking supplements. You may also benefit from extra vitamin C because it increases your ability to absorb iron from plant food. And vitamin B12-enriched grains or supplements are a must to supply the nutrients found only in fish, poultry, milk, cheese and eggs.

I'm a couch potato who plans to start exercising

When you do head for the gym, take it slow, and take an extra dose of vitamin E. A study at the USDA Center for Human Nutrition at Tufts University (Boston) suggests that an 800-milligram vitamin E supplement every day for the first month after you begin exercising minimises muscle damage by preventing reactions with free radicals that cause inflammation. After that, you're on your own: The vitamin doesn't help conditioned athletes whose muscles have adapted to workout stress.

I'm pregnant

Keep in mind that 'eating for two' means that you're the sole source of nutrients for the growing foetus, not that you need to double the amount of food you eat. If you don't get the vitamins you need, neither will your baby.

The RNIs for most of the B vitamins, vitamin K and vitamin E are exactly the same as those for women who aren't pregnant. But when you're pregnant, you need extra:

- ✔ **Vitamin D:** Every smidgen of vitamin D in a newborn's body comes from its mum. If she doesn't have enough D, neither will the baby. Be careful, because too little vitamin D can weaken a developing foetus, but too much can cause birth defects. Check with your doctor who can work out what's right for you according to your weight.

- ✔ **Vitamin C:** The level of vitamin C in your blood falls as your vitamin C flows across the placenta to your baby, who may – at some point in the pregnancy – have vitamin C levels as much as 50 per cent higher than yours. So you need an extra 10 milligrams of vitamin C each day for your own health.

- ✔ **Folate:** Folate protects the child against cleft palate (an opening in the roof of the mouth in which the two sides of the palate didn't join together as the unborn baby was developing) and neural tube (spinal cord) defects. The accepted increase in folate for pregnant women has been 100 milligrams (slightly more than the amount in 4 fluid ounces (113 grams) of orange juice). But new studies show that taking 400 milligrams of folate before becoming pregnant and through the first two months of pregnancy significantly lowers the risk of giving birth to a child with cleft palate. Taking 400 milligrams of folate each day through an entire pregnancy reduces the risk of neural tube defect.

- ✔ **Vitamin A:** Extra vitamin A is needed to enhance the mother's stores and allow for the baby's growth in the later stages of pregnancy. However, high intakes of vitamin A can be harmful and lead to liver damage. The safe level of supplementation for pregnant women (set by the American College of Obstetrics and Gynaecology in 1993) is 1500 micrograms per day.

Book II

Food and Nutrition

I'm breast-feeding

You need extra vitamin A, vitamin E, thiamin, riboflavin and folate to produce sufficient quantities of nutritious breast milk (about 750ml) each day. You need extra vitamin D, vitamin C and niacin as insurance to replace the vitamins you lose by transferring them to your child in your milk.

I'm approaching menopause or getting on a bit

Older women require extra calcium to stem the natural loss of bone that occurs when you reach menopause and your production of the female hormone oestrogen declines. You may also need extra vitamin D to enable your body to absorb and use the calcium. Gender bias alert! No similar studies are available for older men. But adding vitamin D supplements to calcium supplements increases bone density in older people. The current RNI for vitamin D is set at 10 micrograms per day.

Check with your doctor before adding vitamin D supplements. In very large amounts, this vitamin can be toxic.

Older people of both genders are also at risk of deficiency of vitamin C, folate and vitamin B12 because they are less likely to eat enough of the foods that are rich sources.

Mighty Minerals

Minerals are substances that occur naturally in non-living things such as water, rocks and soil. Minerals also are present in plants and animals, but they're imported: Plants get minerals from soil; animals get minerals by eating plants or other animals.

Taking stock of the minerals you need

Think of your body as a house. Vitamins are like tiny little maids and butlers, scurrying about to turn on the lights and make sure that the windows are closed to keep the heat from escaping. Minerals are more sturdy stuff: The bricks and mortar that strengthen the frame, and the current that keeps the lights on.

Introducing the major minerals

The following major minerals are essential for human beings

- Calcium
- Phosphorus
- Magnesium
- Iron
- Zinc
- Sulphur
- Fluorine (as fluoride)
- Sodium
- Potassium
- Chloride

Sodium, potassium and chlorine are also known as the principal electrolytes. We discuss them in Book II Chapter 1.

Calcium

About 1.5 kilograms (3 pounds) of your body weight is calcium, 99 per cent of it packed into your bones and teeth.

The remaining 1 per cent is present in extracellular fluid (the liquid around body cells), where it performs the following duties:

- Regulating fluid balance by controlling the flow of water in and out of cells.
- Making it possible for nerve cells to send messages back and forth from one to another.
- Keeping muscles contracting normally.
- Enabling normal blood clotting.

An adequate amount of calcium is also important for controlling high blood pressure – and not only for the person who takes the calcium directly. At least one study shows that when a pregnant woman gets a sufficient amount of calcium, her baby's blood pressure stays lower than average for at least the first seven years of life, meaning a lower risk of developing high blood pressure later on.

Your best food sources of calcium are milk and dairy products, plus fish such as tinned sardines and salmon where the bones are eaten. Calcium is also found in fortified soya milk, bread and cereals, dark green leafy vegetables, pulses, and some dried fruits, seeds and nuts. However, the calcium in some plant foods is less well absorbed than that from animal foods and is present in smaller amounts meaning that you often need to eat quite large amounts to meet requirements. Tap water is also a reasonable source of calcium in hard water areas.

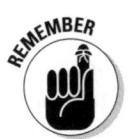

Dietary needs for calcium are highest during periods of rapid bone growth such as infancy and teenage years. Needs during pregnancy are generally covered by increased absorption, but requirements do go up by an extra 550 milligrams per day for breastfeeding mothers. The recommended nutritional intakes (RNIs) are 1000 milligrams per day for 11–18-year-old boys and 800 milligrams per day for girls; and 700 milligrams per day for adults.

In order for your body to absorb calcium, you need an adequate supply of vitamin D from your diet, sunlight, or supplements.

Phosphorus

Like calcium, phosphorus is essential for strong bones and teeth: 85 per cent of phosphorus in your body is in your bones. You also need phosphorus to transmit the *genetic code* (genes and chromosomes that carry information about your special characteristics) from one cell to another when cells divide and reproduce. In addition, phosphorus:

✔ Helps maintain the pH balance of blood (keeps it from being too acidic or too alkaline)

✔ Is vital for metabolising carbohydrates, synthesising proteins, and ferrying fats and fatty acids among tissues and organs

✔ Is part of *myelin*, the fatty sheath that surrounds and protects each nerve cell

Phosphorus is found in almost everything you eat so deficiency is rare. The best sources are high-protein foods such as meat, fish, poultry, eggs and milk. These foods provide more than half the phosphorus in a non-vegetarian diet; cereals, nuts, seeds, pulses, fruit and vegetables also provide respectable amounts.

The RNI for adults is 550 milligrams per day, with an extra 440 milligrams for breastfeeding mothers. Like calcium, requirements are higher during growth spurts: 775 milligrams per day for boys aged 11–18 and 625 milligrams per day for girls.

Magnesium

Your body uses magnesium to regulate energy release, nerve cell function, and muscle contraction. It's also used to make body tissues, especially bone. The adult human body has about 30 grams of magnesium, and three-quarters of it is in the bones. Magnesium also is part of more than 300 different enzymes that trigger chemical reactions throughout your body.

The main sources of magnesium in the typical UK diet are bread and other cereal products especially whole grains followed by beverages such as beer and coffee (no, that's not an excuse for another pint). Milk and meat are also good sources. Many other plant foods are also a rich supply of magnesium, including dark green vegetables (magnesium is part of chlorophyll, the green pigment in plants), seeds, nuts and pulses.

The RNI for adults over 19 is 300 milligrams per day for men and 270 milligrams per day for women. Breastfeeding women are recommended to take an additional 50 milligrams a day. Deficiency is rare but low intakes can occur in people with restricted diets.

Iron

The adult body contains around 4–5 grams of iron, the majority of which is found as a constituent of haemoglobin and myoglobin, two proteins that transport and transfer oxygen to the cells. You find haemoglobin in red blood cells (it's what makes them red). Myoglobin (*myo* = muscle) is in muscle tissue. Iron also is part of various enzymes and is essential for healthy functioning of the immune system.

The best food sources of iron are offal (liver, heart, kidneys), red meat and meat products, eggs and oily fish. These foods contain haem (*haem* = blood) iron, a form of iron that your body can easily absorb.

Whole grains, fortified cereals, green leafy vegetables, dried fruit, pulses, nuts and seeds contain non-haem iron and you don't absorb it so well. Plants contain fibre and substances called *phytates* and *tannins* that bind this iron into compounds, so that your body has a harder time getting at the iron. However, eating plant foods with meat or with foods that are rich in vitamin C (like tomatoes or fruit juice) can enhance the absorption of iron from plant foods.

The RNIs for iron are 11.3 milligrams per day for boys aged 11–18, 8.7 milligrams for men, 14.8 milligrams a day for women aged 11–50, and 8.7 milligrams for women above 50.

Book II

Food and Nutrition

Zinc

The human body has about 2 grams of zinc stored mainly in muscle and bone and that zinc performs a wide range of roles in the body including normal growth and repair, wound healing and healthy immunity. An adequate supply of zinc is vital for making many enzymes and hormones, including growth hormones, insulin and testosterone, the hormone a man needs to produce plentiful amounts of healthy sperm. Without enough zinc, male fertility falters.

Good sources of zinc are red meat and meat products, milk, eggs, fish and shellfish (yes, the old wives' tale is true: Oysters – a rich source of zinc – are useful for men!). Other good sources include wholegrain cereals, green vegetables, pulses and beans, as well as some nuts and seeds. However, like with iron, you absorb the zinc in plants less efficiently than the zinc in foods from animals.

Over the age of 15, the RNI for men is 9.5 milligrams per day and 7 milligrams a day for women. Breast-feeding women should aim for an extra 6 milligrams a day for the first four months and an extra 2.5 milligrams per day until breast-feeding stops.

Fluorine

Fluorine is found mainly in the form of fluoride in both food and water. Your body stores fluoride in bones and teeth. Researchers often classify it as semi-essential since although a deficiency has never been demonstrated in humans it does have some health benefits. For example it's clear that its incorporation into dental enamel hardens it, reducing your risk of getting tooth decay. Low water levels are associated with much higher rates of dental caries. In addition, some nutrition researchers suspect (but haven't proved) that some forms of fluoride can be used to treat osteoporosis.

Sulphur

Although sulphur is often considered an essential nutrient for human beings, it's almost never included in nutritional books or charts. Why? Because sulphur is an integral part of all proteins as well as being found in fats and many body fluids. Any diet that provides adequate protein also provides adequate sulphur and deficiency is very rare.

Small amounts of fluoride occur naturally in all soil, water, plants and animal tissues. You also get a steady supply of fluoride from fluoridated drinking water. About 75 per cent of your intake comes from water and only 25 per cent from food.

Since it's hard to find proof of a biological need for fluoride, no set RNIs exist, but a safe intake for adults and children over 6 is 0.5 milligrams per kilogram of body weight a day.

Introducing the trace elements

Trace elements also are minerals, but you need them in much, much smaller amounts – microgram (mcg) quantities – in other words, just a trace. Trace elements include:

- Iodine
- Selenium
- Copper
- Manganese
- Chromium
- Molybdenum

Iodine

Iodine is a component of the thyroid hormones thyroxine and triiodothyronine, which help regulate cell activities. These hormones are also essential for protein synthesis, tissue growth (including the formation of a healthy nervous system), and bones.

In the United Kingdom the major source of iodine is milk and milk products. This isn't because it occurs naturally but because cows are often given iodine-rich feedstuffs, and milk is processed and stored in machines and vessels cleaned with iodine-based disinfectants.

The best natural sources of iodine are seafood and plants grown near the ocean, including seaweeds. In some other countries people are most likely to get the iodine they need from iodised salt (plain table salt with iodine added). Products found naturally in some vegetables such as turnips, sweet potatoes, cabbage, millet and corn can inhibit the absorption of iodine. However, in practice this only has a significant effect if your iodine intake is unusually low.

For adults the RNI is set at 140 micrograms per day.

Selenium

Selenium was identified as an essential human nutrient in 1979 when Chinese nutrition researchers discovered that people with low body stores of selenium were at increased risk of *Keshan disease*, a disorder of the heart muscle with symptoms that include rapid heartbeat, enlarged heart, and (in severe cases) heart failure, a consequence most common among young children and women of child-bearing age. Selenium deficiency has also been linked to reduced function of the immune system.

Recent studies suggest that selenium may have powerful antioxidant properties enabling it to protect against heart disease and cancer, especially of the lung, prostate, colon and rectum. Studies are promising but benefits from increasing intake or supplementation have not yet been proven. Vitamin E and selenium interact and are able to compensate to some degree for deficiencies in the other.

Fruit, vegetables and cereals grown in selenium-rich soils are themselves rich in this mineral, but in the United Kingdom selenium levels in soil and in many imported crops are relatively low. As a result the best sources of selenium are meat and offal (liver and kidneys), fish, eggs and brazil nuts.

The adult RNIs for selenium are 75 micrograms a day for men and 60 micrograms per day for women, with an extra 15 micrograms per day recommended during breastfeeding.

Copper

Copper is an antioxidant found in enzymes that deactivate free radicals (pieces of molecules that can link up to form compounds that damage body tissues). Copper may therefore be important in helping to protect against cancer and heart disease. Copper also helps to defend the body against infection. Research suggests that copper may even play a role in slowing the ageing process by decreasing the incidence of *protein glycation*, a reaction in which sugar molecules hook up with protein molecules in your bloodstream, twist the protein molecules out of shape, and make them unusable. Protein glycation may result in bone loss, high cholesterol, and cardiac abnormalities. In people with diabetes, excess protein glycation may also be a factor involved in complications such as loss of vision.

Book II

Food and Nutrition

In addition, copper:

✔ Promotes the growth of strong blood vessels and bones

✔ Protects the health of nerve tissue

You can get the copper you need from eating meat , bread and cereals and green vegetables. Other rich sources include s liver shellfish, nuts, tea, coffee and beans, including cocoa beans (bring on the chocolate!). Most other foods apart from milk and dairy products provide some so copper deficiency is rare in the United Kingdom except as a result of severe malnutrition or genetic disorders.

The RNIs for adults are 1.2 milligrams a day, with an extra 0.3 milligrams a day needed during breastfeeding.

Manganese

Manganese is an essential constituent of the enzymes that metabolise carbohydrates and synthesise fats (including cholesterol). Most of the manganese in your body is in glands (pituitary, mammary, pancreas); organs (liver, kidneys, intestines); and bones. Manganese is important for a healthy reproductive system. During pregnancy, manganese speeds the proper growth of foetal tissue, particularly bones and cartilage.

You get manganese from whole grains, cereal products, nuts, fruits and vegetables. Tea is also a good source. There is no RNI, but safe intakes are estimated to be greater than 1.4 milligrams per day for adults.

Chromium

Chromium plays several roles in normal metabolism. It's a necessary partner for *glucose tolerance factor* (GTF), a group of chemicals that enhances the action of insulin (an enzyme from the pancreas) to regulate your use of glucose, the end product of metabolism and the basic fuel for every body cell. It also seems to be involved in maintaining both normal blood sugar and cholesterol levels.

People with a deficiency of chromium can develop impaired glucose tolerance, which is improved by chromium supplementation. As a result this led people to look at a possible role for chromium in the prevention and treatment of diabetes.

Research in the United Kingdom looked at moderate doses of chromium obtained from diet, but found no benefit to glucose tolerance or lipids in adults with type 2 diabetes. Other studies are inconclusive or show no benefit. Advice remains to ensure adequate dietary intake from both animal sources such as red meat and offal, and vegetable sources (wholegrain cereals, nuts and seeds, pulses and yeast).

No RNIs are set but safe levels are above 25 micrograms per day for adults.

Molybdenum

Molybdenum (pronounced mo-lib-den-um) is part of several enzymes that metabolise proteins. You get molybdenum from beans and cereals, but local soil levels determine the amount. Cows eat cereal grains, so milk and cheese have some molybdenum. Molybdenum also leeches into drinking water from surrounding soil. Safe intakes for adults are set in the range of 50–400 micrograms per day.

Munching more minerals: People who need extra

If your diet provides enough minerals to meet the RNIs, you're in pretty good shape, most of the time.

But a restrictive diet, the circumstances of your reproductive life, and just getting older can increase your need for minerals. Here are some scenarios.

You're a strict vegetarian

Vegetarians who avoid fish, meat, poultry and eggs must get their iron from fortified and wholegrain cereals, seeds, nuts, dried fruit, green leafy vegetables, pulses and beans. Because iron in plant foods is bound into compounds that are difficult for the human body to absorb, taking a source of vitamin C such as salad, fruit juice, or fruit with your meal can help you absorb the iron.

Vegans – vegetarians who avoid all foods from animals, including dairy products – have a similar problem getting the calcium they need. Calcium is in vegetables, but it, like iron, is bound into hard-to-absorb compounds. So vegans need calcium-rich substitutes. Good food choices are soya milk fortified with calcium, orange juice with added calcium, tofu processed with calcium sulphate, nuts and seeds.

A similar story applies to zinc. Good vegetarian sources include wholegrain cereals, green vegetables, pulses and beans, as well as some nuts and seeds. However the zinc in plants, like the iron and calcium in plants, is less efficient than the zinc in foods from animals.

Mineral supplements may be useful for some vegetarians with a limited range of foods.

You're a woman

The average woman of reproductive age loses about 20 milligrams iron a month during menstruation. Women whose periods are very heavy lose more blood and more iron and need more than the RNI. Because getting the iron you need from a diet providing fewer than 2000 calories a day may be difficult, you may develop a mild iron deficiency. To remedy this, some doctors prescribe a daily iron supplement.

Women who use an intrauterine device (IUD) may also take iron supplements because IUDs irritate the lining of the uterus and cause a small but significant loss of blood and iron.

You're pregnant

The news about pregnancy is that women may not need to take in extra minerals above and beyond the RNIs. Pregnant women still need minerals not only to build foetal tissues, but also new tissues and increased blood volume in their own bodies. However, most of this seems to be provided by increased absorption as a response to increased demand. You may need nutritional supplements if your usual intake or stores are low.

You're breast-feeding

Nursing mothers need extra iron (met by increased absorption), calcium, phosphorus, magnesium, copper, zinc and selenium to protect their own bodies while producing nutritious breast milk. The same supplements that provide extra nutrients for pregnant women will meet a nursing mother's needs.

You're menopausal

At menopause, your body begins producing less of the bone-protecting hormone oestrogen, and you begin losing bone tissue. You need extra calcium. Severe loss of bone density can lead to osteoporosis and an increased risk of bone fractures, especially if you have a family history of osteoporosis. Women of Caucasian and Asian ancestry are more likely than women of African ancestry to develop osteoporosis. (Men also lose bone tissue as they grow older, but their bones are heavier and denser, and they lose bone tissue less rapidly than women do.)

Twenty years ago, nutritionists thought that you couldn't do anything about age-related loss of bone density – that your body stopped absorbing calcium when you passed your mid-20s. Today, everybody knows that increasing your calcium consumption can slow the loss of bone tissue no matter what your age.

Phabulous Phytochemicals

The latest buzzword in nutrition is *phytochemicals*, a five-syllable mouthful meaning 'chemicals from plants'. Phytochemicals are the substances that produce many of the beneficial effects associated with a diet that includes lots of fruits, vegetables, pulses and grains.

Phytochemicals are everywhere

We've been eating phytochemicals all our lives without knowing it. The following are all phytochemicals:

- ✔ **Carotenoids,** the pigments that make fruits and vegetables orange, red, yellow and green.

- ✔ **Isothiocyanates,** the smelly sulphur compounds that make you turn up your nose at the aroma of boiling cabbage.

- ✔ **Daidzein and genistein,** hormonelike compounds in many fruits and vegetables.

- ✔ **Actein,** a hormonelike compound in black cohosh, a native North American herb used by Native Americans and some modern herbalists as a remedy for female troubles such as hot flushes and other signs of menopause.

- ✔ **Dietary fibre,** the indigestible part of plant foods.

- ✔ **Anthocyanins,** antioxidant pigments such as the colouring agent that makes blueberries blue.

Book II

Food and Nutrition

These and other phytochemicals such as vitamins (yes, vitamins) perform beneficial housekeeping chores in your body. They:

- ✔ Keep your cells healthy.

- ✔ Slow down tissue degeneration.

- ✔ Prevent the formation of *carcinogens* (cancer-producing substances).

- ✔ Reduce cholesterol levels.

- ✔ Protect your heart.

- ✔ Maintain your hormone balance.

- ✔ Keep your bones strong.

Perusing the different kinds of phytochemicals

The most interesting phytochemicals in plant foods appear to be antioxidants, hormonelike compounds, and enzyme-activating sulphur compounds. Each group plays a specific role in maintaining health and reducing your risk of certain illnesses.

Antioxidants

Antioxidants are named for their ability to prevent a chemical reaction called *oxidation*, which enables molecular fragments called *free radicals* to join together, forming potentially carcinogenic compounds in your body.

Antioxidants also slow the normal wear and tear on body cells, so a diet rich in plant foods (fruits, vegetables, grains and beans) is known to reduce the risk of heart disease and may reduce the risk of some kinds of cancer. For example, consuming lots of lycopene (the red carotenoid in tomatoes) has been linked to a lower risk of prostate cancer as long as the tomatoes are mixed with an edible oil, which makes the lycopene easy to absorb.

Hormone-like compounds

Many plants contain compounds that behave like *oestrogens*, the female sex hormones. Because only animal bodies can produce true hormones, these plant chemicals are called *hormone-like compounds* or *phyto-oestrogens* (plant oestrogen).

The three kinds of phyto-oestrogens are:

- Isoflavones, in fruits, vegetables and beans.
- Lignans, in grains.
- Stillbenes, in grapes and wine.

The most valuable phyto-oestrogens appear to be the isoflavones known as *daidzein* and *genistein*, two compounds with a chemical structure similar to *estradiol*, which is the oestrogen produced by mammalian ovaries.

Although questions remain about exactly what dose is best, many studies have shown that isoflavones and lignans are safe and useful for human beings and that regularly consuming foods containing isoflavones and lignans, particularly soya, may reduce the risk of heart disease. On the other hand, coumestans, which are up to 100 times as potent as isoflavones, haven't been proven either safe or effective. These common foods provide isoflavones:

Apples	Fennel	Potatoes
Carrots	Garlic	Red clover
Cherries	Parsley	Soya beans
Dates	Pomegranates	

These foods provide lignans:

- Cereals
- Linseeds

Sulphur compounds

Pop an apple pie in the oven and soon the kitchen fills with a yummy aroma that makes your mouth water and your digestive juices flow. But boil some cabbage and – yuk! What is that awful smell? It's sulphur, the same chemical that identifies rotten eggs.

Cruciferous vegetables (which get their name from the Latin word for cross, in reference to their X-shaped blossoms) such as broccoli, Brussels sprouts, cauliflower, kale, kohlrabi, mustard seed, onions, radishes, swede, turnips and watercress all contain stinky sulphur compounds and non-nutrient substances that seem to tell your body to rev up its production of enzymes that inactivate and help eliminate carcinogens.

The presence of these smelly sulphurs is thought to explain why people who eat lots of cruciferous veggies generally have a lower risk of cancer. This theory is bolstered by a laboratory experiment in which rats given chemicals known to cause breast tumours were less likely to develop tumours when they were given *sulphorathane*, one of the smelly sulphur compounds in cruciferous veggies.

Dietary fibre

Dietary fibre is a special bonus found only in plant foods. You can't get it from meat, fish, poultry, eggs, or dairy foods.

Soluble dietary fibre, such as the pectins in apples and the gums in beans, helps mop up unwanted cholesterol and helps lower your risk of heart disease when part of a healthy diet and lifestyle. Insoluble dietary fibre such as the cellulose in fruit skins bulks up stools (faeces) and prevents constipation; moving food more quickly through your gut so food has less time to create substances thought to trigger the growth of cancerous cells. (Turn to the sections 'Considering carbohydrates' and 'Dietary fibre' for more on dietary fibre.)

Plant sterols

The effects of sterol-enriched foods have hit both the headlines and the supermarket shelves in recent years. Sterols and stanols are naturally occurring substances found in plants and wood pulp. Evidence suggests that plant sterols and stanols may reduce blood cholesterol levels by reducing cholesterol absorption from the gut. The research so far suggests that regularly consuming sterols and stanols added to margarines, yoghurts, milks, and other products may reduce both total cholesterol and LDL (bad) cholesterol. Nutritionists are still studying the long-term effect of eating large amounts of sterols and stanols over a long period of time.

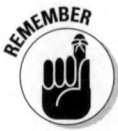

However effective plant sterols might be in reducing cholesterol, it's still vital that you also stay physically active, be a healthy weight, and eat plenty of fruit and vegetables, some oily fish (or a vegetarian supplement), and moderate amounts of saturated fat to protect your heart.

Chapter 3

Exploring How Food Affects Your Health

*Y*ou've probably heard the saying 'you are what you eat', and it's certainly true that many health conditions are linked to poor or inadequate nutrition. In the same way that a car needs good fuel to drive and function well, human bodies need the right nutrients and energy stores to function at peak performance.

In this chapter we explore the link between food and health, and consider how food can affect your mood. If you're one of the many people struggling to control your weight, we help you understand the importance of calories and energy to help maintain your ideal body weight.

Food and Medicine

The science of nutrition emphasises using food to promote health. In other words, a good diet is one that gives you the nutrients you need to keep your body in tiptop condition. However, eating well offers more benefits than simply maintaining normal bodily functions. A good diet may also prevent or minimise the risk of a long list of serious medical conditions including heart disease, type 2 diabetes (an inherited inability to respond to the insulin needed to process carbohydrates), high blood pressure, and cancer.

In this chapter we describe what we know right now about using food to prevent, treat, or cure specific medical conditions. For example:

✔ Eating large amounts of deep green or yellow fruits and veggies coloured with the pigment beta carotene, or red tomatoes and watermelon, which have the red pigment lycopene, may reduce your risk of cancers of the lung, breast, or prostate.

✔ Eating wholegrain cereals high in insoluble dietary fibre (the kind of fibre that doesn't dissolve in your gut) moves food more quickly through your intestinal tract and produces soft, bulky stools that reduces your risk of constipation.

✔ Eating foods such as beans that are high in soluble dietary fibre (fibre that does dissolve in your intestinal tract) seems to reduce the cholesterol circulating in your bloodstream, so preventing it from lodging in and narrowing the walls of your arteries. This reduces your risk of heart disease.

✔ Eating dairy foods (low fat are just as good) and calcium-rich tinned fish, soya products, and green leafy vegetables protects against age-related loss of bone density. It may also help to lower high blood pressure and reduce the incidence of colon cancer.

Not eating certain foods can also be beneficial. Overweight adults who reduce their fat and sugar intake to lose weight may unquestionably prevent a host of medical problems including type 2 diabetes. Similarly, if you're hypertensive, reducing your salt and alcohol intake may help you control your blood pressure.

The joy of food-as-medicine is that it's cheaper and much more pleasant than managing illness with drugs. Given the choice, who wouldn't first opt to try to reduce cholesterol levels with a healthy, low-fat diet, including some oats or beans, rather than with a pill?

Using Food to Prevent Disease

Simply adding a missing nutrient to your diet can cure a deficiency disease. For example, scurvy disappears when people eat foods such as citrus fruits high in vitamin C. But what you probably really want to know is whether specific foods or specific diets can prevent illnesses other than deficiency diseases.

This area of nutrition is awash with anecdotes, but anecdotes aren't science. What the nutrition field needs to judge the claims is evidence from scientific studies. Nutritionists examine groups of people on different diets to see how factors such as eating fish, olive oil, fruit, vegetables and wholegrain cereals (a typical Mediterranean diet), or cutting down on saturated fat, red meat and salt (more common features of the typical UK diet), can affect the risk of specific diseases.

Sometimes, these studies show a strange effect. For example, a recent study suggested that fruit and vegetables protect against most forms of cancer, although seemingly not breast cancer. Sometimes, studies show no effect at all. And sometimes – we like this category best – they turn up results that nobody expected. For example, in 1996, a study was designed to see whether a diet high in selenium would reduce the risk of skin cancer. After four years, the answer was 'Not so you could notice'. But then researchers noticed that people who ate lots of high-selenium foods had a lower risk of lung, breast and prostate cancers. Naturally, researchers immediately set up another study, which happily confirmed the unexpected results of the first.

Eating to reduce the risk of cancer

Book II

Food and Nutrition

Your daily diet is one of the most important factors in determining the risk of cancer – second only to avoiding tobacco smoke. For example:

- ✔ **Fruits and vegetables.** The active anticancer substances in fruits and vegetables include *antioxidants* (chemicals that prevent molecular fragments called free radicals from hooking up to form cancer-causing compounds) and *phyto-oestrogens* (hormone-like chemicals in plants that displace natural and synthetic oestrogens in our bodies).

- ✔ **Foods high in dietary fibre.** Human beings can't digest dietary fibre, but friendly bacteria living in your gut can. Chomping away on the fibre, the bacteria excrete fatty acids that appear to keep cells from turning cancerous. In addition, fibre helps speed food through your body, reducing both the formation and any impact of carcinogenic compounds.

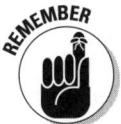

The World Cancer Research Fund (WCRF) *Diet and Health Guidelines for the Prevention of Cancer* are a good start in reducing your risk of cancer. The guidelines are:

- ✔ Choose a diet rich in a variety of plant-based foods.

- ✔ Eat plenty of fruit and vegetables.

- ✔ Maintain a healthy weight and be physically active.

- ✔ Drink alcohol in moderation if at all.

- ✔ Select foods that are low in fat and salt.

- ✔ Prepare and store foods safely.

WCRF Expert Report: Food Nutrition and the Prevention of Cancer: A Global Perspective (1997)

DASHing to healthy blood pressure

In the United Kingdom 16 million people have high blood pressure (also known as hypertension), a major risk factor for heart disease, stroke, and heart or kidney failure. That's one in three of you women readers and two in five of the men.

As you can find out in *High Blood Pressure For Dummies* (published by Wiley), the traditional treatment for hypertension has included drugs (some with unpleasant side effects) combined with specific dietary strategies such as reduced sodium intake, weight loss, alcohol reduction and regular exercise.

International research known as the 'Dietary Approaches to Stop Hypertension' – DASH, for short – has shown that the overall composition of the diet is very important. The DASH diet is rich in fruit and vegetables, whole grains and low-fat dairy products. Poultry, fish and nuts are the main protein sources. This diet can help prevent an age-related increase in blood pressure and lower an already high level, especially when combined with salt reduction. You can find out more about the DASH diet at www. DashForHealth.com.

Easing symptoms of the common cold

Let's move on to foods that make you feel better when you have the sniffles – for example sweet foods. Nutritionists know why sweeteners – white sugar, brown sugar, honey, syrup – soothe a sore throat. All sugars are *demulcents*, substances that coat and soothe the irritated mucous membranes. Lemons aren't sweet, and they have less vitamin C than orange juice, but their popularity in the form of warm drinks for colds and sore throat tablets is unmatched. Why? Because a lemon's sharp flavour cuts through to your taste buds and makes the sugary stuff more palatable. In addition, the sour taste makes saliva flow, and that also soothes your throat.

Food as the Fountain of Youth

Can food help you look, feel, or think younger? Certainly some foods provide nutrients that clearly lessen the natural consequences of growing older. For example:

  ✔ Fruits and vegetables rich in antioxidant vitamins may slow the development of cataracts and help prevent age-related macular degeneration (AMD), a major cause of visual impairment in older adults. Eating a variety of different-coloured fruits and vegetables is especially beneficial.

> ✔ Bran cereals give you the fibre that can rev up your intestinal tract. The contractions that move food through your gut slow a bit as you grow older, which is why older people are more likely to be constipated.

Looking after your skin

Some studies suggest that eating well can also offer some protection to your skin. How soon and how much you develop wrinkles depend in large measure on your exposure to the sun (the more sun, the more wrinkling), plus the genes you inherit from your mother and father, but diet plays a role, too. Eating a diet that provides enough calories to maintain a healthy weight won't prevent wrinkles, but it may help you look younger, as people who are underweight can often have saggy skin.

As you get older the *stratum corneum* (the outer layer of your skin) gets thinner and loses its ability to hold moisture. A diet with sufficient amounts of fat won't totally prevent this drying of the skin, but it does give you a measure of protection. Virtually all sensible nutritionists recommend some unsaturated fat or oil every day such as vegetable oils or the omega 3 fats from oily fish.

Some studies suggest that phytochemicals and dietary antioxidants such as vitamin C and selenium protect against sun damage and the formation of age spots (but by no means all dermatologists support this view). We do know that phytochemicals and antioxidants help against many other chronic health problems, so any effect on the skin can only be a bonus!

Keeping your mind young

Recent research shows that older adults who eat a wide range of nutritious foods perform best in memory and thinking tests. Overall good food habits seem to be more important than any one food or nutrient. No one knows for sure right now why and it's not clear whether making lifestyle changes late in life can help or whether you have to eat carefully over a lifetime in order to reap the benefits.

Diet may help to protect against the onset of dementia (where brain cells are damaged and die faster than normal). In the UK about 650,000 people suffer from dementia; a figure that can only increase given our ageing population. Research suggests that high-fat, especially high-saturated-fat, diets may be detrimental, whereas a Mediterranean-type diet containing antioxidants, B vitamins such as folate, fish, and moderate amounts of alcohol may be protective.

Vegetarianism: From weird to wonderful

Once upon a time non-meat eaters were regarded as really strange people. Today, vegetarianism is commonplace and, it turns out, pretty good for your health, too. Vegetarianism isn't a single diet. At least three basic variations exist:

✔ People who don't eat red meat but do eat fish and sometimes poultry are known as *demi-vegetarians*. (Strictly speaking people who eat fish or poultry are not true vegetarians.) Around 9 per cent of the UK population fit into this group.

✔ People who don't eat meat, fish, or poultry but do eat other animal products such as eggs and dairy products are called *ovo-lacto vegetarians* (*ovo* = egg, *lacto* = milk). This group makes up about 5 per cent of the UK population.

✔ People who eat absolutely no foods of animal origin are called *vegans*. These vegetarians, who eat only plant foods, number around 250,000.

The first two regimens are completely safe from a nutritional standpoint because they contain enough different kinds of food to supply every essential nutrient your body needs.

A vegan diet – no animal products at all – is a bit more tricky. It has no natural vitamin B12, a nutrient found only in foods from animals. Vegans therefore need B12 supplements or foods fortified with it such as breakfast cereals, yeast extracts and meat substitutes.

A vegan diet can also short-change you on calcium and iron. True, many plants have both minerals, but the minerals in the plants are present in forms your body may find harder to absorb. And don't forget protein. The proteins in foods from animals are *complete*, meaning that they provide sufficient amounts of all the essential amino acids your body needs to build new tissue, make enzymes, and do all the good things proteins do. Proteins in plant foods, however, are *incomplete* or *limited*, meaning that they provide insufficient amounts of specific amino acids. To build plant-food dishes with complete proteins you need to combine ingredients such as rice and beans, or peanut butter and bread, which *complement* each other, meaning that each provides the amino acids the other needs more of.

In other words, with a little care and planning, you can get all the nutrients you need from a vegetarian diet that may also:

✔ Lower your risk of heart disease (plants are low in saturated fat)

✔ Reduce your risk of some kinds of cancer (those wonderful antioxidant chemicals in plants)

So bring on the vegetable stir-fry with noodles and serve up the rice and beans!

French research published in 2002 followed almost 2,000 people over seven years and related their diet to their risk of getting dementia. The researchers concluded that people who ate fish at least once a week had a significantly lower risk of being diagnosed with dementia.

Finding Out About Food and Allergies

Approximately 5–8 per cent of all children and only 2 per cent of adults in the UK are affected by true food allergies. Many childhood allergies seem to disappear when children grow older. If those figures seem low to you then you're not alone. Up to 20 per cent of UK adults believe they have a food allergy, but numerous well-conducted trials repeatedly show that the true figure is nearer 2 per cent.

If food allergies are not as common as people think, why read this whole section on them? First, although food allergies are still relatively rare, they're more common now than they were 20 years ago and it doesn't look as if they'll be going away. Food allergies that don't disappear can trigger reactions ranging from trivial (a stuffy nose the next day) to the truly dangerous (respiratory failure). In addition, whenever you're allergic to foods, you're likely to have other allergies that are triggered by such things as dust or pollen or the family cat. So knowing which food does what really pays off. After all, forewarned is forearmed.

Book II

Food and Nutrition

Alerting you to a food allergy

Your immune system is designed to protect your body from harmful invaders, such as bacteria. Sometimes, however, your immune system responds to substances that are normally harmless. A food allergy is just such a response – your body fighting back against specific proteins in foods. Some common allergic reactions to food include:

- Hives (*urticaria*), an acutely itchy, red patch of skin with a pale fluid-filled centre
- Itching
- Swelling of the face, tongue, lips, eyelids, hands and feet
- Rashes
- Headache, migraine
- Nausea and/or vomiting
- Diarrhoea, sometimes bloody
- Sneezing, coughing
- Asthma
- Breathing difficulties caused by tightening (swelling) of tissues in the throat
- Loss of consciousness (anaphylactic shock)

Investigating allergies and intolerances

Your body may respond to a food in one of two ways:

- ✔ **Food allergy:** Specific reaction resulting in an *immunological response* (where the body produces a dramatic reaction in the presence of an allergen) to a food that can be severe or life threatening. Symptoms can be rapid or delayed. Immediate reactions are more dangerous than delayed reactions because they involve a fast swelling of tissues. Immediate reactions may occur within seconds after eating, touching, or – in some cases – even smelling the offending food.

- ✔ **Nonallergic food intolerance:** Reactions to food that can result from a number of causes, but that are not a result of an immunological response. Reactions are usually as a result of histamine release, an interaction with medication, or enzyme deficiency, and often occur after eating a relatively large amount of a specific food. Reactions may occur as long as 24 to 48 hours after you're exposed to the offending food, and the reaction is likely to be much milder, perhaps a slight nasal congestion caused by swollen tissues.

These two responses are often confused. People with a food intolerance can often cope very well with a small amount of a food that in larger quantities would cause them a problem; they can also often manage a problem food when it has been cooked or processed in some way. For instance, people who are intolerant to milk may be fine with yogurt, or people who react to tomatoes can cope with tomatoes cooked in a sauce with pasta.

Avoiding any food unnecessarily can increase your risk of nutritional deficiency. If you have a true food allergy you can't be as flexible. For example, if you're allergic to peanuts you need to steer clear of them in any amount or any form.

Head for Accident and Emergency or call 999 immediately if you – or a friend or relative – show any signs of an allergic reaction that affects breathing.

Understanding how a reaction occurs

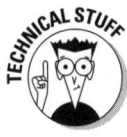

When you eat a food containing a protein to which you are allergic (the allergen), your immune system releases antibodies (IgE) that recognise that specific allergen. The antibodies circulate through your body on white blood cells (basophils) that pass into all your body tissues, where they bind to immune system cells, called mast cells.

Basophils and mast cells produce, store, and release histamine, which causes the symptoms – itching, swelling, hives – associated with allergic reactions. (That's why some allergy pills are called antihistamines.) When the antibodies carried by the basophils and mast cells come in contact with food allergens, boom! You have an allergic reaction.

Food intolerances can cause similar symptoms to food allergies, but the main difference is that the immune system is not involved. Histamine is released as a result after mast cells are activated directly without the need for antibodies.

Often the most important difference between a food allergy and a food intolerance is the way in which they can be diagnosed. A food allergy is far easier to diagnose than an intolerance because you can measure the amount of immunological activity in the blood. With an intolerance you have nothing to measure, but more about that later in the section.

Book II

Food and Nutrition

It's all in the family: Inheriting food allergies

You can inherit a tendency towards allergies, although not the particular allergy itself. If one of your parents has a food allergy, your risk of having the same problem is two times higher than if neither of your parents is allergic to any foods. If both your mother and your father have food allergies, your risk is four times higher. In one truly unusual incident, a transplant patient got a severe peanut allergy along with a new liver from a peanut-sensitive donor. Unlucky or what?

Being aware of the dangers of food allergies

Food allergies can be dangerous. Although most allergic reactions are unpleasant but essentially mild, a small number of people die every year from allergic reactions to food. These people have suffered *anaphylaxis*, a rare but potentially fatal condition in which many different parts of the body react to an allergen in food (or some other allergen), creating a cascade of effects beginning with sudden, severe itching, and moving on to swelling of the tissue in the air passages that can lead to breathing difficulties, falling blood pressure, unconsciousness and death. Many people with true food allergies carry an EPIPEN that contains the hormone epinephrine. If epiniphrine is injected early during an anaphylactic attack it can be life saving.

Considering foods most likely to cause allergic reactions

Here's something to chew on: More than 90 per cent of all allergic reactions to foods are caused by just ten types of food:

- ✔ Milk (cows', goats' and sheep)
- ✔ Eggs
- ✔ Peanuts
- ✔ Tree nuts (brazil nuts, almonds, hazelnuts)
- ✔ Soya bean-based foods (and other legumes such as peas or lentils)
- ✔ Fruit (especially bananas, apples, peaches, plums, cherries and citrus fruits)
- ✔ Fish
- ✔ Shellfish
- ✔ Seeds (especially sesame and caraway)
- ✔ Herbs and spices (especially mustard, paprika and coriander)

The most common foods to cause intolerance reactions are:

- ✔ Cheese (especially matured cheese)
- ✔ Fermented foods such as blue cheese and fermented soya products
- ✔ Yeast extracts
- ✔ Chocolate
- ✔ Red wine
- ✔ Fruits (especially citrus fruits, avocado and banana)
- ✔ Coffee and foods and drinks containing caffeine
- ✔ Wheat

The allergenic food most likely to make headlines seems to be peanuts. People allergic to peanuts may break out in hives just from touching a peanut or peanut butter, and may suffer a potentially fatal reaction after simply tasting chocolate made in a factory where it had touched machinery that had previously touched peanuts.

Testing, testing: Identifying food allergies

Whenever you sprout hives or your skin itches or your eyelids, lips and tongue begin to swell right after you've eaten a particular food, that's a clear sign of a food allergy. Some allergic reactions, however, occur in milder forms, many hours after you've eaten. To identify the culprit, your doctor may suggest an *elimination diet*. This regimen removes from your diet foods known to cause allergic reactions in many people. Then, one at a time, the foods are added back. If you react to one, bingo! That's a clue to what triggers your immune response. An elimination diet is hard work; it takes a lot of effort and requires the support and guidance of a registered dietitian to avoid nutrient deficiency.

A dietitian can also help you find which ingredients appear in the most unlikely foods – for instance, would you ever guess that many brands of ice cream contain wheat? To be absolutely certain of an allergy, your dietitian may challenge your immune system by introducing foods in a form (maybe a capsule) that you can't identify as a specific food. Doing so rules out any possibility that your reaction has been triggered by emotional stimuli – that is, seeing, tasting, or smelling the food.

Two more sophisticated tests – *ELISA* (enzyme-linked immunosorbent assay) and *RAST* (radioallergosorbent test) — can identify antibodies to specific allergens in your blood. But these two tests are rarely required.

Because food allergies and intolerance are so topical, a plethora of therapists with dubious qualifications offer tests with no scientific basis, relieving you of your cash in exchange for an inaccurate diagnosis. Often these tests suggest that you avoid a whole range of foods unnecessarily, putting you at risk of nutritional deficiency. If in doubt, check out the range of reliable and unreliable tests on the Allergy UK Web site www.allergyuk.org.

Coping with food allergies and intolerances

After you know that you're allergic or intolerant to a food, the best way to avoid a reaction is to avoid the food. Unfortunately, that task may be harder than it sounds.

Some allergens are hidden ingredients in dishes made with other foods. For example, people allergic to peanuts have suffered serious allergic reactions after eating chocolate containing traces of nuts. Rye bread may contain some wheat flour, which contains gluten, a protein that is a common food allergen.

Book II

Food and Nutrition

Another problem with food allergies is that you may not even have to eat the food to suffer an allergic reaction. People who react to seafood – fish and shellfish – are known to have developed respiratory problems after simply inhaling the vapours or steam produced by cooking the fish.

If you're someone with a potentially life-threatening allergy to food (or another allergen, such as wasp venom), your doctor may suggest that you carry a syringe prefilled with *epinephrine*, a drug that counteracts the reactions (an EPIPEN). You may also want to wear a medic alert bracelet that identifies you as a person with a serious allergic problem. The food industry is also legally bound to include labels on foods containing some of the most common allergens – especially nuts and peanuts.

How Food Affects Mood

Good morning! Time to wake up, roll out of bed, and crawl into the kitchen for that cup of coffee.

Good day at work? No? Time for a gin and tonic or glass of wine to soothe away the tensions of the day.

Good grief! Your lover has left. Time for chocolate, lots of it, to soothe the pain.

Good night! Time for milk and biscuits to ease your way to sleep.

For centuries, millions of people have used foods in these situations, secure in the knowledge that each food will work its mood magic. Today, modern science knows some of the reasons. Having discovered that emotions are linked to the production or use of certain brain chemicals, nutritionists have identified the natural chemicals in food that change the way you feel.

The following sections describe the chemicals in food that are most commonly known to affect mood.

Alcohol

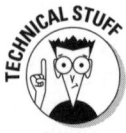

Alcohol is probably the world's most widely used natural sedative. Contrary to common belief, alcohol is a depressant, not a stimulant. If you feel exuberant after one drink, the reason isn't because the alcohol is speeding up your brain. It's because alcohol relaxes your *controls*, the brain signals that normally tell you not to put a street cone on your head or take off your clothes in public.

Alcohol activates the pleasure or reward centres of the brain by triggering the release of both dopamine and serotonin. Many people find that, taken with food and in moderation – defined as 1–2 units a day for a woman and 2–3 units for a man – alcohol can produce a sense of well-being, relaxation and happiness.

Caffeine

On the other hand, caffeine is probably the most widely consumed stimulant in the world. For some people, if they're not used to it, a large dose of caffeine can have a variety of effects. It can:

- Raise your blood pressure
- Speed up your heartbeat
- Stop you sleeping
- Increase urine production

However, doses at the levels commonly consumed have little or no ill effect, especially if you're a regular consumer.

However even in quite low doses, caffeine is mood activating, increasing alertness especially when you're tired. This effect seems to be genuine and not simply the reversal of withdrawal effects when caffeine is withheld. Some people report higher levels of anxiety after exposure to large single doses of caffeine. However, how people react to caffeine is a highly individual affair. Some can drink several cups of normal coffee a day and experience none of the side effects; others tend to get jumpy even on quite low intakes. This may relate to body composition, weight, sex, whatever else they've eaten recently, or even a biochemical difference in the brain. Nobody really knows yet.

Either way, caffeine's effects may last anywhere from one to seven hours. Some researchers believe that children may be particularly sensitive, but insufficient research has yet been carried out to determine the effect of caffeinated fizzy drinks on children's mood. For most adults the average intake of about 300 milligrams caffeine per day seems to be harmless. However, perhaps 10 per cent of the UK population have high intakes, usually defined as greater than about 400 milligrams day for a woman and 500 milligrams day for a man. Use Table 3-1 to work out your own daily level.

Endurance athletes who take caffeine before an event report that it improves alertness and performance, but caffeine is prohibited in sport at high levels. Caffeine can be detected in your urine, and drinking caffeine from a variety of sources (see Table 3-1) can easily add together to produce a positive test result.

Table 3-1	Foods That Give You Caffeine	
Food	*Average caffeine content (mg/Serving)*	*Range (mg/serving)*
Coffee, filter/percolated (200ml)	90	61–126
Coffee, instant (200ml)	58	42–68
Coffee or tea, decaffeinated (200ml)	2	1–4
Tea (200ml)	40	32–56
Cocoa (200ml)	5	1–8
Cola drinks (330ml can)	23	11–71
Chocolate bar (50g)	8	5–17
Stimulant ('energy') drinks (200ml)	48	1–70

Source: Joint Food Safety and Standards Group (1998). Food Surveillance Information Sheet no. 144. Ministry of Agriculture, Fisheries and Food. London

Carbohydrate and protein

Proteins are composed of a series of building blocks known as amino acids. Several amino acids are important in mood. The amino acid tryptophan can be converted in the body to the 'feel-good' neurotransmitter serotonin, which elevates and enhances mood, acting like a natural tranquilliser. Good sources of tryptophan are animal proteins such as lean meat, poultry, fish and dairy products. Nuts, pulses and brown rice are also rich suppliers.

Glucose, the end product of carbohydrate metabolism, is the sugar that circulates in your blood and the basic fuel your body runs on. Sufficient glucose from a high carbohydrate diet also increases the uptake of tryptophan and increases serotonin release from nerve cells in the brain. A combination of tryptophan-rich proteins and carbohydrates is therefore thought to be especially mood enhancing. Wholegrain cereals, pasta, bread, oats, rice, fruit and pulses provide a slow supply of glucose into the bloodstream for a steady release of serotonin to help moderate and stabilise mood.

Women prone to hormone disruption during their monthly cycle have naturally lower levels of serotonin in their brains. A low-carbohydrate diet may increase irritability and make their moods more unsteady.

Less is known about the effects of high fat and sugar intakes. Some researchers suggest that filling up on fatty and fried foods can negatively affect your mood, making you tired and apathetic. If you eat simple sugars on an empty stomach, you absorb the sugars rapidly into your blood, triggering an equally rapid increase in the secretion of *insulin*, a hormone that takes them back out of your blood to the cells that can use it. The result is a rapid decrease in the amount of sugar circulating in your blood, a condition known as *hypoglycae-mia* (hypo = low; glycaemia = sugar in the blood) that can make you feel temporarily jumpy and irritable rather than calm. However, when eaten on a full stomach – dessert after a full meal – simple sugars are absorbed more slowly and may exert the calming effect usually linked to complex carbohydrates (starchy foods).

Some studies show very positive results using a balance of carbohydrate and protein-rich foods to improve mood, but the results aren't always clear cut. Other studies have found no benefit. Not all nutritionists believe the amounts of certain nutrients in the diet (such as tryptophan) are large enough to have an effect. Why not try it for yourself? After all, a good balance of carbohydrates and protein is protective against a whole range of other health problems too!

Using Food to Manage Mood

Nutrition is important in mental function and certainly plays a role in depression. What you eat won't change your personality or alter the course of a mood disorder. But certain foods may be able to add a little lift or a small moment of calm to your day, increase your effectiveness at certain tasks, or make you more alert.

- ✔ One cup of coffee in the morning is a pleasant push into alertness. Seven cups of coffee a day can make you jittery and feel on edge.

- ✔ A glass of wine or a gin and tonic is generally a safe way to relax. Three and you may be getting *too* merry (or moody).

- ✔ A good breakfast on a morning when you have to be on your toes can do wonders for your mood, concentration and performance. Try a bowl of porridge oats or muesli with dried fruit and low-fat milk, or wholegrain toast with lean grilled bacon or baked beans.

- ✔ Got an important lunch meeting? Order starches and protein – pasta or rice with chicken or fish and a fresh tomato and basil sauce; a jacket potato and beans – and add a side salad and fruit for dessert. Your aim is to get the calming carbs with just a little protein and not too much fat.

Calories: The Energisers

Cars burn petrol to get the energy they need to move. Your body burns (*metabolises*) food to produce energy in the form of heat. This heat warms your body and powers every move you make.

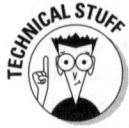

Nutritionists measure the amount of heat produced by metabolising food in units called kilocalories (Kcals). A *kilocalorie* is the amount of energy it takes to raise the temperature of one kilogram of water one degree centigrade at sea level. Energy is also expressed as kilojoules, the standard international (SI) unit for energy, and the more scientifically accurate way to express energy. However, most of us are more familiar with food energy expressed as kilocalories. One kilocalorie is equal to 4.18 kilojoules.

In common use, nutritionists often substitute the word *calorie* for *kilocalorie*. This information isn't scientifically accurate: Strictly speaking, a calorie is really $\frac{1}{1000}$ of a kilocalorie. But the word calorie is easier to say and easier to remember, so that's the term you sometimes see when you read about the energy in food and that's the word we use in this book. And few nutrition-related words have caused as much confusion and concern as the humble calorie. Read on to find out what calories mean to you and to your nutrition.

Counting the calories in food

When you read that a portion of food – say, one banana – has 105 calories, it means that metabolising the banana produces 105 calories of heat that your body can use for work.

You may wonder which kinds of food have the most calories. The answer is that it depends which nutrients they contain.

One gram of...	Has this many calories
Carbohydrates	3.75
Protein	4
Alcohol	7
Fat	9

In other words, a gram of protein or carbohydrate gives you fewer than half as many calories as a gram of fat. That's why high-fat foods, such as crisps, are higher in calories than low-fat foods, such as boiled potatoes.

However, it's not always that simple, as foods usually contain a mix of nutrients. As a good example, take a chicken breast and a beefburger, both high-protein foods. If you serve the chicken without its skin, it contains very little fat, while the beefburger is (we hate to say) full of it. A 100g (3.5oz) skinless chicken breast provides 140 calories, while a 100g (3.5oz) burger has around 270 calories. (These are weights when cooked.)

How many calories do you need?

Think of your energy balance as a bank account. You make deposits when you consume calories from food and drink. You make withdrawals when your body burns up energy on activity. Nutritionists divide the amount of energy you withdraw each day into two parts:

- The energy you need when your body is at rest.
- The energy you need when you are physically active.

To keep your energy account in balance, you need to take in enough each day to cover your withdrawals. As a general rule, infants and adolescents need more energy weight for weight than adults do, because they're continually making large amounts of new tissue. Similarly, an average man burns more energy than an average woman because his body is larger and has more muscle, thus leading to the totally unfair, but totally true fact that a 70 kilogram (11 stone) man can consume about 10 per cent more calories than a 70 kilogram (11 stone) woman of the same age and activity level, and still not gain weight. For the numbers, turn to the next section and Table 3-2.

Book II

Food and Nutrition

Resting energy expenditures

Even when you're at rest, your body is busy burning calories. Your heart beats. Your lungs expand and contract. Your intestines digest food. Your liver processes nutrients. Your glands secrete hormones. Your muscles work gently. Cells send electrical impulses backwards and forwards among themselves, and your brain continually signals to every part of your body.

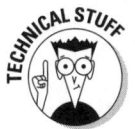

The energy that your resting body uses to do all this stuff is called (quite appropriately) *resting energy expenditure*, abbreviated as REE. The REE, also known as the *basal metabolic rate or BMR*, accounts for a whopping 60 to 70 per cent of all the calories you need each day. To find your resting energy expenditure (REE), you must first know your weight in kilograms (kg). One kilogram equals 2.2 pounds (lbs). So to get your weight in kilograms, first calculate your weight in pounds (1 stone is 14 pounds) then divide the amount in pounds by 2.2. For example, if you weigh 10 stone 10 pounds or 150 pounds, that's equal to 68.2 kilograms (150 ÷ 2.2). Enter that into the appropriate equation in Table 3-2 – and hey presto! You have your REE.

Table 3-2 How Many Calories Do You Need When You're Resting?	
Sex and Age	*Use this Equation to Work Out Your REE*
Males	
0–3 years*	(60.9 × weight in kg) – 54
3–10 years*	(22.7 × weight in kg) + 495

(continued)

Table 3-2 *(continued)*

Sex and Age	Use this Equation to Work Out Your REE
10–17 years	(17.7 × weight in kg) + 657
18–29 years	(15.1 × weight in kg) + 692
30–59 years	(11.5 × weight in kg) + 873
60–74 years	(11.9 × weight in kg) + 700
75+	(8.4 × weight in kg) + 821
Females	
0–3 years*	(61.0 × weight in kg) – 51
3–10 years*	(22.5 × weight in kg) + 499
10–17 years	(13.4 × weight in kg) + 692
18–29 years	(14.8 × weight in kg) + 487
30–59 years	(8. 3 × weight in kg) + 846
60–74 years	(9.2 × weight in kg) + 687
75+	(9.8x W in kg) + 624

*Source: Modified Schofield Equations from Dietary Reference Values for Food Energy and Nutrients for the United Kingdom. Report of the Panel on Dietary Reference Values of the COMA of Food Policy (Department of Health 1991) *The National Research Council, Recommended Dietary Allowances (Washington, D.C.: National Academy Press, 1989)*

Energy for work

Your second largest chunk of energy is the energy you withdraw to spend on physical activity. That's everything from brushing your teeth in the morning to mowing the lawn or working out in the gym.

Your total energy requirement (the number of calories you need each day) is your REE plus enough calories to cover the amount of work you do.

Table 3-3 defines the energy expenditure of various activities ranging from the least energetic (sleeping) to the most (playing football, climbing stairs).

Table 3-3	How Active Are You When You're Active?	
Activity Level	Activity	Average Energy Expenditure (Kcals per Hour) for a Person of 60 kg
Resting	Sleeping, lying down, sitting, standing at rest, reading, writing, listening to radio, watching TV, eating.	60–80

Activity Level	Activity	Average Energy Expenditure (Kcals per Hour) for a Person of 60 kg
Very light	Sewing, dusting, cooking, playing a musical instrument, driving, washing up, ironing, playing snooker, bowling, general office and laboratory work.	90–140
Light	Strolling gently at 2mph, vacuuming, washing and dressing, electrical work, painting and decorating, cricket.	150–200
Moderate	Walking at 3mph, mopping floor, gentle gardening, cleaning windows, table tennis, sailing, golf, garage work, carpentry, bricklaying.	210–260
Heavy	Brisk walking at 4mph, heavy gardening, dancing, moderate swimming, volleyball, slow jogging, labouring, digging, road construction, chopping wood, gentle cycling.	270–350
Very heavy	Walking with a load uphill or cross country, brisk jogging, cycling, football, energetic swimming, tennis, skiing.	360–600

Adapted from Dietary Reference Values for Food Energy and Nutrients for the United Kingdom. Report of the Panel on Dietary Reference Values of the COMA of Food Policy (Department of Health, 1991)

Book II

Food and Nutrition

So how much should you weigh?

A number of charts and tables claim to lay out *standard* or *healthy weights* for adults, but sometimes the figures appear so low that it seems you can't really get there without constant dieting.

We all know overweight people who live long and happy lives and slim ones who leave us sooner than they should. However, people who are overweight have a higher risk of developing some illnesses, such as type 2 diabetes. We're all made so differently that an ideal weight doesn't really exist. However, you need to know the healthy weight range for your height. One good guide is the *Body Mass Index (BMI)*, a number that measures the relationship between your weight and your height and offers some predictive estimate of your risk of weight-related disease. Another way is looking at your waist circumference. We look at both methods in the next sections.

Calculating your Body Mass Index

To calculate your BMI, measure your height in metres (take your shoes off) and figure out your weight in kilograms (definitely take your shoes off!). Now multiply the figure for your height by itself (square it). Divide your weight (in kilograms) by your height (in metres) squared.

For example, if you are 1.6m (5'3") tall and weigh 70kilograms (11 stone) the equations for your BMI look like this:

$$\text{BMI} = \frac{70}{1.6 \times 1.6} = \frac{70}{2.6} = 27$$

Check out Table 3-4 to see how your BMI relates to your weight.

Table 3-4	Classification of Weight Categories Using BMI
Category	*BMI*
Underweight	18.5
Healthy weight	18.5–24.9
Overweight	25–29.9
Moderately obese	30–34.9
Severely obese	35–39.9
Morbidly obese	>40

Current nutritional research suggests that the healthiest BMI is about 21.0. A BMI higher than 28 doubles the risk of illness (especially diabetes and heart disease) and death.

You can see that for each BMI category a range of weights is given. If you have a small frame and proportionately more fat tissue than muscle tissue (muscle is heavier than fat), you're likely to be at the low end of the range. When you have a large frame and proportionately more muscle than fat, you're likely to be at the high end. As a general (but by no means invariable) rule, that means that women – who have smaller frames and less muscle – weigh less than men of the same height and age.

BMI is not a perfect measure of weight because it doesn't measure body fat specifically. If BMI alone is used, very muscular people can be mistakenly classified as obese.

Measuring your waist circumference

Measuring your waist circumference is another useful method for assessing any weight-related health risks such as diabetes and heart disease. Fat stored centrally around the abdomen (tummy), or *central obesity*, is linked more closely to health risks than fat stored around the hips. Recommended cut off points are shown in Table 3-5. If you are in the 'at risk' category, avoid further weight gain. If you are in the 'substantially increased risk' category, we strongly advise you to lose weight. South Asian men seem to be especially at risk from central obesity, so the cut off point for risk starts at a lower waist circumference for this group.

Table 3-5	Waist Circumference Cut-Off Points	
	At Risk	*Substantially Increased Risk*
Men	> 94cm	>102cm
Women	>80cm	>88cm
South Asian men	>90cm	>102 cm

Source: World Health Organisation, 1998

Book II

Food and Nutrition

Controlling your weight effectively

Remember that every body is built differently and we all have different calorie needs. The guidelines in this book are not hard-and-fast rules. However, realistic rules can enable you to control your weight safely and effectively:

✔ **Rule No. 1: Not everybody starts out with the same set of genes – or fits into the same pair of jeans.** Some people are naturally larger and heavier than others. If that's you, and all your weight is within the healthy range, don't waste time trying to fit someone else's idea of perfection. Relax and enjoy your own body. Spot reduction on fatty areas is virtually impossible by dieting.

✔ **Rule No. 2: If you're overweight and your doctor agrees with your decision to diet, you don't have to set world records to improve your health.** Even a moderate loss of weight can be highly beneficial. Losing just 10 to 15 per cent of your body weight can lower high blood sugar, high cholesterol, and high blood pressure, reducing your risks of diabetes, heart disease and stroke. For a 90-kilogram person that's just 9 kilograms!

✔ **Rule No. 3: The only number you need to remember is *3,500*, the number of calories it takes to gain or lose 0.5 kilograms (1 pound) of body fat.** So if you simply:

- Cut your calorie consumption from 3,000 calories a day to 2,500 and continue to do the same amount of physical work, you'll lose 0.5 kilograms a week.

- Go the other way, increasing from 2,500 to 3,000 calories a day, without increasing the amount of work you do, and seven days later you'll be 0.5 kilograms heavier.

Losing weight by controlling calories

Modest calorie restrictions can produce safe and beneficial weight loss. You simply eat a sensible diet that includes a wide variety of different foods containing sufficient amounts of essential nutrients. The Department of Health has an interesting set of estimated average energy requirements for adult men and women based on actual measurements of the amount of daily calories burned by healthy adults of different ages and weights at different levels of activity. Table 3-6 shows the estimated average requirements for energy (kcals/day) for adult men and women based on age, weight and activity level. You can see that if you're active you can take in more calories and still keep your weight steady. If you're less active, you need fewer calories.

But here's a tip for smart calorie counters: Not only does physical activity help to protect against heart disease and cancer, but when you're looking to lose a few pounds, increasing your activity is better than just cutting back on calories.

Table 3-6	**Estimated Average Calorie Requirements for Energy (Kcals/Day) for Adults Based on Age, Weight and Activity Level**				
Weight (kg)	*Inactive*	*Moderately Active*	*Weight (kg)*	*Inactive*	*Moderately Active*
Men 19–29 years			**Women 18–29 years**		
60	2224	2727	50	1722	1961
65	2344	2846	55	1818	2081
70	2440	2990	60	1937	2200
75	2559	3110	65	2033	2320
80	2655	3229	70	2129	2440
Men 30–59 years			**Women 30–59 years**		
65	2272	2751	50	1746	2009
70	2341	2846	55	1818	2081
75	2440	2966	60	1866	2129
80	2511	3062	65	1913	2200
85	2583	3157	70	1985	2272

Weight (kg)	Inactive	Moderately Active	Weight (kg)	Inactive	Moderately Active
Men 60–64 years			**Women 60–64 years**		
74	2380	n/a	63.5	1900	n/a
Men 65–74 years			**Women 65–74 years**		
71	2330	n/a	63	1900	n/a
Men over 75 years			**Women over 75 years**		
69	2100	n/a	60	1810	n/a

Source: Adapted from Dietary Reference Values for Food Energy and Nutrients for the United Kingdom. Report of the Panel on Dietary Reference Values of the Committee on Medical Aspects of Food Policy (Department of Health, 1991). N/a = data not available

The trick is managing your calories and not letting them manage you. Once you know that fats are more fattening than proteins and carbohydrates, and that your body burns food to make energy, you can strategise your energy intake to match your energy expenditure, and vice versa.

Looking to the Future: New Research into Food and Mood

The field of food and mood is growing all the time and fascinating studies hit the scientific journals almost every month. In this section we look at some of the latest research and try to sort the fact from the fiction.

Essential fatty acids

Essential fatty acids may also influence the way we feel. The long chain omega 3 group of fatty acids make up an amazing 65 per cent of brain tissue, concentrated mainly in the brain cell membranes. Research suggests that they may affect mood by keeping brain cell membranes flexible and fluid, and enabling neurotransmitters to signal effectively. Low levels of omega 3 are associated with a higher risk of depression – the lower the level, the more severe the mood disturbance. Several respected researchers believe that anyone lacking omega 3 in their diet is at risk of developing low moods and irritability, including children with mood and behaviour disorders. Research also suggests that heart attack victims who were advised to increase their omega 3 intake from oily fish seem to have improved levels of mood over those not given this advice.

You can get essential fatty acids from oily fish, fish oil supplements, and seeds and seed oils such as rapeseed and linseed. Supplementation seems to be helpful in the treatment of at least some groups of depressed patients. Although more research needs to be done in this area, it's perhaps yet another reason to eat those oil-rich fish.

Selenium and folate

Both selenium and folate play a role in determining the levels of neurotransmitters in the brain. Surveys suggest that dietary intakes of both may be marginally low in some groups of the population and that these low intakes may be linked to a higher risk of depression as well as a poorer response to treatment for depression. It's unclear whether these low levels are a result or a cause of low mood, but supplements of selenium and folic acid in some trials seemed to improve mood in those with the lowest levels of these nutrients.

Fruit and vegetables, wholegrain or fortified cereal products contain selenium and folate. Selenium also comes from meat, fish and nuts – especially brazil nuts. Ensure that you have an adequate intake, especially as these nutrients seem to play a variety of other roles in the body including possible protection against heart disease, cancer and dementia.

Chocolate

It may come as no surprise, but a recent Mintel survey showed that consumers were willing to make certain changes to achieve a healthier diet but most were reluctant to give up chocolate, considering it a vital 'mood food' – satisfying their emotional needs when feeling low. So is there any substance to this claim? Well yes, perhaps!

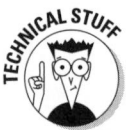

Chocolate products, especially those with a high cocoa content (more than 70 per cent cocoa beans), contain a range of pleasure-enhancing ingredients. Anandamide, also known as 'the bliss molecule', is a neurotransmitter that mimics the euphoric and heightened sensitivity effect of cannabis in the brain. In addition, chocolate contains two chemicals that slow the breakdown of the anandamide already produced in your brain, thus intensifying its effects. (You'd need to eat at least 100 bars of chocolate at one time to get any real marijuana-like effect.)

Chocolate also contains trace levels of phenylethylalanine (PEA) – a stimulant similar to amphetamine that your body releases when you're in love, making you feel good all over. Low levels have been linked to depression. Chocolate also contains caffeine and another stimulant known as theobromine.

Many researchers don't believe that the amounts of these chemicals in chocolate are strong enough for a genuine mood-altering effect in the brain. Researchers found that cocoa-filled capsules containing the same chemicals as chocolate don't satisfy cravings the way chocolate does. They argue that it's only the sweetness and pleasurable feeling of chocolate in the mouth that make us feel so happy. Spoilsports!

Book II

Food and Nutrition

Chapter 4

Taking a Look Inside the GL Diet

The diet industry is worth millions because people are continually searching for that elusive perfect diet. Diet fads come and go; some diets are effective and some are downright dangerous. Industrialised countries face an obesity epidemic with huge implications in terms of individual suffering and medical costs. Therefore, people turn in hope to the latest eating trends fuelling the quest for the perfect diet – diets that seem to become more and more extreme.

Working with patients, training the dieticians of the future, and sifting through the mountain of scientific evidence surrounding different dietary theories means that we can see the problem of finding an effective diet from many different angles.

We work with people who need help improving their diet and lifestyle, and we have access to the evolving science along with the skills to translate new findings into real-life strategies and real foods. As dieticians, we're at the frontline in the battle to find a diet that's satisfying, good for you, and promotes a healthy weight. We have great news for you – we've found it!

Recipes in This Chapter

▶ Scrambled Eggs and Smoky Bacon

▶ Fast Muesli

▶ Breakfast Smoothie

▶ Breakfast to Go

▶ Vitality Salad

▶ Adulterated Hummus with Low-GL Bread and Salad

▶ Chicken and Vegetable Crumble

▶ Mediterranean Bacon Pasta

▶ Salmon and Sweet Potato Fishcakes

▶ Tuna Pasta Bake

▶ Stir-Fry with Chicken

▶ Bite-Size TV Dinner Platter

▶ Punchy Fresh Fruit Salad

▶ Blackberry and Apple Crumble

▶ Snacks in a Bag

▶ Sardines on Toast

▶ Baked Veggie Skewers

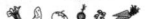

Introducing the Glycaemic Load Diet

In this chapter we introduce you to the *Glycaemic Load Diet* (GL Diet), the most significant breakthrough in nutritional science by far. The GL Diet is balanced and provides all the nutrition you need to be healthy. We share with you why the easy-to-follow low-GL way of eating can give you more energy, reduce your risk of disease, stamp out your food cravings, and enable you to maintain a healthy weight.

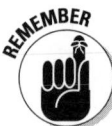

Weight-loss diets often forget about the complete nutritional package you need to achieve not only a healthy weight but a healthy body, too. The GL Diet is sustainable for life – that means it's both safe and nutritionally complete.

Easy to choose, easy to use

The GL Diet is based on eating certain carbohydrates, as part of a healthy diet, that slowly release energy keeping you going for longer, rather than storing the fuel away as fat.

One of the best things about the GL-way of eating is the flexibility that you have with food. Whether or not you're trying to lose weight, you won't feel at all as if you're on a restrictive diet. Think of the GL Diet as an eating plan, rather than a diet – much nicer!

The two most important factors for healthy eating are:

- **Enjoy your food:** Eating is a pleasant aspect of your life. The GL Diet doesn't ban any foods nor make other foods obligatory. Enjoying your food the GL-way means getting a better balance of foods in your diet in order to be healthy and to minimise the risk of disease.

- **Eat a variety of foods:** The greater the variety of foods you eat, the more essential nutrients your diet will contain, especially the necessary vitamins and minerals.

Low-GL food guides

Here are some at-a-glance guidelines:

- **Meat, fish and poultry:** Choose a good mixture of protein foods including lean meats, skinless poultry, and a mix of white and oily fish.

- **Fruit and vegetables:** Pretty much all fruit and veg are great on a low-GL diet (take a look at the Cheat Sheet). Aim to eat a rainbow of different colours to get the best mix of vitamins and minerals.

- **Fats:** Replace saturated fat (such as butter and lard) with polyunsaturated (such as corn oil) and monounsaturated fats (such as olive oil).

- **Nuts and seeds:** All nuts and seeds are good for you and for your low-GL plan in moderate quantities.

✔ **Grains:** Go for the whole grains such as oats, pearl barley, rye and bulgur wheat.

✔ **Pasta, rice and potatoes:** Choose small amounts of pasta and don't overcook it. Mix rice with lentils or beans to lower the GL, and choose small new potatoes or sweet potatoes over large white potatoes.

✔ **Breads:** Pick the grainiest bread possible, because bread with seeds and nuts is lower GL than white or wholemeal bread.

Benefiting from the GL Diet

Here are some of the great physical benefits you can expect from the GL Diet:

✔ Increased energy

✔ Fewer food cravings, because you stay fuller and more satisfied for longer, which helps to control your weight

✔ Fewer mood swings

✔ The opportunity to permanently achieve a healthier weight

✔ A reduced risk of heart disease, diabetes, syndrome X and female hormonal disturbances

Book II

Food and Nutrition

Checking Out the Science Behind GL

Here we take a brief look at the carbohydrate revolution. We mainly give you the facts behind the low-carb hype. We also give you the science behind the GL Diet, so that you can impress all your friends with your technical knowledge but also – and most importantly – so that you can benefit from knowing the science of how the diet works.

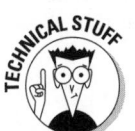

Making the connection between carbs and weight gain

Carbohydrates are composed of carbon, hydrogen and oxygen and are sugar compounds mainly made by plants when plants are exposed to light. Carbs fall into two categories:

✔ **Simple carbohydrates** are carbohydrates with only one or two units of sugar. Some simple sugars, but by no means all, are digested quickly to provide instant energy. Simple sugars include sucrose (table sugar) and lactose (milk sugar).

✔ **Complex carbohydrates,** also known as *polysaccharides*, have more than two units of sugar linked together. Complex carbs are generally digested more slowly than simple sugars and include starches found in potatoes, breads, pasta, rice and cereals. Within this group of carbs is a huge variation in the speed at which they're digested.

✔ **Dietary fibre** aids digestion because it passes through the system without being used for energy (because human digestion can't break the bonds holding the sugar units together).

Your body runs on *glucose* (also a single unit of sugar). All the digestible carbohydrates you get from food provide either glucose or sugar units that are quickly converted to glucose. The glucose is carried into your cells with the help of *insulin*, a hormone produced in your pancreas.

You store a small amount of carbohydrate energy (called *glycogen*) in your muscles and liver. Glycogen is your instant access power store for when you need immediate bursts of energy. These glycogen storage units have limited space and fill up quickly. When your glycogen stores are full, the only way you can store excess energy is as fat. Too much energy from sugar means more energy storage as fat.

Sugar is a really small, simple molecule that needs little digesting before you quickly absorb it into your bloodstream. Your *blood sugars*, which give you the energy your body needs to function properly, are finely balanced. If your blood sugar levels get too high or too low at any given moment, your body has a contingency plan to deal with the problem. The powerful hormone *insulin* helps keep your blood sugars balanced by mopping up excess sugar. When you eat sugary foods, if you don't need a burst of immediate energy, the excess sugar is stored for later use as fat.

Unstable blood sugars make you much more prone to 'grazing' on high-sugar treats (snacking) between meals. A sharp rise in blood sugar when you snack is followed by a quick fall, and you're left feeling hungry and looking for your next sugar fix. All that sugar means just one thing – you guessed it, more fat storage.

Some carbohydrates, such as bread, rice and potatoes, have very similar effects on your blood sugars as the simple sugars; such as the white stuff you put in your coffee. Understanding the principle of how carbohydrates affect us was the basis for a diet revolution – the Glycaemic Index, and then the Glycaemic Load.

Turning to the Glycaemic Index

The *Glycaemic Index (GI)* is a scientific test that measures how long your body takes to convert carbohydrate from the time that you put food into your mouth, to the time that the glucose is stored in your cells. Foods that quickly turn from carbs to glucose (high-GI foods) cause a sharp rise or *spike* in blood sugars and a rapid insulin response. Your blood sugars fall again after the insulin has stored the glucose in your cells, leading to a slump in your energy levels (see Figure 4-1). Foods that slowly convert their carbs into glucose (low- or moderate-GI foods) cause a more gentle production of insulin and provide long-lasting energy.

The nutritionists also found that the carbohydrate foods that turn to glucose in your cells quickly also trigger hunger more quickly, whereas the slow carbs are more satisfying and result in less hunger.

The Glycaemic Index (GI) is an important scientific reference to gauge your body's response to the carbohydrates you consume. Based on the effect that carbs have on your blood sugar, nutritionists classify foods with the Index, and each food is categorised as low-or high-GI.

Stable blood sugars are one of the main factors that make a low-glycaemic diet so helpful in weight control, because stable blood sugars and sustained energy are linked to fewer food cravings.

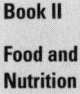

Book II

Food and Nutrition

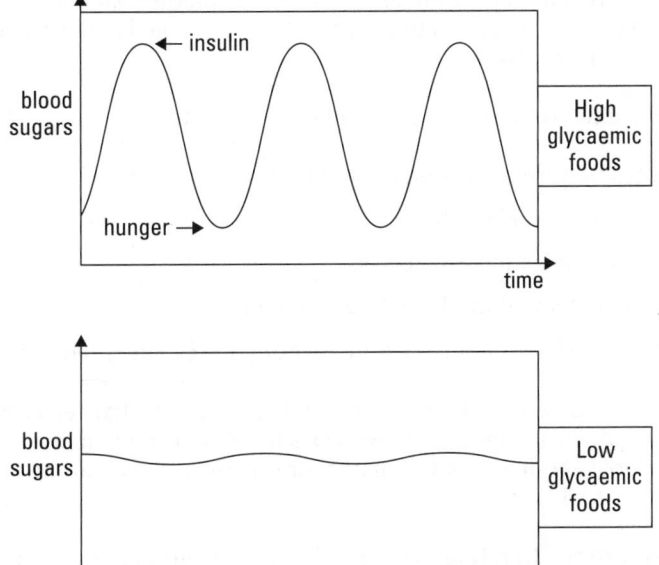

Figure 4-1: A comparison of low- and high-GI food on blood sugar.

The Glycaemic Index is a great foundation for understanding the Glycaemic Load, but GI has flaws that you need to be aware of.

All those GI values can be downright confusing; we've seen people get mixed up about whether the GI means calories, amounts of sugar or even fat. Like counting calories, working out the GI of your meal is impractical and boring. The Glycaemic Index tests the amount of food needed to provide the body with 50 grams of useable carbohydrate, which may be much more or much less than you would ever eat in one sitting. Trying to weigh the ingredients of your meal to get the 50 grams of carbohydrate can give a misleading and confusing result.

Using the Glycaemic Load (GL) to help you to eat healthily is much more sensible and much easier. You don't have to count GLs (unless you really want to) – GL deals with the food on your plate rather than using complex weights and references. The food lists, shopping guide, eating-out guide, and of course the recipes in this book save all the confusion and effort. Eat regularly, take some activity every day, follow our eating plan, and you're living the GL life already!

Welcome to the Glycaemic Load story: real portions, real food

The Glycaemic Load (GL) is derived from a mathematical equation developed by Professor Walter Willet, Chairman of the Department of Nutrition at Harvard Medical School. GL is based on the Glycaemic Index (GI) but also factors in the carb content of an *average portion size*. In other words, GL translates GI into real food portion sizes making the method simpler and more applicable to the way you actually eat. The Glycaemic Load is the final part of the carbohydrate jigsaw.

GL is more effective than GI in a number of ways. GL:

- ✔ Relates to normal portions of food.
- ✔ Means more food choices.
- ✔ Doesn't restrict healthy foods.
- ✔ Means that you don't have to weigh food.
- ✔ Gives the whole picture of how carbohydrates affect blood sugars.

The GL gives you an accurate and sensible picture of what really happens when you eat carbs. Here's how we work it out, but remember, you don't have to worry about any of the maths, or do any of the counting yourself. We've done it all for you.

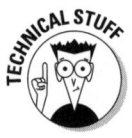

- ✔ First take the GI rating of the food. The website www.glycaemicindex.com gives you all the latest GI-rated foods and their carbohydrate concentration.
- ✔ Divide that number by 100. For example, carrots have a high GI of between 75 and 85, depending on how old the carrots are and how long you cook them for (75 divided by 100 = 0.75).
- ✔ Multiply that number by the actual carbs in an average portion. (100 grams of carrots contains around 7 grams of carbs. $0.75 \times 7 =$ GL of 5.25.)
- ✔ 100 grams of carrots is a normal portion, but to get 50 grams of those crucial useable carbs from carrots for GI testing you need about 750 grams or 1½ pounds of carrots, which might be normal if you're a donkey, but is probably a bit on the heavy side for likes of us humans.

The GL ratings classification is:

✔ Low GL = 10 or less

✔ Moderate GL = 11–19

✔ High GL = 20 or more

The bottom line when it comes to GL and carrots (and loads of other foods for that matter) is that a normal portion of carrots with a GL of 5.25 is low and means that we can eat carrots with confidence as a good, nutritious, healthy food. Now isn't that a more sensible approach than GI?

Medical Benefits of the GL Diet

Adopting a low-GL diet is not just a great eating plan to control your weight. GL focuses on carbohydrate management, but it also embraces all the other aspects of a healthy diet and lifestyle – the GL Diet is much more than simply a weight-loss tool.

Looking at GL and diabetes

Diabetes mellitus, commonly known simply as diabetes, is a condition in which the amount of glucose in your blood is too high or too low because your body can't use glucose properly. Glucose is your body's fuel and you top it up from the food you eat. Insulin is the hormone produced in the pancreas that keeps glucose under control and helps it get to the cells that need the fuel. Insulin works a bit like the thermostat on your central heating system to keep a constant temperature. People with diabetes have problems either producing or using insulin, so they're in danger of having too much or too little glucose in their blood.

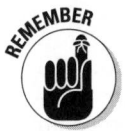

Glucose comes from the digestion of carbohydrate foods, such as bread, rice, potatoes and cereals, and from sugar and sweet foods, as well as from your liver where you make glucose.

Choosing a low-GL diet makes sense for people with diabetes because low-GL foods release sugar into the bloodstream slowly, which in turn helps to control the release of insulin.

Both the European Association for the Study of Diabetes and Diabetes UK, the leading UK charity for people with diabetes, recommend a low-glycaemic, high-fibre diet as a means of maintaining good control of blood sugars and for helping to maintain a healthy weight.

A low-GL diet as part of a healthy lifestyle can help to control your diabetes and reduces your risk of long-term diabetes-related complications.

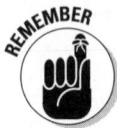

Even small changes in your diet can make a big difference! Two large scientific reviews show that a low-glycaemic diet has a positive effect on blood sugar control in people who already have diabetes, and that swapping just one high-glycaemic food for a low-glycaemic alternative can also have a beneficial effect.

Check out *Diabetes For Dummies* by Dr Sarah Jarvis and Alan L. Rubin (Wiley) if you want to find out more about living with diabetes.

Low GL and high blood pressure

High blood pressure is also known as the silent killer because the condition often goes undetected. *Blood pressure* is the force exerted by blood on the walls of your arteries when your heart beats.

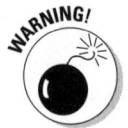

Although high blood pressure can cause headaches, dizziness, and problems with vision, the majority of people with high blood pressure suffer no symptoms at all. However, high blood pressure causes heart attacks, strokes and kidney damage, so have your blood pressure checked by your GP or practice nurse every couple of years or so.

A low-GL diet is unlikely to directly lower blood pressure that is already high. However, people who are overweight and have high blood pressure can expect to see a significant improvement in their blood pressure when they lose as little as five per cent of their body weight.

Reducing the risk of heart disease with low-GL

Coronary heart disease (CHD) occurs when your arteries become narrowed by *atherosclerosis*, a build-up of fatty materials within the walls of your arteries. Atherosclerosis causes a restriction in the supply of blood and oxygen to your heart, particularly when you exert yourself and increase the demands of your heart muscle. Your blood also becomes more prone to clotting.

Atherosclerosis can block the delivery of nutrients to the artery walls, causing them to lose their elasticity. This condition may lead to high blood pressure, which also increases the risk of coronary heart disease.

The main symptom of coronary heart disease is *angina*, caused by insufficient oxygen reaching your heart muscle because of a reduction in blood flow. Angina is a feeling of heaviness, tightness or pain in the middle of your chest that may affect your arms, neck, jaw, face, back or abdomen.

Unfortunately, for many people, the first indication that they have CHD is the on-set of a heart attack. A heart attack happens when the blood supply to a part of the heart muscle is interrupted or stops, usually because of a blood clot in the coronary artery.

Whatever the reason, a low-GL diet has an important role to play in the prevention of heart disease. The GL Diet is an effective measure against heart disease when integrated into a healthy lifestyle:

Book II

Food and Nutrition

- ✔ Be active – 30 minutes a day makes all the difference.

- ✔ Be smoke free. From the moment you stop smoking your risk of a heart attack is reduced, and after one smoke-free year the risk is halved.

- ✔ Keep your alcohol consumption within safe limits. Binge drinking increases your risk of heart attack.

- ✔ Maintain a healthy weight – following the GL Diet and staying active helps take care of that!

Sometimes it's hard to be a woman: Female health and the GL diet

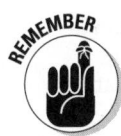

The GL Diet can really help if you suffer from symptoms induced by hormonal change such as *pre-menstrual syndrome* and *polycystic ovary syndrome*. However, don't expect overnight results. From our experience, women usually feel improvements in their symptoms up to three months after a change in their diet. So, stick to the GL Diet and monitor the reduction of your symptoms.

Pre-menstrual syndrome (PMS)

Pre-menstrual syndrome (PMS) is the name given to the disruptive physiological symptoms that appear regularly before a period, but improve when bleeding begins. PMS is a serious medical condition that affects one in three women. PMS is often worse at either end of your reproductive life: around puberty and before the menopause. PMS can be more of a problem after childbirth, during your 30s and 40s, and during times of stress.

More than 150 symptoms are associated with PMS. A woman's individual symptoms can vary from month to month and can appear up to two weeks before a period.

The most common symptoms include:

- ✔ Depression and agitation
- ✔ Breast tenderness
- ✔ Fluid retention and bloating
- ✔ Irritability and mood swings
- ✔ Headaches
- ✔ Skin and hair changes

Polycystic ovary syndrome (PCOS)

Polycystic ovary syndrome (PCOS) affects up to ten per cent of women, although many don't realise that they're suffering from the condition.

Typical symptoms include:

- ✔ Pain from cysts on the ovaries
- ✔ Infertility
- ✔ High blood pressure
- ✔ Acne
- ✔ Central obesity (putting on weight around your middle)
- ✔ Baldness or, conversely, excessive body hair
- ✔ Irregular periods

Scientists don't know the cause of PCOS. However, new research suggests that PCOS may be linked to raised levels of insulin, which stimulate the ovaries to produce too much testosterone. Your body becomes resistant to the effects of insulin, so your pancreas produces higher and higher levels of insulin to get the same effect. Insulin is produced in response to glucose in the blood from food. Peaks of blood sugar from a high-GL diet cause insulin to work even harder in someone with PCOS. Many dieticians working with patients suffering from PCOS recommend a low-GL diet to help control this double-whammy insulin effect.

For more information and advice on PCOS, head to www.verity-pcos.org. uk. See your GP for the many different treatments available for PCOS.

The menopause

The *menopause* is the time when a woman's fertility winds down. The menopause doesn't need to mean new restrictions or physical decline; many women find that the menopause opens new opportunities to them and is a very positive time of their life. Menopause starts to occur in most women around their 50th year, although this can vary. Some women face the menopause much earlier or later than this.

As you go through the menopause, your ovaries produce less of the hormone oestrogen. This reduction triggers the brain to release other hormones in an attempt to make the ovaries work harder. The number and quality of eggs released – and thus fertility – decreases.

Symptoms such as hot flushes, sweats, muscle and bone pains, irritability and poor concentration are all linked to these hormonal surges.

The GL Diet can be beneficial to menopausal women in a number of ways:

- Menopausal symptoms are hormone related, and the GL Diet improves the control of the hormone insulin.
- Stable blood sugars improve poor concentration and irritability.
- Many menopausal women find that they gradually gain weight. The GL Diet is effective at helping to control weight.
- The menopause is a time when a women's risk of heart disease increases, and the GL Diet protects against heart disease.

Book II

Food and Nutrition

Hey, wake up at the back!

Most people experience lapses in concentration when you lose your trail of thought or drift off into your imagination for a few brief moments. Don't worry – that is quite normal! Often, people can really struggle to stay awake, let alone concentrate, at specific times of the day, typically mid-morning and mid-afternoon, and this can be a problem when you're at work or school.

Your brain uses glucose in preference to the other organs in the body that need glucose – in short, if the brain doesn't get fuel then everything else slows down, and that's when you get sleepy.

Studies in the UK show that children who eat a breakfast cereal in the morning perform better and are better able to concentrate. Choosing a low-GL breakfast such as porridge or an oat-based cereal, and eating low-GL meals and snacks throughout the day have a similar effect in contributing to this improved performance.

Eating the low-GL way means that you give your body a steady drip-feed of energy so that you can keep going for longer.

Reasons for Eating the Low-GL Way

The GL Diet is far more than a weight-loss plan. The GL Diet can be part of a healthier, happier lifestyle.

Stabilise your blood sugars

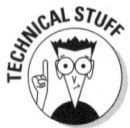

When you eat high-glycaemic foods you experience a rapid increase or a *spike* in glucose (blood sugar). This rise prompts your body to produce *insulin* (a powerful hormone). Insulin flushes the glucose from your bloodstream into your liver and muscles, which store the glucose for later use as energy.

If you constantly eat foods that produce glucose, then you have a continual oversupply in your blood. When your liver and muscles can't store any more, they send the glucose to your fat cells – which expand rapidly! You need to expend energy to use up the stored glucose, but, let's face it, the marathon runners amongst us are in the minority.

Following the glucose spike after eating high-glycaemic foods comes the inevitable rapid fall in blood sugars, which prompts you to redress the balance by eating even more high-glycaemic foods. The cycle is vicious.

Eating low-GL foods means that your blood sugars remain stable because low-GL foods release a steady stream of glucose into the blood rather than a short, sharp glucose rush that you get when you eat high-GL foods. A steady drip-feed of glucose means stable blood sugars and fewer spikes and falls.

Get a handle on your food cravings

Most people feel an overwhelming need to eat in the middle of the morning or the afternoon. All too often, the only food that can satisfy your craving is something sweet or salty and loaded with fat – in other words, high-GL foods. The fall that follows the spike in blood sugars after you've eaten high-GL foods is the point when food cravings occur most often. Eating more high-glycaemic foods starts the blood sugar roller coaster all over again.

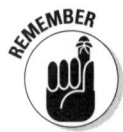

Choosing low-GL foods at meal and snack times means that the blood sugar roller coaster stops in its tracks. When you stop the dramatic rise and fall of your blood sugar levels, your cravings for sweet or fatty foods stop, too. Of course, you'll probably fancy some chocolate or your favourite sweet treat occasionally, and you can still enjoy those foods, some of the time. Eating the GL-way puts you back in control of *when* you choose to indulge.

Control your weight

You don't need to be a mathematician, or even a dietician, to work out that if you eat fewer high-calorie, high-fat, high-sugar foods, your overall calorie or energy intake reduces. Cutting down on these types of foods is the fundamental requirement for weight loss.

You can reduce the amount of sugar in your blood by eating the low-GL way, and you can increase your activity levels to burn fat – the most effective way to lose weight and maintain that loss forever.

Level your moods

When you eat high-GL foods and your blood sugars go up and down like a yo-yo, so too does your mood. Your brain is your control centre – if your brain is starved of energy, the rest of your body stops working. If one minute your brain has excess energy from high-GL food, and the next minute you have an energy slump, you and everyone around you will feel the effect – your bad mood!

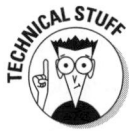

When you're low on fuel you get tetchy, irritable and short-tempered. Many studies show that your *cognitive performance* (how you think and concentrate) is adversely affected when fuel supplies are low (when you're hungry). Ensuring that your brain has a steady and consistent supply of energy is vital.

Following the low-GL plan is all about eating more foods that drip-feed energy, keeping your blood sugars stable, keeping you level-headed, and keeping everyone around you happy.

Balance your hormones

Regularly eating high-glycaemic foods means that the hormone *insulin* (your system for controlling blood sugars) is working in overdrive. Making hormones and putting them to work is no mean feat and takes a lot of energy and resources. Your *endocrine system* (the system that controls your hormones) is involved in just about every aspect of your wellbeing. Your emotional, physical, mental, and even your sexual well-being relies on hormones to stimulate, mediate, and control chemical reactions that keep everything in harmony.

If your insulin is working in overdrive, some of your other hormones are likely to suffer as a result. Eating low-GL foods really can help to balance your hormones because their slow release into your system stabilises your blood sugars and enables insulin to work normally.

No food is banned

Imagine a healthy eating plan where nothing, let alone an entire food group, is banned. How refreshing! Eating healthily means getting a better *balance* of foods in your diet to minimise the risk of disease, and does not put a complete ban on certain foods. A great reason to eat the low-GL way is that you don't have to ban anything.

If you know that a food is high-GL, you can make an informed choice about how you want to handle it. With a high-GL food you can:

- ✔ Eat a little less of it.

- ✔ Eat it a little less often.

- ✔ Mix and match it with other low-GL foods to reduce the overall glycaemic effect.

- ✔ Cook it in a way that reduces its glycaemic effect.

Getting You Started with Some Tasty Delights

Enjoy this sample selection of recipes to get you started. You can see a wider range of recipes in *The GL Diet For Dummies*.

Starting your day with a low-GL breakfast

People who regularly eat breakfast benefit from having more control over their blood-sugar levels. As a result, breakfasters are better prepared for warding off hunger pangs and are less prone to snacking on high-fat, high-sugar foods such as chocolate bars, crisps, cakes and biscuits. Breakfast-eaters also tend to concentrate for longer, which can boost their performance, and even suffer less irritability and stress when compared to those people who skip breakfast.

Scrambled Eggs and Smoky Bacon

Nothing is quite as satisfying as bacon and eggs with toast. However, you can reduce the fat content by using only the egg whites instead of whole eggs.

Preparation and cooking time: *15 minutes*

Serves: *2*

6 rashers (strips) smoked lean bacon

4 large free-range eggs

20 grams / 0.5 ounce / 2 teaspoons butter

2 pieces low-GL bread

Seasoning, to taste

1 Heat your grill to medium-hot temperature, and cook the bacon to your preference (some people like crispy bacon, others a little-less well done!). Break the eggs into a bowl, add seasoning, and whisk together well. When the bacon's almost done, place a small saucepan (skillet) over a medium heat, add the butter, and as soon as it's melted, add the eggs. Whilst the eggs are cooking, stir continuously with a wooden spoon.

2 Toast the bread. When your eggs are just done, turn off the heat, then lightly butter the toast, place the eggs on top, add the bacon, and serve.

Tip: *You can exchange the bacon for smoked salmon, and grill 2 large, flat mushrooms instead of using toast – mix 1 clove of crushed garlic with 2 tablespoons of butter and spread over the mushrooms. Place under a hot grill (broiler) for a couple of minutes, and when ready, top with the scrambled egg.*

Nutrient analysis per serving: Calories 395; Protein 30g; Carbohydrate 12g; Fat 25g; Saturated fat 11g; Fibre 2g; Sodium 1783mg.

Book II

Food and Nutrition

Fast Muesli

You can use any combination of low-GL fresh or dried fruits and your favourite seeds or nuts in this delicious breakfast.

Preparation and cooking time: *7 minutes*

Serves: *1*

1 handful / ¼ cup old-fashioned porridge oats

1 tablespoon raw sunflower seeds

1 tablespoon linseeds / flaxseeds

1 tablespoon crushed walnuts

½ teaspoon ground cinnamon

2 tablespoons dried apricots, chopped

150 grams / 5.5 ounces / ⅔ cup plain bio or Greek-style yoghurt

1 teaspoon honey (preferably runny)

1 Put the oats, seeds, walnuts and ground cinnamon into a non-oiled frying-pan and place over a medium-high heat. Keep stirring the ingredients in the pan for about 3 minutes – don't let them burn!

2 Once ready, transfer the dry-roasted oats and seeds into a bowl, scatter with the apricots, dollop on the yoghurt, drizzle over the honey, and enjoy.

Tip: *Add unsweetened desiccated coconut to the toasting mix for that tropical feel.*

Nutrient analysis per serving: Calories 400; Protein 15g; Carbohydrate 35g; Fat 20g; Saturated fat 3g; Fibre 4g; Sodium 130mg.

Breakfast Smoothie

You can use any low-GL fresh fruit you like in this quick recipe. As an alternative, you can use frozen summer berries, which gives you a colder, thicker smoothie. Allow the frozen fruit to soften slightly before whizzing.

Preparation time: *5 minutes*

Serves: *1*

1 small firm banana

1 nectarine

Handful (quarter of a cup) of blueberries

150 grams / 5.5 ounces / two-thirds of a cup plain bio or Greek-style yoghurt

125 millilitres / 4.5 fluid ounces / half a cup water

1 teaspoon honey (preferably runny)

1 teaspoon grated fresh ginger

Put all the ingredients into a blender and whizz until smooth and creamy. Drink immediately.

Tip: *For a little more protein you can add a measure of vanilla soya or whey protein, which are available from health-food shops (simply follow the directions on the pack for how much to use).*

Nutrient analysis per serving: *Calories 295; Protein 11g; Carbohydrate 60g; Fat 2g; Saturated fat 1g; Fibre 4g; Sodium 130mg.*

Breakfast to Go

This breakfast suggestion really is a case of grab and go, so you have no excuse for missing breakfast if you're in a rush. Oatcakes come in coarse- and fine-texture varieties, so try both to see which you prefer.

Preparation time: *2 minutes*

Serves: *1*

2 oatcakes

1 slice of cheese

1 apple

Handful of grapes

Chuck everything into bag and eat as you go. If you have time, break the slice of cheese in half, pop the cheese on the oatcakes, and slice the apple on top.

Tip: Wrap the oatcakes separately in cling-film to keep them from getting soggy.

Nutrient analysis per serving: Calories 316; Protein 9g; Carbohydrate 46g; Fat 11g; Saturated fat 5g; Fibre 3g; Sodium 460mg.

Doing lunch: A selection of low-GL lunches

Vitality Salad

Avocado is a great extra ingredient in this salad, but it does quickly discolour. Add diced avocado just before eating the salad, or keep the avocado pieces in a separate pot and squeeze some fresh lemon juice over them, which helps prevent the browning process.

Preparation time: *10 minutes*

Serves: *1*

Half a head of your favourite crunchy lettuce

1 generous handful basil leaves, or your favourite herb (about ¼ cup)

1 generous handful fresh spinach or watercress (about 1 cup)

1 carrot, coarsely grated

1 tablespoon raw sunflower seeds, lightly toasted (dry-fried in a hot pan)

1 tablespoon pine nuts, lightly toasted (dry-fried with the sunflower seeds)

40 grams / 1.5 ounces reduced-fat mature cheddar, coarsely grated (about 3 slices)

1 handful sprouted seeds (available from loads of stores in the chilled section, or sprout your own)

Your choice of dressing, to serve

Shred the lettuce, herbs and spinach, and mix with all the other ingredients. Pour your favourite dressing over the salad, and toss just before eating.

Tip: To make a fantastic dressing, dilute 1 tablespoon hummus with 2 tablespoons extra-virgin olive oil and 1 tablespoon balsamic vinegar, and shake thoroughly. Voilà – a thick creamy dressing! Alternatively, simply dress with a mixture of fresh lemon juice, balsamic vinegar and extra-virgin olive oil; or use an extra-virgin olive oil that has been infused with herbs or spices.

Variation: You can add other greens or vegetables to this fabulous salad, such as broccoli, blanched beans, or rocket.

Nutrient analysis (without dressing) per serving: Calories 380; Protein 21g; Carbohydrate 12g; Fat 28g; Saturated fat 6g; Fibre 5g; Sodium 360mg.

Adulterated Hummus with Low-GL Bread and Salad

Hummus is one of our favourite dips. Eating hummus is a great way for people who don't like the texture of whole chickpeas to get a good healthy dose of beany nutrition.

Preparation time: *5 minutes*

Serves: *1*

Grab a small pot of hummus (home-made or shop bought), and mix in any or all of the following ingredients:

Chopped black olives

Chopped red pepper

Chopped spring onions

Toasted pine nuts

Prepare your favourite salad and pop it into your lunch box together with your pot of hummus and a slice of low-GL bread or a couple of oatcakes. Dress the salad just before you eat it.

Nutrient analysis per serving: *Calories 350; Protein 12g; Carbohydrate 17g; Fat 22g; Saturated fat 0.5g; Fibre 4g, Sodium 900mg.*

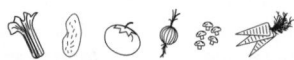

Chicken and Vegetable Crumble

This crumble is perfect for those chilly days when you really want to eat for comfort. The oats in the crumble topping give a lovely nutty flavour.

Preparation time: *10 minutes*

Cooking time: *20 minutes*

Serves: *4*

2 tablespoons extra-virgin olive oil

400 grams / 15 ounces chickpeas (usually 1 tin), drained and rinsed

3 large skinless, boneless chicken breasts, cut into chunks

2 garlic cloves, crushed or grated

1 pinch medium-hot chilli powder

2 courgettes, washed and julienned (chopped into thin strips)

1 carrot, washed and julienned

400 grams / 14 ounces (usually 1 tin) chopped tomatoes

75 grams / 2.5 ounces / ¼ cup mature reduced-fat cheddar cheese, grated finely

75 grams / 2.5 ounces / ¼ cup porridge oats

1 teaspoon chilli powder

Seasoning, to taste

1 Heat the olive oil in a pan over a medium heat. Cook the chicken pieces until browned (about 10–12 minutes), turning occasionally.

2 Add the chickpeas, garlic and chilli, and stir for a minute or two. Add the courgette and carrot, and stir for 30 seconds, then add the tomatoes and stir together. Cook for another few minutes until the chicken pieces are no longer pink in the middle and are properly cooked through. Season generously. Transfer to an oven-proof dish.

3 Mix the cheddar, oats and chilli powder in a bowl and rub together with your fingers to make a savoury crumble. Sprinkle the crumble evenly over the chicken and vegetables mixture, and cook under a hot grill (broiler) until the top is golden.

Tip: Serve on a bed of spinach, which will wilt deliciously under the hot bake.

Nutrient analysis per serving: Calories 425; Protein 41g; Carbohydrate 32g; Fat 16g; Saturated fat 4g; Fibre 6 g; Sodium 270mg.

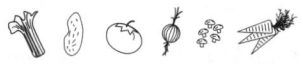

Mediterranean Bacon Pasta

This dish conjures up ideas of a sun-drenched Mediterranean shoreline, and is perfect for a relaxing summer lunch.

Preparation time: 10 minutes

Cooking time: 10 minutes

Serves: 4

200 grams / 7 ounces dried pasta (penne or fusilli)

2 tablespoon extra-virgin olive oil

6 rashers of lean bacon, cut into cubes

1 onion, diced

2 cloves garlic, crushed or grated

400 grams / 15 ounces (usually 1 can) chickpeas, drained and rinsed

60 grams / 2 ounces sundried tomatoes, dried, or in oil, drained chopped roughly

60 grams / 2 ounces pitted black olives, chopped roughly

Large handful fresh basil, chopped roughly

Seasoning, to taste

Parmesan, grated for serving

1 Cook the pasta as per the instructions on the packet until al dente (offers a little resistance when you bite it), drain, and rinse with cold water to stop the cooking process.

2 Heat the olive oil in a frying pan, add the bacon and cook for about 2 minutes. Then add the onion and the garlic to the pan. Cook until the bacon starts to brown, stirring occasionally. Stir in the chickpeas, the sundried tomatoes and the olives.

3 Add the pasta, and stir through to warm. Gently mix in the basil, and serve on warmed plates with plenty of black pepper and parmesan, to taste.

Nutrient analysis per serving: Calories 474; Protein 24g; Carbohydrate 57g; Fat 18g; Saturated fat 4g; Fibre 7g; Sodium 1136mg.

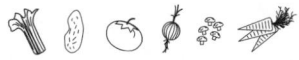

Delectable dinners: Low-GL suppers

Salmon and Sweet Potato Fishcakes

These fishcakes are great to make in advance or in batches to freeze.

Preparation time: *30 minutes*

Cooking time: *5 minutes*

Serves: *4*

1 large free-range egg

400 grams / 14 ounces sweet potato, cut into chunks

400 grams / 14 ounces salmon (tinned or fresh)

Zest of 1 lemon

1 teaspoon wholegrain mustard

2 tablespoons fresh coriander, finely chopped

Freshly ground black pepper

Extra-virgin olive oil, for frying

Mixed salad or steamed low-GL vegetables, to serve

1 Hard boil the egg in cold water in a small pan. Bring to the boil and simmer for 12 minutes. Immerse in cold water, peel, and chop finely.

2 Meanwhile cook sweet potato chunks for 10–12 minutes until tender, drain well, and mash.

3 If you're using fresh salmon, poach the steak or fillet in a frying pan with just enough water to cook it, then remove from the water and flake the salmon into the sweet potato mash. If you are using tinned salmon, then drain, remove any large bones, and crumble into the sweet potato mash.

4 Mix all the ingredients together well in a large bowl, and form into 4 large fishcakes, or 8 smaller ones. Fry over a medium heat in olive oil, and serve immediately with fresh salad or steamed low-GL vegetables.

Nutrient analysis per serving: Calories 289; Protein 21g; Carbohydrate 21g; Fat 14g; Saturated fat 3g; Fibre 2.5g; Sodium 192mg.

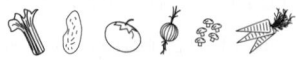

Tuna Pasta Bake

Tuna is a very popular fish that most people enjoy eating. The tuna works well here with a little spice from the horseradish or chilli.

Preparation time: *20 minutes*

Cooking time: *20 minutes*

Serves: *4*

160 grams / 3.5 ounces / 1 cup dried fusilli pasta

2 tablespoons extra-virgin olive oil2 large onions, sliced

2 x 200 grams / 7 ounce cans tuna in brine, drained

3–6 cloves garlic, crushed or grated (you can use less or more to your taste)

2 teaspoons wholegrain mustard

1 teaspoon horseradish or ½ teaspoon hot chilli flakes

Freshly ground black pepper, to taste

400 grams / 14 ounces (usually 1 can) haricot beans, drained and rinsed

400 grams / 14 ounces (usually 1 can) chopped tomatoes 3 tablespoons half-fat soft cheese or low-fat crème fraîche or natural Greek-style yoghurt

1 low-fat mozzarella block (approximately 150 grams / 3 ounces), cut into cubes

Large handful fresh basil, roughly chopped

50 grams / 1.5 ounces / ¼ cup reduced-fat mature cheddar, grated finely

Book II

Food and Nutrition

1 Preheat the oven to 200°C / 400°F / Gas Mark 6. Cook the pasta as per the instructions on the packet, cook until *al dente* (firm to the bite), drain immediately, and running under cold water to stop the cooking process. Set aside.

2 In a large frying pan, heat the olive oil and soften the onions. Add the tuna and the garlic, then stir in the mustard, the horseradish or chilli, and season generously with black pepper. Stir in the haricot beans and allow to cook for a few minutes. Pour over the chopped tomatoes and stir in the soft cheese (or crème fraîche or yoghurt). Remove from the heat, and stir in the cooked pasta, mozzarella and basil. Transfer the mixture into a shallow baking dish, sprinkle with the grated cheddar, and grind over some more pepper.

3 Bake in the oven for 15–20 minutes, until the cheese is golden brown on top. Serve with crisp salad.

Variation: *You can use sausages (with high lean-meat content) or bacon as a substitute for tuna.*

Nutrient analysis per serving: *Calories 548; Protein 47g; Carbohydrate 54g; Fat 17g; Saturated fat 7g; Fibre 8g; Sodium 870 mg.*

Stir-Fry with Chicken

Stir-fry makes for a super quick and healthy meal. If you prefer, use prawns or fish instead of the chicken.

Preparation time: *10 minutes*

Cooking time: *10 minutes*

Serves: *4*

4 chicken breasts, skinned, boned, and cut into strips

1 tablespoon soy sauce

250 grams / 9 ounces dried noodles – mung bean noodles (these are the lowest GL of the 3), buckwheat noodles or rice noodles

2 tablespoons avocado oil, coconut oil or vegetable oil (these oils have a higher 'smoke point' and are better for high-temperature frying)

2 spring onions (scallions), finely sliced

Approximately 600 grams / 20 ounces / 2 to 3 cups fresh vegetables cut into strips (any

combination of carrots, courgettes, baby sweetcorn, mushrooms, bean sprouts, sugar-snap peas, mange tout, sweet peppers, broccoli, cabbage)

2 garlic cloves, crushed or grated

2 tablespoon hoisin sauce

120 millilitres / 1/2 cup stock – chicken or vegetable

1 teaspoon toasted-sesame oil

2 tablespoons toasted sesame seeds (fry in a dry pan until golden)

1 Place the chicken strips in a bowl, sprinkle with the soy sauce, and toss well, making sure that the strips are coated.

2 Put a pan of water on for the noodles and cook as per the instructions on the packet until *al dente* – you want the noodles to be ready at the same time as the stir-fry, not before, so adjust your timing to the cooking instructions.

3 Heat a wok or large frying pan on a high heat, and swirl in the avocado, coconut or vegetable oil. Add the chicken immediately and stir-fry for 3 minutes. Carefully remove from the pan, without taking too much of the oil with it, and keep warm.

4 Stir-fry the onion, vegetables (but not the bean sprouts) and garlic (add the garlic last so you don't burn it). Stir-fry for about 2 minutes – until the veg is crisp yet tender. Pour in the stock, then return the chicken to the wok and stir in the hoisin sauce. If you're using bean sprouts, add them at this stage. Return to simmer and stir for about 3 minutes until the chicken is cooked.

5 Drain the noodles, and toss them in the sesame oil and sesame seeds. Serve immediately in warm bowls.

Variation: To spice up this dish, add a pinch of chilli and Chinese 5-spice or stir in a teaspoon of horseradish for some warm heat. You can use spaghetti for noodles; use Worcestershire sauce in place of soy sauce; and use BBQ or brown sauce in place of hoisin sauce.

Nutrient analysis per serving: Calories 533; Protein 42g; Carbohydrate 57g; Fat 16g; Saturated fat 3g; Fibre 10g; Sodium 755mg.

Bite-Size TV Dinner Platter

Perfect for a night in or when you need nibbles for guests (simply multiply the ingredients). Make a selection of the ideas below, forget the cutlery, and dive straight in!

Total preparation time: *25 minutes*

Total cooking time: *6 minutes*

Serves: *2*

Book II

Food and Nutrition

Spicy avocado spread

1 slice rye bread, cut into quarters

1 small avocado

4 generous dashes Tabasco sauce

1 teaspoon fresh lemon juice

1 teaspoon freshly ground black pepper

Chopped fresh corriander, to serve (optional)

Mash all the ingredients together in a bowl, then spread on the quarters of bread and decorate with coriander.

Hummus and toppings

1 slice rye bread, cut into quarters

1 tablespoon pine nuts, toasted until golden

2 tablespoons hummus

1 teaspoon paprika

1 tablespoon fresh coriander (cilantro), chopped

Spread the hummus equally between the pieces of bread, then sprinkle with the paprika, pine nuts and coriander.

Nutrient analysis per serving: Calories 511; Protein 23g; Carbohydrate 32g; Fat 33g; Saturated fat 5g; Fibre 6g; Sodium 1428mg.

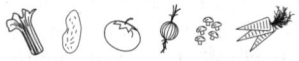

Just desserts: Virtuous low-GL puddings

Dessert is the perfect end to a meal – especially if, like us, you have a bit of a sweet tooth that just has to be satisfied. Unfortunately, delicious puddings are often packed full of sugar and refined flour. We've wracked our brains, drawn upon our culinary skills, and come up some delightful desserts, which fit perfectly into the GL way of eating.

Punchy Fresh Fruit Salad

As well as a scrumptious dessert, this fruit salad makes a great breakfast (without the Cointreau!). Eat the salad with yoghurt or with muesli – or both.

Don't make the fruit salad too far in advance because, even protected by the citrus juice in a covered bowl, the apple and pears can still become a little brown.

Preparation time: *20 minutes*

Serves: *4*

2 nectarines, stoned and cut into chunks

2 pears, cored and cut into chunks

1 punnet (pint) of fresh strawberries, stalks removed and cut in half

1 punnet (pint) fresh blueberries, stalks removed

1 handful seedless grapes

1 apple, cored and cut into chunks

2 oranges, zest and juice

1 lemon, zest and juice

1 small handful fresh mint leaves, taken off the stem and washed

1 tablespoon Cointreau

400 grams / 4 dessertspoons reduced-fat crème fraîche

1 Place the prepared fruit in a large glass serving bowl.

2 Pour the orange and lemon juice over the fruit, and add most of the zest (leaving 1 teaspoon for the cream), the mint leaves and the Cointreau. Stir well, ensuring that all the fruit is covered with the juice, then cover the bowl with cling film.

3 Mix the remaining lemon and orange zest into the crème fraîche and serve it with large spoonfuls of the boozy fruit.

Variation: *Experiment with low-GL fruit combinations; or squeeze over the juice and seeds of a pomegranate instead of one of the oranges.*

Nutrient analysis per serving: *Calories 168; Protein 4g; Carbohydrate 27g; Fat 4.5g; Saturated fat 3g; Fibre 5g; Sodium 20mg.*

Blackberry and Apple Crumble

The perfect pudding for a cold night. This crumble topping works well on savoury vege-table bakes too if you simply omit the fructose.

Preparation time: *10 minutes*

Cooking time: *30 minutes*

Serves: *2–3*

300 grams / 10 ounces blackberries /1¼ cups (fresh or frozen)

1 large cooking apple, peeled, cored, and cut into chunks

3 tablespoons cold water

1 tablespoon fructose

For the crumble:

80 grams / 3 ounces / 1/ 2 cup old-fashioned porridge oats

40 grams / 11/ 2 ounces ground almonds

30 grams / 1 ounce walnuts, crushed

40 grams / 11/ 2 ounces / 4 teaspoons butter

2 tablespoons fructose

1 tablespoon low-fat Greek-style yoghurt, low fat crème fraîche or reduced-fat cream, to serve

Book II

Food and Nutrition

1 Preheat the oven to 190°C / 375°F / Gas Mark 5.

2 Place the apple in a saucepan with the water and cook rapidly, being careful not to burn them, for about 3–4 minutes. Stir in the blackberries and 1 tablespoon of fructose, and simmer for another couple of minutes. Transfer the fruit to an ovenproof dish and set aside.

3 In a mixing bowl, blend the oats, ground almonds, crushed walnuts and fructose together. Rub in the butter with your fingertips until you have a nice crumbly texture. Sprinkle the crumble evenly over the fruit, and place in the oven for 30 minutes.

4 Serve with a spoonful of crème fraîche, Greek-style natural yoghurt or reduced-fat cream.

Variation: *You can experiment with other low-GL fruits; and add different nuts to the crumble.*

Nutrient analysis per serving if serves 3 : *Calories 400 ; Protein 7g; Carbohydrate 34 g, Fat 27g; Saturated fat 9g; Fibre 3 g; Sodium 10582mg.*

Smart snacks: Low-GL quick bites and healthy nibbles

Snacks in a Bag

These super-quick ideas are delicious and nutritious and will keep you going until you have time for something more substantial.

Dried Fruit and Nuts

A handful of unsalted nuts and 6 dried and chopped apricots are a nutrient packed snack that will keep you on the go until the next meal. They're easily portable and unlike some snacks, not in the least bit messy to eat. Put them in a pot or a re-sealable plastic bag and take wherever you go – you'll never grab snacks full of refined sugar again!

Tip: Nuts are loaded with protein, minerals like zinc, magnesium and selenium, and anti-oxidants like vitamin E. They contain fat but it's mostly the beneficial monounsaturated kind. They are also low-GL. However, both apricots and nuts are high in calories so keep to a small amount of each. Try to find organic apricots because they are less likely to have added preservatives.

Nutrient analysis per serving: *Calories 261; Protein 9g; Carbohydrate 20g; Fat 16g; Saturated fat 2.5g; Fibre 5g; Sodium 97mg.*

Crudités

Take a bag of crudités with you – carrots, cauliflower, celery, apple, broccoli, peppers, and so on – chopped into slices or batons and sealed in a plastic bag to keep them fresh and crunchy.

Tip: Pop them in the fridge where possible, and don't worry if the apple turns a bit brown, it won't harm you.

Nutrient analysis per serving: *Calories 40; Protein 0g; Carbohydrate 7g; Fat 0g; Saturated fat 0g; Fibre 2g; Sodium 25mg.*

Toasted Seeds

Toasted seeds are a miracle food – throw a handful of your favourite seeds such as sunflower seeds, pumpkin seeds, pine nuts, and so on – into a pan, dry toast them, and let them cool, then throw them into a bag and tie in a knot.

Nutrient analysis per handful: *Calories 165; Protein 5g; Carbohydrate 3g; Fat 15g; Saturated fat 1.5g; Fibre 2 grams, 10 milligrams sodium.*

Sardines on Toast

Sometimes the old recipes are the best! Okay, we know this dish isn't exactly original, but take a trip down memory lane by snacking on this tried-and-tested reliable favourite.

Preparation and cooking time: 7 minutes

Serves: 1

1 tin (100g) sardines in olive oil, drained

1 teaspoon Worcestershire sauce

1 slice low-GL toast

30 grams / 1 ounce / 2 tablespoons reduced-fat mature cheddar, coarsely grated

Book II

Food and Nutrition

1 Preheat the grill (broiler) to very hot.

2 Mash the sardines up in a bowl with the Worcester sauce. Spread the mixture on the toast, top with the cheese, and grill until melted. Grind over some fresh black pepper – delicious!

Nutrient analysis per serving: Calories 360; Protein 36g; Carbohydrate 13g; Fat 19g; Saturated fat 6g; Fibre 1.5g; Sodium 1073mg.

Baked Veggie Skewers

These easy and delicious vegetable skewers are perfect with a couple of slices of scrummy hard cheese such as Manchego (a type of ewe's cheese from Spain) or rounds of soft goat's cheese.

Preparation time: *5 minutes*

Cooking time: *40 minutes*

Serves: *Makes 6 skewers*

2 courgettes, cut into 1-inch chunks

1 aubergine, cut into 1-inch chunks

Half a sweet potato, peeled and cut into ½-inch chunks

2 tablespoons extra-virgin olive oil

1 tablespoon balsamic vinegar

1 garlic clove, crushed or grated

Freshly ground black pepper

1 In a bowl, mix the vegetable chunks with the oil, vinegar and garlic.

2 Thread the vegetables onto small skewers (soak wooden skewers in water first to prevent them from burning), and arrange on a baking tray with plenty of room between each skewer.

3 Pop into a medium oven (350 F /180 C/ Gas mark 4) to cook for about 35 to 40 minutes until soft.

Nutrient analysis per stick: *Calories 56; Protein 1g; Carbohydrate 4g; Fat 4g; Saturated fat 0.5g; Fibre 1.5g; Sodium 7mg.*

Chapter 5

Incorporating the GL Diet into Your Daily Life

. . . .

. . . .

*M*aking changes to your diet can be a struggle, so the results need to be worthwhile. The GL Diet gives you an eating plan that helps you safely lose and maintain your weight – and boost your overall health at the same time.

This chapter gives you everything you need to get started on a low-GL eating plan, from shopping and cooking to getting the results you want.

Starting Your Low-GL Plan

You've made up your mind to give low-GL eating a go – congratulations. You can look forward to feeling more energised, experiencing fewer food cravings, and achieving a healthy, stable weight. You're raring to go, but where do you start? And how does low-GL eating fit together with other aspects of a healthy diet?

In this chapter we help you find the answers to both of these questions. We take you step by step through the process of making the dietary change towards including low-GL foods in your daily life. We provide you with some examples of low-GL alternative eating in our sample meal plans, and show you how a low-GL diet fits simply and easily alongside other recommendations for healthy eating.

Changing Your Diet the Simple and Successful Way

Changing your established behaviour patterns is never easy, and changing what you eat is no exception.

We've learnt from experience that you need strategies to help you make and maintain dietary changes. The following list is a summary of your action plan for undertaking this change:

- **Establish your goals:** Decide on what you want to change about your diet.

- **Plan your actions:** Settle on what you are going to do to achieve your goals.

- **Overcome the barriers:** Find out how to get around the things that prevent you from changing your diet.

- **Prevent relapse:** Get back on track when you start to waver.

The following sections describe your action plan in more detail, putting you on the path to make eating the low-GL way second nature.

Setting SMART goals

As a first step to changing your current eating plan towards a low-GL diet, you need to decide what changes you want to make and translate these changes into goals that you aim for. Make sure that your goals are *SMART* for maximum effectiveness.

To illustrate what we mean by this term we use goals about fruit and vegetables because they are a vital part of a low-GL way of eating. Make your goals:

- **Specific.** Make your goals clear and not too general. Replace 'Eat more healthily' or 'Eat more fruit and vegetables' with 'Eat five portions of fruit and vegetables a day'.

- **Meaningful.** Make sure that your individual goals have a beneficial effect on your overall diet. For example, having a goal of drinking a carton of fruit juice a day is specific but isn't very meaningful in terms of the overall health benefit. You need five fruit and vegetable portions a day. Juice of any type only counts once (check out the section 'What's a portion?').

- **Acceptable.** You don't have to eat anything you don't like simply because the nutritional content is good for you, or because someone tells you that you ought to eat it. With the low-GL way of eating no food is compulsory and better still, no food is banned. The GL Diet is all about eating normal food, with nothing odd or unpleasant – and no cabbage soup!

✔ **Realistic.** The goals you set for yourself need to stretch you but not so much that you can't achieve them. As a golden rule, avoid setting any goal that begins with the words 'I will never' or 'I will always'. Tell yourself 'I will always have fruit instead of dessert' and you're setting yourself up for failure because you feel as if you're denying yourself. Instead, tell yourself 'I will enjoy a small dessert when I feel I've deserved it and not feel guilty about it'. Be kind to yourself and build some flexibility into your goals. Allow yourself some treats along the way.

✔ **Tailored to you.** We don't know about you, but in our opinion, to have any chance of lasting, a realistic dietary change has to fit properly into your lifestyle, not vice versa. If you don't have time available every day to shop for or prepare fresh fruit and vegetables, an alternative goal is to ensure that you stock up once a week on a combination of fresh fruit and veg, ready-to-use products, and a selection of frozen and canned fruit and vegetables.

Book II

Food and Nutrition

Planning action

Now that you've set your goals, think hard about how you're going to achieve them. For example, to help you achieve the goal of eating five different servings of fruit and vegetables a day, think about fulfilling this target by:

✔ **Changing the *quantity* of the food, or types of food you eat.** You can increase the amount of fruit and veg you eat at a meal. If you usually have one vegetable with your evening meal, add another. If you usually have one piece of fruit in your lunch box, try two. This simple step increases your fruit and veg quota with very little effort.

If you love high-GL foods, such as white varieties of bread, pasta and rice, eat them in smaller portions or simply less often.

✔ **Changing the *frequency* of eating certain foods.** You can increase how often you eat fruit and vegetables. If you don't have fruit or vegetables at every meal, try doing so for a few days and see how easy making this change can be. Have a glass of juice with breakfast, or add some sliced fruit to your cereal. Pop a couple of tomatoes into your lunch box or make sure that you serve a salad with pasta at dinner. Similarly, you can *reduce* the frequency of eating certain foods. If you usually have a chocolate bar every day as a snack, save it for a treat on Fridays. You'll enjoy it all the more.

Keep a food diary for a few days so you can check back to see how you're doing.

✔ **Changing the *types* of foods you eat.** You can change the types of foods you eat within a food group. Don't get stuck using the same fruit and vegetables – try including a wide variety of low-GL choices and you're more likely to reach the goal of eating five portions a day.

Replace high-GL refined white bread, pasta and rice with low-GL wholegrain varieties such as seeded breads, brown basmati rice, bulgur wheat or couscous. If you love potatoes, try new potatoes or sweet potatoes instead (or have a smaller portion).

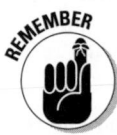

Pulses and beans are wonderful low-GL foods, and can be considered a vegetable towards part of your five-a-day, though multiple portions can only count once (see the section 'What counts towards my five a day?').

Small changes *do* count. Making several small improvements to your diet over time has an amazing ripple effect as the benefits of your efforts accrue and really start to make a difference to your health.

Overcoming barriers to change

Changing your diet isn't just about knowing what you should and shouldn't eat – the healthy choice also has to be an easy choice, otherwise your eating plan becomes difficult to sustain. Think carefully to identify the barriers that may stop you from changing your diet and maintaining healthy eating in the long term.

Your barriers and their possible solutions may include:

✔ **Your lack of time to shop.** If you have dificultly carrying home all the fruit and vegetables your family needs, and your local corner shop doesn't carry much stock, you can set up a supermarket home-delivery service (check out the Web sites of the major supermarkets). Even better, you can register for a local organic fruit and vegetable box scheme, which delivers seasonal produce weekly to your door. Check out 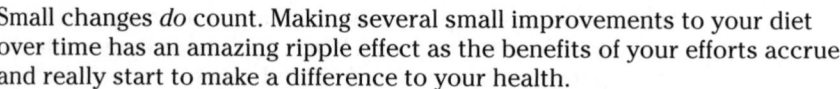www.alotoforganics.co.uk/cats/organic-vegetables.php for a list of vegetable delivery services.

✔ **Your lack of time to cook.** If you're pushed for time during the week, set aside some time to cook in bulk and then freeze the meals. You can simply reheat the meals as you need them. Stock up on convenience items such as quick-cook grains, fresh pasta and sauces, chunky vegetable soups and canned pulses. If you're really rushed, you can improve the GL of a ready meal or shop-bought pizza by serving with an extra portion of canned, frozen or fresh vegetables, or a bag of salad.

✔ **Your lack of cooking skills.** Eating well doesn't necessarily involve following complex recipes. We include some quick and easy recipes in Book II, Chapter 4. Keep a look-out for other quick, low-GL recipes in magazines or on the Internet. If you use good quality fresh ingredients you can often put together a delicious dish with minimal preparation.

✔ **Your lack of money to spend on fresh ingredients.** Buying fruit and vegetables and even meat and fish in season is always cheaper. Look out for special offers and bulk buys that you can freeze or store. Farmer's markets and food co-ops are great places to shop economically. If you have green fingers you can even try growing your own in the garden or on an allotment. (Gardening is great exercise too!)

✔ **Your likes and dislikes.** Why not experiment and try a new food once a week? Try a new vegetable as an accompaniment or in a soup; a new pulse or bean in a salad; or one of the more unusual low-GL grains instead of potatoes or bread. Not every food will be a success but over time you can build up a whole new range of low-GL additions to your diet.

Take the time to explore your own barriers and the options available to you. Lateral thinking and planning can really help you overcome your obstacles to change.

Book II

Food and Nutrition

Seeking support

You're more likely to succeed with your dietary change, as with any other behavioural change, if you get support from friends and family. A low-GL way of eating is naturally healthy and suitable for anyone, so ask the rest of your household or workplace to get on board with the GL Diet.

If you have a colleague at work who's also a low-GL convert, try taking turns to make a packed lunch for the pair of you.

Dealing with relapse

For most people, a normal part of dietary change is to experience an occasional relapse back into old, unhealthy habits, whether for a meal, a day, or a whole week of Christmas parties. The important thing is to accept that your diet won't always be perfect and put the relapse behind you.

Try to work out what may trigger a relapse, to help prevent you going through the whole cycle again. Were you feeling stressed after a bad day at work or bored at home with nothing to do? After you pinpoint your triggers to unhealthy eating habits you can take steps to avoid the triggers in the future. Plan how else you can deal with stress or boredom. Eat regular meals and low-GL snacks so that you avoid getting so hungry that you give in to food cravings. If you know that a particular food shop always tempts you in, avoid walking past it.

Experiencing relapse is a normal part of dietary change, so forgive yourself, and get back on track as soon as you can.

A Day in the Life of Low-GL: Sample Meal Plans

The preceding sections show you how to set and stick to goals. This section shows you how a few minor changes to your daily diet can make a huge difference to your health, well-being and weight. Are you ready to leap straight into a low-GL lifestyle? The following sample daily eating plans illustrate how simple actions can help you instantly lower the GL of your diet.

Case study one

Jane is a 30-year-old mother of two young children. Breakfast is a rushed meal prior to getting the kids off to school. Lunch is usually a snack at home. Jane nibbles the kids' snacks or a couple of high-GL rice cakes during teatime with the kids. Dinner is a cooked meal including a vegetable, accompanied by a bottle of wine, which she shares with her husband.

Take a look at Table 5-1 to understand how adjusting the quantity, reducing the frequency, and changing the types of food she eats during the day (see the section 'Planning action') can improve Jane's diet.

Table 5-1	Jane's Pre-GL and Post-GL Diet	
Meal	*High GL*	*Low GL*
Breakfast	Cornflakes with raisins and semi-skimmed milk	All bran with dried apricots or berries and semi-skimmed milk
Lunch	Spaghetti hoops on two slices white toast	
	Tinned rice pudding with jam	Large portion of baked beans on one slice soya and linseed toast
		Fruit yoghurt mixed with nuts and toasted oats
Dinner	Roast chicken, large jacket potato and peas. Canned peaches in syrup with condensed milk	

Meal	High GL	Low GL
	Half a bottle of sweet white wine	Roast chicken, medium-sized baked sweet potato, peas, carrots and broccoli. Fresh fruit salad with reduced-fat single cream
	1–2 glasses dry white wine	
Snacks	Rice cakes, Mars bar, potato crisps	Rye crisp breads with reduced-fat soft cheese spread, cashew nuts, dried apple rings, fresh fruit

Book II

Food and Nutrition

Case study two

Tony is a 55-year-old office worker. Tony likes a good breakfast before work but usually just grabs a sandwich at his desk for lunch. Dinner is a takeaway or sit-down meal at a local Indian restaurant, at least a couple of times a week.

A few simple changes, as outlined in Table 5-2, can really improve Tony's diet.

Table 5-2	Tony's Pre-GL and Post-GL Diet	
Meal	**High GL**	**Low GL**
Breakfast	Cocopops with milk Croissants with jam	Porridge with milk and 1 teaspoon fructose Multigrain bread with grilled tomatoes and mushrooms
Lunch	Large cheese baguette Tortilla chips Can of fizzy drink	Open sandwich of cheese on sourdough bread with a side salad Unsalted peanuts and an apple Can of diet drink or flavoured water
Dinner	Lamb madras, large portion white rice, naan bread, poppadoms and mango chutney	Lamb and lentil curry, side dish of spinach (saag) with cucumber raita and a small chappati
Snacks	Hot chocolate, coffee, biscuits, pretzels	Tea, coffee, fresh fruit, homemade soup, oatcakes with hummus or peanut butter, plain popcorn

Write down your own typical daily eating plan, or list what you had to eat yesterday. Use this list as a starting point to pinpoint simple changes to lower the GL of your diet.

Finding Balance: How the GL Diet Fits into Healthy Eating

As registered dieticians, any eating plan we follow, or recommend to anyone else, must be varied enough to avoid the risk of dietary deficiency and balanced enough to prevent diet-related illness, such as heart disease and cancer. The low-GL way of eating consists of wonderful variety of healthy foods. You don't need to buy any special 'low carb' foods, you don't need to pop any pills, and you don't need to take any nutritional supplements.

If you *only* take into account the GL aspect of your diet, you can find yourself eating meals that are low in refined carbohydrate, whole grains and cereal fibre, and high in saturated fat. However, this section acts as a checklist for helping you follow a balanced diet alongside the principles of low GL eating. We also answer some of the most commonly asked questions about healthy eating.

Facing the fats

Everyone needs a certain amount of fat in their diet to provide essential fatty acids and absorb fat-soluble vitamins, and to make food tasty and palatable. Fats come in two main types: saturated and unsaturated.

- ✔ **Saturated fats** generally come from animal sources with two exceptions, coconut and palm oil. Saturated fats are usually solid at room temperature. Research shows that saturated fat raises blood cholesterol and so increases the risk of heart disease, and most people get far too much in their diet. Reducing your intake of butter, cream, full-fat dairy products, cakes, biscuits and pastry helps restrict saturated fat intake. Cutting down on fatty meats and meat products and replacing them with lean cuts or alternatives such as poultry, game, fish, soya, Quorn (a meat substitute made from mushroom-like protein), nuts and pulses also lowers your saturated fat intake.

- ✔ **Unsaturated fats** are commonly derived from plant foods and fish and are in liquid form as oils. Unsaturated fats can help lower blood cholesterol and so protect against heart disease. They come in two main types: *polyunsaturated oils* from sunflower, corn and soya oils, as well as from seeds, nuts and fish; and *monounsaturated fats*, found in rapeseed and olive oil, some nuts and avocados. On a low GL diet, choose unsaturated oils and spreads for cooking and salad dressings.

A special kind of fat – omega-3

The particular type of polyunsaturated fat found in fish, known as *omega-3,* can help lower your blood pressure, reduce blood clotting, and help your heart beat in a normal rhythm, all of which help reduce the occurrence of heart attacks, especially in people at high risk such as people with high blood pressure or high cholesterol levels.

Recent evidence also suggests that a deficiency in omega-3 may play a role in the occurrence of mental health problems such as depression, dementia (including Alzheimer's disease), and even learning and behaviour problems in some children.

What is an oily fish and how much should I eat?

A variety of low-GL oily fish all provide omega 3, whether canned, frozen, fresh or smoked, including:

- ✔ Anchovies
- ✔ Herring
- ✔ Kippers
- ✔ Mackerel
- ✔ Pilchards
- ✔ Salmon
- ✔ Sardines
- ✔ Trout
- ✔ Tuna

Fresh or frozen tuna counts as oily, but canned tuna is not very rich in omega-3.

For clear-cut health benefits, aim to eat a portion of oily fish at least once a week, or more if you're at risk of heart disease. A portion is about 140 grams or 1 small can.

What if I don't eat fish?

Vegetarians can get omega-3 from omega-3 enriched eggs or spreads (check the label). Organic milk is also a relatively good source of omega-3. Oils and seeds such as flaxseeds, linseeds, rapeseed, and some nuts including peanuts, pecans, almonds and walnuts as well as green leafy vegetables all contain omega-3, although at much lower levels.

Book II

Food and Nutrition

If you simply don't enjoy eating fish, try taking omega-3 capsules made from fish-body oil (not the same as cod-liver oil). Aim for around 0.5–1 gram of omega-3 fat per day. Stick to the recommended dose shown on the label. Certain brands are especially formulated for children.

Fitting in the fruit and vegetables

A good intake of fruit and vegetables is central to a low-GL eating plan. As well as being low GL, fruit and vegetables contain a whole cocktail of *phytochemicals* or beneficial nutrients that protect against heart disease and cancer. Studies clearly show the health benefits that can be gained from eating at least five different portions of fruit and vegetables a day.

What counts towards my five a day?

All types of fresh, frozen, tinned and dried fruit and vegetables can contribute towards your five a day quota. However, fruit juice, dried fruit and pulses only count once each day because they contain fewer of the protective nutrients. Five glasses of orange juice won't cut it!

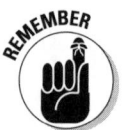

Potatoes don't count towards one of your five portions. Potatoes are classed as a starchy carbohydrate instead, along with bread and other cereals. Potatoes, other than baby new potatoes, are also high-GL. All other vegetables are low in GL.

To get the best mix of phytochemicals, eat a variety of colours and create a rainbow of fruit and veg in your diet.

What's a portion?

The following examples show you what counts as one portion:

- 2–3 small fruits, such as kiwis, satsumas, plums, figs or apricots
- 1 medium fruit, such as an orange, pear, nectarine, banana or apple
- 1 slice of larger fruit, such as pineapple, melon or papaya
- 1 handful of berries, such as strawberries, cherries or grapes
- 3 tablespoons of cooked or tinned fruit
- 1 tablespoon of dried fruit, such as apricots
- A glass (150 millilitres) of 100 per cent fruit juice
- 3 tablespoons of cooked beans or pulses
- 3 heaped tablespoons of cooked vegetables
- 1 small bowl of salad
- Half an avocado or grapefruit

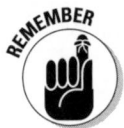

Encourage children to eat at least five different fruits and vegetables each day, but in smaller portion sizes – around a handful.

Can I take a dietary supplement instead?

Unfortunately, we do not recommend taking dietary supplements as a substitute to eating a healthy balanced diet. Pills containing isolated vitamins or minerals do not have the same benefits as actually eating the fruits and vegetables themselves.

Daily dairy

Most dairy foods are low-GL but they can also be high in saturated fat. The best dairy choices are the reduced-fat varieties, such as semi-skimmed milk, low-fat yoghurt, and lower fat cheeses. Low-fat dairy products are just as high in nutrients, such as calcium, as the full-fat varieties.

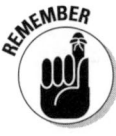

Dairy foods are the primary source of calcium, providing you with the richest and best-absorbed form of this vital element in your diet. You need an adequate quantity of calcium to maintain strong bones and help prevent osteoporosis or brittle bones in later life. Recent studies show that dairy foods also play a role in helping to lower blood pressure and possibly even help to control body weight.

How much dairy do I need?

Aim for 2–3 servings per day of lower fat varieties of milk, cheese or yoghurt. A serving is:

- ✔ 1 carton (150 grams / 5 ounces) natural or low-fat Greek-style yoghurt

- ✔ ⅓ pint skimmed or semi-skimmed milk

- ✔ 1 ounce (30 grams) cheese (lower fat types include: feta, mozzarella, ricotta, Brie, Camembert, Gouda, Edam, soft goat's cheese and reduced-fat hard cheese)

Useful amounts of calcium can also come from cottage or curd cheese, quark (a soft cheese), fromage frais, and low-fat soft cheese and cheese spreads.

What if I don't eat dairy foods?

You can find limited amounts of calcium in tinned bony fish, such as sardines or pilchards, in a variety of nuts, in sesame seeds, green leafy vegetables, dried fruit such as figs, and tap water (if you live in a hard-water area). Higher calcium alternatives include calcium-enriched soya products such as milk, cheese and yoghurts, soya-bean curd (tofu), calcium-fortified water, or even a daily calcium supplement.

Don't forget fibre

Fibre is a type of carbohydrate. Two types of fibre keep your body healthy:

- **Soluble fibre** helps to lower cholesterol levels, control blood-sugar levels, and promotes healthy gut bacteria. A low-GL diet is naturally high in soluble fibre found in fruit, vegetables, pulses, oats and oat bran.

- **Insoluble fibre** helps keep the bowel healthy, protecting against bowel cancer and preventing constipation. Whenever possible, ensure that you choose unrefined wholegrain versions of starchy foods such as bread, pasta, rice or other cereal products. Low GL providers of insoluble fibre include rye or mixed wholegrain or seeded bread, brown basmati or wild rice, wholewheat pasta, and other whole grains, such as pearl barley, bulgur wheat and quinoa.

Water, water everywhere

Water carries nutrients around your body, helps you get rid of waste products (via urine), and controls your body temperature (through sweat). Ideally, you need to drink 6–8 glasses or cups of fluid a day; more if the weather's very hot or if you're very active.

The good news is that any fluid, not just water, can contribute towards your total fluid intake. Low GL drinks include milk, coffee, tea, sugar-free squash, low calorie fizzy drinks and diluted fruit juices. But not all liquids are equally rehydrating. Very strong coffee and the alcohol in beer, wine and spirits, act as *diuretics*, chemicals that make you urinate more.

A word about salt

Most people eat too much salt in their diet – around 9 grams (one and a half teaspoons) per day. High salt intake may be associated with high blood pressure, so try to keep your intake below 6 grams (1 teaspoon) of salt per day on your low-GL plan. Salt is a chemical compound called *sodium chloride*. All forms of salt, including sea and rock salt, are sodium chloride.

Around three quarters of the salt you eat is hidden in processed foods including cereal products, sauces, ready meals and takeaways. To help reduce your total intake, check the label for lower salt varieties when buying these foods as part of your low GL diet.

To assess the salt content of a food from the label, simply multiply the sodium by 2.5. So a food product labelled as containing 0.5 grams of sodium has 1.25 grams of salt.

Take a look at the recipes in this book, and you'll see that we use no added salt. We also give you the sodium content in the nutritional analysis of each recipe.

You can cut down on adding salt to your food during cooking and while at the table by using any type of fresh or dried herbs and spices, including black pepper, instead. For dishes that require salt, you can use a salt substitute made from potassium chloride, commonly available in supermarkets.

Cruising with Confidence: Low-GL Shopping and Eating on the Run

Book II

Food and Nutrition

Any eating plan worth its salt must fit easily into your lifestyle to be successful. That's why we've taken out the effort of shopping for low-GL ingredients, and put together handy checklists and shopping tips for wherever you go to buy food. We also give you some ideas on how to build a store cupboard of low-GL ingredients, and hints on how to help make sense of food labels.

After the shopping, we take you on a cruise around the fast food outlets and sandwich bars for low-GL choices to grab when you're out and about.

Filling up on fruit and vegetables

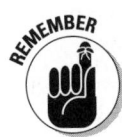

When you choose your fruit and vegetables, think about filling your trolley with a rainbow: The greater the variety of colours you buy, the greater the mix of antioxidant nutrients you get to help protect against cancer and heart disease.

You can choose from a great variety of some of the lower GL fruits and vegetables shown in Tables 5-3 and 5-4.

Table 5-3	Low-GL Fresh Fruit Checklist		
Apples	Fresh figs	Mangos	Peaches
Apricots	Grapes	Melons	Pears
Bananas (the less ripe, the better)	Grapefruits	Nectarines	Pineapples
Berries (all types)	Kiwis	Oranges	Plums
Cherries	Lemons/limes	Papayas	Satsumas

Table 5-4	Low-GL Fresh Vegetable Checklist		
Artichokes	Carrots	Leeks	Pumpkins
Asparagus	Cauliflower	Lettuce	Radishes
Aubergines	Celery	Mange tout	Rocket
Avocados	Courgettes	Mushrooms	Spinach
Bean sprouts	Cucumbers	Okra	Squashes
Broccoli	Endive	Onions	Swedes
Brussels sprouts	Green beans	Peas	Sweetcorn
Cabbage	Kale	Peppers	Tomatoes

Most vegetables have a low GL and you can eat loads of them without a care. Some root vegetables such as parsnips, sweet potatoes, yams and cassava have a moderate GL but they still make excellent alternatives to other starchy carbohydrates with a high GL such as mashed potatoes, jacket potatoes and chips. You can boil, bake or mash these alternative root vegetables. Follow these useful tips for buying fruit and vegetables:

✔ Frozen fruit and vegetables can sometimes have a higher vitamin content than fresh products, which can sit on the shelf or are in transit for some time. Useful purchases include frozen spinach, broad beans, peas and sweetcorn. Berries of all varieties freeze well and are very useful in desserts.

✔ Look for canned fruit and vegetables without added sugar or salt. Low-GL canned veggies include artichoke hearts, water chestnuts, spinach, sweetcorn, mushrooms, peas and, of course, tinned tomatoes.

✔ Beans and pulses are key players in the low-GL diet. Dried varieties need soaking and careful cooking. Tinned varieties are pricier but save you time. Reduce the salt by always draining and rinsing tinned beans and pulses. Select pulses from lentils (red, green, brown or puy), split peas and chickpeas. Low-GL beans include kidney, butter, cannelloni, haricot, aduki, butter, borlotti, flageolet and pinto. And don't forget low-sugar baked beans!

✔ Seeds are powerhouses of nutrients and are low-GL, too. Choose from sunflower, sesame, flax or linseeds, pumpkin, poppy and melon. Pine nuts are wonderful toasted in savoury dishes.

✔ Nuts are another great part of a low-GL diet. Choose unsalted wherever possible, including almonds, Brazil nuts, chestnuts, hazelnuts, macadamia, pecans, peanuts pistachios, cashews and walnuts. You can use ground almonds instead of flour in some baked dishes. Sugar-free peanut butter and reduced-fat coconut milk are useful store cupboard ingredients.

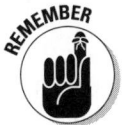

Size matters when buying nuts, seeds, dried fruit and pulses. Be economical and buy in bulk or loose-packed from a local co-op, ethnic or wholefood shop rather than at the supermarket. If stored correctly, these ingredients keep fresh for some time.

Choosing meat, fish and alternatives

All unprocessed meat, poultry, fish and shellfish are naturally low in carbohydrate and so have a low GL. Choose lean cuts without added cereals or breadcrumbs where possible. Table 5-5 is your handy checklist for low-GL choices.

Book II

Food and Nutrition

Table 5-5	Low-GL Meat, Fish and Alternatives Checklist	
Canned or fresh crab	Fresh, frozen or smoked fish (white and oily)	Lean red meat
Canned oily fish	Fresh or frozen shellfish	Offal
Canned tuna	Fresh or frozen squid	Quorn
Chicken portions	Game	Soya mince
Chicken or turkey mince and stir fry pieces	High-meat content, lean sausages	Tofu
Eggs	Lean mince	Whole chicken

Opting for milk and dairy foods

Milk and dairy foods, apart from sweetened and condensed milk, are naturally low in GL but can sometimes be high in saturated animal fat (linked to an increased risk of heart disease). Table 5-6 guides you towards the lower fat choices.

Table 5-6	Low-GL Milk and Dairy Foods Checklist	
Fromage frais	Low-fat single cream	Reduced-fat hard and soft cheese, cottage cheese
Long-life milks and cream	Low-fat sour cream	Skimmed or semi-skimmed milk
Low-fat crème fraîche	Olive oil margarines	Soya milk
Low-fat Greek yoghurt	Parmesan cheese	Yoghurt (bio or natural)

Buying bread, cereals and potatoes

Another food group for your trolley is the starchy foods – bread, cereals and potatoes. The choices you make from this group affect the GL of your diet more than any other food group, so follow our tips with extra care.

Table 5-7	Low-GL Bread, Cereals and Potatoes Checklist	
Bran-based cereals	New potatoes	Sweet potatoes
Brown rice	Oatmeal /porridge oats	Wholegrain, rye, and seeded bread
Buckwheat or kasha	Oat bran	Wholegrain porridge
Bulgur/cracked wheat	Oat cakes	Wholemeal pasta
Couscous	Pearl barley	Yams, celeriac

Here are some tips for when you buy bread, cereals and potatoes:

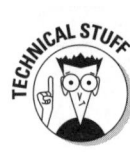

- ✔ Low-GL varieties of bread include those made with 100 per cent wholegrain or wholemeal flour, multi-seeded, soya and linseed, sourdough, rye or pumpernickel.

- ✔ Choose rice a with a high *amylose* content, such as long grain, wild and brown basmati rice, rather than short grain or white sticky rice.

  Rice contains two types of starch: *amylose* and *amylopectin*. The GL of amylose is lower because the molecules are packed tightly together, making it take longer to digest.

- ✔ Wholemeal pasta and fettuccine have a lower GL than most other pasta. Cook your pasta until al dente (still firm when bitten). Mix pasta and rice with beans and pulses to reduce the overall GL, and remember to keep your portions small.

- ✔ For breakfast, choose from wholegrain oats, oat bran, bran-based cereals, or make your own muesli. We give you a lovely recipe for fast muesli in Chapter 4.

- ✔ Try adding pearl barley to stews and casseroles or mixed with rice and pasta as an alternative.

- ✔ Potatoes are a high-GL food. Go for small new potatoes or try mashed or baked celeriac, yam or sweet potatoes, which have a lower GL.

Some stores have an organic or health food aisle where you may find a better range of low-GL grains and cereals than in the main aisles.

Building a store cupboard of low-GL ingredients

Stock up on the low-GL staples shown in Table 5-8 and creating meals from your store cupboard stock will be a doddle. We're not suggesting that you stock up on all these ingredients in one go, but just buy one or two items each week and your store cupboard supplies can soon grow.

Table 5-8	Low-GL Store Cupboard Checklist		
Capers	Gherkins	Passata	Sugar-free jams
Curry pastes	Harissa	Pesto	Sugar-free pickles
Dried herbs and spices	Mustard	Pure fruit spreads	Sundried tomatoes
Dried mushrooms	Natural vanilla extract	Sauces (such as soy)	Tahini paste
Flavoured vinegars	Olives	Sauerkraut	Tomato puree
Fructose	Olive paste (tapenade)	Stock cubes	Vegetable/ olive/seed oils

Book II

Food and Nutrition

Choosing GL-friendly fast food

Sometimes you don't have time to sit down and enjoy a leisurely meal – you just need a pit stop to grab something quick and easy to fill that gap while on the run. Low-GL choices are still possible in this situation – you just need to know where to look.

Eating on the run

Some fast-food outlets now offer healthy salads. However, skip the high-GL crispy croutons and choose a light dressing.

If you simply can't resist having the occasional burger, try a smaller burger, cheeseburger, grilled chicken sandwich or even a bean burger. Add some mustard, low-fat mayonnaise or gherkins. Discard the top off the burger bun and eat as an open sandwich to reduce the amount of bread. Accompany the burger with a large salad instead of fries.

Go for diet drinks or lower fat milkshakes instead full sugar or full-fat options. Fresh fruit, fruit salad and yoghurt are good low-GL dessert options. Even the good old-fashioned fish and chip shops offer some lower GL options. Ask for your chicken or fish without the batter. Mushy peas are a great accompaniment, or try a pickled egg or pickled onion.

Smart sandwich-bar selections

Most sandwich bars and coffee shops offer open sandwiches so you can eat less bread, and some shops even provide a 'breadless' sandwich – lean cold meat, tuna or cheese with salad all wrapped up in lettuce. If bread is the only option, choose the darkest, densest, grainiest bread available.

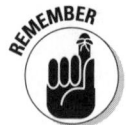

Look out for pumpernickel, rye, seeded, sourdough or stoneground wholegrain bread and ask for thin slices. Ask the staff to use a little light mayonnaise, salad dressing or mustard instead of butter or margarine. Then fill up your sandwich with some of these low-GL choices:

✔ Lean deli meats, such as roast beef, ham, pastrami or bacon

✔ Chicken, duck or turkey

✔ Tuna, prawns, crab, crayfish or smoked salmon

✔ Low-fat cream cheese or cottage cheese

✔ Chargrilled vegetables

✔ Olives, gherkins

✔ Salad vegetables including spinach, peppers, avocado, onions, rocket, tomatoes and cucumber

Many sandwich bars also serve soup, which is a satisfying alternative to a sandwich. Select a soup packed with vegetables and pulses, and eat with a small wholegrain roll.

To accompany your meal, choose a packet of popcorn or nuts instead of crisps. Cashews, almonds, or pumpkin or sesame seeds are good GL-friendly choices. A small (20–30 gram) bar of high-cocoa solids dark chocolate can satisfy a sweet tooth, but only indulge yourself now and then.

Sandwich bar dessert options include yoghurt, fruit salad, berries or fresh fruit. Make sure that you order your coffee without flavoured syrups but for variety try soya milk in your cappuccino or latte. Even better, go for a fruit or herb tea, vegetable juice, a sugar-free smoothie or bottled water.

Replacing Common Ingredients with GL-Friendly Alternatives

This section guides you through some easy tips for making the best low-GL choices when your options are limited. We also give you some general pointers to help you make traditional favourite foods and recipes more GL friendly and best of all, we tell you everything you need to know to keep your GL diet as flexible as possible.

Breaking your potato habit

Don't get us wrong, we're not anti-potatoes! However, the structure of a potato and some of the ways you cook them make potatoes high-GL. Large white potatoes, boiled to a pulp, is a recipe for GL disaster. Follow our tips to help you keep potatoes, and some great alternatives, on the menu.

Smashing mashing

A steaming bowl of smooth, creamy mashed potatoes is surely one of the most comforting foods in the world. Usually, you use large white flowery potatoes to make mashed potato, which is not great news for your GL and stabilising your blood sugars.

But don't write off mashed potato for good. You can make a great chunky potato crush with baby new potatoes. Keep the skins on the potatoes and boil until cooked, then crush them with a fork so that the potatoes are just broken rather than smooth. Add a little butter or low-fat spread and some black pepper. Alternatively, add some natural yoghurt and fresh chopped chives – delicious.

A whole host of other veggies make great tasting, colourful mash. You can use them for topping on dishes such as fish pie or shepherd's pie, or simply use mash as a side vegetable.

The basic recipe is to peel, chop, boil the vegetables in water until cooked, and then, you guessed it, mash! (See? You're a great cook after all!)

Great alternative mash combos include:

- **Cauli mash:** Try this dish before you say a thing! Boil a whole cauliflower, then mash with a little mustard, some crème fraîche and black pepper. This combination is the creamiest mash you'll ever eat!

- **Celeriac and herb mash:** The poor celeriac is probably one of the ugliest veggies you'll ever see, but get past the peeling and simply treat it like mashed potatoes. Add parsley or basil. This slightly aniseed flavoured mash goes brilliantly with rich sauces and gravies.

   ✔ **Carrot and swede mash:** Two vibrant looking and tasting veggies that were just meant to be together.

   ✔ **Carrot and sweet potato mash:** This mash is great for children – bright orange with just a touch of sweetness.

Coasting for a roasting

Simply follow these top tips for keeping the GL lid on your roast:

   ✔ Choose leaner cuts of meat and poultry.

   ✔ Instead of roast potatoes, roast a selection of the following vegetables for a change: carrots, sweet potatoes, celeriac, butternut squash and red onions.

   ✔ Serve plenty of steamed vegetables, and aim for three or four different side dishes of vegetables.

   ✔ Use a teaspoon of cornflour to thicken gravy, and skim off any excess fat from meat juices.

Sweet potatoes also make great baked potatoes. You can cook them in the oven or the microwave and they're delicious with cottage cheese and chives.

Baking cakes

Bet you didn't think you'd find tips for baking cakes in a book with 'diet' in the title! We love food too much to ban anything. Admittedly, if you're trying to lose weight a slice of cake every day is not such a great idea, but remember – the GL Diet is a diet for life, not just a week or so. Now, at some time in your long and healthy life you're sure to have a birthday, or Christmas, right? A special occasion calls for a cake, and we can share a few simple tips to lower the GL of your cakes and desserts.

The main ingredients that you're looking to replace in a cake recipe are the sugar and the white flour. You can make a fantastic sponge cake using equal quantities of 100 per cent wholemeal flour and almond flour. Use fructose instead of sugar but remember that you only need two-thirds of the amount in the recipe because fructose tastes much sweeter than table sugar.

Fructose browns more quickly at high temperatures than regular sugar, so slightly reduce the recommended oven temperature and keep an eye on your cake while cooking.

If you want to make your sponge extra special, swap sugar-filled icing, frosting or jam for delicious fresh fruit such as strawberries and a dash of low-fat crème fraîche.

Rumble for a crumble

Fruit crumbles are a real traditional, old fashioned pudding. Show us a person who doesn't like crumble and we'll eat our . . . crumble! The fruit is good for you, but the traditional crumble topping is full of flour and sugar – not helpful when you're trying to eat low GL.

Here's our tried and tested low-GL crumble topping, which our friends and families love:

225 grams / 8 ounces / 1 cup old fashioned porridge oats

1 teaspoon ground cinnamon

50 grams / 1 ½ ounces / ¼ cup ground almonds

2 tablespoons fructose (fruit sugar)

1 tablespoon butter or olive oil spread

1 Put all the ingredients in a bowl and rub together with your fingertips until you have a crumbly mixture.

2 Then add the crumble to your favourite softened fruit. Apple and blackberry, apple and pear, rhubarb, raspberries, blackcurrants and gooseberries all work brilliantly in a crumble. Soften the fruit by gently heating it in a pan with a little water for a few minutes.

3 Simply bake in a hot oven for 20 to 30 minutes or until golden brown. Serve with low-fat crème fraîche or natural yoghurt.

Cheeky cheesecakes

Cheesecake isn't exactly the best dessert to choose when you're trying to lose weight. However, for the odd special occasion you can make this dish as a low-GL dessert by reducing the amount of sugar and using lots of different fresh fruit in the topping. For the sweet biscuit base try using ground nuts such as almonds with a tablespoon of fructose and a little butter or olive oil spread instead of smashed digestive biscuits. Plain low-fat cream cheese topped with fresh fruit makes a great topping.

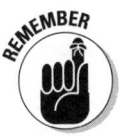

Cheesecake is still a calorie-packed pud, so cut yourself a small portion.

Controlling portion sizes

A trick for limiting the damage is to fill your plate the GL-friendly way.

Imagine dividing your plate into quarters. Now fill two quarters with vegetables, one quarter with protein, and one quarter with carbs. Figure 5-1 shows you how. Simply remember 'veggie veggie protein carbs'.

Book II

Food and Nutrition

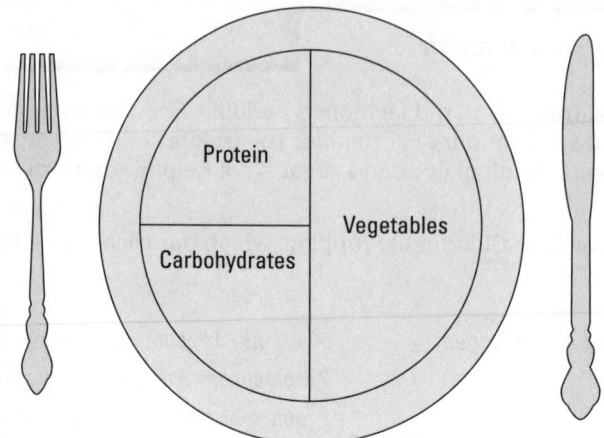

Another way to limit the damage from a less than GL-friendly meal is to reduce the total amount of food you eat. This tip sounds obvious, but you can find exercising portion caution difficult without looking as if you're trying to guess the weight of foods. Try to always serve yourself, rather than allowing your generous host to pile food on your plate.

To judge the overall size of your meal, estimate whether you could fit all the food on your plate into your cupped hands. Have a look at your cupped hands now. Yippee for those of you with big hands!

Your cupped hands represent your stomach. This method is a rough guide but will help you avoid indulging in large quantities of high-GL foods.

Book III
Physical Health: Achieving Fitness

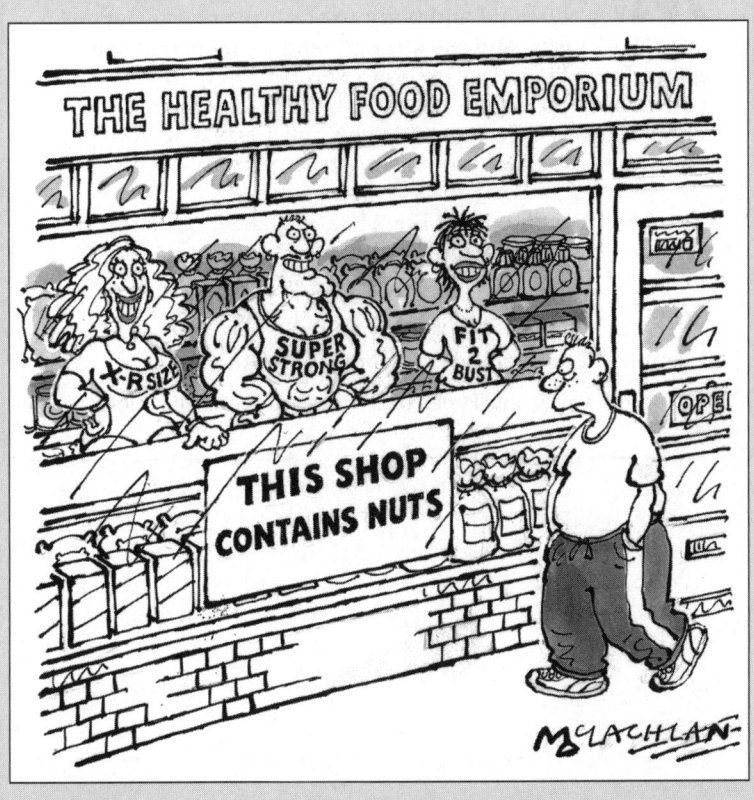

In this book . . .

Maintaining your physical health is necessary for a
healthy mind and body so you have energy for
your daily tasks, and the strength and resilience to keep
going. Book III focuses on how exercise can help you, and
provides ideas to get you started. We also help you
choose which exercises will suit your lifestyle so you
know how to include some activity every day.

Here are the contents of Book III at a glance:

Chapter 1

Enjoying the Benefits of Being Physically Active

*B*eing physically active can have many benefits to your overall health and well-being including looking and feeling good, and having loads more energy.

In this chapter we want you to find out why exercise is worthwhile and start you off with some simple stretches to start relaxing your body and releasing muscle tension. Stretching helps to lengthen muscles ensuring that the joints are held in the correct alignment, promoting improved posture.

Knowing Why You Need to Bother

You already know how important exercise is in your life, but sometimes it is important to remind yourselves of the many benefits to keep you going on your physically active journey.

Even if you're the most committed exerciser, you probably have moments when your best intentions are stifled by excuses not to work out. You're too tired or too busy, the weather is not suitable or your friend's away. Any time you experience any of these moments, remind yourself of the benefits described in this chapter to keep you on target.

Decreasing Your Risk of Medical Problems

Keeping physically active helps to reduce health problems. Some of the health benefits include:

✔ Helping you feel more energetic, happier and more positive.

✔ Boosting your body's immune system to help fight those winter colds.

✔ Keeping your muscles more mobile and stronger, supporting your bones and joints more.

✔ Improving your balance, which is particularly important as you get older, reducing your risks of falls and fractures.

✔ Boosting your sleep and helping you wake less at night.

✔ Reducing the symptoms of premenstrual syndrome, including bloating, lower-back pain, headaches and anxiety.

✔ Easing the symptoms of the menopause.

✔ Strengthening your bones by reducing the decline in bone mass as you age and reducing your risk for osteoporosis.

✔ Relieving arthritic pain.

✔ Easing lower-back pain by strengthening your abdominal and lower back muscles.

✔ Improving your blood pressure.

✔ Reducing the risk of some cancers, including colon cancer and breast cancer.

✔ Lowering your risk of coronary heart disease, by reducing your blood cholesterol.

✔ Reducing your risk of having a stroke.

Controlling your weight

You can of course lose weight by dieting, but you end up losing more muscles and not the evil fat. Combining dieting with weight training helps to prevent your muscles from wasting away and aerobic exercise is the most efficient way to burn calories. Some of the other weight-control benefits of exercise include:

- Burning extra calories helps prevent weight gain as you age.
- You're more likely to keep the weight off.
- You can eat more without gaining weight to enjoy those occasional meals out!

Improving your body shape and your looks

Who would want to turn down the opportunity to have a firmer derrière, and toned arms and legs! The more exercise you do, the more you improve your muscle strength and tone, helping you feel and look younger, and boosting your self esteem. The stimulating effect from exercise promotes a better sense of well-being.

Exploring the psychological benefits

Creating a better sense of well-being is a great benefit from exercise, along with:

- Gaining confidence in yourself.
- Enhancing your memory.
- Reducing stress and depression.
- Calming your mind, and controlling your anger through breathing exercises.
- Feeling happier over the longer term.

Book III

Physical Health: Achieving Fitness

Unlocking social benefits

Walking with a friend is a great way to have fun or even meet new people. Not only are you keeping up to date with news about friends, family or colleagues, you are also helping to get things off your mind and clear your head.

Next time you take a walk, enjoy the following benefits:

- Meet new people.
- Clear your head.
- Widen your network of friends.

Enjoying life more

Having more fun and enjoying life are something you often strive for. Exercise can often make you more creative by coming up with great ideas during exercise. Exercising your body boosts your brain cells and you can find you are productive by being less tired. As you enjoy life more at work and at home you will find your family also gain. You are setting a great example for your children and grandchildren by making exercise a natural part of everyday life.

Check out how you can enjoy life more:

✔ Sharing time with other people.

✔ Stimulating your brain and becoming more creative.

✔ Having more fun.

Considering Why Stretching is a Good Place to Start

Stretching is the key to maintaining your flexibility – in other words, how far and how easily you can move your joints. As you get older, your tendons (the tissues that connect muscle to bone) begin to shorten and tighten, restricting your flexibility. Your movement becomes slower and less fluid. You don't stand up as straight. You walk more stiffly and with a shorter stride. You find it more difficult to step up to a kerb or bend down to pick up rubbish. Stretching your rear thigh, hip and calf muscles can make a big difference.

Flexibility is one of the keys to good posture. When your front neck muscles are short and tight, your head angles forward. When your shoulders and chest are tight, your shoulders round inwards. When your lower back, rear thigh and hip muscles are tight, the curve of your back becomes exaggerated. A regular stretching routine also can reduce pain and discomfort, particularly in your lower back. In fact, the pain often disappears when you begin doing simple stretches for your lower-back and rear-thigh muscles.

What's more, flexibility exercises can correct muscle imbalances. Say that your front-thigh muscles are strong, but your rear thighs are tight and weak. (This is a common scenario.) As a result, you end up relying on your front thighs more than you should. Chances are, you won't even notice this, but it will throw off your movement in subtle ways – you may have a short walking stride or bounce too high off the ground. Muscle imbalances can eventually lead to injuries such as pulled muscles. They also contribute to clumsiness, which in itself can lead to injury. Finally, if you indulge in any kind of sport – even going bowling or playing cricket on Sunday afternoons – stretching may help you perform better. The ability to move freely in a wide variety of directions makes you a better athlete.

Before, after, during? Knowing when to stretch

Contrary to popular opinion, stretching is not the first thing you should do when you walk into the gym or arrive at the park for a jog. Don't stretch your muscles until you've at least warmed up thoroughly; we think stretching at the end of your workout, after you've finished your workout but before you shower, is even better. A post-workout stretch is a great way to relax and ease back into the rest of your day, and has been shown to reduce injuries.

Don't stretch before you cool down. Putting your head below your heart right after a workout can cause fainting and nausea. Wait until your heart rate dips below 100 or you aren't feeling breathless before you lie down to stretch.

Following a few rules of stretching

Here are the basic rules for a useful and safe flexibility workout:

- ✔ **Stretch as often as you can – daily, if possible.** Always stretch after every workout, both cardiovascular and strength training. When you stretch on days you don't work out, be sure to warm up with a few minutes of easy movement like shoulder rolls, gentle waist twists, or light cardio activity.

- ✔ **Move into each stretching position slowly.** Never force yourself into a stretch by jerking or snapping into position.

- ✔ **Notice how much tension you feel.** A stretch should rate anywhere from mild tension to the edge of discomfort on your pain meter. It should never cause severe or sharp pain anywhere else in your body. Focus on the area you're stretching, and notice the stretch spread through these muscles.

- ✔ **Never bounce.** No matter which type of stretching you choose, once you have found the most comfortable stretch position, stay there or gradually deepen the stretch. Bouncing only tightens your muscle – it doesn't loosen it. Forceful bouncing increases the risk of tearing a muscle.

- ✔ **As you hold each position, take at least two deep breaths.** Deep breathing promotes relaxation.

A simple stretching routine

In the following sections, we show you a thorough, basic stretching routine to get you started. If you consider stretching too boring, too painful or too complicated, you'll like this section. It features a no-brainer stretching routine that won't pull your hamstrings like a rope in a tug of war. In this section, we demonstrate classic stretches because they're the type most fitness experts recommend. After you have mastered these moves, the workout should take about five minutes.

Keep in mind that this is just a starting point. We think it's a great idea to learn additional stretches; there are literally hundreds to choose from. Varying your flexibility routine allows you to stretch your muscles at a number of angles. Plus, you'll be able to give the necessary extra attention to the muscles you use most in your particular workout. For example, if you're a tennis player or rower, you may want to do a few extra upper-body stretches. If you're a runner, do a few additional hamstring and lower-back stretches. If you're a cyclist, emphasise your quadriceps and glutes.

Neck stretch

This stretch is designed to loosen and relax the muscles in your neck.

Stand or sit comfortably. Drop your left ear towards your left shoulder, and gently stretch your right arm down and a few inches out to the side (see Figure 1-1), using your opposite hand to assist the stretch by gently pulling on the side of your head. Repeat the stretch on your right side.

Keep these tips in mind as you perform the neck stretch:

- ✔ Keep your shoulders down and relaxed.
- ✔ Your ear may or may not touch your shoulder, depending on how stiff you are.

Chest expansion

This stretch targets your shoulders, chest and arms and helps promote good posture.

Sit or stand up tall and bring your arms behind you, clasping one hand inside the other (see Figure 1-2). Lift your chest and raise your arms slightly. You should feel a mild stretch spread across your chest.

Keep in mind the following tips as you perform the chest expansion:

- ✔ Resist arching your lower back as you pull your arms upwards.
- ✔ Try to keep your shoulders relaxed and down.
- ✔ Don't force your arms up higher than is comfortable.

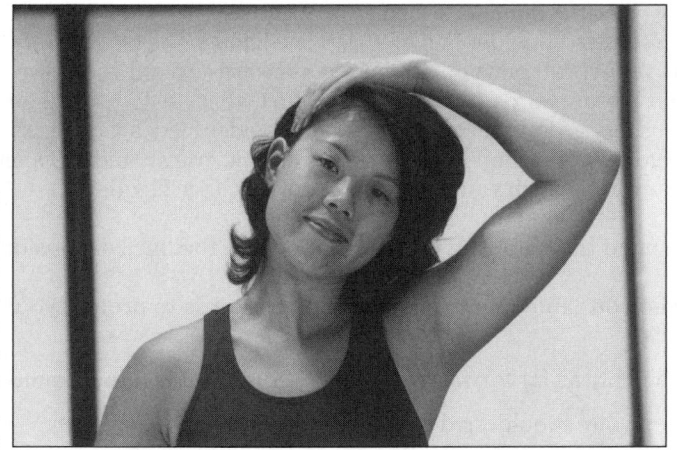

Figure 1-1:
The neck stretch loosens and relaxes the muscles in your neck.

Photograph by Sunstreak Productions, Inc.

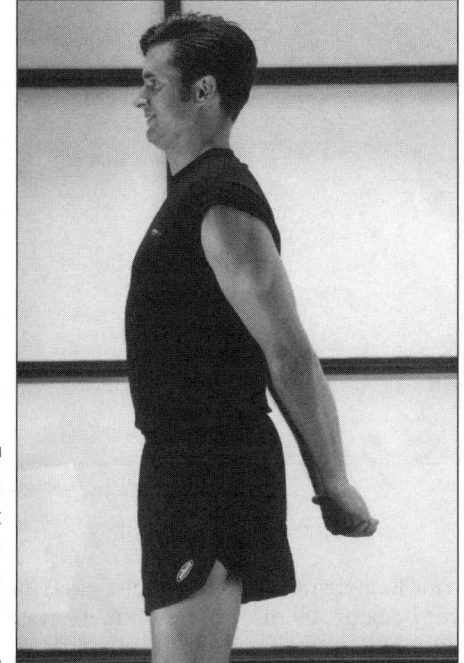

Figure 1-2:
The chest expansion promotes good posture.

Photograph by Sunstreak Productions, Inc.

Back expansion

This move stretches and loosens your shoulders, arms, upper-back and lower-back muscles.

Standing tall with your knees slightly bent and feet hip-width apart, lift your arms in front of you to shoulder height. Clasp one hand in the other. Drop your head towards your chest, pull your abdominals inwards, round your lower back, and tuck your hips forwards so that you create a C shape with your torso. Stretch your arms forwards so that you feel your shoulder blades moving apart and you create an 'opposition' to your rounded back. You should feel a mild stretch slowly spread through your back and shoulders. (See Figure 1-3.)

Keep in mind the following tips as you perform the back expansion:

- ✔ Keep your abdominal muscles pulled inwards to protect your lower back.

- ✔ Lean only as far forward as you feel comfortable and balanced.

- ✔ Keep your shoulders down and relaxed.

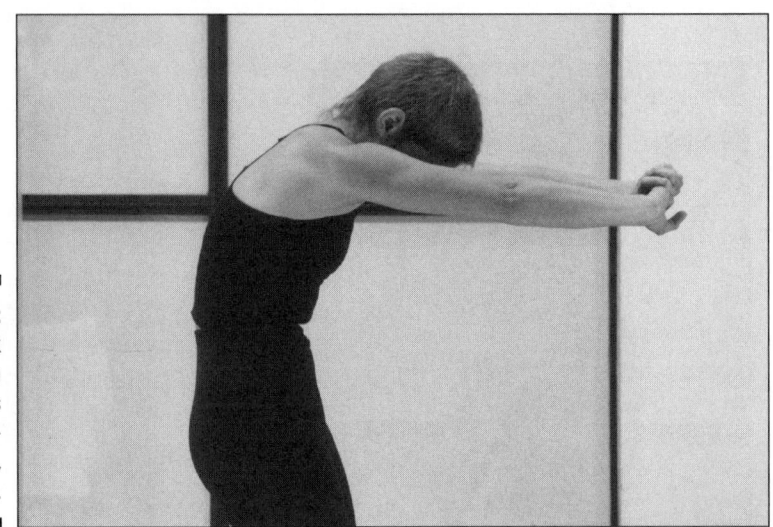

Figure 1-3: The back expansion stretches your shoulders, arms, and back.

Photograph by Sunstreak Productions, Inc.

Standing hamstring stretch

This is a great stretch for your hamstrings (rear-thigh muscles) and your lower back. If you have lower-back problems, do the same exercise while lying on your back on the floor and extending your leg upwards.

Stand tall with your left foot a few inches in front of your right foot and your left toes lifted. Bend your right knee slightly and pull your abdominals gently inwards. Lean forward from your hips, and rest both palms on top of your right thigh for balance and support (see Figure 1-4). Keep your shoulders down and relaxed; don't round your lower back. You should feel a mild pull

gradually spread through the back of your leg. Repeat the stretch with your right leg forward.

Keep in mind the following tips as you perform the standing hamstring stretch:

✔ Keep your back straight and your abs pulled inwards to make the stretch more effective and to protect your lower back.

✔ Don't lean so far forward that you lose your balance or feel strain in your lower back.

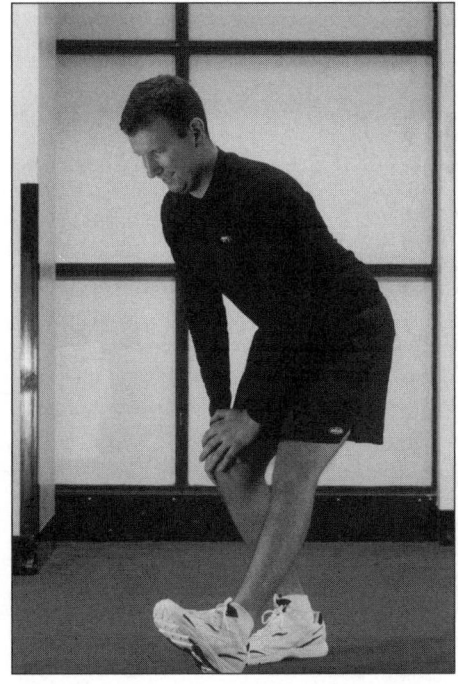

Figure 1-4:
The standing hamstring stretch targets your rear-thigh muscles.

Photograph by Sunstreak Productions, Inc.

Standing quad stretch

This stretch focuses on the quadriceps (front-thigh muscles). Be extra gentle with this stretch if you're prone to knee or lower-back pain. If back pain is an issue for you, you can do a similar stretch while lying on your side, bending your top knee, and bringing your heel towards your buttocks.

Stand tall with your feet hip-width apart, pull your abdominals in, and relax your shoulders. Bend your left leg, bringing your heel towards your bottom,

and grasp your left foot with your right hand (see Figure 1-5) or with your left hand if the opposite hand is too uncomfortable. You should feel a mild pull gradually spread through the front of your left leg. Then switch legs.

Keep these tips in mind as you perform the standing quad stretch:

✔ Hold onto a chair or the wall if you have trouble balancing.

✔ Don't lock the knee of your base leg.

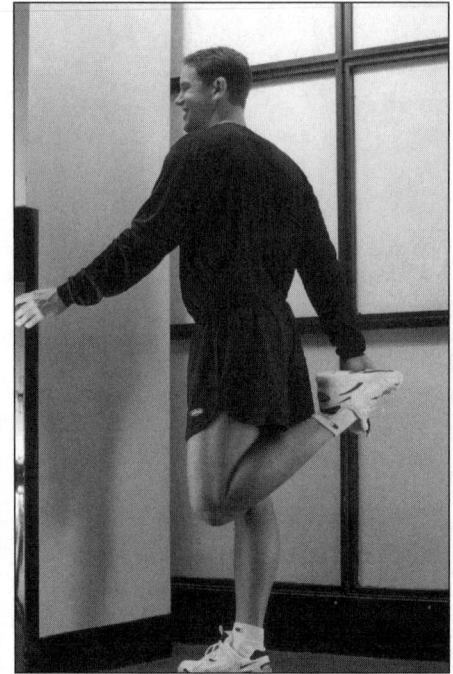

Figure 1-5:
The standing quad stretch targets your front-thigh muscles.

Photograph by Sunstreak Productions, Inc.

Double calf stretch

This stretch offers some relief for the calf muscles, which tend to be tight and bunched up from daily activities such as walking and standing.

Stand with your feet together about 2 feet from a wall that you're facing. Pull your abdominals gently inwards and don't round your lower back. With straight arms, press your palms into the wall and lean forwards from your ankles, keeping your heels pressed as close to the floor as possible (see Figure 1-6). You should feel a mild stretch spread through your calf muscles.

Keep in mind the following tips as you perform the double calf stretch:

- ✔ Keep both heels flat on the floor or as close to the floor as your flexibility allows.

- ✔ Keep your abs pulled in to prevent your lower back from sagging or arching.

- ✔ To increase the stretch, bend your elbows, leaning your chest towards the wall.

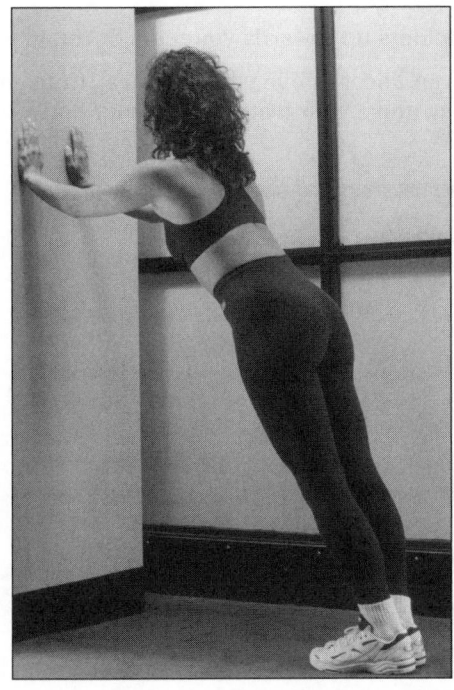

Figure 1-6:
The double calf stretch helps relieve tightness in your calf muscles.

Photograph by Sunstreak Productions, Inc.

Book III

Physical Health: Achieving Fitness

Butterfly stretch

This exercise stretches your inner thighs, groin, hips and lower back. If you are prone to lower-back discomfort, take extra care to lean forward from your hips rather than rounding your lower back. This exercise may also cause some knee discomfort.

Sit up tall with the soles of your feet pressed together and your knees dropped to the sides as far as they will comfortably go. Pull your abdominals gently inwards and lean forward from your hips. Grasp your feet with your hands and carefully pull yourself a small way further forward (see Figure 1-7). You should feel the stretch spread throughout your inner thighs, the outermost part of your hips, and lower back.

Keep in mind these tips as you perform the butterfly:

- ✔ Increase the stretch by carefully pressing your thighs towards the floor as you hold the position.
- ✔ Don't hunch your shoulders up towards your ears or round your back.
- ✔ To reduce stress on your knees, move your feet away from your body. To increase the stretch, move your feet towards your body.

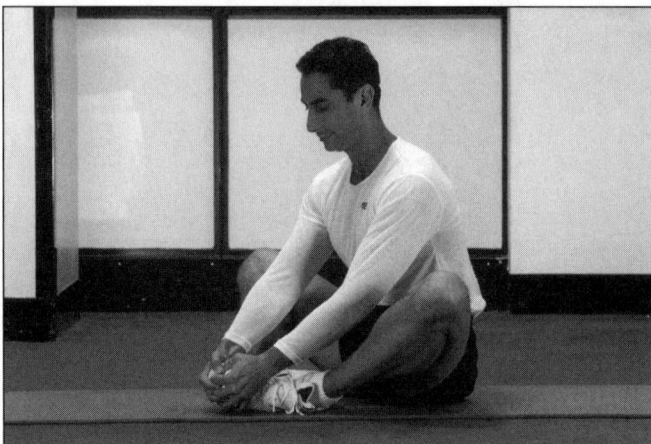

Figure 1-7:
The butter-fly stretch targets your inner thighs, groin, hips and lower back.

Photograph by Sunstreak Productions, Inc.

Chapter 2

Setting Goals and Giving Rewards

· ·

In This Chapter

▶ Establishing fitness goals

▶ Rewarding yourself in small ways

▶ Making fitness a daily habit

· ·

*N*o matter what shape you're in, making a start on a fitness programme is always worthwhile, even if the action is simply sitting down and reading this chapter!

This chapter outlines the basics to help you establish a plan of attack to help make exercise a habit for you. Identifying your personal fitness goals is a great start, with some rewards to entice you along the way.

Establishing Your Plan of Attack

You wouldn't start or expand a business without a plan – a clear-cut idea of where you want to take your company and how you propose to get there. Instead, you would assess your cash flow and expenses, choose a location for your office, decide on your hours of operation, and develop strategies to overcome obstacles.

Your workout programme deserves the same level of attention, whether you're just beginning to map out your fitness plan or looking to expand and improve your current fitness routine. This chapter helps you develop your plan of attack. We show you how to set realistic goals and track your progress, and we offer strategies for sticking to your plan so that your workout programme is successful.

Setting goals

Before you embark on a new exercise programme – or attempt to invigorate your existing one – clarify why you want to get fit. Maybe heart disease runs in your family and you want to avoid carrying on that tradition. Maybe you can't keep up with your grandchildren.

Research shows that goal-setting works. In typical studies, scientists give one group of exercisers a specific goal, such as doing 60 sit-ups. Meanwhile, they tell a second group of exercisers simply, 'Do your best.' The exercisers with specific goals tend to have significantly more success than the comparison groups. This approach can work for you, too.

When you start an exercise programme, you need to set a few different types of goals. Look at the big picture while giving yourself stepping stones to get there. Having mini-goals makes your long-term goals seem more feasible. Here's a look at the different types of goals you should set.

Long-term goals

Make sure your long-term goals are realistic. If you're starting your swimming programme today, jumping into the freezing cold waters of the English Channel and swimming all the way to France is not exactly what we recommend for a six-month goal. On the other hand, don't be afraid to dream. Choose a goal that really sparks you – something that may be out of reach at the moment but is not out of the realms of possibility. People are often surprised by what they can accomplish. We had a client who was 60 years old when he started training for a trek up Alaska's Mount McKinley. We eventually had the guy walking uphill for up to 90 minutes on the treadmill with a heavy pack and hiking boots. After six months of training, the man successfully completed his trek. He was the oldest one on the trip, but he wasn't the slowest. His success inspired him to train for many other hiking events.

Judge for yourself what's realistic. Some people rise to the occasion when they set goals that seem virtually impossible. Other people get discouraged by setting extremely high expectations. If you're a beginner, we recommend setting moderately challenging goals. If you reach your goals earlier than you expect, that's the time to choose more ambitious ones. Here are some concrete examples of long-term goals that may spark your imagination:

- Complete a 50-mile bike ride in four months' time.
- Lose three per cent body fat in 10 weeks.
- Do one full pull-up.
- Reduce your cholesterol count 5mmols/litre.
- Fit into that pair of jeans.
- Walk one mile in under 15 minutes.

Short-term goals

Six months is a long time to wait for feelings of success. In order to stay motivated, you need to feel a sense of accomplishment along the way. When Suzanne was cycling from the John O' Groats to Lands End, she didn't dream about reaching Lands End every day; she focused on a goal that seemed more manageable, like finishing each day and enjoying a nice hot bath. She also planned to meet different friends at regular intervals to make the goal seem more manageable. Set short-term goals for one week to one month. Here are some examples:

- Take two step aerobics classes a week for one month.
- Improve your one-mile walk time by 20 seconds.
- Use the cross trainer four times this week for 30 minutes each time.
- Cycle 60 miles a week for the next four weeks.

Immediate goals

Immediate goals refer to goals for each week, day or workout. This way, when you walk into the gym, you don't waste any time figuring out which exercises to do. Here are examples of immediate goals:

- Spend a full ten minutes stretching at the end of a workout.
- Do upper-body weight exercises and 20 minutes on the cross trainer.
- Run two miles.
- Cycle a hilly 20-mile course.

Book III

Physical Health: Achieving Fitness

Backup goals

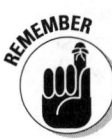

You always need a Plan B, in case something happens and you're not able to reach your primary goal as soon as you want to. By setting backup goals, you have a better chance of achieving something, and you don't feel like a failure if your long-term goal doesn't work out. Suppose your long-term goal is to lose more than half a stone by eating healthier and walking three miles a day. Your backup goal could be increasing your stamina enough to walk three miles in less than an hour. Or say that you're training for a 10-kilometre run in the spring, but you sprain an ankle and have to stop running. If one of your backup goals is to strengthen your upper body, you can still keep on track while your ankle heals.

Finding ways to reward yourself

You let your kids watch their favourite DVD when they come home with good marks, right? You give your golden retriever a doggy treat when he fetches the ball? So, be nice to yourself, too. Attach an appropriate reward to each of your goals. If you lose three per cent body fat over the next two months, buy yourself a nifty sports watch. If you lift weights three days a week for a month, treat yourself to a massage. Sure, it's bribery, but it works. Short-term rewards are particularly important because there's always a chance that you may not make it all the way to your long-term goal. You need to give yourself credit for making it even halfway. (By the way, triple-decker fudge cake isn't what we have in mind for a reward. Try to make sure your reward is as healthy as your goal.)

Writing everything down

Setting goals and rewards is pretty easy; forgetting what they are is even easier. To keep yourself honest – and motivated – consider recording your goals and accomplishments on paper. One friend of ours sticks his goals on the inside of his gym locker. Some people program their computers to flash their goals on screen twice a day. A member of Liz's Thursday night Internet chat group posts her fitness and weight-loss accomplishments on the message board every week, along with a note thanking other members for their encouraging comments. (And this idea of sharing your goals with others, even someone in the cubicle next door, is a powerful motivator and may keep you from giving up.) Losing 30 pounds was a big milestone for this woman and touched off quite a buzz among the regulars. Other members of the group read these messages avidly and live vicariously through her progress; many have been inspired to start their own fitness programmes. Here are some other ways that you can monitor your progress.

Making a goal sheet

Write down your goals on a piece of paper or index card and put it somewhere so that you can see it every day, like stuck on top of your desk or on your refrigerator. Next to every goal, write down the corresponding reward. This strategy isn't just for amateurs. Many world-class athletes use it, too. Figure 2-1 shows a sample goal sheet that you can fill out each week. Underneath each heading, write down your goal and your target date.

Keeping a workout log

Whatever your goals are, keeping track of your workouts in a *workout log* (also called a *workout diary* or *training diary*), as shown in Figure 2-2, can help you get better results. You can look back at the end of each week and say, 'I did that?' And you may be inspired to accomplish even more. Keeping a log shows you whether your goals are realistic and gives you insight into your exercise patterns. If you're losing weight, building strength or developing stamina, you won't have to wonder what works, because you'll have a blow-by-blow description of everything you've done to reach your goals.

Long-Term Goals	Long-Term Rewards
Backup Long-Term Goals	
Short-Term Goals	Short-Term Rewards
Weekly Goals	Weekly Rewards
Workout Goals	Daily Rewards

Figure 2-1:
Make a goal sheet like the one here (or photocopy this one).

Book III

Physical Health: Achieving Fitness

On the other hand, if you get injured or stuck in a rut, you can turn to your diary for clues as to why. You may discover that if you don't eat before you cycle, your usual route takes five minutes longer. Maybe you pull a hamstring every time you run over a certain hilly course. Maybe you're more susceptible to catching a cold if you don't rest at least one day each week.

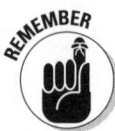

A workout diary keeps you honest. You may think that you're working out four times a week. But when you check through your log, you may realise that you've been overestimating your efforts.

Day of the Week	Date		Conditions	
Goals				
Cardiovascular Training	Time		Distance	Difficulty Rating
Strength Training		Weight	Sets	Reps	Notes
Notes					

Figure 2-2:
A sample
workout log.

Here are some suggestions for filling in the blanks.

Day, date, and conditions

Don't forget to note the day and date. This information helps you assess what you've done in a week; when you look back, you'll know whether you ran those 20 miles in one week or two. Also, you may discover that you always have a bad workout on Fridays because you stay up late Thursday nights to watch *ER*. Maybe Friday is the day for you to take off. Note the day and date of your rest days as well. This way you know how much recovery time you're giving yourself.

In the Conditions box, you may also want to note the weather conditions, including the wind and the temperature, because you work much harder when it's raining or hot. Describe the course you cover (was it hilly or flat?); who you worked out with ('Marge talks too much'); and how you feel before, during and after your workout. These notes may help you trace the root of any training problems that crop up.

Goals for the workout

Write down what you hope to accomplish during your workout, like completing a 20-minute session on the cross trainer or swimming a half-mile. Rather than scribbling a few lines while you're running from the locker room into an aerobics class, fill in this section the night before or, better yet, immediately following your last workout. This makes you stop and think about just what it is you're trying to achieve. If you keep your goals in mind, you may have more enthusiasm for your workout.

Cardiovascular training

Write down the type of activity, whether it's stationary cycling, walking, skating, rowing, and so on. In the Time and Distance sections, note how long your aerobic session lasted and (when applicable) how far you went – for example:

- ✔ **Cardiovascular Training:** 'Jogged on treadmill'
- ✔ **Time:** '20 minutes'
- ✔ **Distance:** '1.8 miles'

Book III

Physical Health: Achieving Fitness

In the Difficulty Rating box, rate your workout on a scale from 1 to 10. Don't base this assessment simply on the number of miles you walked or the number of calories you burned. Instead, rate your workouts according to how hard you push yourself. A 1 rating is an extremely easy day; a 10 is an all-out workout. The purpose of the difficulty rating is to remind you to aim for a healthy mix of numbers. If you rate a 9 on Monday, Tuesday is a good day for a 2 workout. Log a 0 for the days you don't exercise.

Strength training

Jot down the name of each exercise, the amount of weight you lifted, and the number of sets you did. If you don't know the name of an exercise, make it a point to find out. Writing down 'bicep curl' may reinforce the idea that this exercise strengthens your biceps. You may also want to note what changes you need to make during your next weight-lifting session. Suppose you use 25 kilograms on the leg-press machine and have a pretty easy time of it. In your diary, write that you want to try 30 kilograms the next time. Also, note which exercises are particularly easy and which need more attention.

Stretching

Simply note whether you stretched or not. You may also jot down a few words about which muscles felt the tightest and which stretches felt the best.

<u>Notes</u>

Here's your chance to record any details that don't seem to fit into the other categories. For example, you may describe a new leg exercise you tried. Or you may elaborate on which yoga poses you found most difficult. Or you may realise that you always feel great when you work out with a certain friend. Write down whatever you feel is important.

Making Exercise a Habit

Fifty per cent of new exercisers quit within eight weeks. Of course, we want to make sure that you're among the other 50 per cent. The following tips can help you get over the hump and boost the odds that you'll stick with your new programme. We discuss several of these topics in detail throughout the book, but we want you to keep them in mind from the start.

Expect to feel uncomfortable at first

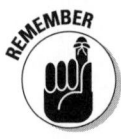

Exercise doesn't need to be painful, but if you've neglected your body, don't expect a free ride. Despite what you hear on infomercials – 'just five minutes a day, and you can do this on the couch while watching TV!' – exercise is a serious commitment. You can't get into shape without exerting some real effort and, perhaps, without experiencing some (but not a lot of) discomfort.

Pace yourself

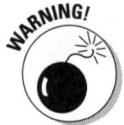

Don't buy every exercise DVD on the market or try every weight machine in the gym the first day. You'll kill your enthusiasm and drop out fast. Always keep yourself hungry for more.

Work out with friends or join a club

An 'exercise buddy' can push you to new heights – or get you outside for a walk on the days when you'd rather stay at home and watch repeats of your favourite TV programme. If you make a date to meet a friend at the gym, you're a lot more likely to show up than if you make a date with yourself.

Take the initiative to find workout buddies by joining an exercise class at your community centre or local gym or a charity event or race that has a training programme.

Mix it up

One common complaint about exercise is that it's boring. But if you change your workouts every couple of months, or even every time you exercise, that excuse pretty much flies out the window. This book is filled with ideas for varying your workouts – experimenting with different weight-training equipment, trying new stretches, and changing the intensity of your cardiovascular programme, doing full-body or body-part workouts, training energy systems, varying the number of repetitions , sets, times, intensity techniques, and so on.

Not only does this strategy keep you motivated, but it also keeps you healthy. Many injuries are the result of repeating the same movement patterns. So if you alternate, say, swimming with running, you're less likely to develop the knee problems that are common to runners or the shoulder injuries that crop up among swimmers.

Buy the right gear and equipment

Cycling isn't going to be fun if you're riding an old clunker that doesn't shift gears properly. Walking isn't going to be comfortable or safe if you're doing it in sandals. You don't need to spend lots of money on top-of-the-line equipment, but investing in the right gear and equipment can sometimes mean the difference between success and failure.

Book III

Physical Health: Achieving Fitness

Here are some tips on shoes, one of the most important fitness purchases:

✔ **Buy the right shoe for your sport.** Walking shoes are more flexible and have firmer heel support than running shoes. Shoes for tennis, golf and basketball have their own special designs; even sprinters and distance runners have different footwear needs. If you dabble in a variety of activities – walking one day, biking the next, and lifting weights the next, *cross training shoes* may suffice (ask for them at your favourite sporting-goods store), but if you spend a lot of time doing one particular activity, invest in shoes designed for that activity.

✔ **Don't go for the cheap option.** Bargain brands may look the same, but today's fitness shoes are highly technical. Beneath those swooshes, stripes and flashy colours, a lot of biomechanical engineering is going on to protect your feet, ankles and other joints. A decent pair of sports shoes may be quite expensive but you save money down the line: One thing that's always more expensive than a good pair of shoes is a visit to an orthopaedist.

✔ **Make sure the shoes feel good from the moment you put them on.** Forget this 'breaking in' business. Try on several pairs of shoes, and take each one for a test run around the shopping centre. Bounce up and down in them; mime a few quick volleys.

Cut yourself some slack

Recognise that people come in all shapes and sizes, and everyone improves at a different pace. Getting inspiration from other people is great, but don't let anyone else's accomplishments diminish your own. Be proud that you've worked up to walking three miles every other day, even if your neighbour runs ten miles a day.

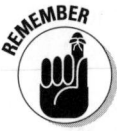

And don't get angry with yourself if you miss a few days – or even a few months – of exercise. Expect to be up and down a bit in your motivation, which means you won't always exercise with the same consistency and frequency. If you let it slip, just try again. You have the rest of your life to get this right.

Chapter 3

Taking an Active Approach to Fitness

*1*n this chapter we take you on a crash course to understand aerobic and cardiovascular exercise. We explain how you can work out what exercise is safe for you, how long to exercise for, when to rest, and how to maintain your fluid intake. We also show you the key elements of designing a fitness plan to boost your health and maximise your fitness.

Cardio Crash Course

If you hang around people who exercise, you're going to hear the word *cardio* pretty often. Someone may say, 'I prefer to do cardio after I lift weights' or 'My gym has great cardio equipment.' *Cardio* – which means 'for your heart' in medical jargon – is short for cardiovascular exercise, the kind that strengthens your heart and lungs and burns lots of calories.

In Book III Chapter 1, we list all kinds of reasons to pursue this sort of exercise – everything from lowering your blood pressure, to sleeping more soundly, to trimming that spare tyre. This section explains how exactly to get those benefits – in other words, what type of exercise counts as cardio. We introduce you to terms such as *aerobic*, *anaerobic* and *target heart rate zone*. After you understand the basic concepts involved in cardio exercise, use the cardio plans near the end of this section to design a cardio workout programme based on your goals.

Two cardio rules that you can't break

You wouldn't try to sell someone a stereo without a few pleasant introductory words to your potential customer, right? You need to ease him into things with a couple of jokes or at least a 'Good morning. How can I help you?' And certainly you wouldn't turn your back on him the minute he handed over his credit card; you'd congratulate him on the purchase and wish him a nice day. Well, the same principles apply to exercise. No matter what type of cardio workout you do – whether it's walking, playing football or mountain-biking – you need to ease into it with a warm-up and ease out of it with a cool-down.

Warming up

A *warm-up* simply means 5 to 15 minutes of aerobic exercise at a very easy pace. For example, runners may start out with a brisk walk or a slow run. If you're going on a hilly bike ride, start with at least a few miles on flat terrain. Be aware that stretching is not a good warm-up activity.

People who are out of shape need to warm up the longest. Their bodies take longer to get into the exercise groove because their muscles aren't used to working hard. If you're a beginner, any exercise is high-intensity exercise. As you get more fit, your body adapts and becomes more efficient, thereby warming up more quickly.

Many people skip their warm-up because they're in a hurry. Cranking up the exercise bike or hitting the weight room right away seems like a more efficient use of time. Bad idea. Skimp on your warm-up, and you're a lot more likely to injure yourself. Besides, when you ease into your workout, you enjoy it a lot more. A trainer we know says: 'If you don't have time to warm up, you don't have time to work out!'

What exactly does warming up do for you? Well, for one thing, a warm-up warms you up – literally. It increases the temperature in your muscles and in the tissues that connect muscle to bone (tendons) and bone to bone (ligaments). Warmer muscles and joints are more pliable and, therefore, less likely to tear. Warming up also helps redirect your blood flow from places such as your stomach and spleen to the muscles that you're using to exercise. This blood flow gives you more stamina by providing your muscles with more nutrients and oxygen. In other words, you tire more quickly if you don't warm up.

Finally, warming up allows your heart rate to increase at a safe, gradual pace. If you don't warm up, your heart rate will shoot up too quickly, and you'll feel like you're walking through a knee-high snowdrift.

What does *aerobic* mean, anyway?

The term *cardio* is often used interchangeably with *aerobic*. Aerobic exercise is any repetitive activity that you do long enough and hard enough to challenge your heart and lungs. To get this effect, you generally need to use your large muscles, including your bottom, legs, back and chest. Brisk walking, cycling, swimming ,a session on the stepper or cross trainer at the gym count as aerobic exercise.

Movements that use your smaller muscles, like those leading into your wrists and hands, don't cut it. Channel surfing with your remote control can certainly be repetitive, sustained and intense – particularly when performed by certain husbands and boyfriends we know – but it's not aerobic.

Aerobic means with air, and *cardio*, coined in the late 1960s by fitness pioneer Dr Kenneth Cooper, means heart. When you exercise aerobically, your body needs an extra supply of oxygen, which your lungs extract from the air.

Think of oxygen as the fuel in your car: When you're waiting at a traffic light, you don't need as much fuel as when you're driving along a motorway. During your aerobic workouts, your body continuously delivers oxygen to your muscles.

However, if you push yourself hard enough, eventually you switch gears into using less oxygen: Your lungs can no longer suck in enough oxygen to keep up with your muscles' demand for it. But you won't collapse, at least right away. Instead, you begin to rely on your body's limited capacity to keep going without oxygen. During this time, you're exercising *anaerobically,* or without air.

Anaerobic exercise refers to high-intensity exercise like all-out sprinting or very heavy weight lifting. After about 90 seconds, you begin gasping for air and you feel a burning sensation in your legs. That's when your body forces you to stop.

Book III

Physical Health: Achieving Fitness

Cooling down

After your workout, don't stop suddenly and make a dash for the shower or collapse on the couch. Ease out of your workout just as you eased into it, by walking, jogging or cycling lightly. If you've been using a cross trainer or stepper at Level 5 for 20 minutes, you could cool down by dropping to Level 4 for a couple minutes, then to Level 3, and so on. This *cool-down* should last 5 to 10 minutes – longer if you've done an especially hard workout.

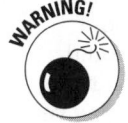

The purpose of the cool-down is the reverse of the warm-up. At this point, your heart is jumping, and blood is pumping furiously through your muscles. You want your body to redirect the blood flow back to normal before you rush back to the office. You also want your body temperature to decrease before you hop into a hot or cold shower; otherwise, you risk fainting. Cooling down prevents your blood from pooling in one place, such as your legs. When you suddenly stop exercising, your blood can quickly collect, which can lead to dizziness, nausea and fainting. If you're really out of shape or at high risk for heart disease, skipping a cool-down can place undue stress on your heart.

How hard do you need to push?

To reap the benefits of cardio exercise, how much huffing and puffing do you need to do? Not as much as you probably think. Sure, you won't benefit much from walking on the treadmill as if you're strolling down the supermarket aisles; they don't call it working out for nothing. On the other hand, exercising too hard can lead to injury and make you more susceptible to colds and infections; plus, you may get so burned out that you want to set fire to your exercise bike. Also, the faster you go, the less time you can keep up the exercise. Depending on what you're trying to accomplish, you may gain just as much, if not more, from slowing things down and going farther.

To get fit and stay healthy, you need to find the middle ground: a moderate, or aerobic, pace. You can find this middle ground in a number of different ways. Some methods of gauging your intensity are extremely simple, and some require a foray into arithmetic. This section looks at three popular ways to monitor your intensity.

The talk test

The simplest way to monitor how hard you're working is to talk. You should be able to carry on a conversation while you're exercising. If you're so out of breath that you can't even string together the words 'Help me, Mummy!' you need to slow down. On the other hand, if you're able to belt out 'Livin' La Vida Loca' at the top of your lungs, that's a pretty big clue that you need to pick up the pace. Basically, you should feel like you're working, but not so hard that you feel like your lungs are about to explode.

Perceived exertion

If you're the type of person who needs more precision in life than the talk test offers, you may like the so-called *perceived exertion* method of gauging intensity. This method uses a numerical scale, typically from 1 to 10, that corresponds to how hard you feel you're working – the rate at which you perceive that you're exerting yourself.

An activity rated 1 on a perceived exertion scale would be something that you feel you could do forever, like sit in bed and watch *Chariots of Fire*. A 10 represents all-out effort, like the last few metres of an uphill sprint, about 20 seconds before your legs buckle. Your typical workout intensity should fall somewhere between 5 and 8. To decide on a number, pay attention to how hard you're breathing, how fast your heart is beating, how much you're sweating, and how tired your legs feel – anything that contributes to the effort of sustaining the exercise.

The purpose of putting a numerical value on exercise is not to make your life more complicated but rather to help you maintain a proper workout intensity. For example, suppose you run two miles around your neighbourhood, and it feels like an 8. If after a few weeks running those two miles feels like a 4, you know it's time to pick up the pace. Initially, you may want to have a perceived exertion chart in front of you. Many gyms post these charts on the walls, and you can easily create one at home. After a few workouts you can use a mental chart. Table 3-1 shows a sample perceived exertion chart.

Table 3-1	Perceived Exertion Chart	
Numerical Rating	*Subjective Rating*	*Sample Activities*
0	Nothing at all	Sitting still, reading
1	Very light	Standing in line
2	Light	Taking a leisurely stroll
3		
4	Light/moderate	
5	Moderate	Walking at a moderate pace, gardening
6		
7	Hard	Jogging briskly, cycling over rolling hills
8	Very hard	Running
9		
10	Extremely hard	Sprinting up a steep hill

Book III

Physical Health: Achieving Fitness

Measuring your heart rate

The talk test and the perceived exertion chart are both valid ways to make sure that you're exercising at the right pace. But there's a more precise way: measuring your *heart rate,* the number of times that your heart beats per minute. (Your heart rate is also called your *pulse.*) You can determine this number either by counting the beats at your wrist or neck or by wearing a gadget called a heart-rate monitor. This section discusses both and also lets you know why you want to measure your heart rate and how you can determine your own target heart-rate zone.

Why monitor your heart rate?

Keeping track of your heart rate, by whatever method, sounds like an incredibly advanced thing to do – something way beyond a beginner's needs. But even if you're just starting out, heart-rate monitoring is abundantly effective.

When you're just starting to work out, you may not have a good sense of how hard to push yourself. And with all that 'no pain, no gain' propaganda, you may be working harder than you really need to. Actually, this happens to advanced exercisers and athletes all the time. Left to their own devices, they try to outdo themselves every day. The smart ones use a heart-rate monitor to remind them to slow down. However, for most people, the problem is getting into a higher gear.

Knowing how hard you're working during a workout is far more helpful than simply knowing how fast you're going. For example, running nine-minute miles on a hot, humid afternoon takes a lot more effort than running at the same pace on a cool, overcast morning. If you rely only on your stopwatch, you may push yourself to run nine-minute miles in the heat, when that pace may put excess stress on your body. If you pace yourself according to your heart rate instead, you know when you need to back off.

The same goes for when you're tired. If you've had a particularly hard week at work, your body may not be up to your usual workout. Without checking your heart rate, you may force yourself to do Level 4 on the cross trainer or stepper, when, in fact, your body isn't up to the task. If you monitor your pulse, you may find that, in order to keep up with Level 4, you have to exceed the high end of your training zone – a signal to drop down a notch or two.

By keeping track of your heart rate over a long period of time, you discover some interesting things about your progress. When you're a beginner, your heart has to work a lot harder to keep up with your body's demands for blood and oxygen. If you work out on a regular basis, your aerobic system gradually becomes more efficient. Suppose when you started, Level 1 on the exercise bike used to get your heart up to about 140 beats per minute; now, two months later, your heart rate is 125 beats per minute. This drop means that you need to step up the difficulty of your workout. You can see why keeping good records of your workouts is a good idea.

To find out how much your fitness level is improving, watch how fast your heart rate drops after a workout. Measure your heart rate immediately upon finishing your exercise session and then one minute later. The better shape you're in, the faster your heart rate drops. Ideally, your heart rate should plunge at least 20 beats in the first minute. People in really good shape drop 40 beats or more. Keep track of this measure. You'll see a gradual improvement over a period of weeks and months. (Taking prescription or over-the-counter medication may affect the way your heart and blood pressure respond to exercise. Check with your doctor about this.)

Your *resting heart rate* is the number of times your heart beats per minute when you're just sitting around. When you start exercising, your resting heart rate may be as high as 90. But after a few months of exercising, your resting heart rate may drop 10 or 20 beats. Some top athletes in endurance sports have resting heart rates as low as 30 beats per minute. However, don't compare your heart rate to anyone else's. Your resting heart rate is partly determined by heredity.

Your resting heart rate can also tell you a lot about your recovery from day to day. Keep your monitor by your bed and strap it on first thing in the morning, on a daily basis. Or, take your pulse manually. If your heart rate is ten beats higher than usual, you probably haven't recovered from yesterday's workout.

Your target heart-rate zone

Your heart rate can tell you so much about your body – how fit you are, how much you've improved, and whether you've recovered from yesterday's workout. But how do you know what heart rate to aim for? There's no magic number. Rather, there's a whole range of acceptable numbers, commonly called your *target heart-rate zone*. This range is the middle ground between slacking off and knocking yourself out. Typically, your *target zone* (as it's called for short) is between 50 per cent and 85 percent of your *maximum heart rate*, the maximum number of times your heart should beat in a minute without dangerously overexerting yourself.

The point at which your body switches from using oxygen as its primary source of energy to using stored sugar is referred to as your *anaerobic threshold*. (You may also hear this referred to as the point at which *lactic acid* builds up.) When you're in poor physical shape, your body isn't very efficient at taking in oxygen, and you hit your anaerobic threshold while exercising at relatively low levels of exercise. As you become more fit, you're able to go farther and faster, yet still supply oxygen to your muscles. If a couch potato tries to run an eight-minute-mile pace, he's going to go anaerobic pretty quickly. An elite runner can run an entire marathon at about a five-minute-mile pace and still stay primarily aerobic.

Book III

Physical Health: Achieving Fitness

At the low end of your zone, you're barely breaking a sweat; at the high end, you're dripping like a Derby winner. If you're a beginner, stick to the lower end so you can move along comfortably for longer periods of time and with less chance of injury. As you get more fit, you may want to do some of your training in the middle and upper end of your zone.

So how do you know what your maximum heart rate is? Well, we don't recommend running as hard as you can until you keel over, and then counting your heartbeats for one minute. A safer and more accurate way is to have your maximum measured by a professional such as a physician or exercise specialist. You can also use a number of mathematical formulae to estimate your maximum.

The most time-honoured method for determining maximum heart rate is for men to subtract their age from 220 and for women to subtract their age from 226. Keep in mind that this formula gives you only an estimate. Your true maximum may be as many as 15 beats higher or lower. Also, this formula is generally used for activities during which your feet hit the ground. (To estimate your max for cycling, subtract about five beats from the final result; for swimming, subtract about ten beats.)

Using that easy formula to find your max, find your target heart-rate zone by calculating 50 per cent and 85 per cent of your maximum. Here's the maths for a 40-year-old man:

$$220 - 40 = 180$$

This is his estimated maximum heart rate.

$$180 \times 0.50 = 90$$

This is the low end of his target zone. If his heart beats less than 90 times per minute, he knows that he's not pushing hard enough.

$$180 \times 0.85 = 153$$

This is the high end of his target zone. If his heart beats faster than 153 beats per minute, he needs to slow down.

Okay, so now you know how to figure out your target heart-rate zone. But how do you know if you're in the zone? In other words, how do you know how fast your heart is beating at any given moment? As we mention earlier in this chapter, you can check your heart rate in two ways: taking your pulse manually or using a heart-rate monitor.

Using a heart-rate monitor

You can eliminate the inaccuracy and inconvenience of taking your heart rate by wearing a heart-rate monitor. With a monitor, you don't need to stop exercising or take the time to count anything. At any given moment you can find out your heart rate by glancing at your wrist. A good monitor can cost less than £25. The really fancy ones cost up to £200. They offer features such as a clock, a timer, and an alarm that you can set to beep when you wander out of your target zone.

Most of the cardio equipment in gyms is now 'heart-rate-monitor compatible'. The machines pick up the signal from the monitor, and your heart rate pops up on the display console, so you don't have to wear the wristwatch. This saves you the trouble of bringing your wrist up to your eyeball while you're moving.

The most accurate type of monitor is the *chest-strap variety,* which operates on the same principle as a medical electrocardiogram (ECG). You hook an inch-wide strap around your chest. This strap acts as an electrode to measure the electrical activity of your heart. This information is then translated into a number, which is transmitted via radio signals to a wrist receiver that looks like a watch with a large face. All you have to do is look at your wrist, and you instantly know how many times your heart is beating that moment, whether it's 92 or 164.

Chest monitors are very accurate, but some are subject to interference from electromagnetic waves like those given off by some treadmills and cross trainer or stepper. (Better, newer models come equipped with coded signals that prevent this interference.) Exercising next to someone else who's wearing a monitor may also scramble signals, a sort of electronic equivalent of getting your braces locked with someone else's when you're kissing. You may need at least four feet between users for monitors to function properly, although several companies now offer models with a special device to eliminate interference.

Less accurate than chest monitors are *photo-optic models*, often sold with home equipment. These clip onto your earlobe or fingertip and detect the heartbeat there. Your heart rate shows up on a handheld or clip-on digital screen or special wristwatch. These models cost only about £20, but any movement of your wrist, hand or fingers can cause highly erratic or false readings. Daylight, poor circulation, and high-intensity exercise may also skew the results.

Following a cardio plan for good health

Book III

Physical Health: Achieving Fitness

If your goal is to feel better and live longer, a little aerobic exercise goes a remarkably long way. Research shows that the people who gain the most from aerobic exercise are those who go from being completely slothful to only marginally slothful – not the ones who go from being fit to super fit. The people in the bottom 20 per cent of the population, fitness-wise, are 65 per cent more likely to die from heart attack, stroke, diabetes or cancer than the highly fit people in the top 20 per cent. However, when those couch potatoes move up just one notch on the fitness scale, by simply adding a daily 30-minute walk, they're only 10 per cent more likely to die from these causes than super-fit people.

If you have no designs on walking the Pennine Way or losing more than three stones, you may want to know the minimum amount of exercise that can make a difference in your health. Here are some answers.

How often you need to do cardio for good health

Research suggests that you can lower your risk of heart disease just by walking for 20 minutes three times a week. This typically is enough exercise to increase your energy level and stamina too, although not enough to cause much in the way of fat loss. If you're a beginner, we recommend working out five or six days rather than three days a week (keeping the workouts short) simply so that you get into the habit of exercising.

How long your workouts should last for good health

If your goal is to improve your health, you don't need to do all your exercise in big chunks. Studies show that doing three ten-minute bouts of aerobic exercise has nearly the same health benefits as doing one half-hour session.

How hard you need to push for good health

If you're simply looking to feel better and improve the quality of your everyday life, being active is the key, even if you don't always reach your target zone (see the 'Your target heart-rate zone' section earlier in this chapter). However, to realise the maximum health benefits – significantly lowering your heart-disease risk, for example – it's wise to work out in your target zone the majority of the time. Plus, even if you have modest goals, you may want to crank up your intensity just to keep things interesting.

Be aware that, when you're a beginner, any exercise you do is high-intensity exercise. As you get more fit, you need to adapt your routine to match your increasing strength and lung power. When Liz's mum started working out, she couldn't complete 10 minutes on the treadmill at 2 mph. After three months, she was able to do 20 minutes at 4 mph – an improvement that in the beginning would have seemed inconceivable.

Following a cardio plan for weight loss

If your goal is permanent fat loss, the 'cardio plan for good health' isn't going to cut it. You simply won't burn enough calories to make a significant impact. Here's why: In order to lose half a kilo in one week, you need to create a 3,500-calorie deficit; in other words, you need to burn off 3,500 more calories than you eat. A 30-minute power walk on flat ground burns about 120 calories. (See the 'The activities that burn the most calories' section later in this chapter.) So, to burn off half a kilo of fat by walking, you'd have to hoof it for more than two hours a day.

Don't worry – we're not suggesting that you exercise two hours every day! In fact, we think the best way to lose fat is to create a calorie deficit by burning calories through exercise and cutting calories you eat. For example, over the course of a week, you may cut 250 calories per day by switching from mayonnaise to mustard on your sandwich at lunch and snacking on low-calorie yoghurt instead of enjoying the extra creamy fruity dessert. Meanwhile, you could burn an extra 250 calories a day by taking a one-hour walk or a half-hour jog.

Here are some general cardio guidelines for weight loss. We suggest that you consult a registered dietician and certified fitness trainer to come up with a plan best suited to your specific goals and schedule.

How often you need to do cardio for weight loss

Here's the cold, hard truth: You probably need to do five or six workouts a week.

How long your workouts should last for weight loss

Here's another dose of reality: You should aim for at least 45 minutes of exercise, a mix of cardio and strength training, six days per week. Again, you don't need to do all this sweating at once, but for the pounds to come off, the calories you burn need to add up.

How hard you need to push for weight loss

To make a serious dent in your fat-loss programme, we suggest that you work out in your target zone most of the time.

During low-intensity aerobic exercise, your body does use fat as its primary fuel source. As you get closer to your breaking point, your body starts using a smaller percentage of fat and a larger percentage of carbohydrates, another fuel source. However, picking up the pace allows you to burn more total calories, as well as more fat calories.

Here's how: If you go in-line skating for 30 minutes at a leisurely roll, you might burn about 100 calories – about 80 per cent of them from fat (so that's 80 fat calories). But if you spend the same amount of time skating with a vengeance over a hilly course, you might burn 300 calories – 30 per cent of them from fat (that's 90 fat calories). So at the fast pace, you burn more than double the calories and 10 more fat calories.

Book III

Physical Health: Achieving Fitness

Of course, going faster and harder is not always better. If you're just starting out, you probably can't sustain a faster pace long enough to make it worth your while. If you go more slowly, you may be able to exercise a lot longer, so you'll end up burning more calories and fat that way.

The activities that burn the most calories

'Maximise your workout and burn over 1,000 calories per hour!' That's a claim you may see in advertisements for treadmills, cross trainers, steppers and other cardio machines. And it's true. You can burn 1,000 calories per hour doing those activities – if you crank up the machine to the highest level and if you happen to have bionic legs. If you're a beginner, you'll last about 30 seconds at that pace, at which point you'll have burned 8.3 calories, and the paramedics will be scooping you off the floor and hauling your wilted body away on a stretcher.

There's a better approach to calorie burning: Choose an activity that you can sustain for a good while – say, at least 10 or 15 minutes. Sure, running burns more calories than walking, but if running wipes you out after a half mile or bothers your knees, you're better off walking.

Table 3-2 gives calorie estimates for a number of popular aerobic activities. The number of calories you actually burn depends on the intensity of your workout, your weight, your muscle mass, and your metabolism. In general, a beginner is capable of burning 4 or 5 calories per minute of exercise, while a very fit person can burn 10 to 12 calories per minute.

The table includes a few stop-and-go sports such as tennis and basketball. Activities like these are not aerobic in the truest sense, but they can still give you a great workout and contribute to good health and weight loss. The numbers in this chart apply to a 10-and-a-half-stone person. (If you weigh less, you'll burn a little less; if you weigh more, you'll burn a little more.)

Table 3-2	Calories Burned during Popular Activities			
Activity	*15 min.*	*30 min.*	*45 min.*	*60 min.*
Aerobic dance	171	342	513	684
Bicycling at 12 mph	142	283	425	566
Bicycling at 15 mph	177	354	531	708
Bicycling at 18 mph	213	425	638	850
Boxing	165	330	495	660
Circuit weight training	189	378	576	756
Gardening	85	170	255	340
Golf (carrying clubs)	87	174	261	348
In-line skating	150	300	450	600
Jumping rope, 60–80 skips/min.	143	286	429	572
Karate, tae kwon do	192	834	576	768
Kayaking	75	150	225	300
Rowing machine	104	208	310	415
Running 10-minute miles	183	365	548	731
Running 8-minute miles	223	446	670	893
Ski machine	141	282	423	564
Slide	152	304	456	608

Activity	15 min.	30 min.	45 min.	60 min.
Swimming free-style, 35 yds/min.	124	248	371	497
Swimming free-style, 50 yds/min.	131	261	392	523
Tennis, singles	116	232	348	464
Tennis, doubles	43	85	128	170
Walking, 20-minute miles, flat	60	120	180	240
Walking, 20-minute miles, hills	81	162	243	324
Walking, 15-minute miles, flat	73	146	219	292
Walking, 15-minute miles, hills	102	206	279	412
Water aerobics	70	140	210	280

Book III

Physical Health: Achieving Fitness

Following a cardio plan to maximise your fitness

When you get the hang of this exercise thing, you may find that you want more of a challenge. Instead of being satisfied with a boost in energy and a decrease in heart-disease risk, you may want to test yourself in a five-kilometre run or a weeklong hiking trek in the Lake District.

The best approach is to increase no more than 10 per cent each week. So, if you walk 150 minutes one week, walk no more than 165 minutes the next.

Treat getting into good cardiovascular shape like a really important ongoing project. You may struggle through the first session, maybe even the first five to ten. But if you stick with it three times a week for at least six weeks, you'll start to notice dramatic changes. At that point, you'll recover much more quickly from your workouts. Instead of going home and crashing on the sofa, you may feel ready to go bowling or out for a walk.

How often you need to do cardio for maximum fitness

Five days a week is a good goal to aim at. Most people feel best with two days off a week; everyone should take at least one day of complete rest. In the 'Giving it a rest' section later in this chapter, we explain how to tell whether you need more rest.

How long your workouts should last for maximum fitness

Depending on your sport and your goal, you probably need to mix in at least a couple long workouts – an hour or more – per week. Just make sure you don't increase the length of your workouts by more than 10 per cent a week; otherwise, your risk of injury becomes pretty high.

How hard you need to push for maximum fitness

Even when you're training to get in your best shape ever, you don't want to go all-out every day. (In fact, only serious athletes peaking for an event should ever go all-out – and even then, only once or twice a week.) Your target zone includes a large range of intensity levels. On some days, stay near the bottom of the range and go for a longer workout; on other days, push harder and go for a shorter workout. Try any or all of the training techniques described in the next section.

Four ways to boost your fitness

You can play plenty of games to challenge your body. This section discusses four training techniques that you can try after about a month or two of training at 50 to 60 per cent of your maximum heart rate. The less conditioning you start with, the more cautious you should be. Try:

- **Interval training:** With *interval training,* you alternate short, fairly intense spurts of exercise with periods of relatively easy exercise. For example, say you're out cycling. After warming up for 15 minutes or so, you may try cycling all-out for 30 seconds and follow this with a few minutes of easy pedalling until your heart rate slows down a little, to about 120 or fewer beats per minute. Then you do another tough 30-second interval, and so on. In essence, you're switching between the low and high ends of your target zone.

  When you first try interval training, keep the high-intensity periods short – 15 to 30 seconds. Follow these periods with at least three times as much active rest (so, 45 to 90 seconds). *Active rest* means that you keep moving between intervals instead of stopping dead. So after you do that 30-second bike sprint, pedal slowly for about 90 seconds. You may need even more recovery than that, especially if you're a beginner. As you become more accustomed to higher levels, you can increase the length of the high-intensity intervals as you decrease the length of the low-intensity intervals. Eventually, you can aim for a 1:1 hard-to-easy ratio, measuring intervals in terms of time or distance.

✔ **Fartlek:** This charming word means 'speed play' in Swedish. *Fartlek* is basically interval training without an exact measure of time or distance. You just do your intervals whenever you feel like it. You may try sprinting to every other telephone pole. Or set your sights on that horse standing in the field down the road and pick up your pace until you reach him.

✔ **Uphill battles:** You can add hills to walking, biking, running or skating workouts. You have to work harder when you come to a hill, but ultimately you're rewarded with extra strength and stamina. As a bonus, going uphill can burn twice as many calories as exercising on flat land. One fun drill is to do hill repeats. Find a long, fairly steep hill and then sprint up it and jog down it, repeating this sequence four to eight times.

Here's a trick to make hill workouts seem easier: Pick a landmark that's partway up the hill, such as a bush or post box. Pretend that you have a rope in your hands and cast it over your landmark. Now pull yourself up the hill with your imaginary rope. When you reach your landmark, cast your rope onto something farther up the hill and keep doing this until you reach the top.

✔ **Tempo workouts:** *Tempo workouts* help you learn to move faster. During a tempo drill, you move at a pace that you consider challenging but not brutal, keeping that pace for four to ten minutes. Do that a couple of times each workout. In between, exercise at your normal pace. If you're new to tempo training, begin with short tempos and gradually increase their length. Anyone training for a local road race or a 'bike-a-thon' will find tempo work helpful.

Training for a specific event

Thinking of training for a five- or ten-kilometre race, a half-marathon, a hundred-mile bike ride or a triathlon? Ideally, you want to spend at least 16 weeks (about 4 months) preparing for your event. Take the first 6 to 10 weeks just getting used to running, cycling, swimming, and so on, slowly building up your weekly mileage by 10 per cent each week. Starting at about 9 to 11 weeks, begin using the techniques listed in the 'Four ways to boost your fitness' section earlier, mixing them into your routine. For example, one week, you might do uphill training one day; the next week, you might try a tempo workout on a Monday and a fartlek on a Thursday. In between, you run, cycle or swim at a more moderate pace or take a day off, allowing your body time to recover before your next workout. By 16 weeks, you should be ready for the big day.

For more specific information about training for a running event, check out Wiley's *Marathon Training For Dummies,* by Tere Stouffer Drenth, which includes information on racing at distances from five kilometres to marathons.

Book III

Physical Health: Achieving Fitness

Giving it a rest

For most people, exercising too much is about as big a problem as saving too much money. However, some beginners – in their zeal to make up for 20 years of neglecting their bodies – vow to exercise every day for the next 20 years. This is not a good idea. If you're trying to get fit, your workouts are only part of the equation; rest is just as important.

Aim for a balance between hard days and easy days. If you do an intense interval day on Monday, do an easy workout Tuesday. If you do two tough days in a row, your legs may feel like someone inserted lead pipes in them while you were sleeping. Everyone should rest at least one day a week. (Just don't let that one day off slip into three years.) And when we say take a rest day, we mean no exercise. Nothing at all. An easy day does not count as a rest day. In addition to taking a day or two off each week, you may also want to take an easy week every month or two. So if you usually jog 15 miles a week, cut back to 7 just for the week. Drastic cutbacks can help re-motivate you and give your body the break it may need.

There's no magic formula to determine exactly how much rest is best for your goals and fitness level. But here's a good rule: If you're doing everything right, you should be able to wake up in the morning and say, 'I know my workout's going to be really good,' rather than, 'How on earth am I going to make it to the gym?'

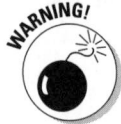

Exercisers of all levels are susceptible to overtraining. For an elite athlete, overtraining might be running 80 miles in a week; for a beginner, running 8 miles might be too much. Here are some signs that you've overdone it:

- ✔ **Your resting heart rate sounds like a pneumatic drill drilling through concrete.** In other words, if your heart rate is way above what it normally is – say, about 10 beats – take it very easy or take a day or two off.

- ✔ **You feel chronically sore or weak.** If you lift a ketchup bottle and it feels like a half-kilo dumbbell, stay at home.

- ✔ **You get chronic colds and infections.**

- ✔ **You're not sleeping well.**

- ✔ **You're irritable, anxious or depressed.** It's not a good sign if your response to locking your keys in your car is smashing the window to retrieve them instead of calling a dealer.

- ✔ **You can't concentrate or you feel disoriented.** If you make a right-hand turn signal while you're on an exercise bike, it's time for a rest.

What happens if you stop exercising?

Aerobic conditioning is a use-it-or-lose-it proposition. A couple of days of inactivity won't set you back, but if you continue to slack off, your improvements fade in a matter of weeks. Research indicates that most of the benefits from aerobic training are lost within two weeks to three months.

But there's good news, too. You can preserve your hard-earned fitness even if you go through a period when you don't exercise as much as usual. Suppose you're a tax accountant. You get into a really good routine of jogging on the treadmill four days a week for a half-hour, and you keep up the routine for four straight months.

Then, suddenly, tax return time arrives, and for two months you're buried in Inland Revenue forms. Well, instead of abandoning exercise altogether, which would practically guarantee that you lose all your conditioning, you can cut back and still maintain your fitness for up to 12 weeks.

Instead of running 30 minutes 4 days a week, you could get by with 30 minutes twice a week or 15 minutes 4 times a week. The only requirement is that you keep up your usual pace. When you get back to your regular routine after dealing with the tax returns, you may find that you've lost no fitness at all – or maybe just a tiny bit.

Knowing why drinking lots of fluids is important

Staying hydrated isn't just important for when you work out. More than 75 per cent of your body is made up of water – even bone is more than 20 per cent water. When you don't drink enough water, your blood doesn't flow properly, and your digestive track doesn't run smoothly. New research even suggests that drinking plenty of water can reduce the risk of breast, colon and urinary tract cancers.

You've probably heard that you need to drink 8 glasses of water a day – 9 to 13 if you exercise. Here's where that number comes from: You typically lose about 2.5 litres of water per day – 500 ml to sweating and evaporation, 500 ml to breathing, and 1.5 litres to waste removal. You can replace up to 500 ml through the water in the foods you eat, but you have to make up the remaining 2 litres by drinking fluids, water being the best choice.

Recent research suggests that you need a much higher fluid intake, from 3 to 6 litres per day. The low end is if you're eating lots of fruits and vegetables (and you are, aren't you?), because those foods are high in fluids. The high end is if you're working out for many hours per day and in hot weather (which we, incidentally, don't recommend). Your fluid intake can come from many sources, as outlined in the following list:

✔ **Water:** Good old-fashioned water is far and away the best way to get your fluids. Water is critical for proper functioning of your organs, so you want to get the majority of your fluids by drinking water. Keep a water bottle with you at all times: on your desk, in your handbag and in your car.

If you don't like the taste of water, you can try filtering your water: Brita and other companies make low-cost filter systems. If you're still not thrilled with the taste of water, try squeezing a slice of lemon into each glass or having a flavoured bottled water instead.

✔ **Sports beverages:** Sports drinks include Gatorade, Powerade, Lucozade and so on, and if you've never tried them, they're actually quite palatable. Most supermarkets also have their own range of sports drinks. The advantage of a sports drink over water is that it includes *electrolytes* like potassium, magnesium, calcium and sodium that you lose as you sweat. Sports drinks can also keep you from getting a stomach-ache after exercising.

The disadvantage is that sports drinks are pretty high in calories, and if you get in the habit of thinking of sports drinks like water, you can easily gain weight. If you really feel you need to include a sports drink after workouts, try to limit your daily intake to 350 ml, just after you finish exercising.

Sports drinks are expensive if you buy them in individual bottles. To save money, buy the powdered version at your local supermarket. You simply mix the powder with water, and you pay less than one-tenth the price with exactly same flavour. You can dilute sports drinks in extra water to reduce calories and sugar content.

✔ **Carbonated sodas and carbonated sports drinks:** Carbonated beverages, including sugary sodas, add calories to your diet without adding any vitamins or other nutrients, and they don't contain the electrolytes that sports beverages offer. Be aware that all carbonated beverages, even carbonated water, also contain phosphates, which can interfere with calcium absorption and may lead to bone-density problems. A treat now and then isn't going to hurt you, though.

✔ **Juice:** 100-per-cent orange juice is rich in potassium, vitamin C and other important vitamins. However, it's high in calories and doesn't really fill you up, so go easy on it. One small glass per day (about 200 ml) is about all you need. You get a better effects by eating the whole fruit, so if you're choosing between the fruit and the juice, go with the fruit – it's more filling than juice and provides additional nutrients.

✔ **Semi-skimmed or skimmed milk:** Two or three 200–300 ml glasses of low-fat or skimmed milk are an excellent source of calcium, but you may not be able to stomach a glass of milk right after working out. If not, try drinking a glass of skimmed milk just before bed (warm it up in the microwave, if you like). In addition to helping you get much-needed calcium, milk has protein, which may help you fall asleep quickly.

✔ **Coffee and tea:** Coffee and tea are hot, tasty beverages, but a better choice is water. However, coffee and tea are fluids that count in your daily total of 2 litres, and if you look forward to your mug(s) of coffee or tea everyday, you don't need to stop drinking it completely. Just limit the total number of mugs, because caffeine can have a dehydrating effect, negating some of the benefits of drinking the fluids in the first place.

Don't rely on thirst to tell you when to drink. By the time your mouth feels parched, you're already mildly dehydrated. Prevent dehydration by drinking all day long. Keep a water bottle at your desk, and always carry a bottle when you work out. You know that you're not drinking enough if your urine is dark and low in volume rather than clear and plentiful. Keep in mind that vitamin supplements can make your urine dark or fluorescent yellow; in this case, volume is a better indicator.

Book III

Physical Health: Achieving Fitness

Chapter 4

Exploring Types of Exercise to Suit Your Lifestyle

*I*n this chapter we cover some of the most popular forms of exercise from the huge range of exercise activities to choose from, so hopefully you can find a type of exercise you like and that suits you. We discuss what you need and offer training strategies and safety tips to help you.

Walking (Those Boots were Made for It)

Can you really get fit by walking? Absolutely – as long as you walk long enough, hard enough and often enough. A recent study found that, among people who are successful in maintaining long-term weight loss, nearly 80 per cent walk as their main physical activity.

The beauty of walking is that it's simply a matter of putting one foot in front of the other. Sure, walking burns fewer calories per minute than jogging, but most people last longer on a walk than a run, so you can make up for the deficit. Plus, compared to runners, walkers enjoy a relatively low injury rate.

Essential walking gear

Although the rest of the animal kingdom does fine without the benefit of special equipment, human feet don't have adequate padding to meet the demands of walking in the modern world. You need a good pair of walking shoes to avoid foot, ankle, knee, hip and lower-back problems.) Replace your shoes when the tread begins to wear thin or when the sides start to cave inwards or outwards.

Walking shoes need to be more flexible than running shoes because you bend your feet more when you walk, and you push off from your toes with more oomph. Also, because your heels bear most of your weight when you walk, you need a firm, stable *heel counter,* the part of the shoe that wraps around your heel to keep your foot in place.

If you plan to hike or walk over rugged terrain, look for a walking shoe with treaded soles and added heel and ankle support. If you're focusing on speed walking or high mileage, go for a little more cushioning in the *midsole,* the area between the tread and the inside of the shoe.

Walking the right way

Okay, we lied to you: There actually is more to walking than simply putting one foot in front of the other. The biggest mistake walkers make is bending forward, a sure way to develop problems in your lower back, neck and hips. Your posture should be naturally tall. You needn't force yourself to be ramrod straight, but neither should you slouch, overarch your back, or lean too far forward from your hips. Relax your shoulders, widen your chest, and pull your abdominals gently inwards. Keep your head and chin up and focus straight ahead.

Meanwhile, keep your hands relaxed and cupped gently, and swing your arms so that they brush past your body. On the upswing, your hand should be level with your breast bone; on the downswing, your hand should brush against your hip. Keep your hips loose and relaxed. Your feet should land firmly, heel first. Roll through your heel to your arch, then to the ball of your foot, and then to your toes. Push off from your toes and the ball of your foot.

Run through a mental head-to-toe checklist every so often to see how you're doing. To find out more about fitness walking (yes, there's plenty more to tell), read *Fitness Walking For Dummies* (published by Wiley).

Fitness walking tips for novices

Although walking is the most basic of all fitness activities, novice fitness walkers can still benefit from the following pointers:

> ✔ **Increase your workout time gradually.** Most people can start off with five 10- to 20-minute walking sessions a week; after about a month, they can increase each workout by 2 or 3 minutes per week until walking 30 to 45 minutes is comfortable. (Five days a week may sound like a lot, but an almost-daily walk makes it easier to get into the habit.)

✔ **Walk as fast as you comfortably can.** If you walk very fast – at a 12-minute-mile to 15-minute-mile pace – you can burn twice as many calories as when you walk at a 20-minute-mile pace. You may not be able to move at such supersonic speeds in the beginning, but as you get fit, you can mix in some fast-paced intervals.

✔ **If you're walking on the side of a road, walk against traffic so you can watch cars approach.** On pavements or footpaths, walk any way you want.

✔ **Add some hills.** Walking over hilly terrain shapes your bottom and thighs and burns extra calories (about 30 per cent more calories than walking on flat terrain, depending, of course, on the steepness of the hills).

✔ **Sneak in a walk whenever you can.** Leave your car at home and hoof it to the train station. Take a 15-minute walk during your lunch break. Traverse the airport on foot rather than on that automatic walking belt. It all adds up.

Increasing the Pace with Running

Like walking, running is a workout that you can take with you anywhere. You don't need a rack on your car or a suitcase full of equipment; you just open the door and go. Plus, as any pathological runner will tell you, nothing is quite as satisfying as getting a good run under your belt. You work up a great sweat, you burn lots of calories, and your muscles feel pleasantly invigorated after you've finished.

No single type of exercise is better than all the rest. It's merely a question of what's best for you. Many runners develop frequent, chronic injuries. Many people have joints that simply will not tolerate all that pounding. If you're not built to run, don't argue with your body. You can get in great condition in other ways. And if you're a beginner, hold off on running until you've built up stamina and strength.

Essential running gear

Treat yourself to a good pair of running shoes (women will also want a supportive jogging bra, too).

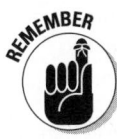

The shoe that's best for you depends on your weight, the shape of your foot, your running style, and any special problems you may have, such as weak ankles or bad knees. Try on several models in the shop, and take each one for a test drive around the shopping centre or at least run a couple of laps around the shop.

Your running shoes should be fairly flexible, especially across the ball of the foot. Hold the shoe at both ends and bend it; it should break right at the ball of the foot. You want cushioning, but not so much that you can't feel your foot hitting the ground. Look for a stable *heel counter* (the part of the shoe that wraps around your heel to keep your foot in place). If your foot slides around a lot, that can mean trouble down the road.

Running the right way

Runners have a habit of looking directly at the ground, almost as if they can't bear to see what's coming next. Keeping your head down throws your upper-body posture off-kilter and can lead to upper-back and neck pain. Lift your head and focus your eyes straight ahead.

Relax your shoulders, keep your chest lifted, and pull your abdominal muscles in tightly. Don't overarch your back and stick your bottom out; that's one of the main reasons runners get back and hip pain.

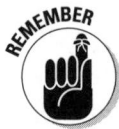

Keep your arms close to your body, and swing them forward and back rather than across your body. Don't clench your fists. Pretend you're holding a butterfly in each hand; you don't want your butterflies to escape, but you don't want to crush them, either.

Lift your front knee and extend your back leg. Don't shuffle along like you're wearing cement boots. Land heel first and roll through the entire length of your foot. Push off from the balls of your feet instead of running flat-footed and pounding off your heels. Otherwise, your feet and legs are going to object long before your cardiovascular system does.

If you experience pain in your ankles, knees or lower back, stop running for a while. If you don't, you could end up having to sit on the sidelines for months.

Running tips for novices

These tips help you get fit and avoid injury.

- ✔ **Start by alternating periods of walking with periods of running.** For example, try two minutes of walking and one minute of running. Gradually decrease your walking intervals until you can run continuously for 20 minutes. If you have the inclination, you can build from there. Of course, sticking with a walk/run routine is fine; you're less likely to injure yourself that way.

- ✔ **Vary your pace.** Different paces work your heart, lungs and legs in different ways.

✔ **Always run against traffic when running on the side of a road.** This allows you to see oncoming cars and dive for the side of the road, if necessary. If you're running on steeply cambered (angled away from the centre line) country roads and the road is flat, you can run in the middle of the road to save wear and tear on your legs. But as you head up or down hills, get as far over to the side (that is, away from the road) as possible to avoid speeding cars mowing you down. Consider carrying a lightweight mobile phone for emergencies.

✔ **Don't increase your mileage by more than 10 per cent a week.** If you run 5 miles a week and want to increase, aim to do 5½ miles the following week. Jumping from 5 miles to 6 miles doesn't sound like a big deal, but studies show that if you increase your mileage by more than 10 per cent, you set yourself up for injury.

Cycling: Road and Mountain

Talk to a group of cyclists and, chances are, you're talking to a group of ex-runners. Cycling is perfect for people who can't take the relentless pounding of running or find the slow pace a real drag. Cycling is the best way to cover a lot of ground quickly. Even a novice can easily build up to a 20-mile ride.

Cycling can be a hassle. You can't just grab your shoes and head out the door. You need your helmet, water bottle, gloves, sunscreen and glasses. And even with all your protective gear, you can never be too cautious. Cycling is a low-impact sport – unless you happen to impact the ground, a car, a tree, a rut or another cyclist.

Essential cycling gear

If you haven't owned a bike since grammar school, prepare yourself for a shock. *Mountain bikes,* the fat-tyre bikes with upright handlebars, are somewhat less expensive than comparable *road bikes,* the kind with the curved handlebars. Don't take out a second mortgage to buy a fancy bike, but if you have any inkling that you may like this sport, don't skimp, either. You'll just end up buying a more expensive bike later.

Generally, the more expensive the bike, the stronger and lighter its frame. A heavy bike can slow you down, but unless you plan to enter the Tour de France, don't get hung up on a matter of ounces. Cheaper bikes are made from different grades of steel; as you climb the price ladder, you find materials such as aluminium, carbon fibre and titanium. The price of a bike also depends on the quality of the *components* – the mechanics that enable your bike to move, shift gear and brake.

Book III

Physical Health: Achieving Fitness

Cheaper bikes come with *toe clips* (pedal straps) that enable you to pull up on the pedal as well as push down. But you can pull up even more efficiently with clipless pedals, which lock into cleats affixed to the bottom of your cycling shoes. These pedal systems are like ski bindings: You're locked in, but your feet pop out easily when you fall. To clip out, you simply twist your foot to the side.

Beginners usually have an accident or two with clipless pedals because they haven't developed the instinct to twist sideways. Suzanne once tipped over with both feet clicked into her pedals. We'll spare you the details of her injury, but let's just say that she ended up at the gynaecologist.

Find a bike dealer you trust and be aware that bike prices are negotiable. Ask the salesman to throw in a few free extras, like a bike computer to measure your speed and distance or a seat bag to carry food and tools.

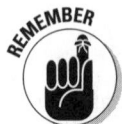

Don't even think about pedalling down your street without a helmet snug atop your noggin. Cycling gloves make your ride more comfortable and protect your hands when you crash. Glasses are important to protect your eyes from the dust, dirt and gravel.

Buy a pair of padded cycling shorts and a brightly coloured cycling jersey so that you can easily be seen. Unlike cotton T-shirts, jerseys wick away sweat so that you won't freeze on a downhill after you worked up a big sweat climbing up. Plus, jerseys have pockets in the back deep enough to hold lots of snacks. Always carry a water bottle or wear a hydration pack. Finally, carry gear to change a flat tyre – and learn how to use it. There's no cycling equivalent of the AA to come and save you.

Cycling the right way

To protect your knees from injury, position your seat correctly (ask your salesperson for advice) and pedal at an easy cadence. *Cadence* refers to the number of revolutions per minute that you pedal. Inexperienced cyclists tend to use a higher gear than they can handle, which forces them to turn the pedals in slow motion; their legs tire prematurely, their knees ache, and they cheat themselves out of a good workout. Get in the right gear so that you're pedalling at a comfortable cadence.

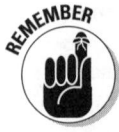

Road cycling can wreak havoc on your lower back because you're in a crouched position for so long. Relax your upper body and keep your arms loose. Grasp your handlebars with the same tension as you'd use to hold a child's hand when you cross the street. Pedal in smooth circles rather than simply mashing the pedals downward. Imagine that you have a bed of nails in your shoes, and you have to pedal without stomping on the nails.

Cycling tips for novices

You can learn a lot about cycling – and get faster in a jiffy – by riding with a club or friends who have more experience. Here are some pointers to start your cycling career:

- ✔ **Remember that you are a vehicle and are required to follow the rules of the road.** Ride with traffic, not against it.

- ✔ **Stop at all signs and lights, and use hand signals.** Don't trust a single car – ever. Assume that the driver doesn't see you, even if he happens to be staring you in the face.

- ✔ **When you go off-road, start on wide paths or cycle tracks rather than narrow 'single-track' paths that require technical skills.** And don't think that you're immune to injury because there are no cars. More crashes happen on mountain tracks than on the road because there are more obstacles and riders get careless and cocky.

- ✔ **Head into a turn at a slow enough pace so that you maintain control, and never let your eyes wander from the road or track.** Never squeeze the brakes – particularly the front brake – with a lot of pressure. You'll go flying over the handlebars, a manoeuvre we would not recommend.

Diving Into Swimming

Swimming is truly a zero-impact sport. Although you can strain your shoulders if you overdo it, there's absolutely no pounding on your joints, and the only thing you're in danger of crashing into is the wall of the pool. You can get a great aerobic workout that uses your whole body. Plus, water has a gentle, soothing effect on the body, so swimming is helpful for those with arthritis or other joint diseases.

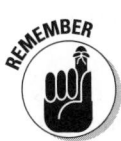

Swimming is great for people who want to keep exercising when they're injured and for people who are pregnant or overweight. That extra body fat helps you glide along near the surface of the water, so you don't expend energy trying to keep yourself from sinking like a stone.

Swimming the right way

You'll probably spend the bulk of your workouts doing the front crawl, also called *freestyle*. It's generally faster than the other strokes, so you can cover more distance. Don't cut your strokes short; reach out as far as you can, have your hand enter thumb-first so it slices the water like a knife, and pull all the way through the water so your hand brushes your thigh. Use an S-shaped sculling movement, where your hand moves out, then in, then out again

Book III

Physical Health: Achieving Fitness

across your body/thigh and out of the water. Elongate your stroke so that you take fewer than 25 strokes in a 25-metre pool. The fewer the strokes, the better. Top swimmers get so much power from each stroke that they take just 11 to 14 strokes per length of a 25-metre pool.

Kick up and down from your hips, not your knees. Don't kick too deeply or allow your feet to break the water's surface. Proper kicking causes the water to 'boil' rather than splash.

Breathe through your mouth every two strokes, or every three strokes if you want to alternate the side that you breathe on. You need as much oxygen as you can get. Beginners sometimes make the mistake of taking six or eight strokes before breathing, which wears them out quickly. To breathe, roll your entire body to the side until your mouth and nose come out of the water – imagine that your entire body is on a skewer and must rotate together. Don't lift your head out of the water to breathe – you'll spend a lot of energy doing that, and it'll slow you down in the water.

Swimming tips for novices

Even if you're the queen of your aerobics class or a champion at cycling uphill, you may still tire quickly in the pool at first. More than almost any other aerobic activity, swimming relies on technique. The following tips can help you get the most out of your swimming workouts.

- ✔ **Take a few lessons if you haven't swum in a while.** Beginners waste a lot of energy flailing and splashing around rather than moving forward.

- ✔ **Break your workout into intervals.** For example, don't just get into the pool, swim 20 laps, and get out. Instead, do 4 easy laps for a warm-up. Then do 8 sets of 2 laps at a faster pace, resting 20 seconds between sets. Then cool down with two easy laps, and maybe a few extra laps with a float. Mix up your strokes, too. The four basic strokes – freestyle, backstroke, breaststroke and butterfly – use your muscles in different ways.

- ✔ **If swimming is your bag, join a swim club.** Swimming clubs, often located at your local leisure centre, are geared towards adult swimmers of all levels. A coach gives you a different workout every time you swim and monitors your progress. Best of all, you have fellow swimmers to work out with. Don't worry about being slow; the coach will group you in a lane with other people your speed. If you have a competitive spirit, you can compete in club competitions, where you swim against others who are roughly your speed.

- ✔ **If you find swimming a big yawn but enjoy being in the water, try water running or water aerobics.** Water running is a pretty tough workout because the water provides resistance from all directions as you move your legs. It's an excellent workout for injured runners because, even though it's non-impact and easy on your joints, it helps maintain aerobic conditioning. Don't assume that water aerobics is for little old ladies in flowered caps. With the right instructor and exercise programme, you can get a challenging water-aerobics workout. Water running can be even tougher.

Circuit Training for Fitness and Fun

Circuit training is a unique method of working out that combines cardiovascular exercise with strength training. Circuit training includes a warm-up, followed by a succession of strength-building exercises at *stations* (in between which you walk fast or run), followed by a cool down. (Note that a station can be just a spot where you do push-ups; it doesn't have to be anything fancy.) You get to decide how long your total workout will be, how many stations you'll include, and what exercises you'll do at those stations. Workouts are fun, the time flies by, and within just a few weeks of doing circuits two days per week, most people notice a big difference in the strength of their arms, legs, abdomen and buttocks.

Setting up stations and knowing which exercises to do

Have you even seen a circuit-training area at your local park? Along a trail, stations appear periodically, and at those stations are instructions for doing push-ups or pull-ups or a variety of other strengthening exercises.

You don't need to use the stations set up at your local park, though. Your local gym may have a circuit-training class or may have a self-paced circuit routine that you can do in your own time. You can also easily set up stations in your own home. If you have a weight machine, you're way ahead of the game and can do most of the weight-lifting exercises there. But if you don't, gather up the following inexpensive equipment and set up stations in your exercise room, spare bedroom, (dry) basement, garage, garden (in good weather), or any other place you can think of:

- A sit-up mat or thick towel (for sit-ups, push-ups, crunches, Pilates exercises)

- One pair each of 0.5–7-kilogrm weights (for curls, shrugs, upright rows, punches, and so on)

- A weight bar with however much weight you can handle for squats

- A sturdy chair or ledge (for chair dips)

- A pull-up bar secured in a doorway (for pull-ups, hanging abs)

- A stairway or step (for step-ups, single-leg squats, toe raises)

Arrange each of these so that they're 10 to 20 feet apart; a circle or square can work, but so can a zigzag pattern, as long as you have some room to walk quickly or run between stations. If you need to place the stations closer than this – say, right next to each other – that's fine. Just do jumping jacks, jump rope, or run in place with high knees for ten seconds between exercises.

For detailed coverage of all these exercises, get a copy of *Weight Training For Dummies,* 2nd Edition (published by Wiley).

At each station, you can do several different exercises, as described in the following sections. However, you can easily forget what exercise you're supposed to do when you get to a station, so we suggest putting a sheet of paper at each station that lists, in order, the one, two or three exercises that you're planning to doing there.

Arm-strengthening stations

Because the warm-up, cool down, and movement between stations work your leg muscles, many people emphasise arm-strength stations in their circuit routines, focusing as many as half of the total number of stations on their arms.

This list is not meant to be exhaustive. If you get results from other arm-strengthening exercises, put those on your circuit. This list is also not meant to imply that you'll include all these exercises in your circuit. You can pick and choose from the list, as best suits your needs.

Dumbbell biceps curl

This exercise, as you may expect, works the biceps. Hold a dumbbell in each hand and stand with your feet as wide apart as your hips. Let your arms hang down at your sides with your palms forward. Pull your abdominals in, stand tall, and keep your knees relaxed. Curl both arms upwards until they're in front of your shoulders. Slowly lower the dumbbells back down and repeat.

Punches

Punches work your shoulders and upper arms. Take a dumbbell in each hand, put each hand in front of its respective shoulder, and stand with your legs wider than shoulder-width apart, abdominals pulled in. Take your right hand, cross it over your body, and punch out to the left. To keep your knees healthy, roll up to your toes on your right leg as you punch out your right arm. Repeat with your left side and vice versa.

Upright rows

Upright rows work the shoulders. While standing, hold a dumbbell in each hand and put the ends of the two weights together, holding your hands right in front of your thighs. Pull your abdominals in. Keeping the weights together, pull your hands up to your collarbone. Lower and repeat.

If you've had any shoulder (specifically, deltoid) injuries, steer clear of upright rows. Instead, do shoulder presses.

One-arm dumbbell row

This exercise works the lats (the widest part of your back just behind your armpit) and biceps. Stand to the right of your weight bench, holding a dumbbell in your right hand with your palm facing in. Place your left knee and your left hand on top of the bench for support. Let your right arm hang down and a bit forward. Pull your abdominals in and bend forward from the hips so your back is naturally arched and roughly parallel to the floor, and your right knee is slightly bent. Tilt your chin towards your chest so that your neck is in line with the rest of your spine. Pull your right arm up until your elbow is pointing to the ceiling, your upper arm is parallel to the floor, and your arm brushes against your waist. Lower the weight slowly back down and repeat.

Push-ups

Push-ups work all the upper-body muscles. Facing the ground, rest your body on your hands and tiptoes, and keep your back and legs perfectly straight. Pull in your abdominals, lower your chest to the ground, and raise your chest back up again by pushing against the ground until your elbows are nearly locked. Repeat. As push-ups become easier for you, try elevating your feet, which makes this exercise much harder.

Shrugs

Shrugs work your trapezius and upper-back muscles. Plant your feet shoulder-width apart. Take a dumbbell in each hand, relax your arms by letting them hang down at your sides, and relax your shoulders. Pull in your abdominals. Without bending your elbows, raise and lower your shoulders. Repeat.

Dumbbell chest press

Working the chest, triceps and shoulders, this exercise is an all-time favourite. Lie on a bench with a dumbbell in each hand and your feet flat on the floor. Push the dumbbells up so that your arms are directly over your shoulders and your palms up. Pull your abdominals in, and tilt your chin towards your chest. Lower the dumbbells down and a little to the side until your elbows are in line with or just slightly below your shoulders. The weights should be directly above the elbow joints, which should create a 90-degree angle. Push the weights back up in a triangular motion to where the weights are directly above your chest, taking care not to lock your elbows or allow your shoulder blades to rise off the bench. Repeat. You can also substitute the bench press if you have a weight machine handy.

Dumbbell shoulder press

Shoulder presses work your shoulders, as well as your triceps and upper back. Hold a dumbbell in each hand and sit on a bench with back support. Plant your feet firmly on the floor about hip-width apart. Bend your elbows and raise your upper arms to shoulder height so that the dumbbells are at ear level. Pull your abdominals in so that there is a slight gap between the small of your back and the bench. Place the back of your head against the pad. Push the dumbbells up and in until the ends of the dumbbells touch lightly directly over your head, and then lower the dumbbells back to ear level. Repeat.

Triceps dips

Triceps dips really work your triceps; in fact, you may find that you can do only one or two dips the first time you attempt this exercise. Use a sturdy chair, ledge, or seat of a weight bench. Extend your legs with your heels on the ground and rest your hands on the outside edge of the chair with your elbows locked. Pull in your abdominals; keep your shoulders back, down, and not rounded; and pull your chest up. Bending your elbows, lower your bottom to the ground and then push yourself back up until your elbows lock again. Repeat.

If you find that you can't lower yourself all the way to the ground and still come back up, lower just half the distance to the ground and do as many that way as you can.

Triceps kickback

Not to be exceedingly obvious, but this exercise works your triceps! Stand to the right of your weight bench, holding a dumbbell in your right hand with your palm facing in. Place your left lower leg and your left hand on top of the bench. Lean forwards at the hips until your upper body is at a 45-degree angle to the floor. Bend your right elbow so that your upper arm is parallel to the floor, your forearm is perpendicular to it, and your palm faces in. Keep your elbow close to your upper arm. Pull your abdominals in and relax your knees. Keeping your upper arm still, straighten your elbow behind you until your entire arm is parallel to the floor and one end of the dumbbell points down. Slowly bend your arm to lower the weight. Repeat. On the second circuit, do the exercise with your left arm.

Leg-strengthening stations

Because your warm-up, cool down, and travel between stations is leg-intensive, you don't need to include a lot of leg-strengthening exercises in your circuit routine. The exercises in this section, however, are some of our favourites.

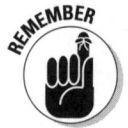

If you have a weight bench with attachments at your disposal, you can add leg extensions, leg curls, leg presses, and any other exercises the machine supports.

Step-ups

Step-ups work nearly every muscle in your leg, as well as your bottom muscles. To do this exercise, you need a step – one of the steps on the bottom of a stairway can work well. However, buying a step-aerobics platform and placing two sets of risers underneath the platform (to a height of 10 to 12 inches) may be more convenient (because it's portable). You simply keep walking or running up and down the one step. Step up on one step and then bring the other leg up on that step, too. Then step back down, following with the other leg. Then up the step again, then back down, and so on.

Single-leg squats

Single-leg squats work your bottom and upper legs and help develop balance. Stand on your right leg at the edge of the step, so that the instep of your right foot comes right to the edge of the step and your left leg is dangling off the step. Pull in your abdominals and bend your right leg on the step at the knee as you push your hips back, sinking into your right heel, until the heel of your left leg just touches the ground. Lead with your right heel, not your toes; straighten the leg on the step. Repeat. On the second circuit, use the other leg.

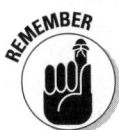

The heels of both feet should be along the same horizontal line. Also, you may need to hang on to something (perhaps a railing) to keep yourself from falling.

Standing calf raise

Standing calf raises work your calves and shins and help develop balance. Stand on the edge of a step or, if you have a step-aerobics platform, place two sets of risers underneath the platform. Stand tall with your abdominals pulled in, the balls of your feet firmly planted on the step, and your heels hanging over the edge. Rest your hands against a wall or a sturdy object for balance. Raise your heels a few inches above the edge of the step so you're on your tiptoes. Hold the position for a moment, and then lower your heels below the platform, feeling a stretch in your calf muscles. Repeat. On the second circuit, use the other leg.

If you find one-legged calf raises too challenging at first, try doing this exercise with both legs.

Lunge

Lunges are amazing for your bottom, hips and upper legs. Stand upright with your feet shoulder-width apart. Take a large step forward, and plant your foot on the ground. Keeping your front knee completely stable and your upper body perfectly vertical, lower your body straight down until your back knee nearly touches the ground. Raise your body straight up and repeat with another step. Keep repeating.

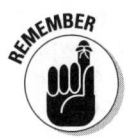

Don't allow your torso to lean forward and be sure to evenly distribute your body weight on both legs. Think of your torso as having a pole placed directly down the centre, like a horse on a merry-go-round, and go up and down, not back and forth. Also keep in mind that the farther you step out, the more emphasis is placed on the bottom and hamstrings; the more shallow your step, the more emphasis is placed on the quads. Finally, when you're in the down position, both knees should form a 90-degree angle, and you should be able to see the tip of your shoe or toes.

Book III

Physical Health: Achieving Fitness

Working your abdomen, bottom and lower back

These exercises help you develop great abs, a nice bottom, and a healthy lower back. This list is not anywhere near all-inclusive, however. In fact, setting up Pilates stations to work your core is an excellent circuit-training option. For more Pilates exercises, check out Book IV. To get the full lowdown, pick up a copy of *Pilates For Dummies* by Ellie Herman (published by Wiley).

Basic crunch

Crunches primarily work the upper region of the abs. In Pilates they're called Upper Abdominal Curls. Lie on your back with your knees bent and feet flat on the floor, hip-width apart. Place your hands extended out towards your knees, across your chest, above your head, or behind your head so your thumbs are behind your ears – depending on what's comfortable for you. Don't lace your fingers together. Hold your elbows out to the sides but rounded slightly in. Tilt your chin slightly, leaving a few inches of space between your chin and your chest. Relax your back into a neutral spine (neutral spine helps maintain the natural curve in the spine. There should be space between the lower back by the lumber spine and the floor – see Book IV Chapter 7 for more on neutral spine). Maintaining the natural curve prevents lower back and neck strain. Gently pull your abdominals inwards whilst maintaining the neutral spine position. Curl up and forward so that your head, neck and shoulder blades lift off the floor. Hold for a moment at the top of the movement and then lower slowly back down. Repeat.

Hanging abs

Hanging abs work the lower region of the abs. Using a pull-up bar or hanging-ab apparatus (ask about it at your gym), hang from the bar, pull in your abdominals, and then lift your knees towards your chest, tucking the pelvis under and causing your spine to round. Lower your legs slowly back to the hanging position. Repeat.

Oblique curls

These curls work the *obliques,* the sides of your core area midsection. Lie on your right side with your arms crossed in front of you. Bending sideways at your waist, lift your upper body off the ground a few inches. You may need to brace your feet under a bar or sturdy piece of furniture. Repeat. On your second circuit, lie on your left side.

Back extension

Back extensions are a great exercise for your lower back. Lie on your stomach, looking down at the floor, arms straight out in front of you, palms down, and legs straight out behind you. Pull your abs in, as if you're trying to create a small space between your stomach and the floor. Lift your left arm and right leg about an inch off the floor, and stretch out as much as you can. Hold this position for five slow counts and then lower your arm and leg back down. Repeat the same move with your right arm and left leg. Continue alternating sides until you complete the set.

Squat

Squats work your bottom and upper legs. Either with your hands on your hips or holding dumbbells with your arms down at your sides (you can also hold your arms out in front of your torso or your fists in at your chest to create a counterbalance, or put them in the overhead position to challenge your posture), stand with your feet as wide apart as your hips and place your weight slightly back on your heels. Let your arms hang down at your sides. Pull your abdominals in and stand tall with square shoulders. Sit back and down, as if you're sitting into a chair. Lower as far as you can without leaning your upper body more than a few inches forward. Don't lower any farther than the point at which you're parallel to the floor, and don't allow your knees to shoot out in front of your toes. When your thighs are parallel to the floor, straighten your legs and stand back up. Don't lock your knees at the top of the movement.

Moving through sample stations

The beauty of circuit training is that you can set up the stations any way you want. You can do each exercise once in the circuit, or you can repeat an exercise two or more times in one circuit. Your circuit can include 5 exercises or 25. You get to decide, see what works for you, tweak the circuit, do it some more, and so on.

Be sure to arrange your circuit so you alternate stations that use similar muscles. In other words, do an exercise for your abdomen, then arms, then legs, then your back, and then go back to abdomen, arms, and so on. Or, if you want to do an arm-intensive circuit, set up a station for your arms, then legs, then arms, then back, then arms, then abdomen, then arms, and so on. Either way, give your muscles a little time to rest before working them again.

Here's a sample way of ordering the exercises. This gives you 21 exercises for your circuit. See the following section for step-by-step instructions on how you work these 21 exercises into a circuit-training workout.

- ✔ Triceps kickbacks
- ✔ Basic crunches
- ✔ Dumbbell biceps curls
- ✔ Step-ups
- ✔ Dumbbell shoulder presses
- ✔ Back extensions
- ✔ Single-leg squats
- ✔ Push-ups
- ✔ Hanging abs

Book III

Physical Health: Achieving Fitness

- ✔ Tricep dips
- ✔ One-arm dumbbell rows
- ✔ Lunges
- ✔ Dumbbell chest presses
- ✔ Obliques curls
- ✔ Upright rows
- ✔ Standing calf raises
- ✔ Shrugs
- ✔ Squats
- ✔ Punches

Putting the Stations Together into a Circuit

After your stations are set up and you've determined an order to follow, follow these circuit-training steps:

1. **For your warm-up, either outside or on indoor equipment, run, walk, cycle, swim, or do any other cardiovascular activity for 5 to 20 minutes, depending on how much you're currently working out each day, and how long you want your overall workout to be.**

2. **When you get back, *immediately* begin your circuit-training workout.**

   You can stop for a quick drink of water, if you absolutely need it. But don't walk around or chit-chat with neighbours or anything like that. Do your warm-up, and then go right to the first station, where you want to ease into your first few strength exercises by using slow, methodical movements.

3. **Set the timer on your watch for 20 to 45 seconds (start on the low end, and gradually build up) and before you begin doing an exercise at the first station, start the timer.**

4. **When your watch beeps, briskly walk or run to the next station, set the timer again, and immediately begin doing the next exercise.**

5. **When the watch beeps again, proceed to the next station, and so on.**

6. **Repeat the entire circuit (all the exercises) at least once.**

   You can do as many circuits as you choose. If you've set up five stations with three different exercises you're going to do at each, and you've set your timer for 30 seconds, the circuit routine is going to take you 7½ minutes, plus walking/running time between stations, so the entire circuit may take you 10 minutes. Given this scenario, you could do three circuits, which gives you a 30-minute workout, plus your warm-up and cool down, which gives you a grand total of 50 to 75 minutes of exercise! Not bad.

7. **When you finish the last circuit, immediately begin your 10- to 15-minute cool down.**

8. **Stretch immediately after finishing your cool down.**

Why Lifting Some Weights is Good for You

Maybe you've never considered yourself the weight-lifting type. Maybe you suspect that the size of one's muscles is inversely proportional to the size of one's brain. Maybe when you see a hulking guy on the street, you think, 'He may be able to bench-press my minivan, but I can read a menu in French.'

The truth is, weight-lifting is an incredibly smart thing to do. It's not just a form of narcissism, and it's not just for body-builders. These days, even 80-year-olds are pumping iron. In this section, we explain why you should, too. We also dispel popular weight-training myths and tell you what kind of results you can reasonably expect. If you think lifting weights seems too boring, too dangerous, too troublesome, or too likely to transform you into Hulk Hogan, we hope this section changes your mind.

First, a quick note: Throughout this section, we use the terms *weight-lifting*, *weight training*, and *strength training* interchangeably, even though you don't necessarily need weight to build strength. *Resistance training* means the same thing, but we spare you that bit of verbiage.

Book III

Physical Health: Achieving Fitness

Five important reasons to pick up a dumbbell

People who start lifting weights regularly will tell you how much more fit, powerful and energetic they feel . . . but enough about feelings. There's plenty of good, solid evidence that strength training does all that and more. We bet that at least one of the following reasons will get you to hoist some iron.

Stay strong for everyday life

If you don't exercise you will lose strength as the years go by. Strength is one of the easiest physical abilities to retain as you get older. Just by lifting a small amount of weight you can boost your muscle strength.

Keep your bones healthy

Keeping your bones healthy can help prevent osteoporosis. Osteoporosis is very common. It is a disease of severe bone loss that causes fractures of the back, hip and wrist, in particular.

Osteoporosis isn't something that happens to you overnight, like becoming eligible for an over-60 discount at the cinema. Most people start out with strong, dense bones – imagine them as poles of steel. But around age 35, most people – men included – begin to lose about ½ to 1 per cent of their bone each year. (For women, bone loss accelerates after menopause – 1 to 2 per cent a year for the first five years and then about 1 per cent annually until age 70. Then the loss slows back to ½ per cent a year.) If you do everything right, however, you can decelerate this bone loss significantly – by about 50 per cent. If you've already lost a lot of bone, you may even be able to build some of it back. Strength training alone can't stop bone loss, but it can play a big role. Also important are calcium, vitamin D, and aerobic exercise such as walking and jogging. (Swimming and cycling don't work because your body weight is supported, either by the water or the bike; when you have to support your own self, your bones respond by building themselves up.)

Strong muscles and strong bones go hand in hand. The more weight you can lift, the more stress you can put on your bones; this stress is what stimulates them. The first astronauts to spend time in space experienced significant bone-density loss. In space, not only does no one hear you scream, but you're weightless – there's no load placed on your muscles and bones. Today's astronauts prevent bone loss by exercising several hours a day.

Prevent injuries

When your muscles are strong, you're less injury-prone. You're less likely to step off a kerb and twist your ankle. Plus, you have a better sense of balance and surefootedness, so you're less apt to take a tumble during a weekend game of tag rugby. Research shows that one out of every three people over age 65 falls at least once a year. Almost 10 per cent of older people who fall are hospitalised for an injury, and about half of those cases involve broken bones.

Look better

Now let's talk about pure, unadulterated vanity. Aerobic exercise burns lots of calories, but weight-lifting firms, lifts, builds and shapes your muscles. A marathon runner may be able to go the distance, but he won't turn any heads on the beach if he has a concave chest and string-bean arms. (He might also be a faster runner if he pumped up a bit.)

We want to be clear here: There's no such thing as spot reducing – that is, selectively zapping fat off a particular part of your body. But you can pick certain areas, such as your bottom or your arms, and reshape them through weight training. And if you have wide hips or a thick middle, you can bring your body more into proportion by doing exercises that broaden your shoulders and back.

Weight training also makes you look better by improving your posture. With strong abdominal and lower-back muscles, you stand up straighter and look more svelte even if you haven't lost an ounce.

Speed up your metabolism

The only way to increase your metabolism is to build muscle, which you can best accomplish by lifting weights.

How does this work? First, a couple of definitions: Your *metabolism* refers to the number of calories you're burning at any given moment, whether you're watching your favourite television programme or riding a bike. But when most people use the term, they're referring to your resting metabolism: the number of calories your body needs to maintain its vital functions. Your brain, heart, kidneys and other organs are cranking away 24 hours a day, and your muscle cells are constantly undergoing repair. All these processes require energy in the form of calories simply to keep you alive.

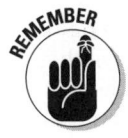

But here's the key: Your resting metabolic rate depends primarily on your amount of *fat-free mass* – everything in your body that's not fat, including muscle, bones, blood, organs and tissue. The more fat-free mass you have, the more energy your body expends in order to keep going. So, you want to be muscular. You can't do anything to increase the size of your liver or brain, but you certainly can make yourself more muscular, and lifting weights is the primary way to do just that.

Keep in mind, however, that packing on a few more kilos of muscle isn't going to turn your body into a calorie-burning inferno. For every half-kilo of muscle you gain, your body may burn an extra 30 to 50 calories per day. That's not a lot, especially if you compensate by eating an extra chocolate bar. One Mars Bar contains 280 calories; a Cadbury's cream egg is 174 calories. However, in the long run, even that small metabolic boost can be significant. If you burn an extra 25 calories per day, you can burn 9,125 calories in a year – enough to lose nearly 3 pounds, or at least prevent a 3-pound weight gain. And if you add 10 pounds of lean muscle, you can burn an additional 300 to 500 calories per day!

If that's not impressive, consider the flip side: If you don't lift weights, your metabolism will slow down every year, as your muscles slowly waste away. And with a more sluggish metabolic rate, you'll gain weight even if you eat the same amount of food. How's that for an incentive to hit the weights room?

One final point: The metabolism-boosting benefits of weight-lifting are particularly important if you're cutting calories to lose weight. Dieting alone tends to cause a loss of muscle as well as fat; if you lift weights while cutting back on your calorie intake, you can preserve muscle – and maintain your metabolism – while losing fat.

Building muscle: Some ideas to keep you going

People can have a lot of misconceptions about weight training. Many people have no idea what changes to expect when they begin lifting weights, so they ask some not-so-stupid questions, like the ones that follow.

Knowing how long it takes to get stronger

You may be able to lift more weight after just one weight-lifting workout. This isn't because you've built up more muscle; it's mainly because your weight-training skills have improved. The first time you try the bench press, you waste a lot of energy trying to balance the bar, keep it steady, and move it in a straight line. But after you get the hang of the process – typically after one weight-lifting session – you're able to put all your energy into lifting the weight.

Another reason you develop strength after just a few weeks of working out is that, in a sense, your muscles have memory. Your nerves, the pathways that link your brain and muscles, learn how to carry information more quickly – much like the speed-dial feature on your telephone. So after learning an exercise, your brain tells your muscles: 'You know what this is. Go for it.'

During the first six to eight weeks you lift weights, most of the strength you gain is due to skill and muscle memory. After that time, your muscles begin to grow. In other words, the sizes of your muscle fibres increase – you don't actually grow more muscle cells. Be aware that some muscles gain strength faster than others do. In general, large muscles, like your chest and back muscles, grow faster than smaller ones, like your arm and shoulder muscles. Most people can increase their strength by between 7 and 40 per cent after about ten weeks of training each muscle group twice a week.

Understanding why some people have greater strength than others

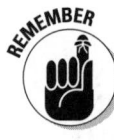

Every body type has a different capacity for building strength and muscle. All the training in the world won't change your body type. If you start out short and narrow, weight training won't miraculously make you tall and broad. Weight training may, however, make you a more fit, muscular version of short and narrow.

Calculating how long it will take before your body looks better

Most people start to see changes after six weeks of weight-lifting, but we can't give you an exact answer. Results depend on your body type, your starting point, and the amount of time and effort you devote to lifting weights. In general, those who have the furthest to go make the most dramatic changes.

Everyone notices the biggest improvements in the muscles that they use the least. The *triceps* are a classic example: You don't use them much in everyday life, so when you start targeting them with weights they become firmer fairly fast. The same goes for shoulders. Most people don't tend to carry much fat on their shoulders, so shoulders shape and tone relatively quickly.

Weight training can speed up your metabolism and give you more muscle tone, better posture, and better body proportions. In addition, lifting weights enhances your aerobic efforts. With stronger muscles, you have more staying power on the cross trainer or stepper, and you're less likely to have a setback due to injury from your aerobic workouts. For example, you may be working out really well when, suddenly, you feel a little twinge in your knee. You lay off for a couple days, which turns into a couple years. You may be able to prevent this whole incident by strengthening your knees. Plus, adding weight training to your new exercise programme gives you more variety and helps keep you motivated.

To obtain much more detailed information about the variety of exercise classes available through gyms and sports centres, using exercise DVDs, or home gyms, please refer to *Fitness For Dummies*.

Book III

**Physical
Health:
Achieving
Fitness**

Book IV
Exploring Yoga and Pilates

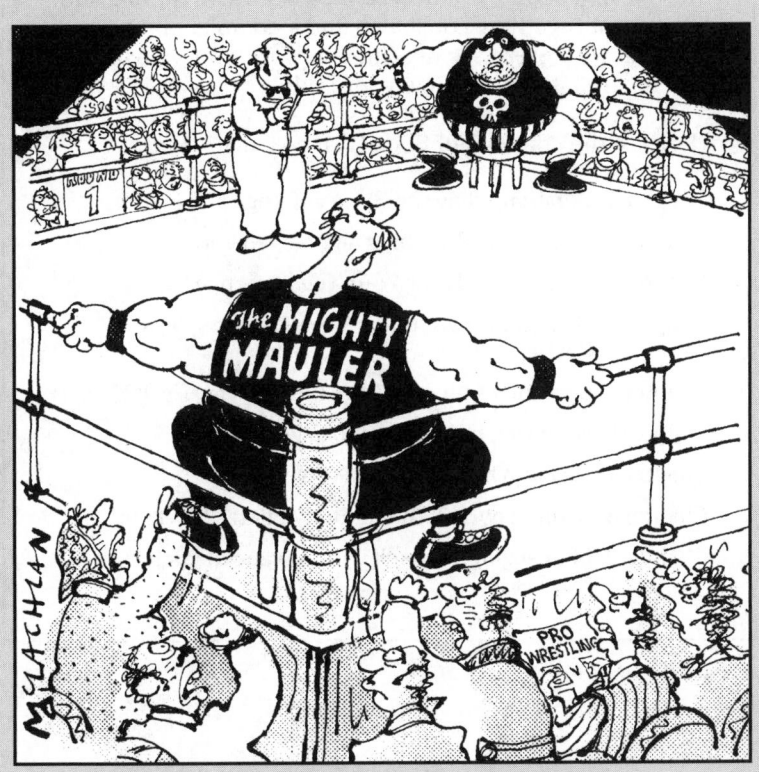

'Good Lord, Fiona, that's
my yoga teacher!'

In this book . . .

Yoga and Pilates have been around for many years so you may have tried some of the exercises before. Book IV takes you through the basic exercises to get you started, and shows you how to incorporate breathing and movement together. You'll also find a complete body workout with exercises designed to work every muscle and to strengthen and tone your body.

Here are the contents of Book IV at a glance:

Chapter 1

Understanding the Basics of Yoga and Pilates

*B*oth Yoga and Pilates incorporate an extensive series of exercises and movements to tone and strengthen the body, and relax and calm the mind.

Understanding some of the basic principles of Yoga and Pilates is useful so you know how the exercises and approaches can benefit you. In this chapter we explore the origins of Yoga and Pilates, the different styles and the basic principles so you can get started on the exercises.

Yoga: What You Need to Know

Yoga originated 5,000 or so years ago in India and reached the rest of the world some 100 years later. It includes physical exercises that look like gymnastics – some of which have even been incorporated into Western gymnastics. These exercises help you become or stay fit and trim, control your weight, and reduce your stress level. Yoga also offers a whole range of meditation practices, including breathing techniques that exercise your lungs and calm your nervous system or charge your brain and the rest of your body with delicious energy.

Moreover, you can use Yoga as an efficient system of health care, one that has proven its usefulness in both restoring and maintaining health. Yoga continues to gain acceptance within the medical establishment. More and more physicians are recommending Yoga to their patients, not only for stress reduction but also as a safe and sane method of exercise, as well as physiotherapy (notably for the back and knees).

But Yoga is more even than a system of preventative or restorative health care. Yoga looks at health from a broad, holistic perspective that's only now being rediscovered by avant-garde medicine. This perspective appreciates the enormous influence of the mind – your psychological attitudes – on physical health.

The word *Yoga* comes from the ancient *Sanskrit* language spoken by the traditional religious elite of India, the *brahmins*. Yoga means 'union' or 'integration' and 'discipline', so the system of Yoga is called a *unitive* or *integrating discipline*. Yoga seeks unity at various levels. First, Yoga seeks to unite your body and mind.

Here's how Yoga can help you with your personal growth:

✔ Yoga can put you in touch with your real feelings and balance your emotional life.

✔ Yoga can help you become less fragmented inwardly and more whole and real. In other words, it can help you understand and accept yourself and feel comfortable with who you are. You won't have to 'fake it' or reduce your life to constant role-playing.

✔ Yoga can greatly improve your links with other people. That is, you become more able to empathise and communicate with others.

Yoga is a powerful means of psychological integration. It makes you aware that you're part of a larger whole, not merely an island unto yourself. Humans can't thrive in isolation. Even the most independent individual is greatly indebted to others. Once your mind and body are happily reunited, this union with others comes about naturally. The moral principles of Yoga are all embracing, encouraging you to seek kinship with everyone and everything.

Finding your niche: Five basic approaches to Yoga

Since the late nineteenth century when Yoga was introduced to the Western hemisphere from its Indian homeland, it has undergone various adaptations. Today, Yoga is practised in five major ways:

✔ As a method for physical fitness and health maintenance

✔ As a sport

✔ As body-oriented therapy

✔ As a comprehensive lifestyle

✔ As a spiritual discipline

We take a look at these five basic approaches in the upcoming sections.

Yoga as fitness training

The first approach, Yoga as fitness training, is the most popular way that Westerners practise Yoga. It's also the most radical revamping of traditional Yoga. More precisely, it's a revision of traditional *Hatha Yoga*. Yoga as fitness training is concerned primarily with the physical body – its flexibility, resilience and strength. This is how most newcomers to Yoga encounter this great tradition. Fitness training is certainly a useful gateway into Yoga, but later on, some people discover that Hatha Yoga also includes moral and spiritual practices that are designed to lead to enlightenment. From the earliest times, Yoga masters have emphasised the need for a healthy body. But they've also always pointed beyond the body to the mind and other important aspects of being.

Yoga as a sport

This second approach, Yoga as a sport, is especially prominent in some Latin American countries but is widely controversial. Its practitioners, many of whom are excellent athletes, master hundreds of extremely difficult Yoga postures to perfection and demonstrate their skills and beautiful physiques in international competitions. But this new sport, which also can be regarded as an art form, has drawn much criticism from the ranks of more traditional Yoga practitioners. They feel that competition has no place in Yoga. Yet this athletic orientation has done much to put Yoga on the map in some parts of the world. We see nothing wrong with good-natured Yoga competitions as long as self-centred competitiveness is held in check.

Yoga as therapy

The third approach, Yoga as therapy, applies yogic techniques to restore health or full physical and mental functioning. In recent years, some Western Yoga teachers have begun to use yogic practices for therapeutic purposes. Although the idea behind Yoga therapy is very old, its name is fairly new. Yoga therapy is, in fact, a whole new professional discipline, calling for far greater training and skill on the part of the teacher than is the case with ordinary Yoga. Commonly, Yoga is intended for those who don't suffer from disabilities or ailments requiring remedial action and special attention. Yoga therapy, on the other hand, addresses these special needs. For example, Yoga therapy may be able to help you find relief from certain ailments such as chronic back pain, asthma, rheumatism, and many others.

Yoga as a lifestyle

The fourth approach, Yoga as a lifestyle, enters the proper domain of Yoga. Yoga once or twice a week for an hour or so is certainly better than no Yoga at all. And Yoga can be enormously beneficial even when practised only as fitness training. But you unlock the real potency of Yoga when you adopt it as a lifestyle. This means *living* Yoga – practising Yoga every day, whether it's physical exercises or meditation. Above all, it means applying the wisdom of Yoga to everyday life and to live *lucidly*, that is, with awareness. Yoga has much to say about what and how you should eat, how you should sleep, how you should work, how you should relate to others, and so on. It offers a total system of conscious and skilful living.

Don't think that you have to be a yogic superstar to practise lifestyle Yoga. You can begin today. Just make a few simple adjustments in your daily schedule and keep your goals vividly in front of you. Whenever you're ready, make further positive changes – one step at a time.

Yoga as a spiritual discipline

Lifestyle Yoga is concerned with healthy, wholesome, functional and benevolent living. Yoga as a spiritual discipline, the fifth and final approach, is concerned with all that *plus* the traditional ideal of *enlightenment* – that is, discovering your spiritual nature.

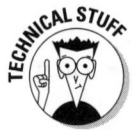

The word *spiritual* has been abused a lot lately, so we need to explain how it's used here. *Spiritual* relates to *spirit* – your ultimate nature. In Yoga, it is called the *atman* (pronounced *aht-mahn*) or *purusha (poo-roo-shah)*.

According to Yoga philosophy, the *spirit* is one and the same for everyone. It's formless, immortal, superconscious and unimaginably blissful. It is one and the same in all beings and things. It is transcendental because it exists beyond the limited body and mind. You discover the spirit in the moment of your enlightenment.

What all approaches to Yoga have in common

The five approaches to Yoga share at least two *fundamental practices:* the cultivation of awareness and relaxation.

- *Awareness* is the peculiarly human ability to pay close attention to something, to be consciously present, to be mindful. Yoga is attention training.

  To see what we mean, try this exercise: Pay attention to your right hand for the next 60 seconds. That is, feel your right hand and do nothing else. Chances are, your mind is drifting off after only a few seconds. Yoga consists in reining in your attention whenever it strays.

- *Relaxation* is the conscious release of unnecessary and therefore unwholesome tension in the body.

Both awareness and relaxation go hand in hand in Yoga. Without bringing awareness and relaxation to Yoga, the exercises would be merely exercises – not *yogic* exercises.

Conscious breathing is often added to awareness and relaxation as a third foundational practice. Normally, breathing happens automatically. In Yoga, awareness is brought to this act, which then makes it into a powerful tool for training the body and the mind.

Understanding the many different types of Yoga

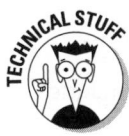

Hatha Yoga has undergone many transformations over the past decades. There are many styles of Hatha Yoga today, including the following:

- ✔ **Viniyoga** – works with a 'sequence process'. Or *vinyasa karma*. The emphasis is on practising a posture based on one's individual needs and capacity: Regulated breathing is an important aspect and the breath is carefully co-ordinated with the postural movements.

- ✔ **Iyengar Yoga** – this style is characterised by precision performance and the aid of various props, such as cushions, benches, wood blocks, straps and even sand bags.

- ✔ **Ashtanga Yoga** – this is a more athletic style of Hatha Yoga.

- ✔ **Kripalu Yoga** – this is a three-stage Yoga incorporating initially postural alignment, co-ordination of breath and movement with postures held only for a short time. In the second stage, meditation is included and postures are held for prolonged periods. In the final stage, the practice of postures becomes a spontaneous 'meditation in motion'.

- ✔ **Integral Yoga** – this style integrates the various aspects of the body-mind through a combination of postures, breathing techniques, deep relaxation and meditation.

- ✔ **Sivananda Yoga** – this style includes a series of 12 postures, the Sun Salutation sequence, breathing exercises, relaxation and *mantra* chanting.

- ✔ **Ananda Yoga** – this is a gentle style designed to prepare the student for meditation, and its distinguishing features are the affirmations associated with postures.

- ✔ **Bikram Yoga** – this approach is fairly vigorous and requires a certain fitness level for participation.

- ✔ **Kundalini Yoga** – its purpose is to awaken the serpent power *(kundalini)* by means of postures, breath control, chanting and meditation.

Book IV

Exploring Yoga and Pilates

✔ **Somatic Yoga** – this is an integrated approach to the harmonious development of body and mind, based both on traditional yogic principles and modern psycho-physiological research. This gentle approach emphasises visualisation, very slow movement into and out of postures, conscious breathing, mindfulness, and frequent relaxation between postures.

As with starting any new exercise programme, consult your doctor before embarking on your Yoga or Pilates journey, especially if you suffer from heart conditions, back pain or serious illness or injury.

The Basics on Pilates

Pilates exercises borrow from Yoga, dance and gymnastics, but also include lots of original movements that distinguish them from these other techniques. The Pilates method consists of a repertoire of over 500 exercises, to be done on a mat or on one of the many pieces of equipment Joseph Pilates invented. Don't worry about having to use complicated equipment – you can get a terrific workout at home with just a simple exercise mat.

The Pilates method works to strengthen the centre (see the section 'Centring' in this chapter), lengthen the spine, build muscle tone and increase body awareness and flexibility.

The Pilates method is also an excellent rehabilitation system for back, knee, hip, shoulder and repetitive-stress injuries. Pilates addresses the body as a whole, correcting the body's asymmetries and chronic weaknesses to prevent re-injury and to bring the body back into balance.

Pilates mat work uses a series of exercises

Pilates exercises are usually done in a series. Series are organised by levels. There are beginning, intermediate and advanced series.

We recommend starting with pre-Pilates (see Book IV Chapter 7). The pre-Pilates exercises give you a deep understanding of the concepts that make up all Pilates exercises. After you understand these concepts, you can apply them to the Beginning Series. After you've mastered the Beginning Series, move on to the Intermediate Series, and so on. As you progress in the method, the series get longer and harder. An intermediate workout includes exercises from the Beginning Series, plus new and harder intermediate exercises. Sometimes you will just do a more difficult version of the same exercise when you advance in levels.

Joe Pilates: A short history of the man

Born in Germany in 1880 with a sunken chest and asthma, Joseph Hubertus Pilates spent his life obsessed with restoring his health and body condition. Over time, he overcame his frailty and became an accomplished skier, diver, gymnast, yogi and boxer, maintaining top physical form well into his seventies. While in an British internment camp during World War I, Pilates rigged springs above hospital beds to allow patients to rehabilitate while lying on their backs. This setup later evolved into the Cadillac, one of the main pieces of equipment in the Pilates method.

In 1923, Pilates emigrated to the United States. He settled in New York City, where he opened a studio on Eighth Avenue in Manhattan and started training and rehabilitating professional dancers. Ballet master George Balanchine and modern dance diva Martha Graham were two of his students.

Originally Pilates developed a series of mat exercises designed to build abdominal strength and body control. He then built various pieces of equipment to enhance the results of his expanding repertoire of exercises. His motivation for building the equipment was to replace himself as a spotter for his clients. He developed 20-odd contraptions, some of which look a little like medieval torture devices. They were constructed of wood and metal piping, and used combinations of pulleys, straps, bars, boxes and springs. His philosophy led him to develop a regimen that 'develops the body uniformly, corrects wrong postures, restores physical vitality, invigorates the mind, and elevates the spirit'. Way ahead of his time, he viewed fitness holistically, emphasising the body working as a whole unit.

Over the decades, Pilates developed over 500 exercises, which he originally called Contrology but which have since come to be known as the Pilates method.

Going through a series in order and trying to complete the whole series when you work out is important. Joseph Pilates was a genius when it comes to understanding muscle balance in the body. The series he developed make sense to the body when done in the correct order. Usually, you start a series with an exercise that warms up the spine, then you do a few exercises that bend the spine in one direction, followed by an exercise that reverses that movement, and so on. You don't have to understand the science behind why these exercises are in the order that they're in (you would need a PhD in kinesiology to fully understand the reasons). Just trust in the method and in the order of the exercises. The longer we study and practise Pilates, the more we appreciate the intelligence of the man who created it.

Pilates builds the powerhouse

Pilates exercises, as a whole, develop strong abdominal, back, bottom and deep-postural muscles. Pilates focuses on the muscles that support the skeletal system and act as the powerhouse of the body.

Book IV

Exploring Yoga and Pilates

Powerhouse is a term that comes from Joe Pilates himself. (See the sidebar 'Joe Pilates: A short history of the man' in this chapter for information about the man who developed Pilates exercises.) The abdominals, bottom, back and inner thigh muscles, when working together, constitute the powerhouse. This is where many of the Pilates exercises can be initiated or the area that is being challenged in many exercises. These muscles are the main stabilising muscles of the body and are very important for preventing injury to the back.

The powerhouse is especially useful when performing back-strengthening exercises, as in back extensions. For example, if you lie on your stomach and squeeze your legs together, imagine pulling your stomach up off the mat so that you could slide a piece of paper underneath your navel. Then tuck your pelvis under by pressing your pubic bone into the mat and complete this movement by squeezing the low bottom muscles. The engagement of these three muscle groups – the abs, the bottom and the inner thigh – means you're working the powerhouse. If you were to rise up into a cobra or back extension (other Pilates movements) with your upper body, you would try to use this powerhouse to resist the swaying and compression in your low back.

Why should you care about this powerhouse?

- ✔ The powerhouse muscles protect your back from potential injury, and if you already have a weak or problematic back, then strengthening the powerhouse will probably alleviate your problems.

- ✔ Working from the centre of the body when doing any movement takes the load off the joints and the spine and helps your body work more efficiently.

- ✔ A strong powerhouse is a sexy thing. Who doesn't enjoy a toned tummy, back and inner thigh?

The eight great principles of Pilates

Joseph Pilates wrote a book called *Return to Life* in which he mapped out the eight principles that inspired the Pilates method. Understanding these principles helps you gain a deeper understanding of the philosophy underlying Pilates. Pilates, more than other exercise programmes, requires *mental* focus. If you don't understand the concepts behind Pilates, it ends up being merely a series of fancy sit-ups and stretches.

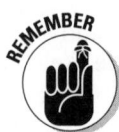

What drives people to continue doing Pilates for years and years is the tremendous transformation they see in their bodies when they delve deeper into the work. You could do Pilates for ten years and still find some revelation about your body or about how to deepen the effects of an exercise. This aspect distinguishes Pilates from the basic workout.

When you do Pilates exercises with the eight key concepts in mind, you gain many more levels of meaning and effectiveness. The following eight concepts give you an idea of just what to think about when doing the exercises.

Control

Joseph Pilates originally called his method 'Contrology' (it wasn't until his students took over teaching for him that people started referring to the method as Pilates). So one of the most fundamental rules when doing Pilates is to control your body's every movement. This rule applies not only to the exercises themselves but also to transitions between exercises, how you get on and off the equipment, and your overall attention to detail while working out.

When doing mat exercises, control comes into play with the initiation and ending of each movement. When you put on the brakes in a controlled manner, you train the muscles to hold themselves in a lengthened state. Over time, the muscles grow long as well as strong. Long and strong muscles – isn't that what we all want? When training clients, we try to encourage smooth and even movements. In our minds we think of getting the muscles to co-operate with each other.

Also, when focusing on control of a movement, the body is forced to recruit helper muscles (called *synergists*), which are usually smaller than the main muscles. When many muscles work together to do one movement, or when muscles work synergistically, the body as a whole develops greater balance and co-ordination. Also, the big muscles won't get too big and bulky because they don't have to do all the work by themselves. Thus you become a long and lean machine.

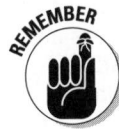

Inner control allows you outer freedom without fear of injury.

Breath

People often hold their breath when performing a new and difficult task. When you hold your breath, you tense muscles that can ultimately exacerbate improper posture and reinforce tension habits. That is why consistent breathing is essential to flowing movement and proper muscle balance. Every Pilates exercise has a specific breathing pattern assigned to it.

Most people breathe at half of their lung capacity. Shallow breathing is an unfortunate side effect of a sedentary and stressful life. Deep inhalation and full exhalation exercises the lungs and increases lung capacity, bringing deep relaxation as a pleasant side effect. Breathing while moving is not always an easy assignment; but when you do, beautiful things can happen. Focused breath can help maximise the body's ability to stretch, and through this release of tension, you'll gain optimal body control.

Breathing is an essential aspect of Pilates and distinguishes it from other exercise forms. Like Yoga, Pilates has specific breathing cues to go with every exercise.

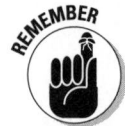

General rule of Pilates breathing: Breathe out on the hardest part of the exercise! For example, if you're throwing a ball, it helps to breathe out as you release the ball. In the same way in Pilates we suggest that you exhale on the hardest work.

Flowing movement

If you were to glance quickly at someone doing Pilates, you might think the person was doing Yoga. But when doing Yoga, you generally hold your position for at least a moment (if not for what seems like an eternity) before moving to the next posture. And although Pilates borrows some of its movements from Yoga, rarely do you ever hold a position for a long time in Pilates. In this way, Pilates is more like dance, in that the flow of the body is essential. The essence of Pilates movements is to allow your body to move freely and, at the end of each movement, to finish with control and precision. This way of moving brings flexibility to the joints and muscles and teaches the body to elongate and move with even rhythm. Flowing movement integrates the nervous system, the muscles and the joints and trains the body to move smoothly and evenly.

Precision

Precision is a lot like control but has the added element of spatial awareness. When initiating any movement, you must know exactly where that movement starts and where it will end. All Pilates exercises have precise definitions of where the body should be at all times, such as the angle at which the legs are moving, which way the elbows are pointing, the positioning of the head and neck, and even what the fingers are doing! The little things count in Pilates.

Centring

Again and again, we need to remind our clients to 'pull the navel to the spine' – in other words, pull in your tummy! This is the first and ultimate Pilates cue. Pulling the navel in towards your spine is how you bring your deep abdominal muscles into action, and all Pilates exercises are done with the deep abdominals engaged to ensure proper centring. Most Pilates exercises focus on developing abdominal strength either directly or indirectly. Never forget to pull the stomach in or you'll be reprimanded by the Pilates gods!

Stability

The focus on stability when performing the exercises is part of the beauty of Pilates and what makes it such a perfect rehabilitation system. In fact, many

Pilates mat exercises are meant to focus primarily on torso stability. *Stability* is the ability to *not* move a part of the body while another part is challenging it. For instance, when raising your arm up as high as you can in front of you, try not to arch your back. In order to accomplish this, you must use your abdominal muscles so that the rib cage doesn't rise up as the arm rises above the shoulder level. Maintaining stillness in the spine as you move the arms and legs requires torso stability accomplished mainly by the abdominal muscles.

Range of motion

Range of motion is a medical term that refers to how much movement a part of the body can do. For instance, how high you can kick your leg out in front of you gives you an idea of how much range of motion you have in your hip. Range of motion can be affected by the muscles, bones and other tissues such as ligaments and fascia (connective tissue). Basically, range of motion is just another way of describing flexibility.

Pilates exercises tend to require the body to move to its fullest length, thereby increasing the range of motion, or flexibility, of your limbs. People whose muscles are very tight will begin to notice an increase in flexibility after doing a few hours of Pilates exercises. If you're very tight, you may need to do some specific stretching exercises in addition to the Pilates exercises. You may find yourself limited by your tightness and unable even to get into the position required to perform a particular exercise. If you find this to be true, you may need to modify the exercise at first, until you gain the flexibility to do the exercise in its classic form.

Opposition

You can lift your arms thinking only of lifting your arms. Or you can think 'down to go up' as you lift your arms, first pulling the shoulders down the back and then raising the arms, focusing on lifting the arms from the back muscles instead. This is opposition in action. When lifting your arm from your back rather than from your arm, you're actually stabilising the shoulder as you lift the arm. We often say to our clients, 'Think down to go up' when they're raising their arms, or 'up to go down' when we're explaining how to roll down the spine. These are both examples of opposition when moving.

Dancers naturally use opposition when they move, and that is what gives them the illusion of floating in the air while simultaneously being weighted to the ground. Opposition as a tool for imagery in moving is generally a way to trick someone into using core muscles rather than the peripheral muscles. This approach brings in more muscles to do a movement (known as synergy) and makes the movement more efficient for the body and ultimately more healthy.

Book IV

Exploring Yoga and Pilates

As Pilates instructors, we use opposition often and in many ways to get clients to find a balance in their bodies. The other example of 'up to go down' when bending over is essential to save your back from eventual demise. The next time you bend down to pick something up, imagine pulling up from your low stomach as you bend forward. Doing so will protect your back by engaging the opposing muscles (the abdominals). Using opposition is a beautiful way to manipulate your body as you perform movements with ultimate elongation and proper body mechanics. You'll see more examples of opposition when you go through the exercises, and the concept will be easier to understand after you've done a few.

What you need to get started

The good news is that you don't need much! Just the basics:

- **A firm mat.** The mat only needs to be as long as your spine and as wide as your body. This mat should be firm enough to support your back when rolling on the floor. You will hurt your vertebrae if you only use a towel or a Yoga mat. We like to use either a gymnastic mat or a fold-up foam mat.

- **Comfy clothes.** Wear what you would wear to a Yoga class, dance class or stretch class. Nothing should bind you – no buttons or tight waistbands. Wearing something form-fitting is nice because it lets you see if your tummy is bulging out or not.

- **Bare feet.** Socks tend to slip on the floor, so we recommend bare feet.

In addition, a small ball is great, although it's not necessary. A small ball is a great cheap tool to have, especially when you're first starting out.

Keeping your eyes on the prize: How you benefit from Pilates

Yeah, yeah, I've heard it a hundred times. When you try and make Pilates a part of your routine, you find that you just don't have time . . . or you don't have the energy . . . or it's too much work! Well, the time for excuses is over. Just in case you need more motivation, this section shows you the rewards you can reap from Pilates – if you keep your eyes on the prize.

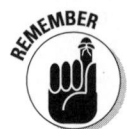

Finding your centre

Most people at some time in their lives experience back pain, and the most common reasons for back pain are poor posture and weak tummy muscles.

A key focus for Pilates is how to pull your navel in towards the spine. By performing this simple action, you engage your deep abdominal muscles. Strengthening these muscles can transform your posture and alleviate back pain. All Pilates exercises are done with this basic centring concept.

An hour-long Pilates mat class, can fire up your abdominal muscles and makes you want to scream. As you become more advanced in the Pilates method, your core strength develops a great deal more. You may notice a greater ease in your body and will probably find increased endurance for lifting, walking and performing daily activities. Your posture improves, and people will see a change in your physicality. Your back pain may just up and go away, as well as other bodily aches and pains like knee, shoulder and hip problems. Developing core strength affects your whole being and gives you a new sense of power.

Mastering the mental component

Pilates teaches you how to be *in* your body: how to properly sit and stand, how to bend and lift, and how to move from the centre of the body. This increased body awareness and core strength helps to improve form in other sports as well, and brings more grace and efficiency to everyday life activities.

People who bring focus and mental presence to their workouts advance more quickly through the exercises and see improvements more readily. Like dance, Pilates demands that your body perform many actions at once. A movement is never just a movement; you must execute it with optimal form, precision and control. Each person has the potential to reach his own level of perfection. Achieving this goal requires focus and attention, and it can be frustrating for those who don't want to be so present in their body.

Helping your spine, the axis of life

The spine has two main functions: first, to be rigid and hold you upright and strong against the elements; and second, to be flexible and allow you to bend over, twist around, and reach in many directions. Most of the time, the spine does an excellent job. The spine is very susceptible to injury because it moves so much and in so many different ways. The risk of injury increases as you get older and the shock-absorbing structures begin to deteriorate. The spine also gets much stiffer as you age, making it more difficult to move about the way you want. Pilates is one of the best methods of exercise to address both spinal stability and spinal rigidity.

Book IV

Exploring Yoga and Pilates

A Pilates exercise usually serves one purpose at a time. One exercise may aim at increasing flexibility in the spine, while another may focus on developing core stabilisation and strength. A balanced workout addresses both concerns, giving the spine more resilience. Joe Pilates loved to use the cat as a model for spinal strength and mobility. He used to say if you do Pilates for

20 minutes a day, your spine will be like a cat's and you will be able to move freely through your life. Meow!

Improving your sex life

Pilates can help your sex life. Increasing body awareness and discovering how to isolate muscles in your pelvic floor can only increase your pleasure and give you more control during sex. (Your pelvic floor muscles include the muscles that control the sphincters of your urethra, anus, and the muscles of the vagina.) And of course, gaining flexibility in the hips and legs, and increasing strength in your pelvis and bottom will give you more choices on what positions you can attempt, and more physical endurance for longer rounds! It will also prevent pulled muscles and injuries if you enjoy more athletic sexual experiences.

Looking good: Pilates and the body beautiful

You may have heard of all the Hollywood stars who are doing Pilates: Madonna, Robin Williams, Sharon Stone, that woman who plays Xena, and many more. Bette Midler even had a Cadillac on her short-lived TV show. You know that if those stars are doing Pilates, it must be doing something good for their vanity! Read on to discover the specifics.

Pilates and weight loss

Many people come to Pilates to lose weight and have a body like a dancer's. Is this realistic? Yes and no.

Aerobic exercise facilitates fat loss, and Pilates is not aerobic until you get to the advanced levels and are able to transition seamlessly from one exercise to another. If you're doing no exercise at all now, you may lose fat doing Pilates . . . because, hey, it's exercise and it will increase your metabolism. But if fat loss is a primary concern to you, try combining Pilates with dance, walking, swimming, cycling, or some gym-based aerobic machine.

Pilates is resistance training, so it strengthens and tones your whole body. You see marked changes especially around the stomach, bottom and thighs. Most importantly, Pilates can make you appear taller and thinner by giving you beautiful posture and grace and ease of movement.

The Pilates way of moving

'Extend your fingertips long and away!' 'Stretch your leg out to its fullest length!' These are common commands of a good Pilates trainer. You should always be accentuating the extension of the limbs, and challenging your body to gain more and more length. This way of moving lengthens the muscles and opens the joints, training your body as dancers train theirs. When you practise elongating the muscles, your muscles remember to stay long and open after you leave the Pilates studio. You can increase flexibility and literally become a longer human being.

The Pilates triad: Abdominals, bottom and inner thigh

What makes Pilates different from a lot of other exercise forms is that you're always using every part of your body. Even if you're doing a bicep curl, you don't let the rest of your body go to jelly; you're holding in your stomach, squeezing your bottom, and pulling your inner thighs together at the same time. When doing Pilates exercises, you almost always work on the triad of abdominals, bottom, and inner thigh, no matter what else is going on. Over time, this combination of muscle usage changes the look ad shape of your middle.

Don't dingle dangle! Pilates and the upper body

Joseph Pilates was a gymnast, and many of the intermediate and advanced exercises reflect this fact. Many Pilates exercises demand a great amount of upper body strength and stability, much like a gymnastics routine. This focus on strengthening the back and upper body sets Pilates apart from most forms of exercise. Most people (especially women) have little upper-body strength. When women start Pilates, they are pleasantly surprised by the tone and definition they gain in their arms and back as they progress in the work. See Figure 1-1 for an example of a Pilates-toned upper body.

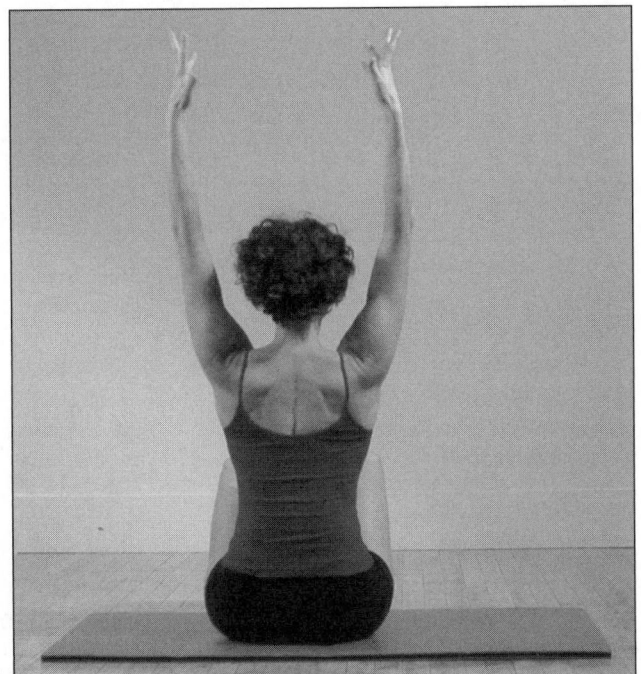

Figure 1-1: Pilates strengthens and tones the upper body.

Book IV

Exploring Yoga and Pilates

Chapter 2

Integrating Breathing and Movement

A key principle of Yoga is to combine an exercise or movement with breathing. Conscious breathing allows the body to move more effectively and relax more into the exercise, linking your mind and body together.

This chapter provides you with the guidelines to use breathing effectively during your Yoga practice. We also introduce the value of meditation to provide you with a deeper level of Yoga practice.

Breath and Movement Simplified

The masters of Yoga discovered the usefulness of the breath thousands of years ago and in Hatha Yoga have perfected a system for the conscious control of breathing. In this section, we share their secrets with you. In the ancient Sanskrit language, the word for *breath* is the same as the word for *life – prana* (pronounced *prah-nah*) – which gives you a good clue about how important Yoga thinks breathing is for your well-being.

Here we show you how to use conscious breathing in conjunction with the Yoga postures, and we also introduce several breathing exercises that you do while being seated on a chair or, if you are up to it, while assuming one of the Yoga sitting postures. Always combine moving in to and out of the postures with proper breathing, because the mix greatly enhances the effect on your physical health and mental tranquillity. Yoga without *prana* would be like putting an empty pot on the stove and hoping for a delicious meal.

Breathe your way to good health

Think of your breath as your most intimate friend. Your breath is with you from the moment you're born and stays with you until you die. In a given day, you take between 20,000 and 30,000 breaths. Most likely, though – barring any respiratory problems – you are barely aware of your breathing. This is like taking your best friend so for granted that the relationship gets stale and is put at risk. To be sure, allowing breathing to occur automatically isn't necessarily to your advantage, because automatic doesn't always mean optimal. In fact, most people's breathing habits are quite poor and to their great disadvantage. They accumulate a lot of stale air in their lungs, which become as unproductive as a stale friendship. Poor breathing is known to cause and increase stress. Conversely, stress shortens your breath and increases your level of anxiety.

You can help alleviate stress through the simple practice of yogic breathing. Among other things, breathing loads your blood with oxygen, which, by nourishing and repairing your body's cells, maintains your health at the most desirable level. Shallow breathing, which is widespread, doesn't oxygenate the ten pints of blood circulating in your arteries and veins very efficiently. Consequently, toxins pile up in the cells. Before you know it, you feel mentally sluggish and emotionally down, and eventually organs begin to malfunction. Is it any wonder that the breath is the best tool you have to profoundly affect your body and mind?

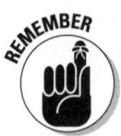

Bad breath is improved by brushing your teeth regularly and occasionally sucking on a mint. Bad breathing, however, is a bad habit that requires a bit more to change: You must retrain your body through breath awareness.

In Yoga, consciously regulated breathing has the following three major applications:

- ✔ Using it in conjunction with the various postures to achieve the deepest possible effect and to prepare the mind for meditation.

- ✔ Using it as breath control (called *pranayama,* pronounced *prah-nah-yah-mah*), to invigorate your vitality.

- ✔ Using it as a healing method, in which you consciously direct the breath to a particular part or organ of the body to remove energetic blockages and facilitate healing; this is Yoga's gentle version of acupuncture.

Taking high-quality breaths

Before you jump right in and make drastic changes to your method of breathing, take a few minutes to assess your current breathing style. You may find it helpful to keep a log of your breathing habits over the course of a couple of days, noting how your breathing changes as situations around you occur. Check your breathing by asking yourself the following questions:

✔ Is my breathing shallow (my abdomen and chest barely move when I fill my lungs with air)?

✔ Do I often breathe erratically (my breathing rhythm is not harmonious)?

✔ Do I easily get out of breath?

✔ Is my breathing laboured at times?

✔ Do I generally breathe too fast?

If your answers to any of these questions is yes, you make an ideal candidate for yogic breathing. Even if your didn't answer yes, practicing conscious still benefits your mind and body.

By the way, men take an average of 12 to 14 breaths per minute, while women take 14 to 15. Breathing at a markedly faster pace – usually associated with *chest breathing* – qualifies as hyperventilation, which leads to carbon dioxide depletion (your body needs some of the gas to maintain the right acid-alkaline balance of the blood).

Relaxing with a couple of deep breaths

Think about the many times you've heard someone say, 'Now just take a couple of deep breaths and relax.' This recommendation is so popular because it really works! Pain clinics across the country use breathing exercises for pain control. Childbirth clinics teach Yoga-related breathing techniques to both parents to aid the birthing process.

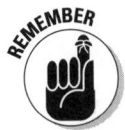

Yogic breathing is like sending an email to your nervous system with the message to relax.

One easy way to experience the effect of simple breathing is to try the following exercise:

1. **Sit comfortably in your chair.**

2. **Close your eyes and visualise a swan gliding peacefully across a crystal-clear lake.**

3. **Now, like the swan, let your breath flow along in a long, smooth and peaceful movement. Ideally, inhale and exhale through your nose.**

   If your nose is plugged up, try the combination of nose and mouth, or just the mouth.

4. **Extend your breath to its comfortable maximum for 20 rounds; then gradually let your breath return to normal.**

5. **Afterwards, take a few moments to sit with your eyes closed and notice the difference in how you feel overall.**

   Can you imagine how relaxed and calm you would feel after 10 to 15 minutes of conscious yogic breathing?

Practising safe yogic breathing

As you look forward to the calming and restorative power of yogic breathing, take time to reflect on a few safety tips that can help you enjoy your experience.

✔ If you have problems with your lungs (such as a cold or asthma), or if you have a heart disease, consult your doctor first before embarking on breath control even under the supervision of a Yoga therapist (unless she happens to be a doctor as well).

✔ Don't practise breathing exercises when the air is too cold or too hot.

✔ Avoid practising in polluted air, including the smoke from incense; whenever possible, practise breath control outdoors or with an open window: Negative ions are positive for your health, at least in moderation. These ions are electrically charged atoms with a negative charge. Positive ions are produced by your TV and computer and have been connected with fatigue, headaches and respiratory problems.

✔ Don't strain your breathing – remain relaxed while doing the breathing exercises.

✔ Don't overdo the number of repetitions. Stay within our guidelines for each exercise.

✔ Don't wear any constricting trousers or belts.

Reaping the benefits of yogic breathing

In addition to relaxing the body and calming the mind, yogic breathing has an entire spectrum of other benefits that work like insurance, protecting your investment in a longer and healthier life. Here are six important gains of controlled breathing:

✔ It steps up your metabolism (the best manager of weight increase).

✔ It uses muscles that automatically help improve your posture so that you can prevent the stiff, slumped carriage characteristic of many older people.

✔ It keeps the lung tissue elastic, which allows you to take in more oxygen food for the 50 trillion cells in your body.

✔ It tones your abdominal area, which is a common site for health problems – many illnesses begin in the intestines.

✔ It helps strengthen your immune system.

✔ It reduces your levels of tension and anxiety.

Breathing through your nose

No matter what anybody else tells you, yogic breathing is typically done through the nose, both during inhalation and exhalation. For the traditional yogis and yoginis, the mouth is meant for eating and the nose for breathing. We know at least three good reasons for breathing through the nose:

✔ It slows down the breath because you are breathing through two small openings instead of the one big opening in your mouth: Slow is good in Yoga.

✔ The air is hygienically filtered and warmed by the nasal passages. Even the purest air contains at least dust particles and at worst all the toxic pollutants of a metropolis.

✔ According to traditional Yoga, nasal breathing stimulates the subtle energy centre – the so-called *ajna-cakra* (pronounced *ah-gyah-chuk-rah*) which is located near sinuses in the spot between the eyebrows. This very important location is the meeting place of the left (cooling) and the right (heating) current of vital energy (*prana*) that act directly on the nervous and endocrine systems.

Folk wisdom knows that every rule has an exception, which is definitely the case with the yogic rule of breathing through the nose. A few classical yogic techniques for breath control require you to breathe through the mouth. When presenting a mouth-breathing technique, we alert you to that fact.

What if I can't breathe through my nose?

Some people may suffer from various physiological conditions that prevent you from breathing through the nose. Of course, Yoga is flexible. If you have difficulty breathing when lying down, try sitting up. The time of day can also make a difference in your ability to breathe. For example, you may be more congested or allergic in the morning than in the afternoon. You, of course, can detect the differences. If you're still not sure how to settle on a comfortable breathing method, first try inhaling through the nose and exhaling through the mouth and, failing this, just breathe through your mouth and don't worry for now. Worry is always counterproductive.

The Mechanics of Yogic Breathing

Most people are either shallow-chest breathers or shallow-belly breathers. Yogic breathing incorporates a complete breath that expands both the abdomen and the chest on inhalation either from the abdomen up or the chest down. Both are valid techniques.

Yogic breathing involves breathing much deeper than usual, which in turn brings more oxygen into your system. Don't be surprised if you feel a little light-headed or even dizzy at the beginning. If this happens during your Yoga practice, just rest for a few minutes or lie down until you feel like proceeding. Remind yourself that there's no rush.

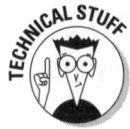

In both chest and abdominal breathing, the abdomen draws in on exhalation. From a mechanical standpoint, yogic breathing moves the spine and works the muscles and organs of respiration, which primarily include the diaphragm, intercostal (between the ribs) and abdominal muscles, and the lungs and heart. When the diaphragm contracts, it is pulled down, which creates more space for the lungs during inhalation. The chest noticeably widens. When the diaphragm relaxes, it moves back into its upward curve, forcing the air out of the lungs.

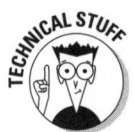

The diaphragm is a vaulted muscle sheath that separates the lungs and heart from the stomach, liver, kidneys and other abdominal organs. It's attached all around the lower border of the rib cage and, by a pair of powerful muscles, to the first to fourth lumbar vertebrae. The diaphragm and the chest muscles activate the lungs, which don't have muscles themselves.

Appreciating the complete yogic breath

If shallow or erratic breathing put your well-being at risk, the complete yogic breath is your ticket to excellent physical and mental health. If you do no other Yoga exercise, the complete Yoga breath – integrally combined with relaxation – will still be of inestimable benefit to you. It's your secret weapon, except Yoga doesn't believe in the use of force.

Belly breathing

Before you jump into practising the complete yogic breath, try out this exercise:

1. **Lie flat on your back and place one hand on your chest, the other on your abdomen. (See Figure 2-1.)**

Place a small pillow or folded blanket under your head if you have tension in your neck or if your chin tilts upwards. Place a large pillow under your knees if your back is uncomfortable.

2. **Take 15 to 20 slow, deep breaths.**

During inhalation, expand your abdomen, during exhalation contract your abdomen, but keep your chest as motionless as possible. Your hands will act as motion detectors.

3. **Pause for a couple of seconds between inhalation and exhalation keeping the throat soft.**

Figure 2-1:
Belly breathing exercises the diaphragm and prepares you for the complete yogic breath.

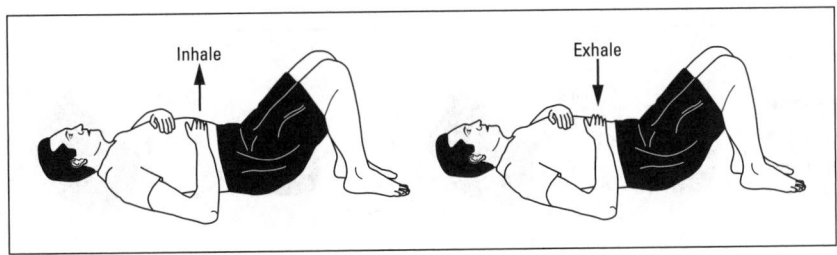

Inhale   Exhale

Belly-to-chest breathing

In belly-to-chest breathing, shown in Figure 2-2, you really exercise your chest and diaphragm muscles, as well as your lungs, and treat your body with oodles of oxygen and life force (*prana*). Your cells will be humming with energy and your brain will be very grateful to you for the extra boost. You can use this form of breathing before you begin your relaxation practice, before and where indicated during your practice of the Yoga postures, and in fact whenever you feel so inclined throughout the day. You don't necessarily have to lie down, as stipulated for the following exercise. You can be seated or even walking. After practising this technique for a while, you may find that it's become second nature to you.

1. **Lie flat on your back with your knees bent and feet on the floor at hip width, and relax.**

Place a small pillow or folded blanket under your head if you have tension in your neck or if your chin tilts upwards. Place a large pillow under your knees if your back is uncomfortable.

2. **Inhale while expanding the abdomen, and then the ribs, and finally the chest.**

Pause for a couple of seconds.

3. **Exhale while releasing chest and shoulder muscles, gently and continuously contracting or drawing the abdomen in.**

Pause again for a couple of seconds.

4. **Repeat the sequence.**

You can greatly enhance the value of this and other exercises by fully participating with your mind. *Feel* the air fill your lungs. *Feel* your muscles work. *Feel* your body as a whole. *Visualise* precious life energy entering your lungs and every cell of your body, rejuvenating and energising you. To help you experience this exercise more profoundly, keep your eyes closed. You can also place your hands on your abdomen and feel it expand upon inhalation.

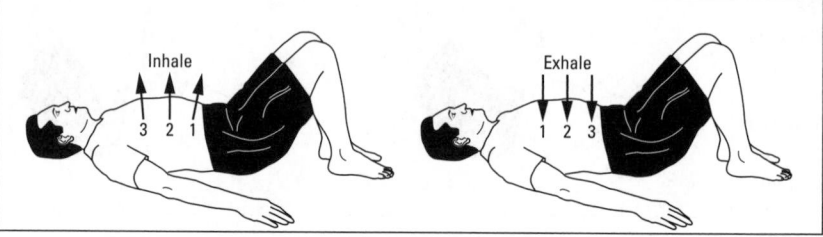

Figure 2-2:
This is the classic Yoga breath.

Taking a pause

During your normal shallow breathing, you will notice a slight natural pause between inhalation and exhalation. This pause becomes very important in yogic breathing. Even though the duration is usually only one or two seconds, this pause is a natural moment of stillness and meditation. If you pay attention to this pause, it can help you become more aware of the unity between body, breath and mind – all of which are key elements in your Yoga practice. With the help of a teacher, you can also learn to lengthen the pause during various Yoga postures to heighten its positive effects.

Partners in Yoga: Breath and Postural Movement

In Hatha Yoga, breathing is just as important as the postures, which we describe in Book IV Chapter 3. How you breathe when you're moving into, holding, or moving out of any given posture can greatly increase the efficiency and the benefits of your practice.

The more you use breathing consciously, the more benefits you gain for your healthand your general well-being. Here are some basic guidelines:

- ✔ Let the breath surround the movement. The breath leads the movement by a couple of seconds; that is, you initiate breathing (both inhalation and exhalation), and then you make the movement.

  - • When you inhale, the body opens or expands.
  - • When you exhale, the body folds or contracts.

- ✔ Both inhale and exhale end with a natural pause.

- ✔ In the beginning, let the breath dictate the length of the postural movement. For example, if you are raising your arms as you inhale and you run out of breath before you reach your goal, just pause your breathing for a moment and then bring your arms back down as you exhale. With practice, your breath will gradually get longer.

- ✔ Let the breath itself be your teacher. When your breath sounds laboured, it's time to back off or come out of a posture.

- ✔ Try to sense the breath flowing into the area you're working on with any given posture.

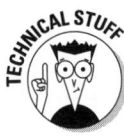

Breathing in four directions

You can move your body in four natural directions:

- ✔ **Flexion:** Bending forwards.
- ✔ **Extension:** Bending backwards.
- ✔ **Lateral flexion:** Bending sideways.
- ✔ **Rotation:** Twisting your body.

Normally, when people move they tend to hold or strain their breath. In Yoga, you simply follow the natural flow of the breath. As a rule, adopt this pattern:

- ✔ Inhale when moving into back bends (as shown in Figure 2-3a).
- ✔ Exhale when moving into forward bends (see Figure 2-3b).
- ✔ Exhale when moving into side bends (see Figure 2-3c).
- ✔ Exhale when moving into twists (as shown in Figure 2-3d).

Book IV

Exploring Yoga and Pilates

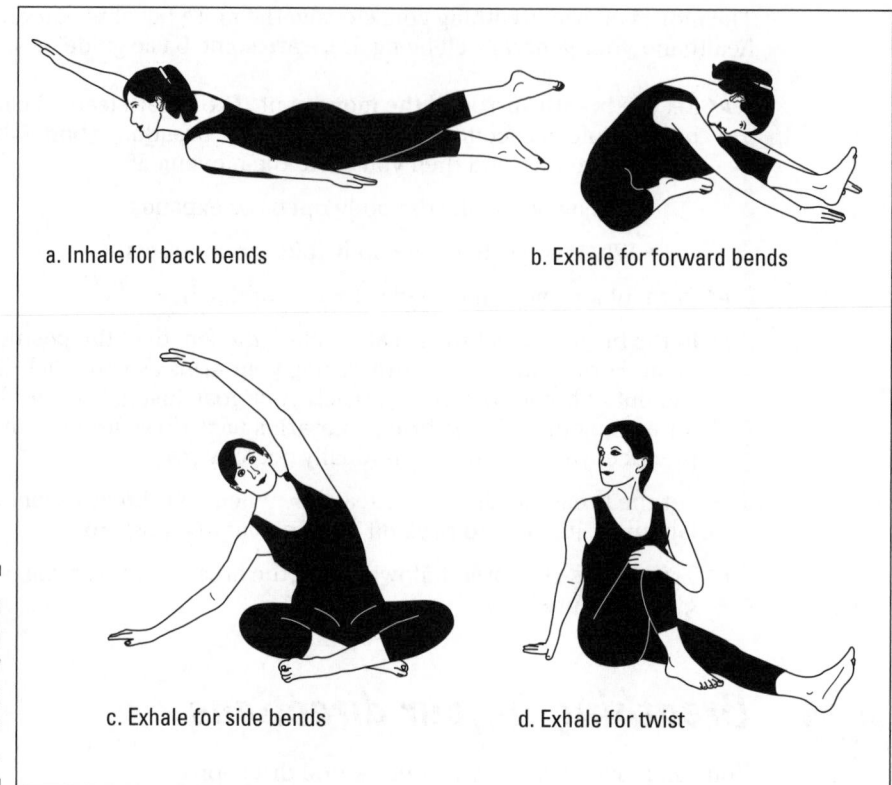

a. Inhale for back bends

b. Exhale for forward bends

Figure 2-3:
Breathing
properly
during
postures is
important.

c. Exhale for side bends

d. Exhale for twist

Understanding the roles of movement and holding in Yoga postures

Most Yoga books talk about *stationary* or *held* Yoga postures (*asanas*). We suggest that before learning to hold a posture, you first become acquainted with moving in and out of most of the postures we recommend in this book. Always, of course, follow the rules of breath and movement given in the immediately preceding section on inhalation and exhalation. Then, when you can move in and out of a given posture easily and confidently, try holding the posture for a short period *without* retaining or straining your breath. You can tell you're straining when your face is turning into a grimace or you feel it going red like a tomato. Learning to move into and out of the postures before adding the element of holding is important for three reasons:

- ✔ It helps to prepare your muscles and joints by bringing circulation to the area. It's like 'juicing your joints' which adds a safety factor.

- ✔ It helps you experience the intimate connection between body, breath and mind.

✔ In the case of stretching postures, moving into and out of a given posture before holding the posture supports the concept of *Proprioceptive Neuromuscular Facilitation* (PNF). If you tighten a muscle before stretching it either by gentle resistance (isotonic) or by pushing against a fixed force (isometric), the subsequent stretch is deeper than just using a static pose. Scientific research now supports this phenomenon; numerous physiotherapy texts refer to it as PNF.

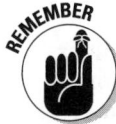

We often ask you to hold a posture for 6 to 8 breaths, which translates to roughly 30 seconds. Keep breathing when you hold a posture – don't hold your breath.

How do I start combining breath with movement?

The arrows in the following exercise and wherever they appear in this book tell you the direction of postural movement and the part of the breath that goes with the movement. *Inhale* means inhalation; *Exhale* means exhalation; *breaths* means the number of breaths defining the length of a postural hold.

1. **Lie on your back comfortably, with your legs straight or bent.**

   Place your arms at your sides near your hips with the palms turned down (see Figure 2-4a).

2. **Inhale through your nose and after one or two seconds begin to slowly raise your arms up over your head – in sync with inhalation – until they touch the ground behind you (see Figure 2-4b).**

   Leave your arms slightly bent.

3. **When you reach the end of inhalation, pause for one or two seconds even if your arms don't make it to the floor. Then exhale slowly through your nose and bring your arms back to your sides along the same path (as in Step 1).**

4. **Repeat this movement with a nice slow rhythm.**

   Remember, open or expand as you inhale, fold or contract as you exhale.

Book IV

Exploring Yoga and Pilates

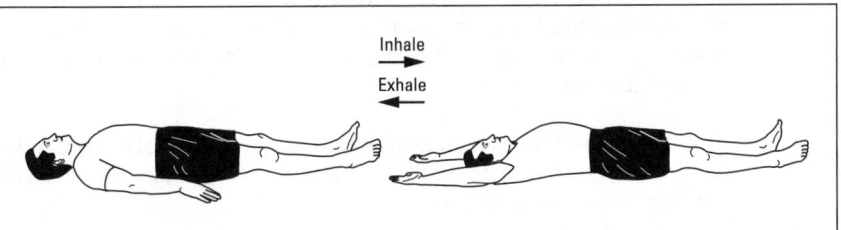

Figure 2-4:
The breath surrounds the movement.

Inhale

Exhale

After you become comfortable with this exercise, combine it with each of our recommended breathing techniques: Use either focus breathing, belly breathing or belly-to-chest breathing. You can decide which technique you prefer as you begin combining breathing with movement.

Sounding off: Yogic breathing

Sound, which is a form of vibration, is one of the means that Yoga employs to harmonise the vibration of your body and mind. In fact, the repetition of special sounds is one of the older and more potent techniques of Yoga. Here, we show you how to try this technique in conjunction with conscious breathing. A good way to start is to use the soft-sounding syllables *ah, ma* and *sa*. (We're not asking you to chant, although chanting can be a great and useful experience as well.) Try the following exercise while sitting in a chair or on the floor:

1. **Take a deep breath, and then as you exhale make a long *ah* sound in a way that you find pleasing and comfortable.**

   Continue the same sound for as long as your exhalation lasts. Then take a resting breath in between and repeat the exercise a total of five times.

2. **Relax for a few moments and next do five repetitions with the sound *ma*.**

   Relax again and conclude by using the sound *sa* five times. After you complete the full cycle, just sit quietly for a few minutes and notice how relaxed you feel.

Sound, or sonar, breathing stimulates the energetic centre at the throat and is quite relaxing.

Practising breath control the traditional way

Hatha Yoga includes various methods of breath control, all of which belong to the more advanced practices and traditionally follow extensive purification of body and mind. Some Western teachers have incorporated these methods into their beginners' classes, but our experience shows us that they are best taught at the intermediary to advanced levels. The following method is suitable for beginners, if you practise it with the necessary modifications and precautions.

Traditional Hatha Yoga emphasises holding the breath – not a good idea for beginners. In this section, we focus on techniques that are safe for any healthy person to practise.

Alternate nostril breathing

Researchers have demonstrated in the lab what Yoga masters have known for hundreds, if not thousands, of years: We don't breathe evenly through both nostrils. In a two-to-three-hour cycle, the nostrils become alternately dominant. It appears that left-nostril breathing is particularly connected with functions of the left cerebral hemisphere (notably verbal skills), while right-nostril breathing seems to connect more with the right hemisphere (notably spatial performance).

The technique called *alternate nostril breathing* goes by various others names, including *nadi-shodhana* ('channel cleansing', pronounced *nah-dee-shod-hah-nah*). Here's how you do it at the beginning level:

1. **Sit comfortably, with your back straight, on a chair or in one of the yogic sitting postures.**

2. **Check which nostril has the most air flowing through it and begin alternate breathing with the open nostril.**

   If both are equally open, all the better. In that case, begin with the left nostril.

   You can check which nostril is dominant simply by breathing through one nostril and then the other and comparing the two flows.

3. **Place your right hand so that your thumb is on the right nostril and the little and ring fingers are on the left nostril, with the index and middle fingers tugged against the ball of the thumb.**

   Note: According to some authorities, you should place the index and middle fingers on the spot between the eyebrows (known as the 'third eye'). We recommend the other method if it feels comfortable to you.

4. **Close the blocked nostril and, mentally counting to 5, inhale gently but fully through the open nostril – don't strain (see Figure 2-5).**

5. **Open the blocked nostril and close the other nostril and exhale, again mentally counting to 5.**

6. **Inhale through the same nostril to the count of 5, and exhale through the opposite nostril, and so on.**

   Repeat 10 to 15 times.

As your lung capacity improves, you can make your inhalations and exhalations longer, but *never* force the breath. Gradually increase the overall duration of the exercise from, say, 3 minutes to 15 minutes.

Book IV

Exploring Yoga and Pilates

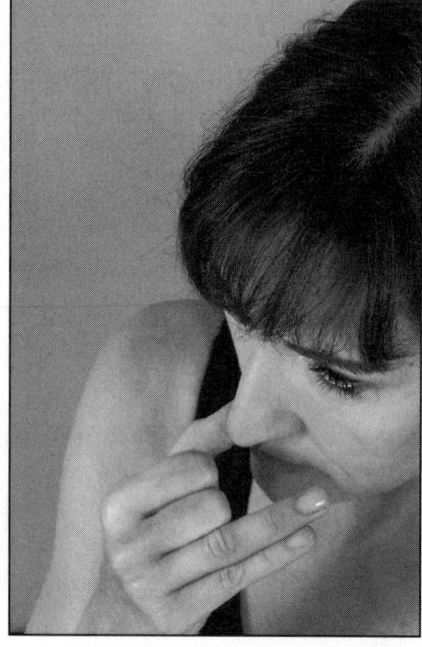

Figure 2-5:
The hand
position for
the alter-
nate nostril
breathing.

Meditation and the Higher Reaches of Yoga

Meditation is a mental process involving focused attention, or calm awareness, which is also called mindfulness.

Many forms or styles of meditation exist, but two basic approaches stand
out: *meditation with a specific focus* and *objectless meditation*. The latter is
pure mindfulness, without narrowing attention to any particular sensation,
idea or other phenomenon. Most beginners find this kind of meditation very
difficult, although some are drawn to it. We recommend that you start out
with meditation on a specific object. The following categories of objects are
suitable for this exercise:

- ✔ A bodily sensation, such as breathing, which makes an excellent focus.
- ✔ A bodily location, such as one of the seven cakras or energy centres (see
  the next section).
- ✔ A process or action, such as eating, walking or washing up.
- ✔ An external physical object, such as the flame of a candle.

✔ A *mantra* (be it a single sound, a phrase or a chant).

✔ A thought, such as the idea of peace, joy, love or compassion.

✔ Visualisation – a special form of meditation involving your creative imagination to picture light, emptiness, your spiritual teacher, a saint or one of the many deities of Hindu or Buddhist Yoga.

Experiment with all these various focal points for meditation until you find what appeals to you the most. Then stick with it. For instance, if you choose to visualise a particular saint or deity, you benefit by always using the same figure in your daily visualisation practice.

Following a few guidelines for successful meditation

Think of your meditation as a tree that you must water every day – not too much and not too little. Trust that one day your nurturing will bring the tree to bear beautiful blossoms and delicious fruit.

Here are seven vital tips to make your meditation tree grow:

✔ **Practise regularly:** Try to meditate every day. If this isn't possible, meditate at least a few times a week.

✔ **Cultivate the correct motivation:** People meditate for all kinds of reasons: health, wholeness, peace of mind, clarity, spiritual growth. Be clear in your own mind why you are sitting down to meditate. The best motivation for meditation (and Yoga practice in general) is to live to your full potential *and* to benefit others by your personal achievements.

In Buddhism, this motivation is known as the *bodhisattva* ideal. The *bodhisattva* (literally 'enlightenment being') seeks to realise enlightenment (the ultimate spiritual state) for the benefit of all other beings. As an enlightened being, you can be far more efficient in helping others in their own struggle for wholeness and happiness.

✔ **Meditate at the same time:** Take advantage of the fact that your body-mind is a creature of habit. After a few weeks of meditating at the same time during the day (or the night), you'll find yourself looking forward to your next meditation session. Traditionally, Yoga practitioners prefer the hour of sunrise, but this time isn't always practical.

Inevitably, you'll have moments when meditation is the last thing you want to do. In that case, resolve to sit quietly for at least five minutes. Often, this break is enough to get you in the mood for full-fledged meditation. If not, don't beat yourself over the head; just go on to something else and try again later or the next day.

Book IV

Exploring Yoga and Pilates

✔ **Meditate in the same place:** Choose the same time, same place, for the same reason: Your body-mind enjoys what is familiar. Use this fact to your advantage by setting aside a room or a corner of a room that your mind can associate with meditation.

✔ **Select an appropriate posture for meditation and do it correctly:** Sit up straight, with your chest open, and your neck free (see the following section for instructions about posture). Don't recline while meditating – you fall asleep – and don't meditate on your bed, even in a sitting position. Your mind is likely to associate the experience with sleep. If you're not used to sitting on the floor, try sitting on a straight-backed chair or on a sofa with a cushion behind your back. If you can comfortably sit on the floor, you have a variety of yogic postures to choose from.

✔ **Select a meditation technique and stick with it:** In the beginning, you may want to try out various techniques to see which appeals to you the most. But after you find a good technique for your particular needs, don't abandon it until it bears fruit (in terms of increased peace of mind and happiness), a meditation teacher advises you to change to a different technique, or you feel really drawn to a different technique.

✔ **Begin with short sessions:** Meditate 10 to 20 minutes at a time at first. If your meditation naturally lasts longer, then simply rejoice in the fact. But don't ever force yourself if the timing creates conflict or unhappiness in you. Also, beware of over-meditating. Often, what beginners regard as a 'nice long meditation' is just self-indulgent daydreaming. Make sure that your meditation contains an element of alertness. When you start drifting off into a comfortable space, you can be sure that you're no longer meditating. Like the practice of the Yoga postures, your meditation must have an *edge* (that is, you must push against the limitations of your mind but without frustrating yourself).

✔ **Be alert, yet relaxed:** Inner alertness, or mindfulness, is not the same as tension or stress. Make sure that your body is relaxed by regularly practising some relaxation exercises. Cats are good examples of this alertness. Even when a cat is completely relaxed, its ears move around like radar dishes catching every little sound in the environment. The more relaxed you are, the more alert your mind can be.

✔ **Don't burden yourself with expectations:** Entering meditation with a desire to grow spiritually and to benefit from the experience is certainly acceptable. However, don't expect every meditation to be wonderful and pleasant.

✔ **Prepare properly for meditation:** As a beginner, don't expect to be able to jump from the fray of your daily activities straight into meditation. Allow your mind a little time to unwind before you sit for meditation. Have a relaxing bath or shower or at least wash your face and hands.

✔ **Be prepared to practise meditation for a lifetime:** You don't grow a tree overnight. On the yogic path, no effort is ever wasted. Therefore, don't give up if your meditation is not what you think it should be after a month or two. Don't conclude too hastily that meditation isn't working or that the technique you're using isn't effective. Instead, correct your understanding about the nature of meditation and then persist. Your very effort to meditate counts.

Be wary of weekend workshops that promise immediate success, if not enlightenment itself. Meditation and enlightenment are lifelong processes.

✔ **Keep your meditation experiences to yourself:** In their enthusiasm, beginners understandably want to share their new discoveries with everyone. Resist the temptation to market your revelations to others, which turns most people off and won't do you any good either. Sharing your meditation experiences indiscriminately with others is like telling your friends (or anyone who will listen) about your intimate love life. It's in poor taste. Therefore, Yoga masters recommend silence on such matters.

✔ **At the end of your meditation, integrate the experience with the rest of your life:** Just as going straight from overdrive into a meditative gear is not prudent, you need to resist jumping up from meditation to return to your other activities. Instead, make a conscious transition into and out of meditation. At the end of the session, briefly recall your reasons for meditating and your overall motivation. Be grateful for any energies and/or insights your meditation generates. Equally importantly, don't feel negative about a difficult meditation experience. Rather, be grateful for *any* experience. Sometimes important insights surface during meditation, and then your challenge is to translate these messages into daily life. When you continually perform this kind of integration, your meditation will deepen more quickly as well.

Breathing mindfully

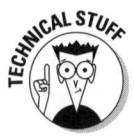

Particularly taught in Buddhist circles, mindful observation of the breath is a meditation exercise that any beginner can try. The breath is the link between body and mind. Since ancient times, the Yoga masters have made good use of this connection. Mindful breathing, or breathing meditation, is a simple and effective way of exploring the calming effect of conscious breathing.

1. **Sit up straight and relaxed.**

2. **Remind yourself of your purpose for meditation and resolve to sit in meditation for a given period of time.**

   We recommend at least 5 minutes for this exercise. Gradually extend the duration.

Book IV

Exploring Yoga and Pilates

3. **Close your eyes or keep them half open while looking down in front of you.**

4. **Breathing normally and gently, focus your attention on the sensation created by the breath flowing in and out of your nostrils.**

   Carefully observe the entire process of inhalation and exhalation as it occurs at the opening of your nostrils.

5. **To prevent your mind from wandering, you can count in inhalation/exhalation breath cycles from 1 to 10.**

Note: Don't be concerned if you notice that your attention has wandered. In particular, don't be judgemental about any thoughts that may pop into your head. Instead, re-dedicate yourself to the process of observing your breath.

The sacred syllable OM

The best known traditional mantra, used by Hindus and Buddhists alike, is the sacred syllable *om* (pronounced *ohmmm*). It's said to be the symbol of the absolute reality, the Self or spirit. It's composed of the letters *a, u, m,* and the nasal humming of the letter *m*. *A* corresponds to the waking state; *u* corresponds to the dream state; *m* corresponds to the state of deep sleep; and the nasal humming sound represents the ultimate reality.

Chapter 3

Getting Ready for Your Yoga Practice

So you're ready to take the plunge into some Yoga practice. The philosophy of Yoga combines together exercise, movement, breathing techniques and relaxation. After a little practice you'll start to feel some of the many health benefits.

In this chapter we introduce some safe and sound principles to help you get started with your Yoga practice. We introduce you to some warm-up exercises to start your body moving. The Sun Salutation is one of the key Yoga exercises and we introduce it in this chapter along with some props you can use to enhance your movement further.

Empowering Yourself with Yoga

Outside agents like doctors, therapists or remedies can help us through major crises, but we ourselves are primarily responsible for our own health and happiness. In particular the source of lasting happiness lies within us. Yoga reminds us of this truth and helps us mobilise the inner strength to live responsibly and wisely.

Maintaining health and happiness

What is health? Most people answer this question by saying that health is the opposite of illness. But health is *more* than the absence of disease. It's a positive state of being. Health is wholeness. To be healthy means not only to possess a well-functioning body and a sane mind but also to vibrate with life, to be vitally connected with one's social and physical environment. To be healthy also means to be happy.

Taking an active role in your own health

Most people tend to be passive in health matters. They wait until something goes wrong, and then they rely on a tablet or a doctor to fix the problem. Yoga encourages you to take the initiative in preventing illness and restoring or maintaining your health. Taking control of your health has nothing to do with self-diagnosis (which can be dangerous); it's simply a matter of taking responsibility for your health. A good physician will tell you that healing is greatly facilitated when the patient actively participates in the process. For example, you may take various kinds of medication to deal with a gastric ulcer, but unless you learn to eat well, sleep adequately, avoid stress and take it easier, you're bound to have a recurrence before long. You must change your lifestyle.

Following your bliss

Yoga suggests that the best possible meaning you can find for yourself springs from the well of joy deep within you. That joy or bliss is the very nature of the spirit, or transcendental Self. Joy is like a 3-D lens that captures life's bright colours and motivates you to embrace life in all of its countless forms. Yoga points the way to happiness, health and life-embracing meaning.

Balancing your life with Yoga

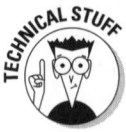

Hindu tradition explains Yoga as the discipline of balance. This is another way of expressing the ideal of unity through Yoga. Everything in you must harmonise to function optimally. A disharmonious mind is disturbing in itself but, sooner or later, it also causes physical problems. An imbalanced body can easily warp your emotions and thought processes. If your relationships with others are strained, you cause distress not only for them but for yourself as well. And when your relationship to your physical environment is disharmonious, well, you trigger serious repercussions for everyone.

A beautiful and simple Yoga exercise called 'The Tree' is meant to improve your sense of balance and promote your inner stillness. Even when conditions force a tree to grow askew, it always balances itself out by growing a branch in the opposite direction from which it's being forced to lean. In this posture, you stand still like a tree, perfectly balanced.

Yoga helps you apply this principle to your life. Whenever life's demands and challenges force you to bend to one side, your inner strength and peace of mind serve as counterweights. Rising above all adversity, you can never be uprooted.

Preparing Yourself for a Yoga Session

Before you start, pause, take a deep breath, exhale slowly, and then ask yourself: 'What do I want from my Yoga experience?' You may find your own answer by taking a few moments to ponder the following questions:

- ✔ Do I simply want to try Hatha Yoga because it's a trendy thing to do?

- ✔ Am I hoping to find a way to decompress (clear the mind and alleviate stress)?

- ✔ Is physical fitness my main interest?

- ✔ Do I simply want to have a more flexible body?

- ✔ Does meditation intrigue me?

- ✔ Do the spiritual aspects of Yoga interest me?

- ✔ Do I have health concerns, such as lower back problems or hypertension, that I expect Yoga to help handle?

After you're clear about your motivation and expectations, don't just think it – *ink it*: Write down your goals so that you can really focus on your specific needs. For example, you may want to be able to cope with stress better. This is your *goal*. In order to achieve it, you have to take your particular situation into account. If you are a super-busy mum and have only half an hour of slack time at night during the week and perhaps a full hour on Sundays, you obviously have to keep your Yoga programme very simple. This is your *need*.

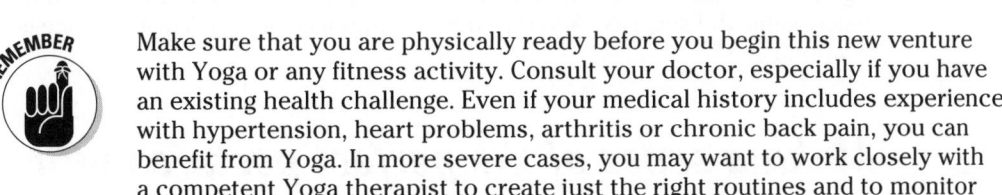

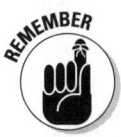

Make sure that you are physically ready before you begin this new venture with Yoga or any fitness activity. Consult your doctor, especially if you have an existing health challenge. Even if your medical history includes experience with hypertension, heart problems, arthritis or chronic back pain, you can benefit from Yoga. In more severe cases, you may want to work closely with a competent Yoga therapist to create just the right routines and to monitor your progress.

Book IV

Exploring Yoga and Pilates

Making time for Yoga

For centuries, the traditional times for Yoga practice have been sunrise and sunset, which are thought to be especially auspicious. These days, busy lifestyles can toss out lots of obstacles to your best intentions: Be pragmatic and arrange your Yoga practice at your convenience. Just keep in mind that statistically, you have a 30 per cent greater chance of accomplishing a fitness goal if you practise in the morning. More important than holding tight to a preset time is just making sure that you work Yoga into your schedule *somewhere* – and sticking with it.

Practising at roughly the same time during the day can help you create a positive habit, which may make it easier to maintain your routine.

Eating before Yoga practice

Whether you're attending a Yoga class or practising on your own, the guidelines for eating before Yoga practice are similar to the advice given for most physical activities. With even the lightest meal, such as fruit or juice, allow at least one hour before the class. For larger meals with vegetables and grains, allow two hours, and for heavy meals with meat, three to four hours. Eating right after the class is okay; you may notice that this snack or meal turns into a pleasant social event with class-mates. (If the socialising aspect sounds like fun, remember that you're not likely to enjoy the same opportunities with private lessons.)

Enjoying a Safe and Sound Yoga Practice

As you travel through yogic postures, you begin to build awareness of the communications taking place between your body and your mind. Do you feel peacefully removed from the raging storm of life around you, comfortable and confident with your strength, motion and steadiness? Or are you painfully in tune with the passage of time, sensing a physical awkwardness or strain in your movements? Listening to your own rhythms – and acknowledging their importance – can help make your Yoga experience an expression of peace, calm and security. And that positive message is what Yoga practice is all about.

Making sense of the perfect posture myth

Some modern schools of Hatha Yoga claim that they teach 'perfect' postures that you can slip into as easily as a tailor-made suit. But how can a perfect posture exist when we are all different? Should a 15-year-old athlete perform a posture or an entire postural routine following the same guidelines that apply to a 60-year-old retired person? Surely not. Besides, these schools disagree amongst themselves about what constitutes a perfect posture. So, to spell it out, the perfect posture is perfectly mythical.

Posture, as explained by the great Yoga master Patanjali 2000 years ago, has only two requirements: A posture should be *steady* and *comfortable*. What could be more plain and simple? Although Patanjali was thinking primarily, perhaps even exclusively, in terms of meditation postures, his formula applies to all postures equally.

- ✔ **Steady posture:** A steady posture is a posture that's held stable for a certain period of time. The key isn't freezing all movement, though. Your posture becomes steady when your mind is steady. As long as your thoughts run wild and your negative emotions are not held in check, your body also remains unsteady. As you become more skilled in self-observation, you begin to notice the ever-revolving carousel of your mind and you become sensitive to the tension in your body. That tension is what Yoga means by 'unsteadiness'.

- ✔ **Comfortable posture:** A posture is comfortable when it is enjoyable and enlivening rather than boring and burdensome. A comfortable posture increases the principle of clarity – *sattva* – in you. But please don't confuse comfort with slouching. *Sattva* and joy are intimately connected. The more *sattva* is present in your body-mind, the more relaxed and happy you will be.

Listening to your body

No one knows your body like you do. The more you practise Yoga, the better you can become at determining your limitations with each posture: Each posture presents its own unique challenge. Ideally, you want to feel encouraged to explore and expand your physical and emotional boundaries without risking strain or injury to yourself.

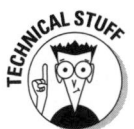

Some teachers speak of practising at the *edge*. The edge is the point of intensity where a posture challenges you but does not cause you pain or unusual discomfort. The idea is to gradually – very slowly and carefully – push that edge farther back and open up new territory. To be able to practise at the edge, you must cultivate self-observation and pay attention to the feedback from your body.

Each Yoga session is an exercise in self-observation without being judgemental. Listen to what your body is telling you through its ongoing communications. Signals constantly travel from your muscles, tendons, ligaments, bones and skin to your brain. Train yourself to become aware of them. You want to be in dialogue with your body instead of indulging in a monologue

Book IV

Exploring Yoga and Pilates

that focuses on your own mind without awareness of your body. Pay particular attention to signals coming from the neck, lower back, jaw muscles, abdomen and any known problem areas of your body (such as a 'difficult' knee or a 'chronic' shoulder muscle).

To gauge the intensity of a difficult Yoga posture, use a scale from 1 to 10, with 10 being at the threshold of pain. Imagine a flashing red light and an alarm bell going off after you pass level 8. Notice the signals and heed them. Especially watch your breath. If your breathing becomes laboured, it's usually a good indication that, figuratively speaking, you are going over the edge. You are the world's foremost expert on what your body is trying to tell you.

Beginners commonly experience trembling when holding certain Yoga postures. Normally, the involuntary motion is noticeable in the legs or arms and is nothing to worry about, as long as you aren't straining. The tremors are simply a sign that your muscles are working in response to a new demand. Instead of focusing on the feeling that you've become a wobbly bowl of jelly, make your breath a little longer if you can and allow your attention to go deeper within. If the trembling starts to go off the Richter scale, then you need to either ease up a little or end the posture altogether.

Moving slowly but surely

All postural movements are intended for slow performance. Unfortunately, most of the time, we're on automatic. Our movements tend to be unconscious, too fast, and not particularly graceful. We stumble, bump into things, and are generally unaware of our bodies. The yogic postures oblige you to adopt a different attitude. Among the advantages of slow motion are:

- ✔ You enhance your awareness, which enables you to *listen* to what your body is telling you and to practise at the *edge* (see the earlier section, 'Listening to your body').

- ✔ You lower the risk of straining or spraining muscles, tearing ligaments, or overtaxing your heart. In other words, your practice becomes much safer.

- ✔ You experience relaxation more quickly.

- ✔ You don't get out of breath, and your breathing overall is improved.

- ✔ You enable more muscle groups to come into action to share the workload.

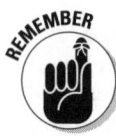

For the best results, practise your postures at a slow, steady pace while calmly focusing on your breath and the postural movement. Resist the temptation to speed up, but instead savour each posture. Remember to relax and be present here and now. If your breathing becomes a little bit laboured or you begin to feel fatigued, just rest until you're ready to go on.

Understanding the Philosophy of Postures

Postures, or *asanas* (pronounced *ah-sah-nah*) in Sanskrit, are probably the part of Yoga that you're most familiar with. They're those poses that look impossible, but that are done with ease by many Yoga students. Beyond stretching and increasing strength and flexibility, Yoga postures help you get in tune with yourself, your body and your environment. Through *asanas,* you can begin to see yourself as at one with your environment.

Yogic postures are more than mere bodily poses. They are also expressions of your state of mind. An *asana* is poise, composure, carriage – all words suggesting an element of balance and refinement. The postures demonstrate the profound connection between body and mind.

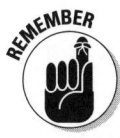 According to traditional Yoga manuals, the main purpose of *asana* is to prepare the body to sit quietly, easily and steadily for breathing exercises and meditation. The way we sit is, in fact, an important foundation technique for these practices; when you perform them properly, the sitting postures act as natural 'tranquillisers' for the body, and when the physical vehicle is still, the mind soon follows.

 If your knees are more than a few inches higher than your hips when you sit cross-legged on the floor, it's an indication that your hip joints are tight. If you try to sit for a long while like this for meditation or breathing exercises, you may very well end up with an aching back. Don't feel bad, you're not alone. Accept your current limitations in this area and use a prop, like a firm cushion or thickly folded blanket, to raise your buttocks off the floor high enough to drop your knees to at least level with your hips.

Getting Ready for Exercise with Warm-Ups

Any physical exercise requires adequate warm-up, and Yoga is no exception. The purpose of warm-up exercises is to increase circulation to the parts of your body you're about to use and also to make you more aware of those areas of your physical self. What's different about the Yoga warm-up is that it is done slowly and deliberately, with conscious breathing and awareness. Here are some of the benefits of yogic warm-up:

   ✔ It brings awareness and presence of mind.

   ✔ It allows you to test your body before executing the postures.

✔ It increases the temperature and blood supply to your muscles, joints and connective tissue.

✔ It prepares your body for more challenging demands and reduces the possibility of muscle tear or strain.

✔ It enhances the supply of oxygen and nutrients, thus providing more stamina for the practice.

✔ It prevents muscle soreness.

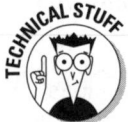

Yoga warm-up postures are also called *preparation poses,* which are usually done *dynamically* and are always performed before other exercises begin. In general, the safest Yoga warm-ups before you begin are simple forward bends and easy sequences that fold and unfold the body. Figure 3-1 shows some of our recommended warm-up exercises. You may select from the various reclining, sitting and standing positions. Warm-up doesn't have to be monotonous or dull!

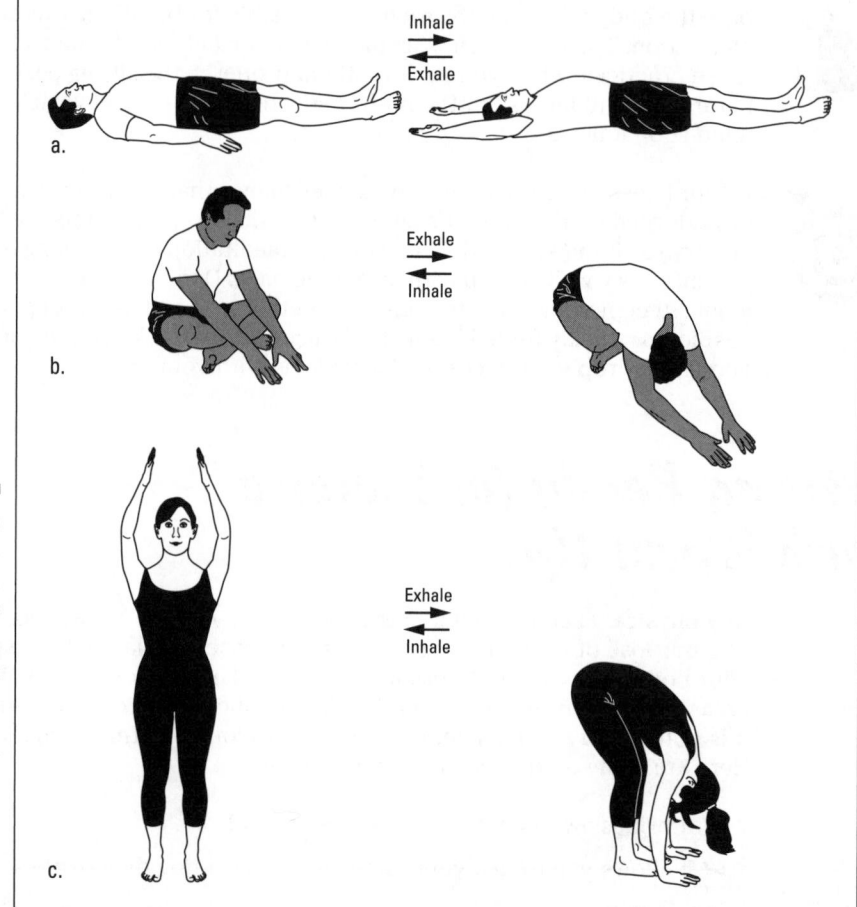

Figure 3-1:
Simple forward bends and easy sequences make great preparation poses whether you're lying down (a), sitting (b) or standing (c).

Asana by any other name

The term *asana* simply means 'seat'. It can denote both the surface on which the Yoga practitioner sits and the bodily posture. Some postures are called *mudras* (pronounced *moo-drahs*) or 'seals', because they're especially effective in keeping the life energy *(prana)* sealed within the body. This leads to greater vitality and better mental focusing. Life energy is everywhere, both inside and outside our bodies, but it must be properly harnessed within the body in order to promote health and happiness.

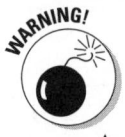

If you have disc problems in your lower back, forward bends may not be a good way to warm-up. Check with your doctor.

In addition to warming up at the beginning of a session, preparation postures are used throughout a given routine to precede and enhance the effect of the main postures (see Figure 3-2 for some samples). For example, the leg lift is used to stretch the hamstrings just before a seated forward bend. The bridge posture works well just prior to a shoulder stand.

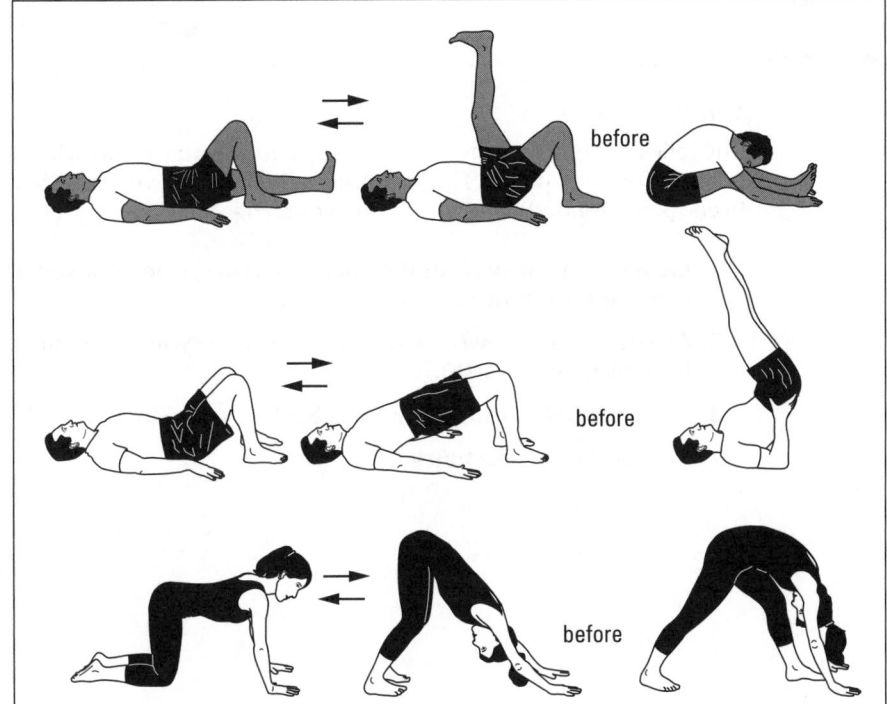

Figure 3-2: Certain postures help you prepare for specific main poses.

Book IV

Exploring Yoga and Pilates

Avoid warming up with more complex postures such as shoulder stands, deep twists or advanced back bends (shown in Figure 3-3). Also, we suggest avoiding a heavy cardiovascular workout before a strenuous Yoga practice because you can experience muscle cramps.

Reclining postures

Most Yoga practitioners enjoy reclining (supine) exercises because they are intrinsically relaxing. When you pair them with warm-ups, you're enjoying the benefits of having your cake and eating it too. The combination effectively allows you to warm-up specific muscles or muscle groups while keeping the other muscles at rest.

Figure 3-3:
Avoid
warming
up with
complex
postures
like these.

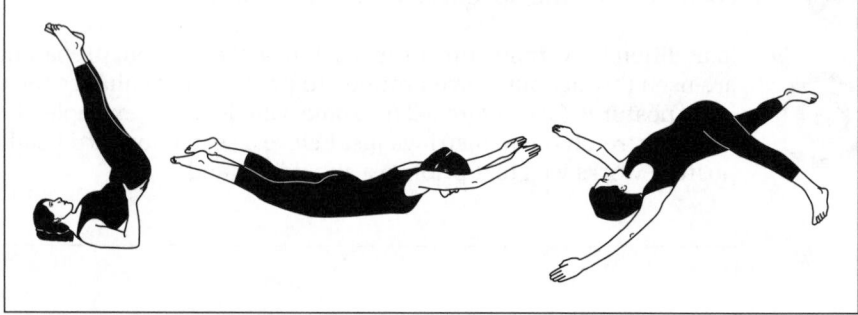

Lying arm raise

The following eight warm-up exercises require you to start with the corpse posture (or dead pose). These exercises help revive you even if you are dead tired (pun intended) when you start your Yoga session.

1. **Lie flat on your back in the corpse posture, arms relaxed at your sides, palms turned down (see Figure 3-4a).**

2. **As you inhale, slowly raise your arms over your head and touch the floor (see Figure 3-4b).**

3. **As you exhale, bring your arms back to your sides.**

4. **Repeat six to eight times.**

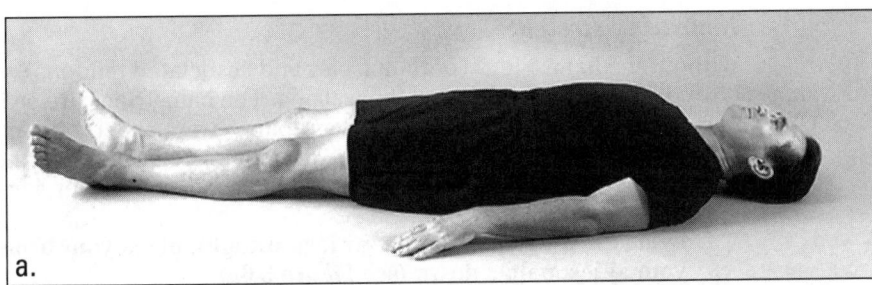

a.

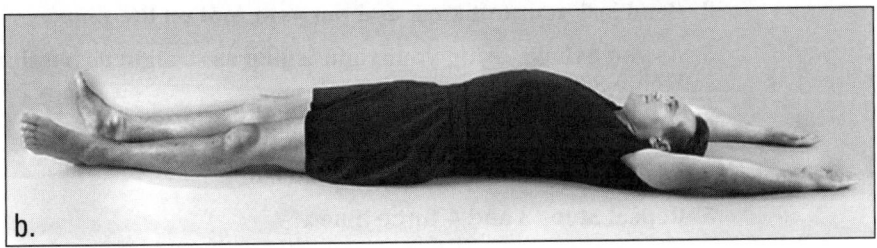

Figure 3-4:
Arm raises
stretch the
back and
warm up the
neck.

b.

Knee-to-chest

Use this exercise for either warm-up or compensation. The knee to chest pose is also a classic in low back programmes.

1. **Lie on your back, knees bent, feet flat on the floor.**

2. **As you exhale, bring the your right knee into your chest. Grip your shin just below your knee (see Figure 3-5a).**

   If you have knee problems, hold the back of your thigh rather than your shin (see Figure 3-5b).

3. **If you can do so comfortably, straighten your left leg on the floor.**

   If you have back problems, though, keep your left knee bent.

4. **Stay on each side for 6 to 8 breaths.**

Book IV

Exploring Yoga and Pilates

Figure 3-5:
Use this
pose to tune
your back.

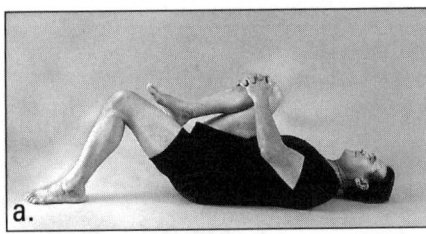

a.

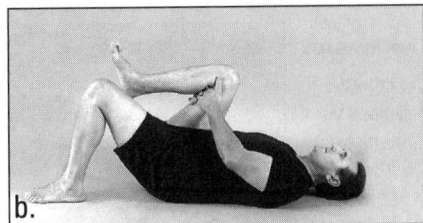

b.

Hamstring stretch

Without the hamstrings (both muscles and associated tendons), you would have to let your fingers do all the walking. The hamstrings are an important part of your anatomy, and it pays to prepare them properly for exercise. When the hamstring muscles aren't warmed up, you can injure them quite easily, especially when you are prone to over-exertion (never a good idea).

1. **Lying on your back with your legs straight, place your arms along your sides, palms down (see Figure 3-6a).**

2. **Bend just your left knee and put your foot on the floor.**

3. **As you exhale, bring your right leg up as straight as possible (see Figure 3-6b).**

4. **As you inhale, return your leg to the floor.**

   Keep your head and your hips on the floor.

5. **Repeat Steps 3 and 4 three times.**

   Then with your hands interlocked on the back of your raised thigh, just above your knee, hold your leg in place (see Figure 3-6c) for 6 to 8 breaths and repeat the sequence on the other side.

Lift your head up on a pillow or folded blanket if the back of your neck or your throat tenses when you raise or lower your leg.

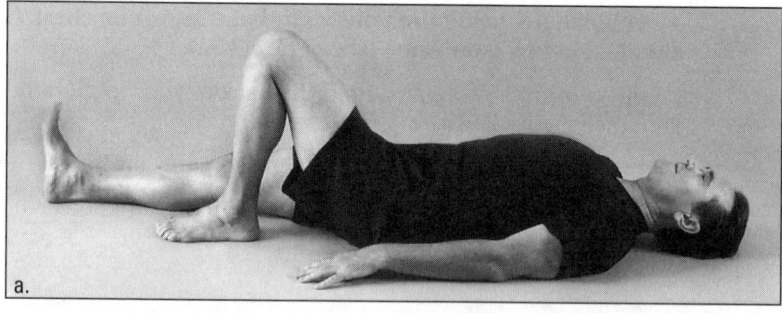

Figure 3-6: Unlock your hamstrings and you open the door to many Yoga postures.

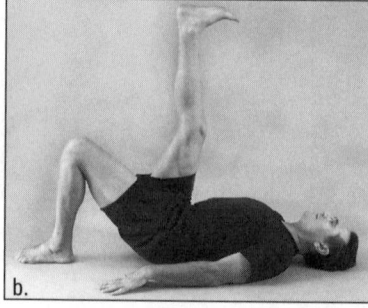

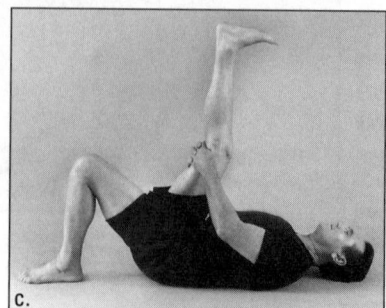

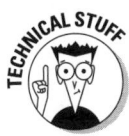

Dynamic bridge – dvipada pitha

You can use this exercise for warm-up and compensation. The Sanskrit term *dvipada* means 'two-footed' and *pitha* means 'seat', which is a synonym for *asana*. The pronunciation is *dvee-pah-dah* and *peet-hah*, respectively.

1. Lie on your back, knees bent, feet flat on the floor at hip width.

2. Place your arms at your sides, palms turned down (see Figure 3-7a).

3. As you inhale, raise your hips to a comfortable height (see Figure 3-7b); as you exhale, return your hips to the floor.

4. Repeat Steps 3 and 4 six to eight times.

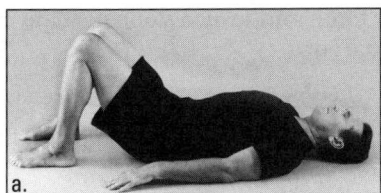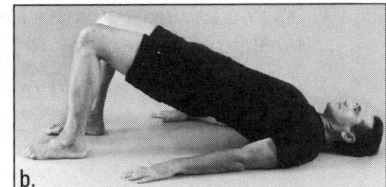

Figure 3-7:
A frequently used posture for preparation, compensation or as a main pose.

Bridge variation with arm raise

This posture is another good candidate for warm-up and compensation.

1. Lie on your back, knees bent, feet flat on the floor at hip width.

2. Place your arms at your sides, palms turned down (refer to Figure 3-8a)

3. As you inhale, raise your hips to a comfortable height and, at the same time, raise your arms overhead to touch the floor (see Figure 3-8b).

4. As you exhale, return your hips to the floor and your arms to your sides.

5. Repeat Steps 3 and 4 six to eight times.

Book IV

Exploring Yoga and Pilates

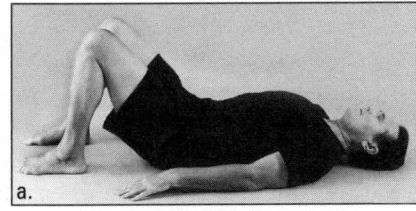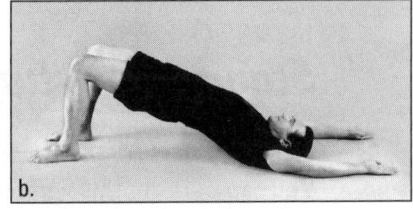

Figure 3-8:
A nice variation for the bridge posture.

Dynamic head-to-knee

Dynamic head-to-knee is a slightly more vigorous kind of warm-up.

Do not perform this sequence if you're having neck problems.

1. **Lie flat on your back in the corpse posture, arms relaxed at your sides, palms turned down (refer to Figure 3-4a).**

2. **As you inhale, raise your arms slowly overhead and touch the floor (see Figure 3-9a).**

3. **As you exhale, draw your right knee towards your chest, lift your head off the floor, and then grasp your right knee with your hands.**

   Keep the top of your hips on the floor. Bring your head as close to your knee as possible, but don't force it (see Figure 3-9b).

4. **As you inhale, release your knee and return your head, arms and straightened right leg to the floor.**

5. **Repeat Steps 1 to 4 on the left side.**

6. **Repeat Steps 2 to 5 six to eight times on each side, alternating right and left.**

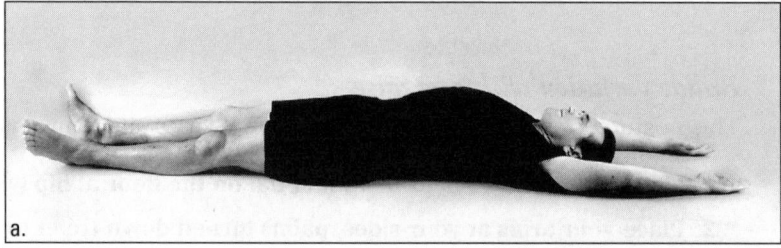

a.

Figure 3-9:
Use this
sequence
before a
slightly
more
physical
routine.

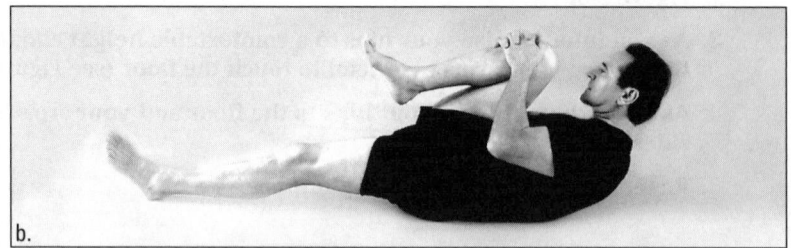

b.

Standing postures

Standing arm raise

You can perform this versatile warm-up almost anywhere when you want to enjoy a complete break from sitting. Try it at the office and start a new trend.

1. **Stand tall, but relaxed, with your feet at hip width (see Figure 3-10a).**

2. **Hang your arms at your sides, palms turned back.**

   Look straight ahead.

3. **As you inhale, raise your arms forward and then up overhead (see Figure 3-10b).**

4. **As you exhale, bring your arms down and back to your sides.**

5. **Repeat Steps 3 and 4 six to eight times.**

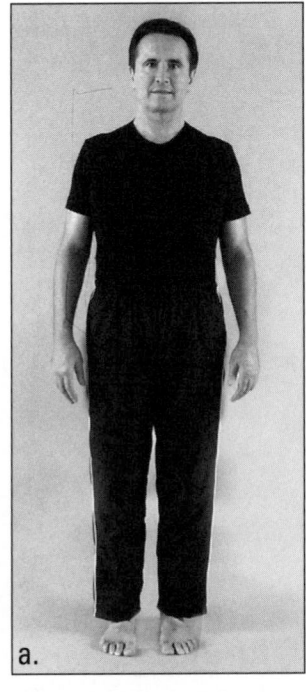
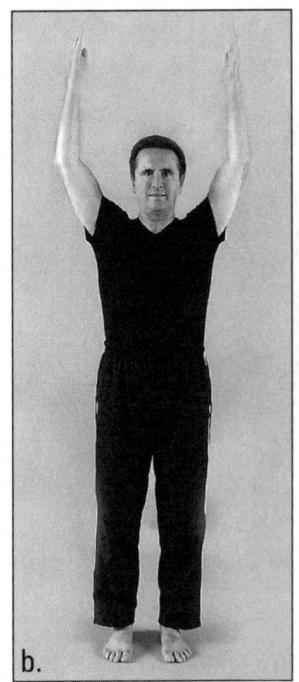

Figure 3-10: Release the most frequent site of tension — the neck and shoulders.

a.   b.

Head turner

Think of your entire upper body, all the way out to your hands, as part of your wing span. Sequences like the head turner, which combine breath and movement in the parts of the upper body, stretch, strengthen and heal your entire wingspan.

1. **Stand tall, but relaxed, with your feet at hip width.**

2. **Hang your arms at your sides, palms turned back.**

   Look straight ahead.

Book IV

Exploring Yoga and Pilates

3. **As you inhale, raise your right arm forward and up overhead as you turn your head to the left (see Figure 3-11).**

4. **As you exhale, bring your arm down and turn your head forward.**

5. **As you inhale, raise your left arm forward and up overhead while turning your head to the right.**

6. **Repeat Steps 3 to 5 six to eight times on each side, alternating right and left.**

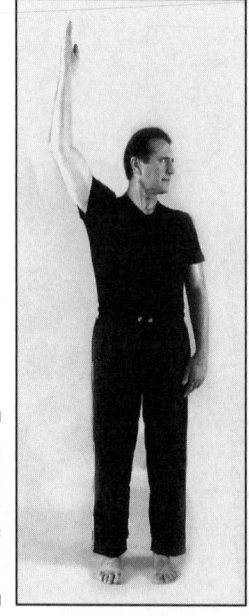

Figure 3-11:
This posture is great for minor stiff necks.

Shoulder rolls

You can use shoulder rolls in many types of exercise routines. The major difference here is that we move slowly, with awareness, co-ordinating with the breath.

1. **Stand tall, but relaxed, with your feet at hip width.**

2. **Hang your arms at your sides, palms turned back.**

   Look straight ahead.

3. **As you inhale, roll your shoulders up and back (see Figure 3-12); as you exhale, drop the shoulders down.**

4. **Repeat Steps 3 and 4 six to eight times.**

   Reverse the direction six to eight times.

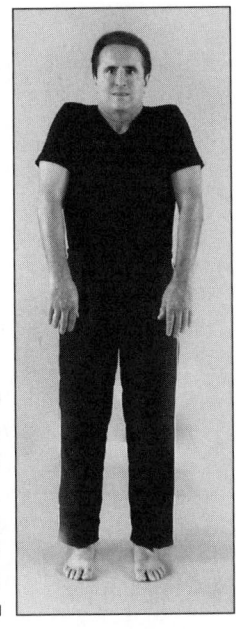

Figure 3-12:
Move
slowly,
co-ordinating
breath and
movement.

Dynamic standing forward bend

You can use this exercise for warm-up and compensation.

1. **Stand tall, but relaxed, with your feet at hip width.**

2. **Hang your arms at your sides, palms turned back.**

3. **As you inhale, raise your arms forward and up overhead (refer to Figure 3-10b).**

4. **As you exhale, bend forward and when you feel a pull in the back of your legs, bend your legs and arms slightly – this is called 'Forgiving Limbs' (see Figure 3-13).**

5. **As you inhale, roll up slowly, stacking the bones of your spine one at a time from bottom to top, and then raise your arms overhead.**

   Finally, release the arms back to your sides.

6. **Repeat Steps 3 to 5 six to eight times.**

Rolling up in Step 5 is the safest way to come up. If you do not have back problems, after a few weeks you may want to try two more advanced techniques: As you come up, sweep your arms out and up from the sides like wings then overhead; or, as you inhale, extend your slightly bent arms forward and up until they are parallel with your ears. Then raise your upper back, then your lower back until you are all the way up and your arms are overhead.

Book IV

Exploring
Yoga and
Pilates

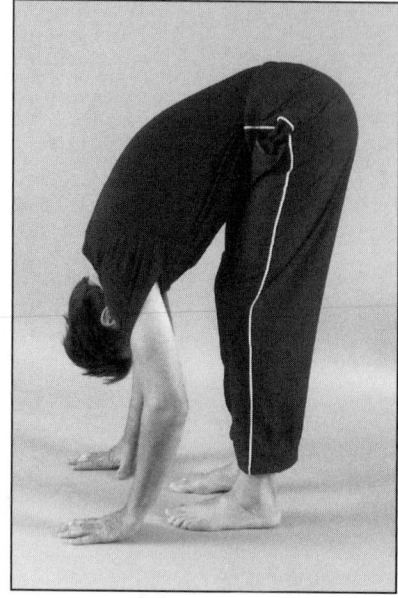

Figure 3-13:
How you come back up is just as important as how you go down.

Sitting postures

Most Westerners are used to sitting on furniture rather than the floor, but try these postures and after a few tries you should loosen up and be able to do them easily.

Sitting fold

The sitting fold is a very simple way to warm up or prepare your back for forward bends or to compensate after sitting twists.

1. **Sit on the floor with your legs crossed in the easy posture,** *sukhasana.* **(see Book IV Chapter 4).**

2. **Place your hands on the floor in front of you, palms down (see Figure 3-14a).**

3. **As you exhale, slide your hands out along the floor and bend forward at the hips.**

   If possible, bring your head down to the floor or just come as close as you comfortably can (see Figure 3-14b).

4. **As you inhale, roll your torso and head up and return to the starting position.**

5. **Repeat Steps 3 and 4 four to six times, then switch your legs and repeat four to six times.**

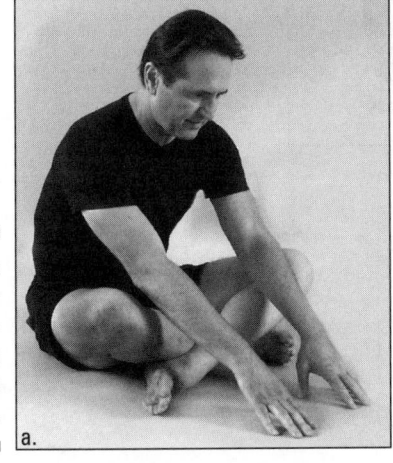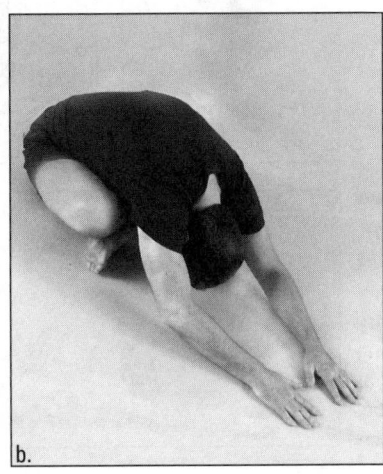

Figure 3-14:
Slide your hands forward on the ground as you exhale.

a. b.

Sitting wing-and-prayer

The wing-and-prayer is an excellent way to decompress the upper spine and open the chest.

1. **Sit on the floor with your legs crossed in the easy posture (see Book IV Chapter 4)**

2. **Join your palms in the prayer position, thumbs at the breastbone (see Figure 3-15a).**

3. **As you inhale, raise your joined hands overhead.**

   Follow your thumbs with your eyes (see Figure 3-15b).

4. **As you exhale, bring your hands back to your breastbone (refer to Figure 3-15a).**

5. **As you inhale, separate your hands and stretch your arms like wings to your sides at shoulder height.**

   Look straight ahead (see Figure 3-15c).

6. **As you exhale, join your palms again at the breastbone (refer to Figure 3-15a).**

7. **Repeat Steps 3 to 6 six to eight times.**

Book IV

Exploring Yoga and Pilates

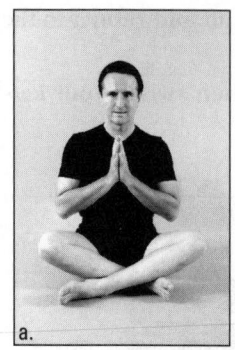
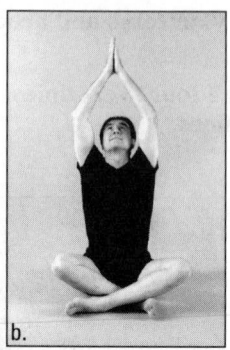
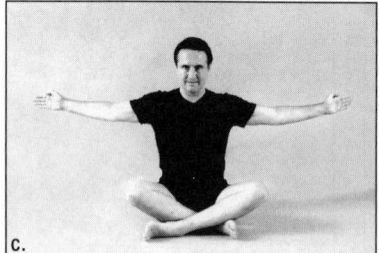

Figure 3-15:
For a quick break, you can also try this sitting in a chair at the office.

Introducing the Sun Salutation

Respected for its excellent effects, the sun salutation is reputed to provide an array of benefits, including:

- ✔ Stretching your spine and strengthening the muscles that support it
- ✔ Strengthening and stretching your arms and legs
- ✔ Improving your posture, co-ordination and endurance
- ✔ Complementing the delicate balance between muscle tension and muscle relaxation
- ✔ Linking body, breath and mind
- ✔ Granting (in most of its forms) aerobic benefits
- ✔ Improving the functioning of your lungs and the delivery of oxygen to your muscles (including the heart)
- ✔ Working well (with modifications) for people of all ages, from children to retired people

The Yoga masters also claim that the sun salutation has deeper psychological and spiritual implications, because it stimulates subtle vital energies leading to states of higher awareness. It's no wonder that so many Yoga videos on the market today include the sun salutation.

Travelling through the 7-step kneeling salutation

If you aren't quite ready to tackle the 12-step sun salutation, the following 7-step variation can give you many benefits and also help you get in shape for the standing variety of *surya namaskara*. Figure 3-16 shows you the various steps involved with this routine. Use any of the Yoga breathing techniques from Book IV Chapter 2.

1. **Sit on your heels in a bent-knee position, bring your back up nice and tall, and place your palms together in the prayer position, with the thumbs touching the sternum in the middle of your chest (see Figure 3-16a).**

2. **As you inhale, open your palms and slightly raise your arms forward, then up and overhead. Raise your buttocks away from your heels, arch your back, and look up at the ceiling (see Figure 3-16b).**

3. **As you exhale, bend forward slowly from the hips. Place your palms, forearms, and then your forehead on the floor and pause with your hips up (see Figure 3-16c).**

4. **Slide your hands forward on the floor until your arms are extended. Then slide your chest forward, bending your elbows slightly, and arch up into the cobra posture, as we describe in Book IV Chapter 5 (see Figure 3-16d).**

5. **As you exhale, turn your toes under, raise your hips up, extend your legs, and bring your chest down. Keep both hands on the floor (see Figure 3-16e).**

6. **As you inhale, bend your knees to the floor and look straight ahead (see Figure 3-16f).**

7. **As you exhale, sit back on your heels and return your hands to the saluting position as in Step 1 (see Figure 3-16g).**

8. **Repeat the entire sequence three to twelve times. Move slowly, pausing after the inhalation and the exhalation.**

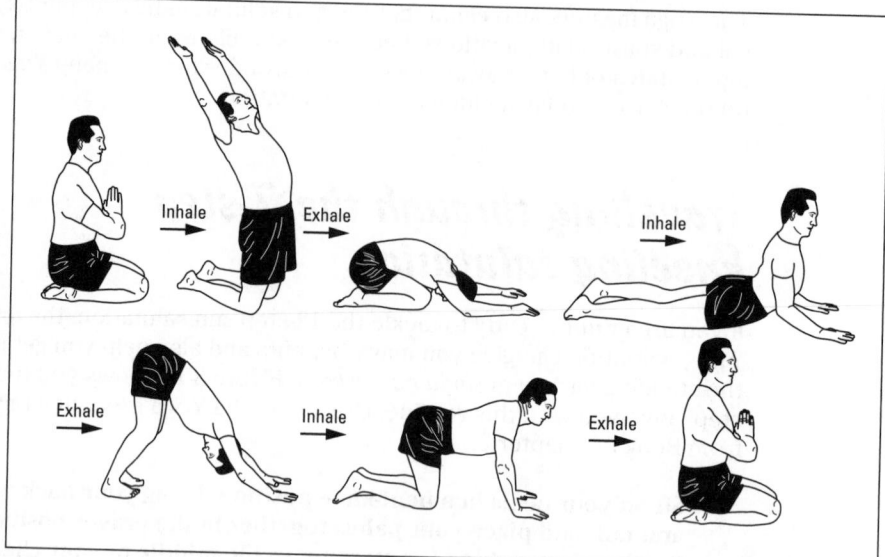

Figure 3-16: Just follow your breath – inhale when you are opening, exhale when you are folding.

Embarking on the 12-step sun salutation

To enjoy the greatest benefit from your Yoga postures, execute them with full participation of your mind. When you stand, really stand; plant your feet firmly on the ground. When you bend, bend with complete attention. When you stretch, stretch with full attention. Your mind not only makes your practice elegant, but also potent.

Use Figure 3-17 as a posture guide to help you through this routine. Use any of the Yoga breathing techniques from Book IV Chapter 2.

1. **Start in a standing position with your feet at hip width. Place your palms together in the prayer position with your thumbs touching the sternum in the middle of your chest (see Figure 3-17a).**

2. **As you inhale, open your palms slightly and raise your arms forward, then up and overhead. Arch your back and look up at the ceiling (see Figure 3-17b).**

3. **As you exhale, bend forward from the hips, soften your knees ('Forgiving Limbs' posture), and place your hands on the floor. Bring your head as close as possible to your legs (see Figure 3-17c).**

4. **As you inhale, bend your left knee and step your right foot back into a lunge.**

Make sure that your left knee is directly over your ankle and your thigh is parallel to the floor, so that your knee makes a right angle. Look straight ahead (see Figure 3-17d).

5. **As you exhale, step your left foot back beside the right and hold a push-up position. If your arms give out, bend your knees to the floor and pause on your hands and knees (see Figure 3-17e).**

6. **Inhale and then as you exhale, lower your knees (from the push-up), chest and chin to the floor. Keep your buttocks up in the air (see Figure 3-17f).**

7. **As you inhale, slide your chest forward along the floor and then arch back into the cobra posture (see Figure 3-17g).**

8. **As you exhale, turn your toes under, raise your hips up, extend your legs, and bring your chest down. Keep both hands on the floor (see Figure 3-17h).**

9. **As you inhale, step your right foot forward between your hands and look straight ahead (see Figure 3-17i).**

10. **As you exhale, step your left foot forward, parallel to and level with the right. Soften your knees and fold into a forward bend, as in Step 3 (see Figure 3-17j).**

11. **As you inhale, raise your arms either forward and up overhead from the front, or out and up from the sides like wings, and then arch back and look up, as in Step 2 (see Figure 3-17k).**

12. **As you exhale, return your hands to the prayer position, as in Step 1 (see Figure 3-17l).**

13. **Repeat the entire sequence three to twelve times. First lead with the right foot, and then alternate with the left foot, for an equal number of times (each side counts as half a round).**

Move slowly, pausing after the inhalation and the exhalation.

If you have back problems, lifting up from the forward bend (in Step 11) with your arms either to the front or sides may cause you some discomfort. If so, you can try the 'roll up': Keep your chin on your chest and roll up, stacking the vertebrae one at a time, with your arms hanging at your sides. When you are fully upright, bring the arms forward, up, and overhead from the front, arch your back just a little, and look up.

If both the 7-step and the 12-step sun salutations are too difficult for you, repeat Steps 1–3 only of the 12-step version until you are ready to do more.

Book IV

Exploring Yoga and Pilates

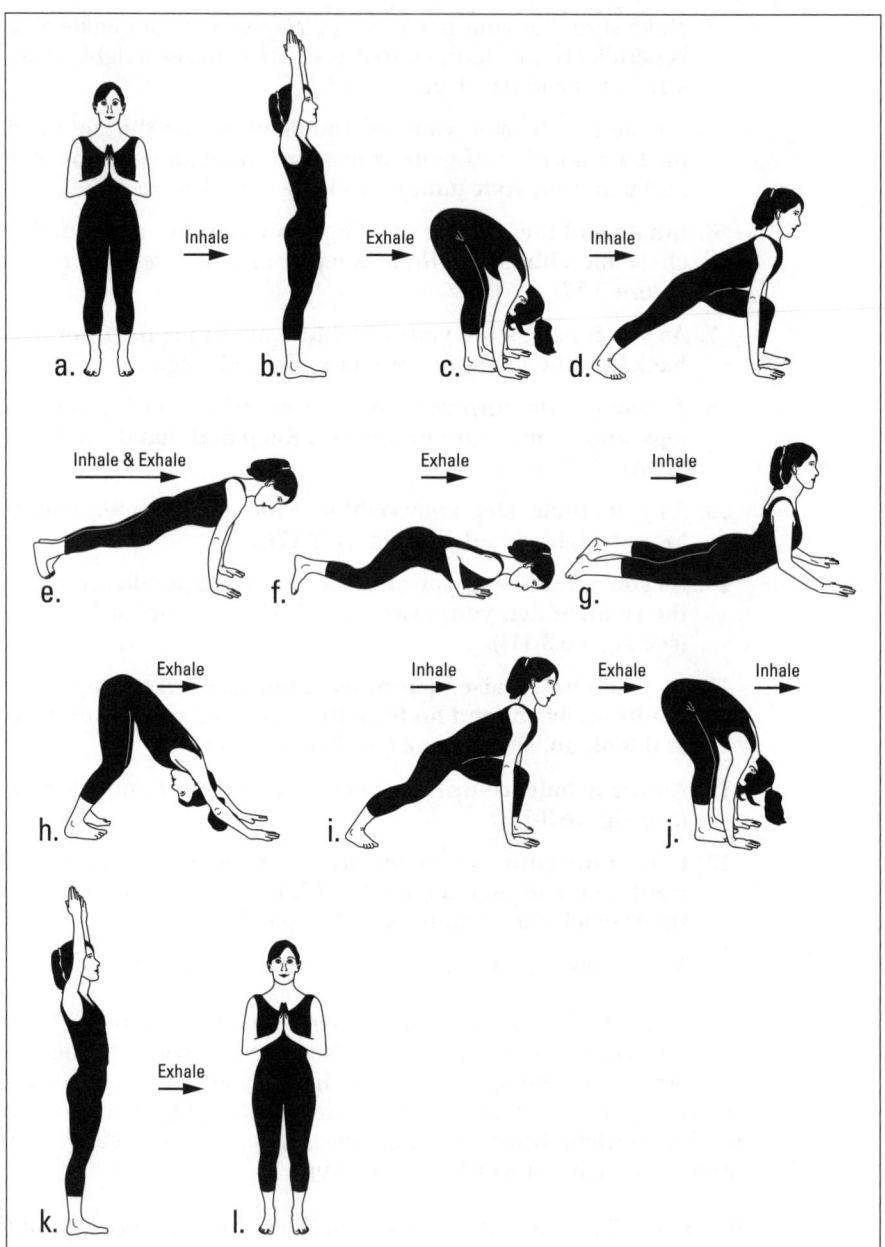

Figure 3-17:
Try different Yoga breathing techniques as you do the sun salutation.

Incorporating some props into your Yoga practice

In your Yoga practice, you can use props as extensively as you want or not at all. In any event, don't dismiss props as 'silly' or 'gimmicky'. Determine on your own how props can help support your yogic practice. Rather than try to look like a magazine-cover or calendar Yoga model, listen to your own body's needs. A folded blanket under your hips can make all the difference when you want to sit cross-legged for more than a couple of minutes; or a wall can be a welcome support for your legs or back while doing particular postures.

Working with a wall

Walls are everywhere, they're free and, best of all, they're a versatile prop. You can use a wall in a great variety of postures, whether to support your buttocks and improve the angle of your forward bend, brace the back heel in the standing postures, or to support the backs of your legs in the reclining raised-legs relaxation position. Walls also can support you in the more advanced inverted postures, such as the half shoulder stand. The wall also works well as a frame of reference by which you can check your posture and alignment.

Using a blanket for more than bedding

Besides the obvious use of keeping you warm during relaxation, blankets can prop the hips in sitting postures, the head and neck in lying postures, and the waist in prone back bends like the locust posture. You can also use blankets as protective padding under the knees when kneeling. Always be sure to fold the blanket thickly, or use more than one blanket when the need arises to raise the hips (or head or shoulders). Also, always use firm, flat blankets for props.

Most blankets nowadays are made out of synthetic materials (or a synthetic/wool blend), so don't worry about your allergy. The firmness of the blanket is important. You want something under your knees or neck that won't sink or collapse, as would a padded blanket or quilt.

Book IV

Exploring Yoga and Pilates

Choosing a chair for comfort

A folding metal chair or a sturdy wooden chair without arms can have multiple uses as a prop in Yoga. Many, if not most, beginners have a hard time sitting on the floor for prolonged periods during meditation or breathing exercises, and sitting on a chair is a great alternative to sitting on the floor. Make sure, though, that your feet are not dangling; if they don't easily touch the floor, place your feet on a phone book. Students with back problems often use a chair during the relaxation phase at the end of a Yoga class.

Lying on your back and placing your lower legs up on a chair, combined with guided relaxation techniques from the instructor, can really help to release back tension or pain. You can find numerous books and magazine articles about doing your entire Yoga practice in a chair, with suggestions for ways to take Yoga chair breaks around the house, or in your office for a quick pick-me-up.

Stretching with a strap

You most frequently use a strap with postures that involve stretching the hamstrings, most commonly from a supine reclining (lying on your back) or sitting position. Someone's old karate belt or tie works great, but so does a rolled-up towel or a bathrobe belt.

Chapter 4

Stretching Your Body through Some Yoga Postures

*Y*oga has the benefit of stretching your body through a variety of postures and movements, including sitting, standing, bending, twisting, balancing, inverted and dynamic postures.

In this chapter we introduce dozens of Hatha Yoga postures to give you a rounded and varied exercise programme.

Go Back to the Start with Compensation Exercises

The reason for doing compensating postures is to ensure that you emphasise the positive effects of Yoga postures and neutralise tension and strain. For example, if you do a strenuous back bend like the cobra and experience tightness in your lower back, you want to be sure to follow up with a simple compensating folding posture, such as the child's posture. You not only need to explore the main Yoga postures, but also to understand how to compensate or bring your body back to where you started.

Here are some basic guidelines for using compensation exercises:

✔ Use one or two simple compensating postures to neutralise tension you feel in any area of the body after a Yoga posture or sequence.

- ✔ Compensating postures are normally done dynamically with a few exceptions, but always with conscious breathing (see Book IV Chapter 2).

- ✔ Perform compensating postures that are simpler or less difficult than the main posture, right after the main posture (see Figure 4-1).

- ✔ Do not follow a strenuous posture with another strenuous posture in the opposite direction. Some Yoga instructors teach the fish posture as compensating for the shoulder stand. However, this combination can cause problems especially for beginners, and therefore we recommend the less strenuous cobra posture instead.

- ✔ Practise compensating postures even when you feel no immediate need for them. This tandem plan applies especially to deep back bends, twists and inverted postures.

- ✔ Back bends, twists and side bends are usually followed with gentle forward bends.

- ✔ Many forward bends are self-compensating but sometimes we follow with gentle back bends.

- ✔ Rest after strenuous postures, such as inverted postures or deep back bends, before beginning the compensating postures.

Compensation postures

Use compensation postures to unwind or bring your body back into neutral, especially after strenuous postures. Compensation is part of bringing you back into balance, which is a key concept in Yoga.

The dynamic cat

You can use the dynamic cat for both compensation and warm-up.

1. **Starting on your hands and knees, look straight ahead.**

2. **Place your knees at hip width, hands below the shoulders.**

   Straighten but don't lock your elbows (see Figure 4-2a).

3. **As you exhale, sit back on your heels and look at the floor (see Figure 4-2b).**

4. **As you inhale, slowly return to the starting position.**

   Again, look straight ahead.

5. **Repeat Steps 3 and 4 six to eight times.**

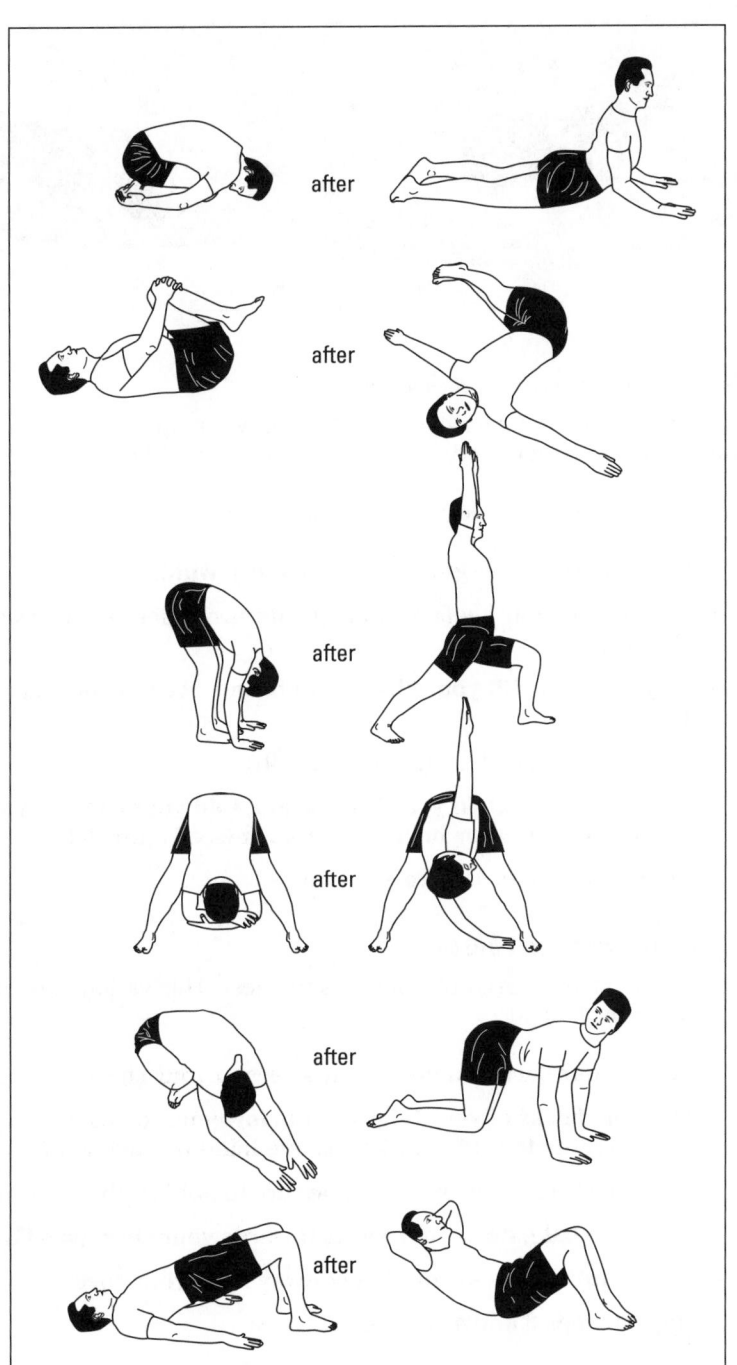

after

after

after

after

after

after

Figure 4-1:
Compensa-
tion pos-
tures for
many of our
main Yoga
postures.

Book IV

Exploring Yoga and Pilates

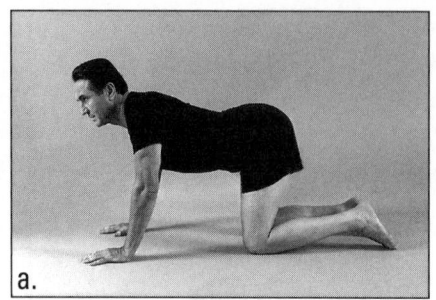
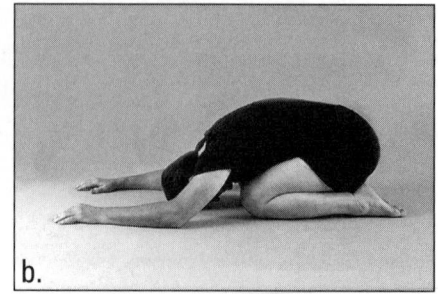

Figure 4-2:
You don't
have to sit
all the way
back, just a
comfortable
distance.

Thunderbolt posture – Vajrasana

This exercise is useful for compensation or warm-up. *Vajra,* pronounced *vahj-rah,* means both 'diamond/adamantine' and 'thunderbolt'.

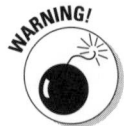

Don't perform the thunderbolt if you have knee problems.

1. **Kneel on the floor, knees and feet at hip width.**

2. **Sit back on your heels, and hang your arms close to your sides (see Figure 4-3a).**

3. **As you inhale, lift your hips back up, and sweep your arms up over your head.**

   Lean back and look up (see Figure 4-3b).

4. **As you exhale, sit on your heels again, fold your chest to your thighs, and bring your arms behind your back (see Figure 4-3c).**

5. **Repeat Steps 2 to 4 six to eight times.**

Dynamic knees-to-chest

You can find many variations of knees to chest. This variation is especially good after back bends.

1. **Lie on your back and bend your knees to your chest (see Figure 4-4a).**

2. **Hold the backs of your thighs just below your knees or cup your hands on the tops of your knees, one hand on each knee.**

   If you have any knee problems, be sure to hold the backs of your thighs.

3. **As you exhale, draw your knees towards your chest (see Figure 4-4b).**

4. **As you inhale, press your knees away from your chest.**

5. **Repeat Steps 3 and 4 six to eight times.**

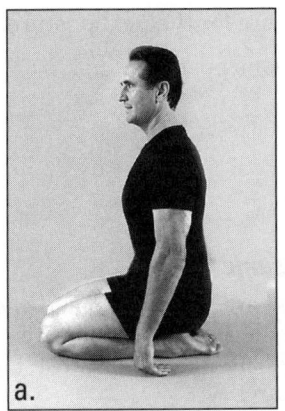
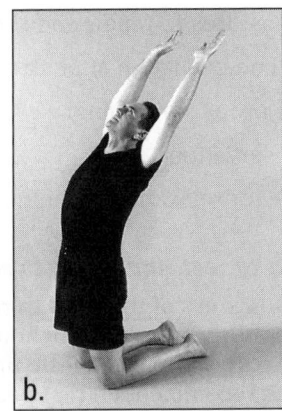

Figure 4-3:
Get into a
nice flow.
Inhale when
you open
and exhale
when you
fold.

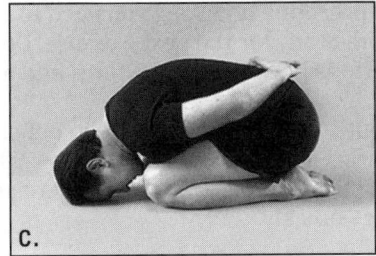

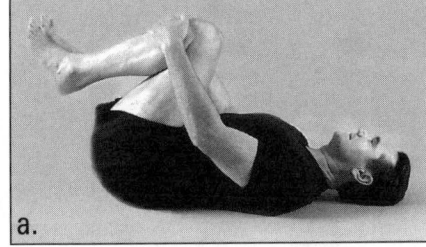
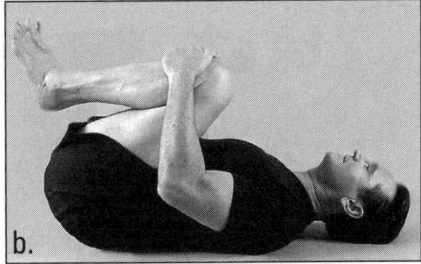

Figure 4-4:
Hold each
leg sepa-
rately.

Rest and relaxation

Rest periods during your routine are an indispensable part of any good Yoga programme. Rest is not just zoning out at the end of a session. In Yoga, a quiet interval is an active tool for enhancing the quality of your practice at the following times, in these ways:

✔ Before the beginning of a class to calm down and establish a union between your body, breath and mind.

✔ Between postures to renew and prepare for the next posture.

✔ As part of compensation after strenuous postures.

✔ To restore proper breathing.

✔ For self-observation.

✔ To prepare for relaxation techniques.

Knowing when to rest and when to resume

The two best indicators of the need to rest are your *breath* and *energy level*. Continue to monitor yourself throughout the session. If your breath is not deep and even, rest. If you feel a little tired after a posture, rest. Figure 4-5 shows you some recommended rest postures.

No die-cast formula can prescribe how long you need to rest. Simply rest whenever you need until you're ready for the next exercise. Don't cheat yourself out of well-deserved rest periods between the postures and at the end of a session.

Of course, if you start out really tired, with a sleep deficit, then you may sleep or need to rest more during your session. If you allow 30 to 60 minutes for your routine, start with rest and some breathing exercises, which can help resuscitate your energies quickly.

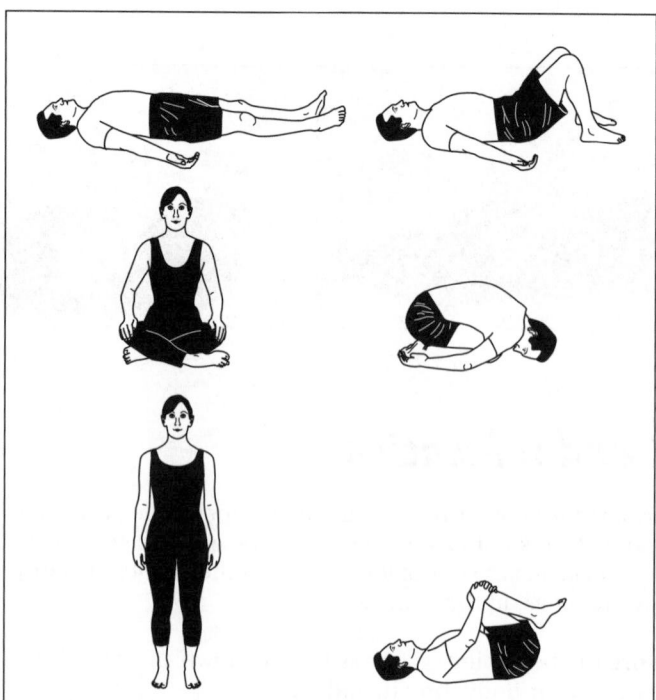

Figure 4-5:
Some rec-
ommended
rest
positions.

Rest postures

You can stay in any rest pose for 6 to12 breaths or as long as it takes to feel rested, which may depend on how much time you have and where you are in the sequence of the routine. Keep in mind that Yoga should never feel like you are in a hurry.

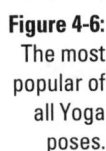

Corpse posture – shavasana

The word *shava*, pronounced *shah-vah*, means 'corpse'; this posture is also called the 'dead pose' or mritasana, from *mrita*, pronounced *mree-tah*, meaning 'dead' and *asana* meaning 'posture'.

1. **Sit on the floor with your knees bent, feet flat on the floor.**

   Press your palms on the floor behind you for support.

2. **Slide your hips forward slightly and lean back onto your forearms.**

3. **Bring your upper back and head to the floor.**

4. **Straighten your legs, and then separate your feet to hip width and turn your feet out.**

5. **Cross your arms over your chest and hug yourself, widening your upper back.**

6. **Release your arms to the floor, rolling out from the shoulders and down to the hands.**

   Turn your palms up (see Figure 4-6).

7. **Slowly turn your head from side to side a few times, coming to rest on the middle of the back of your head.**

8. **Close your eyes and relax.**

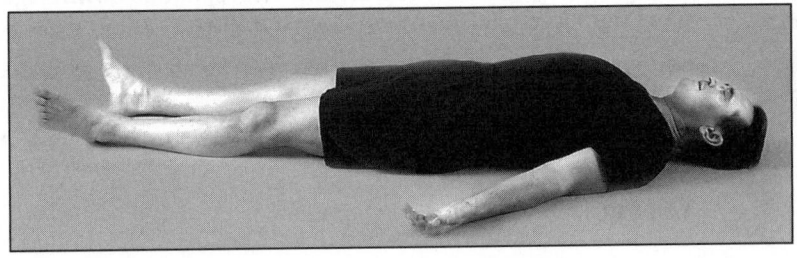

Figure 4-6: The most popular of all Yoga poses.

Book IV

Exploring Yoga and Pilates

Shavasana variation with bent legs

Follow the steps for shavasana but keep your knees bent, feet on the floor at hip width (see Figure 4-7).

TIP

If your back is uncomfortable, place a pillow or blanket roll under your knees. If your neck or throat is tense, place a folded blanket or small pillow under your head.

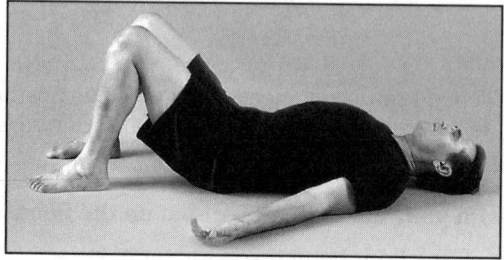

Figure 4-7:
Use this variation for any back problems.

Easy posture – sukhasana

The word *sukha* means 'easy' or 'pleasant'. Compared to some of the other sitting postures, this one is indeed easy as pie.

1. **Sitting on the floor with your legs straight out in front of you, place your hands, palms down, fingers pointing forward, on the floor beside your hips.**

2. **Shake your legs out.**

3. **Cross your ankles, with the left ankle on top and the right ankle on the bottom.**

4. **Press your palms down and cross your legs a little further until your right foot is underneath your left knee and your left foot is underneath your right knee.**

5. **Rest your hands on the top of your knees, palms down, right hand on your right knee, left hand on your left knee.**

   Sit on a folded blanket or cushion if your knees are higher than your hips.

6. **Bring your back, neck and head up nice and tall and look straight ahead (see Figure 4-8).**

   You can keep your eyes open or closed.

Mountain posture – tadasana

The Sanskrit word *tada*, pronounced *tah-dah*, actually means 'palm tree'; hence, this exercise is also called the palm tree posture.

1. **Stand tall, but relaxed, with your feet at hip width.**

   Arms are at your sides, palms turned towards the sides of the legs.

2. **Visualise a vertical line connecting the hole in your ear, your shoulder joint, and the sides of your hip, knee and ankle.**

3. **Look straight ahead, with your eyes open or closed (refer to Figure 3-10a in Book IV Chapter 3).**

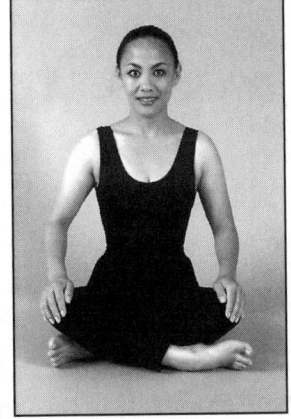

Figure 4-8: Most beginners use this sitting posture.

Child's posture – balasana

The Sanskrit word *bala*, pronounced *bah-lah*, means 'child'.

1. **Start on your hands and knees.**

2. **Place your knees about hip width, hands just below your shoulders.**

   Keep your elbows straight but not locked.

3. **As you exhale, sit back on your heels; rest your torso on your thighs and your forehead on the floor.**

4. **Lay your arms on the floor beside your torso, palms up (see Figure 4-9).**

5. **Close your eyes and breathe easily.**

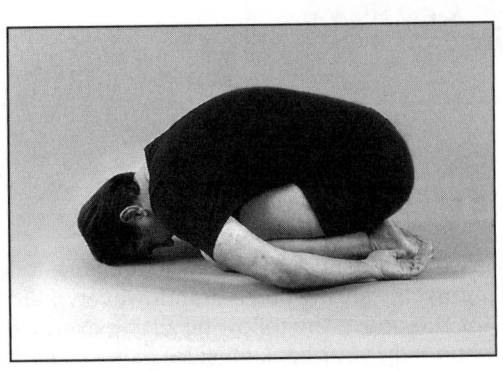

Figure 4-9: This is the position most people first experienced in the womb – very nurturing.

Child's posture with arms in front

Follow the steps for the child's posture, but extend your arms forward at Step 4, spreading your palms on the floor (see Figure 4-10).

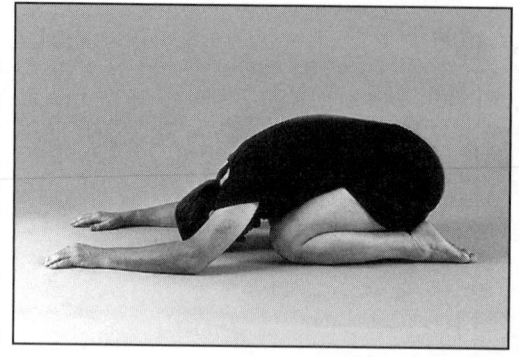

Figure 4-10: With your arms in front, you feel more stretch in your upper back.

Knees-to-chest posture – apanasana

The Sanskrit word *apana*, pronounced *ah-pah-nah*, refers to the downward-going life force or exhalation.

1. **Lie on your back and bend your knees in toward your chest.**

2. **Hold your shins just below the knees (see Figure 4-11).**

    If you have any knee problems, hold the backs of your thighs instead.

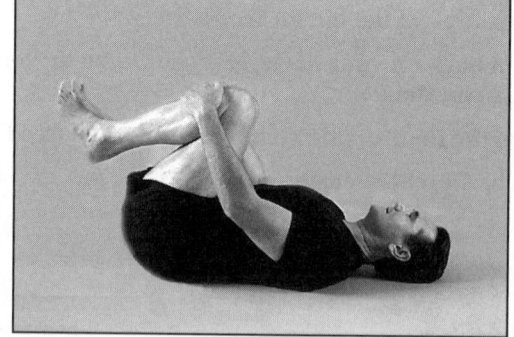

Figure 4-11: Just hold your legs and relax.

Sitting Made Easy

The culture around us greatly influences the way we humans sit. Most Westerners are only comfortable sitting on chairs. However, a lifetime of chair sitting isn't good for the body. The following sitting exercises help to increase your flexibility and help your back muscles gain strength.

The easy posture – sukhasana

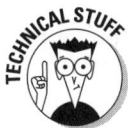

According to Yoga master Patanjali, posture should be 'steady' *(sthira)* and 'easy, pleasant, comfortable' *(sukha)*. The basic Yoga sitting position is called, appropriately, the easy posture *(sukhasana)*; Westerners sometimes call it the *tailor's seat.* We strongly recommend that beginners start their floor sitting practice with the easy posture (see Figure 4-12).

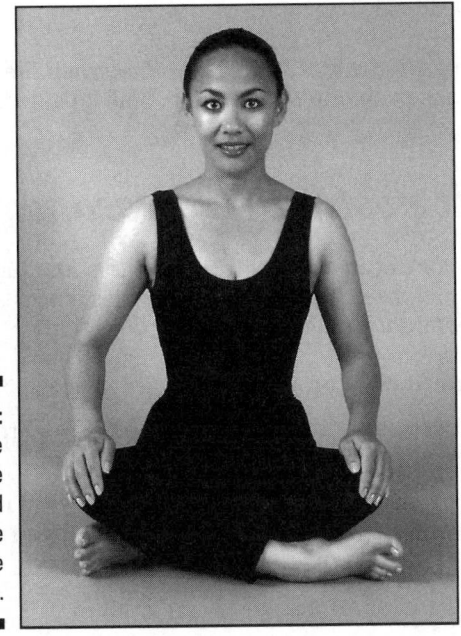

Figure 4-12: Be sure that you're steady and comfortable in the posture.

The easy posture is a steady and comfortable sitting position for meditation and breathing exercises. The posture also helps you become more aware of, and actually increase, the flexibility in your hips and spine and therefore is a good preparation for more advanced postures.

In this posture, and the ones that follow, raising the buttocks off the floor on a firm cushion or thickly folded blanket is helpful, as it allows you to sit comfortably and stably.

1. **Sit on the floor with your legs straight out in front of you.**

   Place your hands on the floor beside your hips, palms down and fingers pointing forward; shake your legs up and down a few times to get the kinks out.

2. **Cross your legs at the ankles with the left leg on top, the right leg below.**

3. **Now press your palms on the floor and slide each foot toward the opposite knee, until the right foot is underneath the left knee and the left foot is underneath the right knee.**

4. **Lengthen the spine by stretching your back in an upward motion and balance your head over your torso.**

Note: In the classic posture, you drop your chin to your chest and extend your arms and lock your elbows; we suggest, however, that you rest your hands on your knees, palms down and elbows bent, and keep your head upright, which is more relaxing for beginners.

Be sure to alternate the cross of the legs from day to day when practising any of the sitting postures because you don't want to become lopsided.

The thunderbolt posture – vajrasana

The thunderbolt posture is one of the safer sitting postures for students with back problems. *Vajrasana* increases flexibility of the ankles, knees and thighs, improves circulation to the abdomen, and is good for digestion.

1. **Kneel on the floor and sit back on your heels.**

   Position each heel under your buttock on the same side and rest your hands on the tops of your knees, elbows bent, palms down.

2. **Lengthen your spine by stretching your back in an upward motion, balance your head over your torso, and look straight ahead (see Figure 4-13).**

Note: In the classic posture, which we don't recommend for beginners, you rest your chin on your upper chest and extend your arms until your elbows are locked and your hands are on your knees.

If you have trouble sitting back on your heels, either because of tightness in your thigh muscles or pain in your knees, put a cushion or folded blanket between your thighs and calves. Increase the thickness of your lift until you can sit down comfortably. If you feel discomfort in the fronts of your ankles, put a rolled-up towel or blanket underneath them.

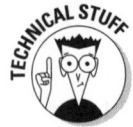

Jnana mudra (pronounced *gyah-nah moo-drah*) meaning "wisdom seal," is one of a number of hand positions used in Yoga. To do this mudra, bring the tip of your index finger to the tip of your thumb to form a circle; extend the three remaining fingers, keeping them close together (as shown in Figure 4-14). This hand gesture makes a nice circuit, sealing off the life energy *(prana)* in your body.

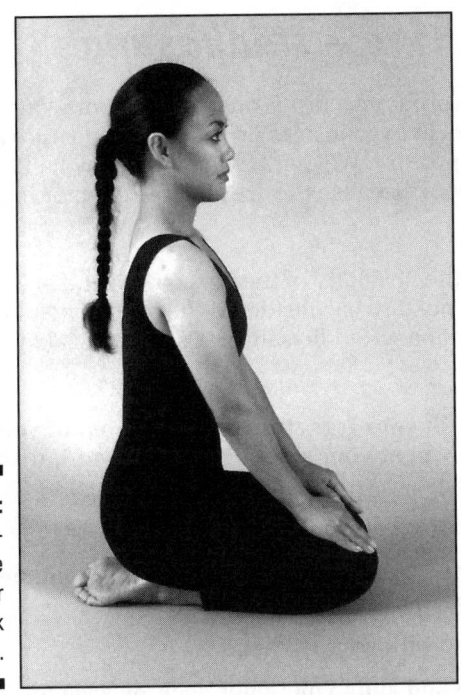

Figure 4-13:
A safe sitting posture for lower back problems.

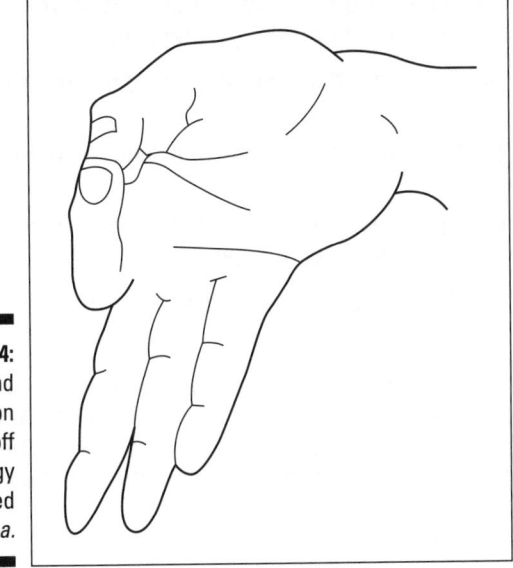

Figure 4-14:
This hand position seals off life energy called *prana.*

The perfect posture – siddhasana

The Sanskrit word *siddha* (pronounced *sidd-hah*), means both 'perfect' and 'adept'. Many Yoga masters in bygone ages preferred this posture and used it often in place of the lotus posture. We don't cover either the half lotus or the full lotus position in this book because they're suitable only for more experienced students.

The *siddhasana* improves the flexibility of the hips, knees and ankles, and strengthens the back. The posture is considered the perfect meditation posture for those practising celibacy. Siddhasana is also beneficial for men with various prostate problems.

1. **Sitting on the floor with your legs straight out in front of you, place your hands, palms down, at your sides, fingers forward, with your hands close to your hips.**

   Shake your legs out in front of you a few times.

2. **Bend your left knee and bring the left heel into the groin, near the *perineum* (the area between the anus and the genitals).**

   Stabilise your left ankle with your left hand.

3. **Bend your right knee and slide your right heel towards the front of your left ankle.**

4. **Lift your right foot and position your right ankle just above your left ankle and bring your right heel into the genital area.**

5. **Tuck the little-toe side of your right foot between your left thigh and calf.**

6. **Place your hands palms down on the same-side knee with arms relaxed.**

7. **Straighten and extend your back and neck, bringing your head up nice and tall; look straight ahead (see Figure 4-15).**

   You can use a cushion to raise your hips, so that they are level with your knees.

Note: In the classic posture, which we don't recommend for beginners, your chin rests on your chest, your arms are straight down, elbows locked, with your palms open in *jnana mudra* (see Figure 4-14) at your knees. The big-toe side of your left foot is pulled up and wedged between your right calf and thigh.

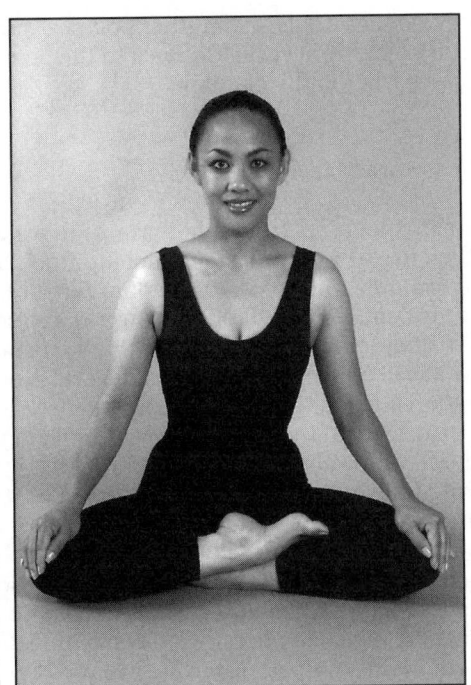

Figure 4-15:
The perfect
posture.

Standing Tall

The standing postures are a kind of microcosm of the practice of *asana* as a whole (except for inversions, or upside-down postures, described in Book IV Chapter 5); you may hear that you can derive everything you need to know to master your physical practice from the standing postures. The standing postures help you strengthen your legs and ankles, open your hips and groin, and improve your sense of balance. In turn, you develop ability to 'stand your ground' and to 'stand at ease', which is an important aspect of the yogic lifestyle.

The standing postures are very versatile. They can be used in the following ways:

✔ As a general warm-up for your practice.

✔ In preparation for a specific group of postures (we like to think of the standing forward bends, for example, as a kind of ramp up to the seated forward bends).

- ✔ For compensation (or to counterbalance another posture, such as a back bend or side bend). See the section 'Go Back to the Start with Compensation Postures earlier in the chapter.

- ✔ For rest.

- ✔ As the main body of your practice.

You can creatively adapt many postures from other groups to a standing position, which you can then use as a learning (or teaching) tool, or for therapeutic purposes. Take, for example, the well-known cobra posture, a back bend that many beginning students find hard on the lower back (see 'Bending over backwards' in Book IV Chapter 5). By performing this same posture in a standing position near a wall, you can use the changed relationship to gravity, the freedom of not having your hips blocked by the floor and the pressure of your hands on the wall, to free your lower back. Then you can apply this newly won understanding about your back in practising the more demanding traditional form of the cobra posture or any other posture that you choose to modify at the wall.

Note: When you try the postures on your own, follow the instructions for each exercise carefully, including the breathing. Always move into and out of the posture slowly and pause after the inhalation and exhalation. Complete each posture by relaxing and returning to the starting place.

When you bend forward from all of the standing postures, start with the legs straight and then soften your knees when you feel the muscles pulling in the back of your legs.

When you come up out of a standing forward bend, choose one of three ways:

- ✔ The easiest and safest way is to roll the body up like a rag doll, stacking the vertebrae one on top of other.

- ✔ The next level of difficulty is to bring your arms up from the sides like wings as you inhale and raise your back.

- ✔ The third and most desirable way, if possible, is to start with the inhalation and extend your arms forward and up along side of the ears. Then continue raising the upper, mid and lower back until you're straight up and your arms are over head.

Mountain posture (tadasana) – building block for other stances

The mountain posture is the foundation for all the standing postures. *Tadasana* aligns the body, improves posture and balance, and facilitates breathing. Although this exercise is commonly called the mountain posture, the name for this position is actually 'palm posture', from the Sanskrit word *tada* (pronounced *tah-dah*). Some authorities also refer to this exercise as the tree posture.

1. **Stand tall but relaxed with your feet at hip width.**

   Hang your arms at your sides, palms turned toward your legs.

2. **Visualise a vertical line connecting the hole in your ear, your shoulder joint and the sides of your hip, knee and ankle.**

   Look straight ahead, with your eyes open or closed (see Figure 4-16).

3. **Remain in this posture for 6 to 8 breaths.**

Note: In the classical version of this posture, the feet are together, and the chin *rests* on the chest.

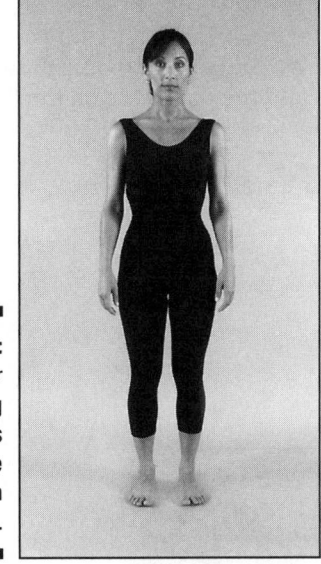

Figure 4-16:
Start your
standing
postures
with the
mountain
posture.

Book IV

Exploring
Yoga and
Pilates

Standing forward bend – uttanasana

The standing forward bend stretches the entire back of the body and decompresses (makes space between the vertebrae) the neck (see Figure 4-17). In the upright posture, the cervical spine and the neck muscles have to work hard to balance the head. Because we generally don't pay enough attention to this part of our anatomy, we tend to accumulate a lot of tension in the neck, which can lead to headaches. This posture frees the cervical spine and allows the neck muscles to relax. It also improves overall circulation and has a calming effect on the body and mind.

Be very careful of all forward bends if you are having a disc problem. If you are unsure, check with your doctor or other health professional.

1. **Start in mountain posture (refer to Figure 4-16) and, as you inhale, raise your arms forward, and then up overhead (see Figure 4-17a).**

2. **As you exhale, bend forward from your hips.**

   When you feel a pull in the back of your legs, soften your knees and hang your arms.

3. **If your head is not close to your knees, bend your knees more.**

   If you have the flexibility, straighten your knees but keep them soft.

   Relax your head and neck downward (see Figure 4-17b).

4. **As you inhale, roll up slowly, stacking the bones of your spine one at a time from bottom to top, and then raise your arms overhead.**

5. **Repeat Steps 1 to 4 three times, and then stay in the folded position (Step 3) for 6 to 8 breaths.**

Note: In the classical posture, the feet are together and the legs are straight. The forehead presses against the shins, and the palms are on the floor.

Figure 4-17: Bending your knees can help stretch your back.

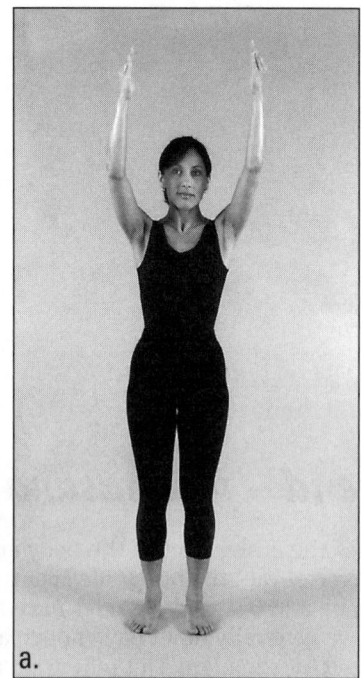

a.

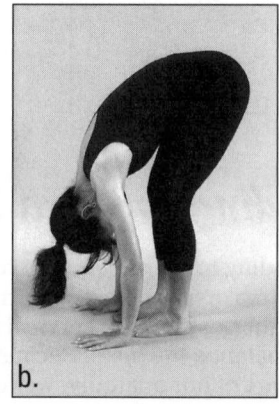

b.

Rolling up in Step 4 is the safest way to come up. If you do not have back problems, after a few weeks you may want to try two more advanced techniques: As you come up, sweep your arms out and up from the sides like wings then over your head; Or, as you inhale, extend your slightly bent arms forward and up until they are parallel with your ears. Then raise your upper back, then your lower back until you are all the way up and your arms are overhead.

The Sanskrit word *uttana* (pronounced *oo-tah-nah*) means 'extended'.

Asymmetrical forward bend – parshva uttanasana

The asymmetrical forward bend stretches each side of the back and hamstrings separately. The posture opens the hips, tones the abdomen, decompresses the neck, improves balance, and increases circulation to the upper torso and head (see Figure 4-18).

1. **Stand in the mountain posture, and as you exhale, step forward about a metre (or the length of one leg) with your right foot.**

   Your left foot will turn out naturally, but if you need more stability turn your left foot out more (so that the toes point to the left.)

2. **Place your hands on the top of your hips and square the front of your pelvis; then release your hands and hang your arms.**

3. **As you inhale, raise your arms forward and then overhead (see Figure 4-18a).**

4. **As you exhale, bend forward from the hips, soften your right knee and both arms, and hang down (see Figure 4-18b).**

   If your head is not close to your right knee, bend your knee more. If you have the flexibility, straighten your right knee but keep it soft.

5. **As you inhale, roll up slowly, stacking the bones of your spine one at a time from the bottom up, and then raise your arms overhead.**

   Relax your head and neck downwards.

6. **Repeat Steps 3 to 4 three times, and then stay in Step 4 for 6 to 8 breaths.**

   Repeat the same sequence on the left side.

Note: In the classical version of this posture, both legs are straight and the forehead presses against the forward leg.

Book IV

Exploring Yoga and Pilates

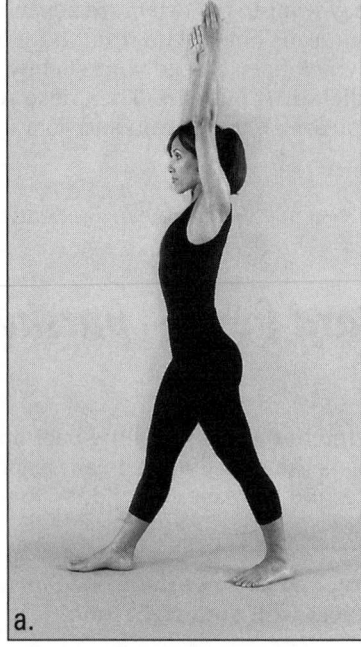

Figure 4-18:
This
exercise
stretches
each side
of the
back and
hamstrings
separately.

a.

b.

Rolling up in Step 4 is the safest way to come up. If you do not have back problems, after a few weeks you may want to try two more advanced techniques: As you come up, sweep your arms out and up from the sides like wings then over your head; Or, as you inhale, extend your slightly bent arms forward and up until they are parallel with your ears. Then raise your upper back, then your lower back until you are all the way up and your arms are overhead.

The Sanskrit word *parshva* (surprisingly, pronounced just like it looks *pahr-shvah*) means 'side' or 'flank'.

Triangle posture – utthita trikonasana

The triangle posture stretches the sides of the spine, the backs of the legs and the hips. This posture also stretches the muscles between the ribs (the intercostals), which opens the chest and improves breathing capacity (see Figure 4-19).

1. **Stand in the mountain posture (refer to Figure 4-16), exhale, and with your right foot, step out to the right about a metre (or the length of one leg).**

2. **Turn your right foot out 90 degrees and your left foot 45 degrees.**

   An imaginary line drawn from the right heel (towards the left foot) should bisect the arch of the left foot.

3. **Face forward and, as you inhale, raise your arms out to the sides parallel to the line of the shoulders (and the floor), so that they form a 'T' with the torso (see Figure 4-19a).**

4. **As you exhale, reach your right hand down to your right shin as close to the ankle as is comfortable for you; then reach and lift your left arm up.**

   Bend your right knee slightly if the back of your leg feels tight (see Figure 4-19b).

   As much as you can, bring the sides of your torso parallel to the floor.

5. **Soften your left arm and look up at your left hand.**

   If your neck hurts, look down at the floor.

6. **Repeat Steps 3 to 5 three times, and then stay in Step 5 for 6 to 8 breaths.**

   Repeat the same sequence on the left side.

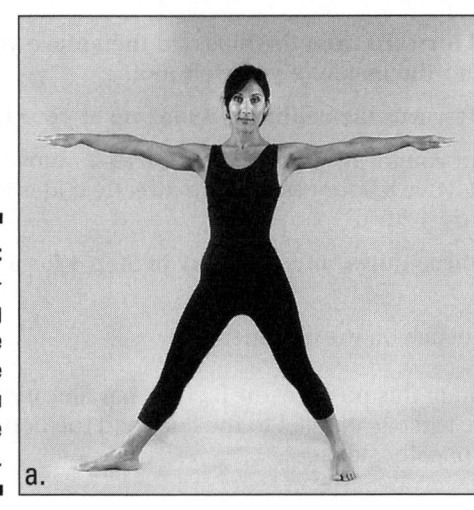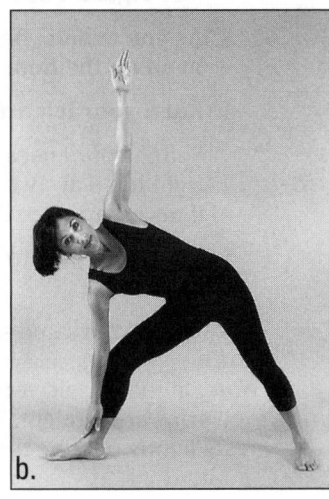

Figure 4-19: The side-bending triangle opens the chest so you can breathe deeply.

a.   b.

Book IV

Exploring Yoga and Pilates

Note: In the classic version of this posture, the feet are parallel, the arms and legs are straight, and the trunk is parallel to the floor. The right hand is on the floor outside the right foot.

The Sanskrit word *utthita* (pronounced *oot-hee-tah*) means 'raised' and *trikona* (pronounced *tree-ko-nah*) means 'triangle'.

Reverse triangle posture – parivritta trikonasana

The action of twists, including the reverse triangle, on the discs between the spinal vertebrae (intervertebral discs) is often compared to squeezing and then releasing a wet sponge: First you squeeze the dirty water out, and then you 'sponge' up the clean water. The twisting-untwisting action increases circulation of fresh blood to these discs and keeps them supple as you grow older. The reverse triangle also stretches the backs of your legs, opens your hips, and strengthens your neck, shoulders, and arms (see Figure 4-20).

1. **Standing in the mountain posture (refer to Figure 4-16), exhale and, with the right foot, step out to the right about a metre (or the length of one leg).**

2. **As you inhale, raise your arms out to the sides parallel to the line of the shoulders (and the floor), so that they form a 'T' with the torso (see Figure 4-20a).**

3. **As you exhale, bend forward from the hips and then place your right hand on the floor near the inside of your left foot.**

4. **Raise your left arm towards the ceiling and look up at your left hand.**

   Soften your knees and your arms. Bend your left knee or move your right hand away from your left foot (and more directly under the torso), if necessary (see Figure 4-20b).

5. **Repeat Steps 2 to 4 three times, and then stay in Step 4 for 6 to 8 breaths.**

   Repeat the same sequence on the left side.

Note: In the classic version of this posture, the feet are parallel and the legs and arms are straight. The torso is parallel to the floor and the bottom hand rests lightly outside the opposite side foot.

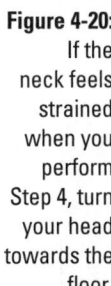

Figure 4-20:
If the neck feels strained when you perform Step 4, turn your head towards the floor.

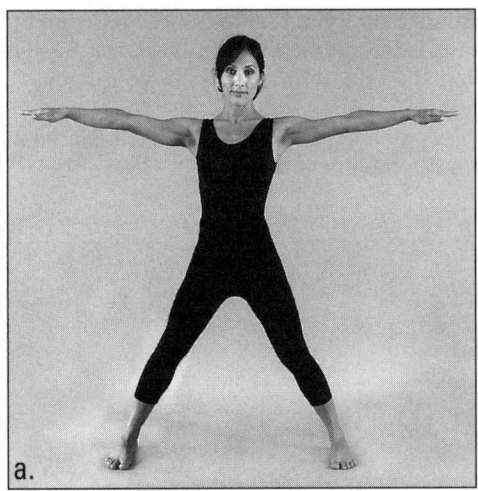

a.

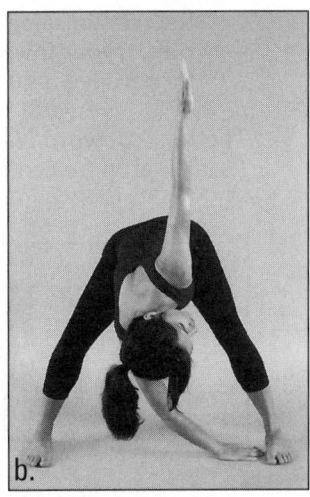

b.

The Sanskrit word *parivritta* (pronounced *pah-ree-vree-tah*) means 'revolved'.

Warrior posture – vira bhadrasana

The warrior posture strengthens your legs, back, shoulders and arms, opens your hips, groin and chest, increases strength and stamina, and improves balance (see Figure 4-21). As its name suggests, this posture instils a feeling of fearlessness and inner strength.

1. **Stand in the mountain posture (refer to Figure 4-16) and, as you exhale, step forward approximately a metre (or the length of one leg) with your right foot (see Figure 4-21a).**

   Your left foot will turn out naturally, but if you need more stability, turn your left foot out more (so that the toes point to the left).

2. **Place your hands on the top of your hips and square the front of your pelvis; then release your hands and hang your arms.**

3. **As you inhale, raise your arms forward and overhead and bend your right knee to a right angle (so that the knee is directly over the ankle and the thigh is parallel to the floor). See Figure 4-21b.**

   If your lower back is uncomfortable, lean the torso slightly over the forward leg until you feel a release of tension in your back.

4. **As you exhale, return to the starting place as in Figure 4-21a. Soften your arms and face your palms towards each other. Look straight ahead.**

5. **Repeat Steps 3 and 4 three times, and then stay in Step 4 for 6 to 8 breaths.**

Book IV

Exploring Yoga and Pilates

Repeat the same sequence on the left side. When you stay in the posture, if your lower back is uncomfortable, lean the torso slightly over the forward leg until you feel a release of tension in your back.

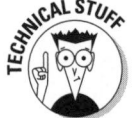

The Sanskrit word *vira* (pronounced *vee-rah*) is often translated as 'hero' and *bhadra* (pronounced *bhud-rah*) means 'auspicious'.

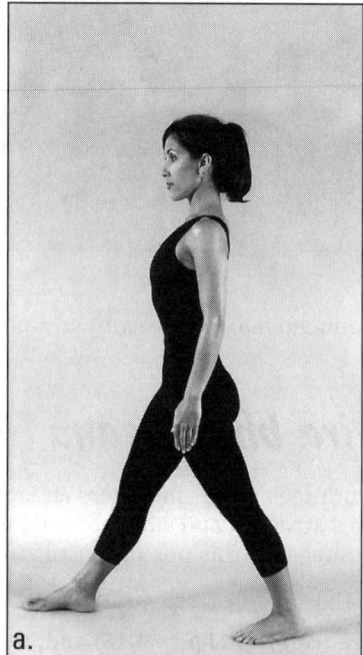
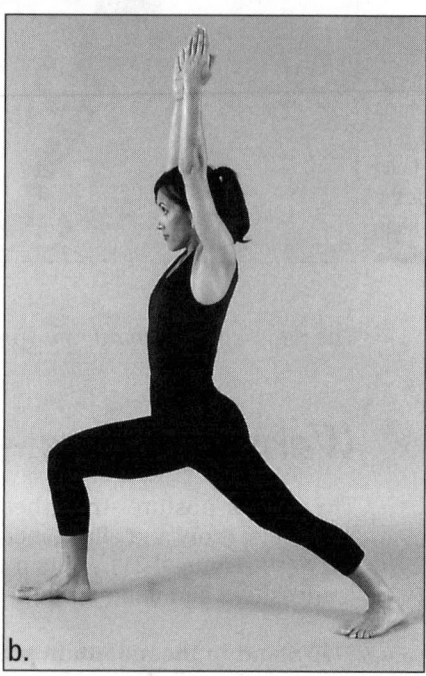

Figure 4-21: The warrior is a position of power and strength.

a.
b.

Standing spread leg forward bend – prasarita pada uttanasana

This posture, also called the wide leg standing forward bend, stretches the hamstrings and the adductors (on insides of the thighs) and opens the hips. The hanging forward bend increases circulation to the upper torso and lengthens the spine.

1. **Stand in the mountain posture, exhale, and, with your right foot, step out to the right about a metre (or the length of one leg).**

2. **As you inhale, raise your arms out to your sides parallel to the line of the shoulders (and the floor) so they form a 'T' with the torso (refer to Figure 4-20.)**

3. **As you exhale, bend forward from the hips and soften the knees.**

4. **Hold your bent elbows with the opposite-side hands, and hang your torso and arms (see Figure 4-22).**

5. **Stay in Step 4 for 6 to 8 breaths.**

Note: In the classic version of this posture, the legs are straight, the head is on the floor (and the chin presses the chest), and the arms reach back between the legs, palms on the floor.

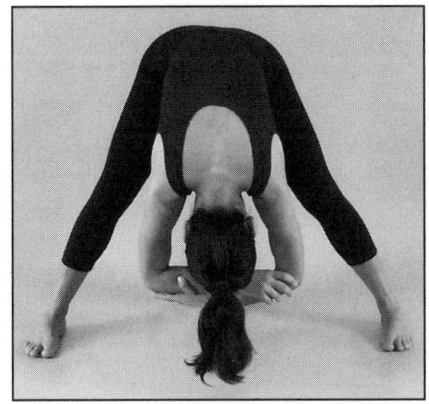

Figure 4-22: A great way to release pressure in the lower back.

The Sanskrit word *prasarita* (pronounced *prah-sah-ree-tah*) means 'out-stretched' and *pada* (pronounced *pah-dah*) means 'foot'.

Half chair posture – ardha utkatasana

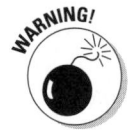

The half chair posture strengthens the back, legs, shoulders and arms, and builds overall stamina. If you find this posture difficult, or have 'problem knees', you may want to skip this position for now and return to it after your leg muscles become a little stronger. Don't overdo this exercise (either by holding the position or by repeating it more than we recommend), or you'll have sore muscles the next day. But there is no harm in experiencing some muscle soreness either, especially if you haven't done any exercise in a long time.

1. **Start in the mountain posture (refer to Figure 4-16), and as you inhale, raise your arms forward and up overhead, palms facing each other (refer to Figure 4-17a).**

2. **As you exhale, bend your knees and squat halfway to the floor.**

3. **Soften your arms but keep them overhead (see Figure 4-23).**

   Look straight ahead.

4. **Repeat Steps 1 to 3 three times, and then stay in Step 3 for 6 to 8 breaths.**

Note: In the classic version of this posture, the feet are together and the arms are straight, with the fingers interlocked and the palms turned upwards. The chin rests on the chest.

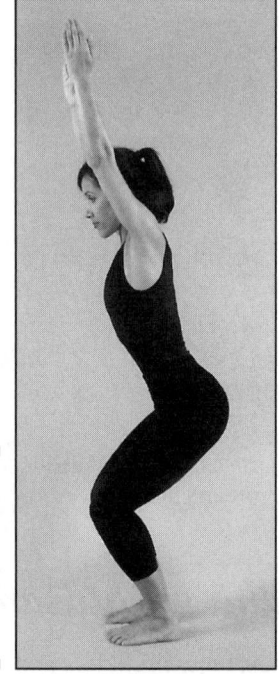

Figure 4-23: The half chair is a great posture for skiers.

The Sanskrit word *ardha* (pronounced *ahrd-ha*) means 'half', while *utkata,* (pronounced *oot-kah-tah*) is translatable as 'extraordinary'.

Balancing Postures for Graceful Strength

A sense of balance is connected with the inner ears. Your ears tell you where you are in space. The ears are also connected with *social space;* if you aren't well-balanced, you may feel – or actually *be* – a bit awkward in your social relationships. Balancing and grounding work can remedy this discomfort. Only when you can stand still – in balance – can you also move harmoniously in the world.

The following postures appear in the order of easier to more advanced exercises. We recommend that if you try the postures individually rather than as part of a sequence, you hold each posture for 6 to 8 breaths. Breathe freely through the nose and pause briefly after inhalation and exhalation.

Balancing cat

Balancing cat strengthens the muscles along the spine *(paraspinals),* the arms and the shoulders, and it opens the hips. The posture enhances focus and concentration and also builds confidence.

1. **Beginning on your hands and knees, position your hands directly under your shoulders, palms spread on the floor, with your knees directly under your hips.**

   Straighten your arms, but don't lock your elbows.

2. **As you exhale, slide your right hand forward and your left leg back, keeping your hand and your toes on the floor.**

3. **As you inhale, raise your right arm and left leg to a comfortable height, or as high as is possible for you (see Figure 4-24).**

4. **Stay in Step 3 for 6 to 8 breaths, and then repeat with opposite pairs (left arm and right leg).**

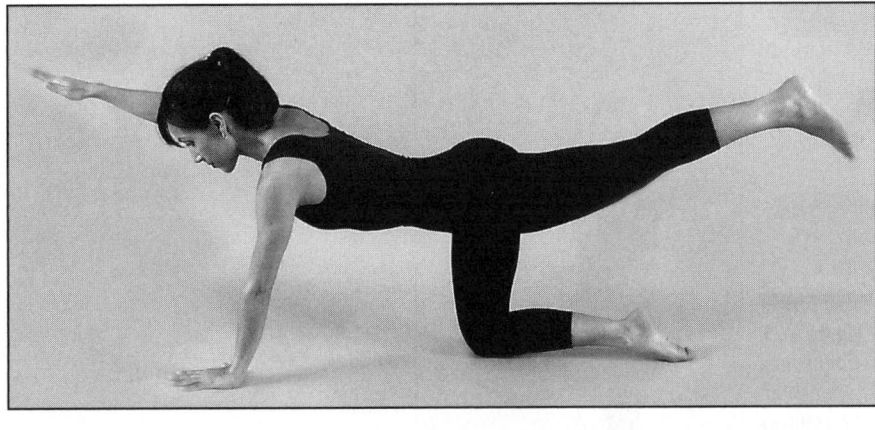

Figure 4-24: Extend your arm and leg fully on the ground before you lift them up.

Book IV

Exploring Yoga and Pilates

This posture is a variation of *cakravakasana* (pronounced *chuk-rah-vahk-ah-sah-nah*). The *cakravaka* is a particular kind of goose, which in India's traditional poetry is often used to convey 'love bird'. Apparently, when these birds have paired up and then are separated, their heartache causes them to call to each other.

The tree – vrikshasana

The tree posture improves overall balance, stability and poise. It strengthens the legs, arms and shoulders, and 'opens' (relaxes and loosens up) the hips and groin. The posture, like the other one-leg balancing poses, enhances focus and concentration and produces a calming effect on the body and mind.

1. **Stand in the mountain posture (see Figure 4-16).**

2. **As you exhale, bend your left knee and place the sole of your left foot, toes pointing down, on the inside of your right leg between your knee and your groin.**

3. **As you inhale, bring your arms over your head and join your palms together.**

4. **Soften the arms and focus on a spot about two metres in front of you on the floor (see Figure 4-25).**

5. **Stay in Step 4 for 6 to 8 breaths and then repeat with the opposite leg.**

Note: In the classical version of this posture, the arms are straight and the chin rests on the chest.

The Sanskrit word *vriksha* (pronounced *vrik-shah*) means 'tree'.

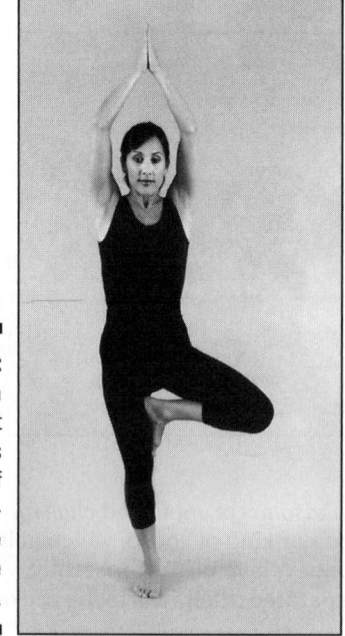

Figure 4-25: Focus on a spot about two metres in front of you: concentrate and breathe slowly.

The standing tree

The standing tree improves overall balance and stability. It strengthens the legs, arms and shoulders, and opens the hips. As with the other one-leg balancing postures, the standing tree enhances focus and concentration.

1. **Stand in the mountain posture (see Figure 4-16).**

2. **As you inhale, raise your arms out to the sides parallel to the line of your shoulders (and the floor) so that they form a 'T' with the torso.**

3. **Steady yourself and focus on a spot on the floor about three metres in front of you.**

4. **As you exhale, bend your left knee, raising it towards your chest.**

   Keep your right leg straight (see Figure 4-26).

5. **Stay in Step 4 for 6 to 8 breaths; then repeat with the right knee.**

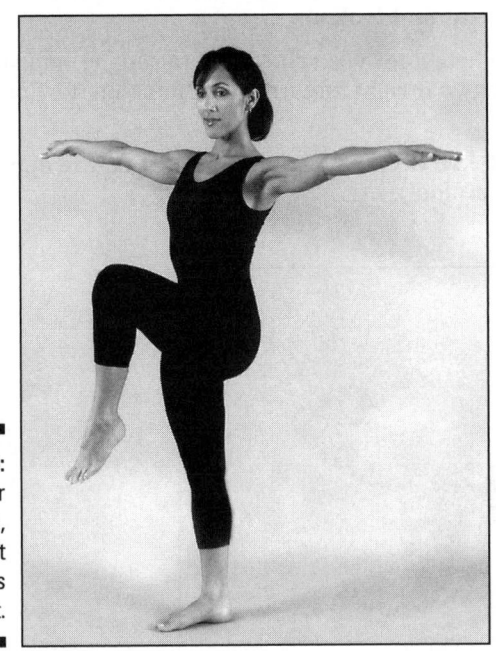

Figure 4-26:
Bend your
left knee,
raising it
towards
your chest.

Scorpion

The scorpion posture improves overall balance and stability. This posture, which is a variation of *cakravakasana*, strengthens the shoulders, improves the flexibility of the hips, legs and shoulders, and enhances focus and concentration.

1. **While on your hands and knees, place your hands directly under your shoulders, palms spread on the floor, and knees directly under your hips.**

   Straighten your arms, but don't lock your elbows.

2. **Place your right forearm on the floor, right hand just behind the left wrist.**

   Reach behind you with your left hand, twisting the torso slightly to the left, and grab your right ankle.

3. **As you inhale, lift your right knee off the floor, raise your chest until it is parallel to the floor, and look up.**

   Find a comfortable height for your chest and raised leg, and steady yourself by pressing your right forearm and thumb on the floor (see Figure 4-27).

4. **Stay in Step 3 for 6 to 8 breaths, and then repeat on the opposite side (left forearm and left foot).**

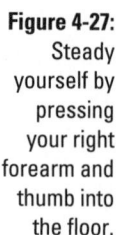

Figure 4-27: Steady yourself by pressing your right forearm and thumb into the floor.

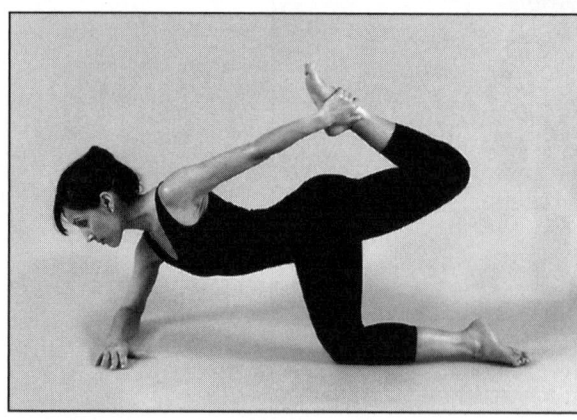

Exercising Those Abs

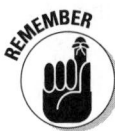

Our yogic postures for the abdominal muscles incorporate a "team approach" that values slow, conscious movement, proper breathing mechanics, and the use of sound. The emphasis here is on the quality of the movement rather than sheer quantity — we believe that a few movements done with diligent attention are much safer and more effective than dozens, even hundreds of mindless repetitions. We also believe that conscious breathing, especially the gentle tightening of the front belly on each exhale, can encourage and then sustain the strength and tone of the abdominals. The use of sound, which we discuss later in this chapter, further enhances this kind of breathing.

Exploring push-downs

Push-downs strengthen the abdomen, especially the lower abdomen. In addition to a floor exercise, you can do push-downs in a seated position by pushing your lower back against the back of your chair. You can perform this exercise sitting in a car, on a plane, or at the office.

1. **Lie on your back, knees bent, feet on the floor at hip width.**

   Rest your arms near your sides, palms down.

2. **As you exhale, push your lower back down to the floor for 3 to 5 seconds (see Figure 4-28).**

3. **As you inhale, release your back.**

4. **Repeat Steps 2 and 3 six to eight times.**

Figure 4-28:
Push your
lower back
down as you
exhale.

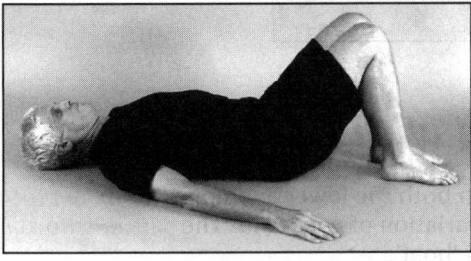

Book IV

Exploring
Yoga and
Pilates

Trying yogi sit-ups

Yogi sit-ups strengthen the abdomen, especially the upper abdomen, the adductors (insides of your legs), the neck and the shoulders.

1. **Lie on your back, knees bent, feet on the floor at hip width.**

2. **Turn your toes in 'pigeon-toed' fashion and bring your inner knees together.**

3. **Spread your palms on the back of your head, fingers interlocked, and keep your elbows wide.**

4. **As you exhale, press your knees firmly, tilt the front of your pelvis towards your navel and, with your hips on the ground, slowly sit up halfway.**

   Keep your elbows out to the sides in line with the tops of your shoulders. Look towards the ceiling. *Don't pull your head up with your arms*; rather, support your head with your hands and come up by contracting the abdominal muscles (see Figure 4-29).

5. **As you inhale, slowly roll back down.**

6. **Repeat Steps 4 and 5 six to eight times.**

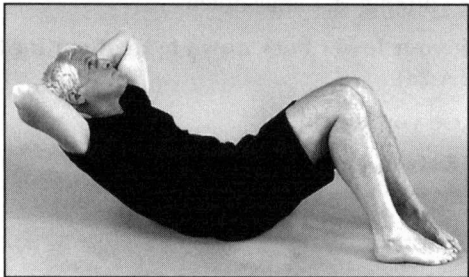

Figure 4-29: Let your eyes follow the ceiling as you sit up.

Strengthening with yogi sit-backs

Yogi sit-backs strengthen both the lower and upper abdomen (see Figure 4-30). This posture is a variation of *navasana*. The Sanskrit word *nava*, pronounced *nah-vah*, means 'boat'.

1. **Sit on the floor with your knees bent, feet on the floor at hip width.**

2. **Place your hands on the floor, palms down, near your hips.**

3. **Bring your chin down and round your back in a 'C' curve (see Figure 4-30a).**

4. **As you inhale, roll slowly onto the back of your pelvis, dragging your hands along on the floor.**

   Keep the rest of your back off the floor to maintain the contraction of the abdominals, but *don't strain* to hold this position; if you feel strain, lift out of the sit-back slightly (see Figure 4-30b).

5. **As you exhale, roll up again, sliding your hands forward.**

6. **Repeat Steps 4 and 5 six to eight times.**

Sit-backs are easier on the neck than most sit-ups. However, if you have lower back problems, be cautious with sit-backs. If you notice any pain in your back, just stop. Work with the other exercises in this chapter instead.

Figure 4-30:
Bring your chin down and keep your back rounded in a 'C' curve.

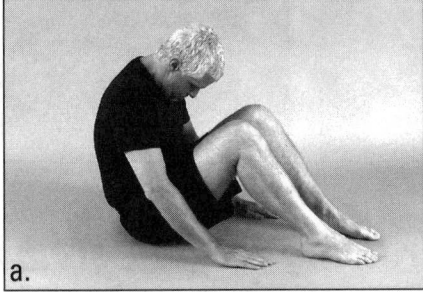
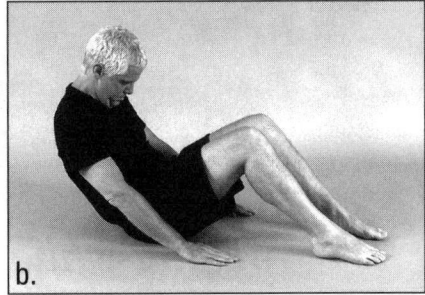

Working with extended leg slide-ups

A variation of *navasana,* the extended leg slide-ups strengthen both the upper and lower abdomen, as well as the neck (see Figure 4-31).

If this pose bothers your neck, support your head by putting both hands behind it. If the problem persists, stop.

1. **Lie on your back with your knees bent and feet flat on the floor at hip width.**

2. **Bend the left elbow and place your left hand on the back of your head, just behind the left ear.**

   Raise the left leg as close to vertical (90 degrees) as possible, but keep your knee slightly bent.

3. **Draw the top of your foot towards your shin to flex your ankle and place your right palm on your right thigh near the pelvis (see Figure 4-31a).**

Book IV

Exploring Yoga and Pilates

4. **As you exhale, sit up slowly halfway and slide your right hand towards your knee.**

   Keep your left elbow back in line with your shoulder and look at the ceiling. Don't throw your head forward (see Figure 4-31b).

5. **Repeat Steps 1 to 4 six to eight times, and then repeat the sequence on the other side.**

Figure 4-31:
Work the abs and the hamstrings.

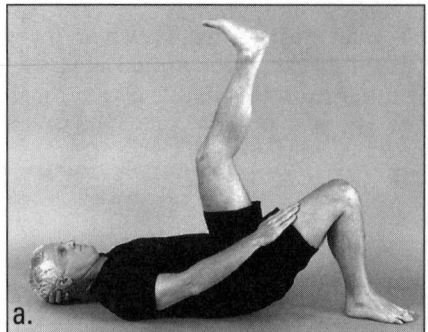
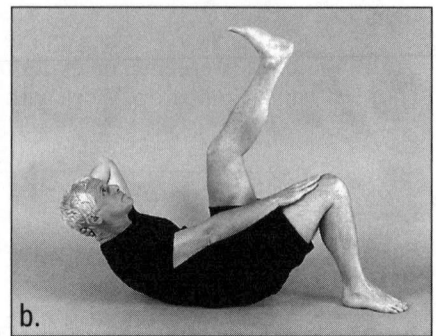

Arching while drawing in your stomach

Arching your back and drawing in your stomach helps to strengthen and tone the abdominal muscles and the internal organs. The posture is especially beneficial for relieving constipation.

1. **Start on your hands and knees, with your hands just below the shoulders and your knees at hip width.**

2. **Inhale deeply through your nose.**

3. **Exhale through your mouth and hump your back like a camel as you bring your chin down.**

   When you have fully exhaled, hold your breath and then pull your stomach in towards your spine (see Figure 4-32).

   Wait two to three seconds with your stomach pulled in and breath restrained, providing you don't end up gasping for air.

4. **As you inhale, return to the starting position.**

5. **Repeat Steps 2 to 4 four to six times, pausing for a breath or two between each repetition.**

Do this exercise only on an empty stomach, and avoid it if you are having stomach pain or cramps of any kind. Avoid this exercise during menstruation.

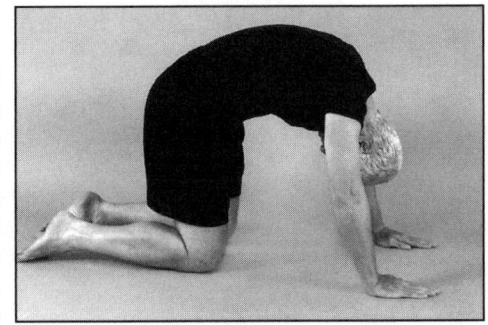

Figure 4-32:
Make sure
you exhale
fully before
you pull
your stom-
ach in.

Chapter 5

Exploring Different Yoga Postures for Health

*P*racticing Yoga regularly can benefit your health as you learn to improve your flexibility and strength.

In this chapter we explore some different postures taking you into some strange positions – from upside down to bending and twisting – to increase your range of movement. The exercises help to strengthen your back, keep your spine supple, and trim your waist . . . so they must be worth the effort!

Turning Attention to the Inversion Postures

Thousands of years ago, the Yoga masters made an amazing discovery: By tricking the force of gravity with the help of inversion exercises, you can reverse the effects of aging, improve your health, and add years to your life.

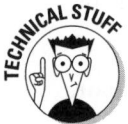

The Sanskrit name for the general category of postural inversions is *viparita karani* (pronounced *vee-pah-ree-tah kah-rah-nee*) or 'reverse process'. This is also the particular name of the three shoulder stand variations we describe in this chapter. Strictly speaking, these inversions are not a regular posture or *asana* at all, but a *mudra* (pronounced *mood-rah*). A *mudra* is far more powerful than a regular *asana,* because it keeps the life energy sealed in your body.

Of all the different types of Yoga postures, inversions are perhaps the most effective for influencing overall change in your body and mind through the endocrine system. In addition to rejuvenating and strengthening your body, the yogic inversions also help you face your fears and actually reverse the tide of stagnation and mental negativity.

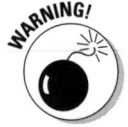

The more advanced inverted postures are a frequent source of injuries for overly enthusiastic beginners working without a teacher. However, you can practise many safe inversions without risk and so receive the tremendous benefits of the yogic 'reverse process'. In this chapter, we treat you to several effective and safe inversion exercises.

Legs up against the wall

Legs up on the wall, which is a variation of *urdhva prasarita padasana,* improves circulation to the legs, hips and lower back and has a calming effect on the nervous system (see Figure 5-1). It also helps alleviate symptoms of PMS in women and prostatitis in men.

1. **Sit sideways with your right side as close to the wall as possible, with both legs extended forward (see Figure 5-1a).**

2. **As you exhale, swing both legs up on the wall and lie flat on your back.**

   Extend your legs up as far as possible. Extend your arms out comfortably at your sides, palms down, and relax (see Figure 5-1b).

3. **Stay in Step 2 for 2 to 10 minutes; use any of the recommended Yoga breathing techniques (see Book IV Chapter 2).**

The dying beetle

A variation of *urdhva prasarita padasana,* the dying beetle posture – excuse the image – improves circulation in the legs, arms, hips and lower back, and has a calming effect on the nervous system. It also improves the range of motion of the ankles, toes, wrists and fingers.

1. **Lying on your back with your knees bent and feet flat on the floor, place your arms at your sides, palms down.**

2. **As you exhale, extend your legs and arms up vertically.**

   Keep the limbs relaxed as you hold them up (see Figure 5-2).

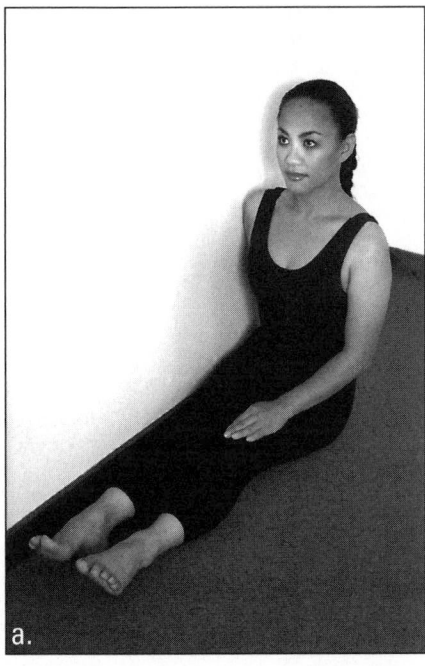 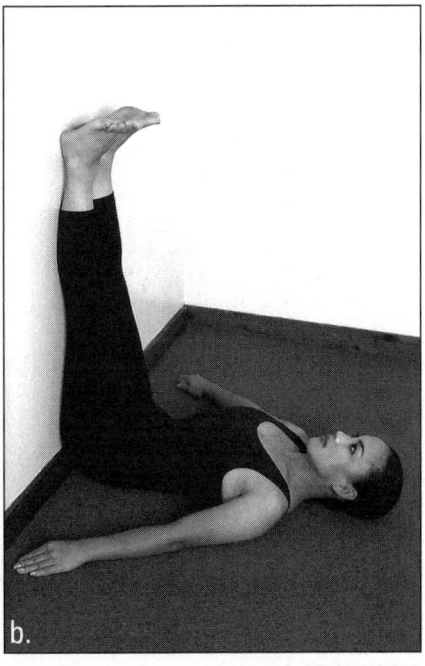

Figure 5-1:
This posture
gives you
a leg up on
gravity.

a.

b.

3. **With your feet, toes, hands and fingers draw circles in the air both clockwise and counterclockwise. If you want, you can make your hands and feet go in different directions at the same time.**

   Breathe freely. Keep your arms and legs up as long as you feel comfortable, and then return to the starting position.

4. **Repeat Steps 2 and 3 three to five times, but do not hold the limbs up for more than a total of 5 minutes; you don't want to tire yourself out or strain your back.**

Avoid this posture if you have lower back problems.

A couple of shoulder stands to get you going

Each of these shoulder stands provides common benefits: improved circulation to the legs, hips, back, neck, heart and head. The postures all stimulate the endocrine glands and improve lymphatic drainage, enhance elimination, and produce a calming and rejuvenating effect on the nervous system. The wall provides a useful prop for the first one; when you're ready, you can then advance with confidence to *viparita karani,* the half shoulder stand.

Book IV

Exploring
Yoga and
Pilates

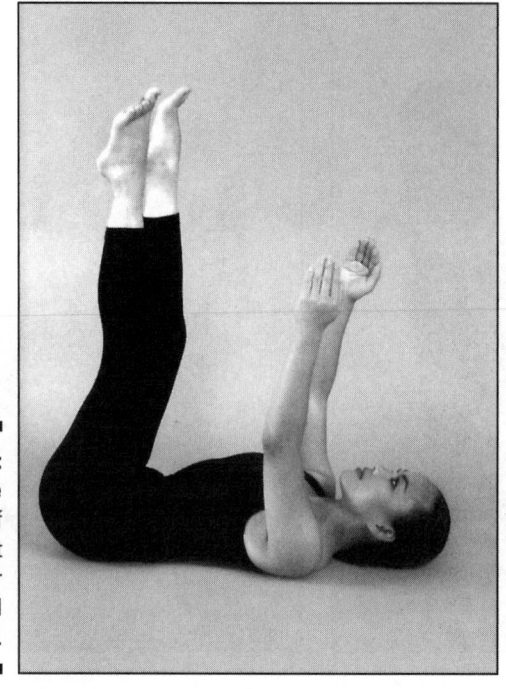

Figure 5-2:
Enjoy the freedom of movement in your ankles and wrists.

Due to the neck's vulnerability, we recommend that you *precede* these postures with a dynamic (or moving) bridge posture (see Book IV Chapter 3) to prepare the neck and *follow* it with a short rest and then a dynamic cobra posture (see the section 'Bending Over Backwards in this chapter) to compensate.

Don't attempt these postures if you're pregnant, have high blood pressure or a hiatal hernia, are moderately overweight, have glaucoma or neck problems, or are in the first few days of your period. Also, do not use a mirrored wall, because you can injure yourself if you fall.

Reverse half shoulder stand at the wall

The reverse half shoulder stand at the wall (see Figure 5-3) is also a variation of *viparita karani*.

1. **Lie on your back with your head towards the wall at a full arms distance from the wall. Bend your knees and place your feet flat on the floor at hip width (see Figure 5-3a). Then bring your arms back and rest your arms along the sides of your body, palms down.**

Finding the correct distance from the wall can depend on the length of your arms. Try these three different measurements: touching the wall with the fingers extended; touching with the knuckles of the fists; and touching with the backs of your hands.

2. **As you exhale, push your palms down, draw your bent knees in and up and raise your hips to a comfortable angle of 45 to 75 degrees.**

   Be sure that your legs are straight but not locked and your feet are directly above your head.

3. **Bend your elbows and bring your hands to the back of your pelvis and then slide your hands up to your lower back.**

   Press your elbows and the backs of your upper arms on the floor for support.

4. **Let your toes slowly and gently touch the wall for support; relax your neck (see Figure 5-3b).**

5. **When you want to come down, first ease your hips to the floor with the support of your hands, and then bend your knees and lower your feet to the floor.**

6. **Stay in Step 4 for as long as you feel comfortable, or up to 5 minutes.**

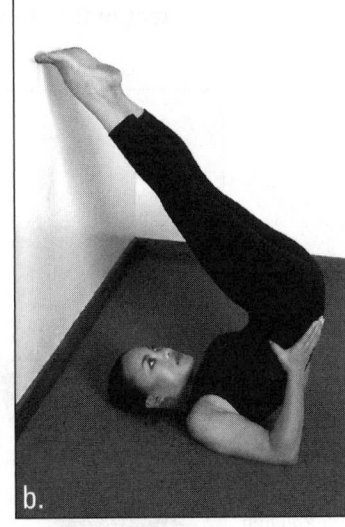

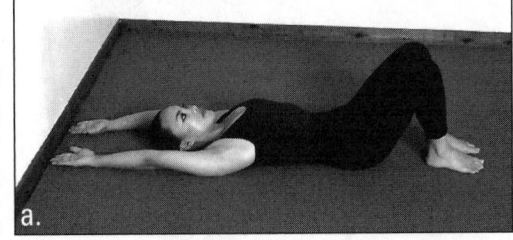

Figure 5-3: Using the wall as a prop.

a.

b.

Half shoulder stand – viparita karani

You can work up to this posture by developing comfort with the reverse half shoulder stand at the wall.

The Sanskrit word *viparita* (pronounced *vee-pah-ree-tah*) means 'inverted, reversed' and *karani* (pronounced *kah-rah-nee*) means 'action, process'. Some authorities call this practice *sarvangasana,* meaning 'all limbs posture'. The word is composed of *sarva* (pronounced *sahr-vah*) and *anga* (pronounced *ahn-gah*) followed by *asana*.

1. **Lie on your back with your knees bent and feet flat on the floor at hip width, rest your arms along the sides of your body, palms down.**

2. **As you exhale, push your palms down, draw your bent knees in and up, and then straighten your legs as you raise your hips (see Figure 5-4a). Then raise your hips to a comfortable angle of 45 to 75 degrees.**

3. **Bend your elbows and bring your hands to the back of your pelvis and then slide your hands up to your lower back. Be sure that your legs are straight but not locked and your feet are directly above your head.**

   Press your elbows and the backs of your upper arms on the floor for support. Relax your neck (see Figure 5-4b).

4. **Stay in Step 3 for as long as you feel comfortable, or up to 5 minutes.**

5. **When you want to come down, first ease your hips to the floor with the support of your hands, and then bend your knees and lower your feet to the floor.**

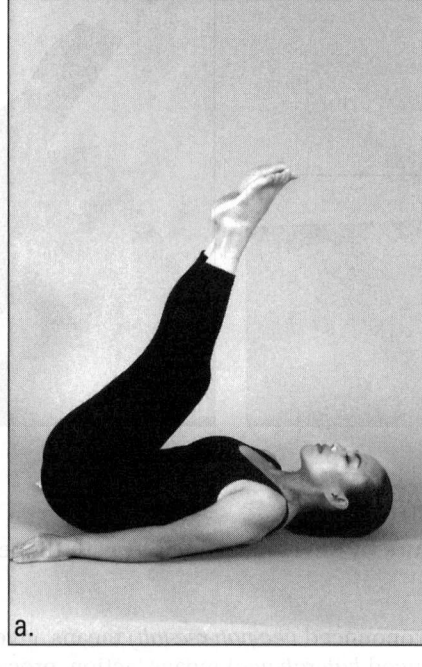
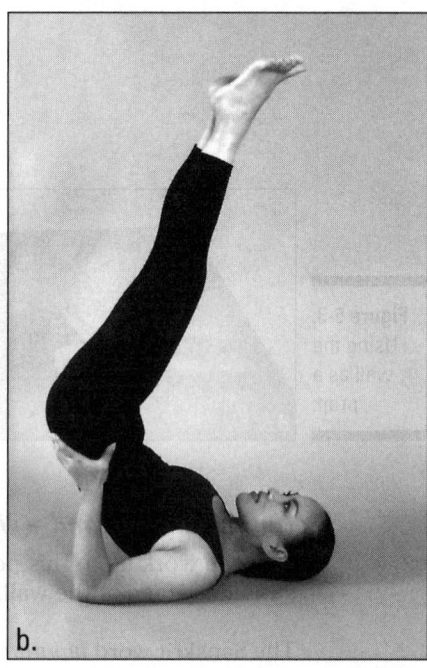

Figure 5-4: You can enjoy the benefits of inversion without compressing your neck.

a.

b.

Bending Over Backwards

Whether you realise it or not, you do a lot of forward bending while going about your everyday business. Putting on a pair of trousers, tying shoelaces, picking things up from the floor, sitting at a desk while typing on a computer keyboard, working in the garden – even many of the sports you play involve varying degrees of forward bending.

The antidote for the cumulative effects of forward bending is the regular practice of Yoga back bends, which stretch the front of the torso (and spine). Appropriately, back bends are performed with an inhalation: the active, opening phase of the breathing cycle. Take a deep inhale right now and notice how your torso (and spine) naturally extends, inviting you to bend backwards. Back bends are known as expansive, 'extroverted' postures that can trigger powerful emotions. The major back bends are usually done towards the middle of a routine, so that you have plenty of time at the start for preparation and compensation afterwards (see Book IV Chapters 3 and 4). In this chapter, we present some of the classic floor back bends.

Cobra 1

The cobra posture increases the flexibility and strength of the muscles of the arms, chest, shoulders and back. Cobra 1 especially emphasises the upper back (see Figure 5-5). The cobra opens the chest, increases lung capacity, and stimulates the kidneys and the adrenals.

1. **Lie on your abdomen with your legs spread at hip width and the tops of your feet on the floor.**

2. **Rest your forehead on the floor and relax your shoulders; bend your elbows and place your forearms on the floor, palms turned down and positioned near the sides of your head (see Figure 5-5a).**

3. **As you inhale, engage your back muscles, press your forearms against the floor, and raise your chest and head.**

   Look straight ahead, as shown in Figure 5-5b. Keep your forearms and the front of your pelvis on the floor as you continue to relax your shoulders.

4. **As you exhale, lower your torso and head slowly back to the floor.**

5. **Repeat Steps 3 and 4 three times; then stay in Step 3 (the last raised position) for 6 to 8 breaths.**

If you have lower back problems, separate your legs wider than your hips and let your heels turn out.

Book IV

Exploring Yoga and Pilates

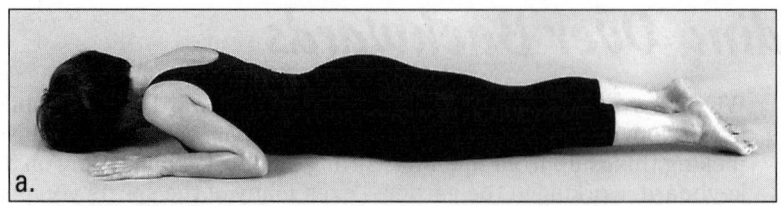

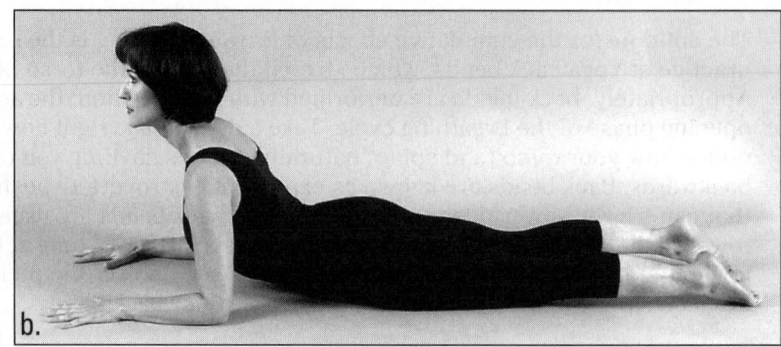

Figure 5-5:
Cobra 1
emphasises
the upper
back and is
less difficult
than
Cobra 2.

This posture is also called The Sphinx. It is a variation of the modified version of *bhujangasana,* which we describe in the next section.

Cobra 2 – bhujangasana

This posture rewards you with most of the same benefits as the Cobra 1, which we describe in the preceding section. In addition, Cobra 2 emphasises flexibility in the lower back (see Figure 5-6).

1. **Lie on your abdomen with your legs spread at hip width and the tops of your feet on the floor.**

2. **Bend your elbows and place your palms on the floor with your thumbs near your armpits.**

   Rest your forehead on the floor and relax your shoulders, as shown in Figure 5-6a.

3. **As you inhale, engage your back muscles, press your palms against the floor, and raise your chest and head.**

   Look straight ahead (see Figure 5-6b). Keep the top front of your pelvis on the floor and your shoulders relaxed. Unless you are very flexible, keep your elbows slightly bent.

4. **As you exhale, lower your torso and head slowly back to the floor.**

5. **Repeat Steps 3 and 4 three times; then stay in Step 3 (the last raised position) for 6 to 8 breaths.**

Note: In the classic posture, the inner legs are joined and the knees are straight. The head is in alignment with the spine and the eyes look forward. The palms are on the floor close to the sides of the torso near the navel, the elbows are slightly bent and the shoulders relaxed.

If you move your hands further forward, the cobra is less difficult; if you move your hands further back, to the sides of your navel, you increase the difficulty.

The Sanskrit word *bhujangasana* is composed of *bhujanga* (pronounced *bhooj-ahng-gah*) meaning 'serpent' and *asana* or 'posture'.

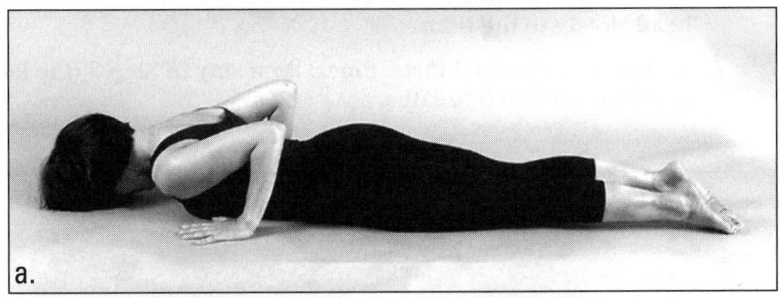

a.

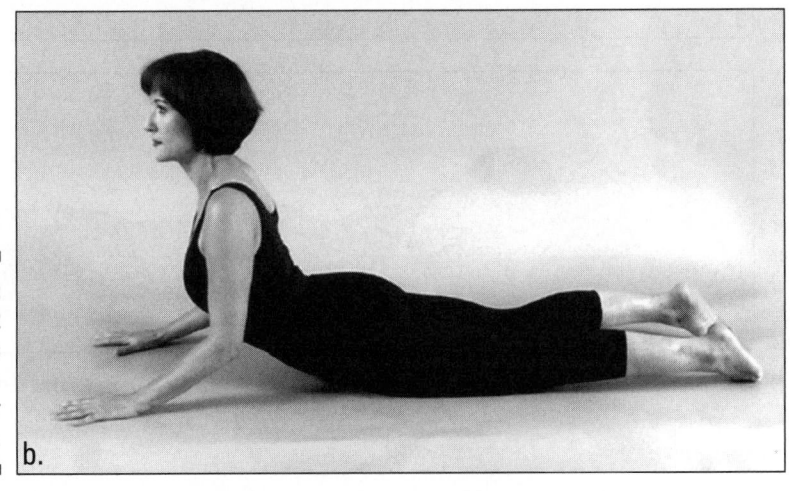

b.

Figure 5-6:
Cobra 2
emphasises
flexibility in
the lower
back.

Book IV

**Exploring
Yoga and
Pilates**

Cobra 3

Cobra 3, which is another version of the classic *bhujangasana,* is unique in that it does not call for placing the hands on the floor. The emphasis is on strengthening both the lower and upper back (see Figure 5-7).

1. **Lie on your abdomen, with your legs spread at hip width and the tops of your feet on the floor; rest your forehead on the floor.**

2. **Extend your arms back, along the sides of your torso, palms on the floor (see Figure 5-7a).**

3. **As you inhale, raise your chest and head, and sweep your arms like wings out to the sides and then all the way forward.**

   Keep your legs on the floor, as shown in Figure 5-7b.

4. **As you exhale, sweep your arms back, and lower your torso and your head slowly to the floor.**

5. **Repeat Steps 3 and 4 three times; then stay in Step 3 (the last raised position) for 6 to 8 breaths.**

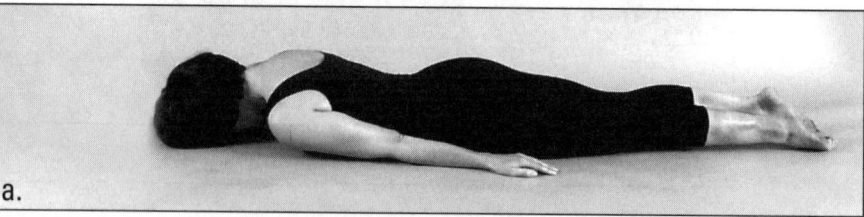

a.

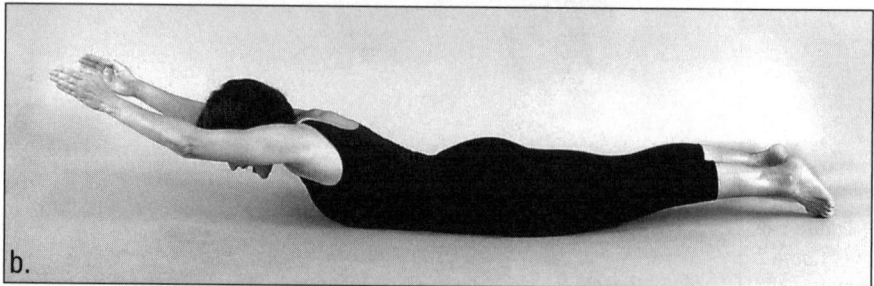

Figure 5-7:
Cobra 3
strengthens
the lower
and upper
back and
the neck.

b.

Bending from Side to Side

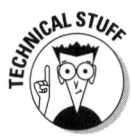

The spinal column can move in four basic ways: It can bend forwards *(flexion),* bend backwards *(extension),* bend sideways *(lateral flexion),* and twist *(rotation).* Of these four, the side bend is most often neglected in Yoga practice. This missed opportunity is unfortunate because side bends help to stretch and tone the muscles along the sides of the abdomen, rib cage and spine, which keeps your waist trim, your breathing full, and your spine supple.

A true side bend fully contracts one side of the body while expanding the other. You can experience the effects of a side bend right now: Whether you're reading these words while sitting on a chair or on the floor, simply lean over with an exhale to your right (or left) side and reach the same-side arm downwards. To realise the full effect of the stretch, reach the opposite-side arm up towards the ceiling. In this section, we cover some safe, creative ways to use side bends on the floor.

Seated side bend

All the side bends have similar benefits. They stretch and tone the muscles along the sides of the torso and increase the flexibility of the spine.

1. **Sit comfortably in a simple cross-legged position (for the easy posture, or *sukhasana*, see Book IV Chapter 4).**

   Place your right palm on the floor, near your right hip.

2. **As you inhale, raise your left arm out to your side and up above your head beside your left ear.**

3. **As you exhale, slide your right hand across the floor out to the right.**

   Let your torso, head and left arm follow, bending sideways to the right (see Figure 5-8).

4. **As you inhale, return to the upright position (as you were at the start of Step 2).**

5. **Repeat Steps 2 to 4 three times; then stay in the bent position (Step 3) for 6 to 8 breaths.**

   Repeat the same sequence on the other side.

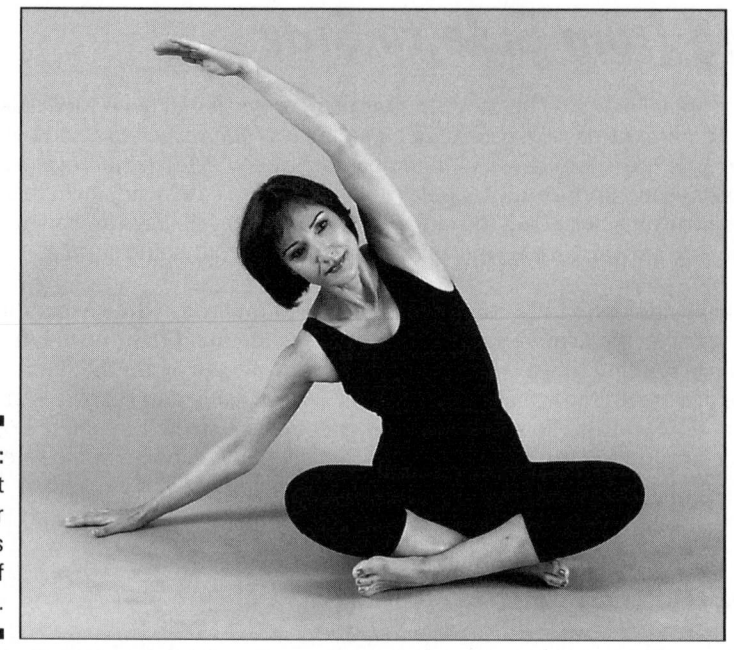

Figure 5-8:
Don't let your buttocks come off the floor.

All-fours side bend

The benefits of this side bend, which is a variation of *cakravakasana,* are the same as for the seated side bend. Many people with back or hip problems have a hard time sitting upright on the floor. The all fours position gives more freedom to the spine and is an easier side bend from the floor.

1. **Start on your hands and knees, with the your knees below your hips and the your hands below your shoulders, palms on the floor.**

    Straighten, but don't lock, your elbows. Look straight ahead.

2. **As you exhale, bend your head and torso sideways to the right and look towards your tailbone (see Figure 5-9).**

3. **As you inhale, return to the starting position in Step 1.**

4. **Repeat Steps 2 and 3 three times; then stay in Step 2 for 6 to 8 breaths.**

    Repeat the same sequence on the other side.

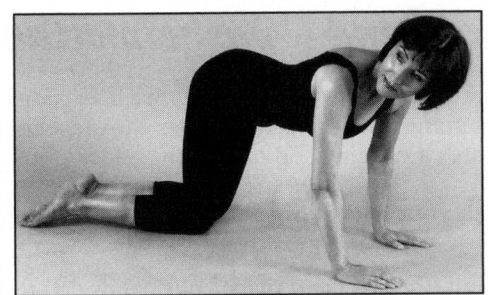

Figure 5-9:
Look back at
what used
to be a tail.

Bending Forward

Of all the ways your torso (and spine) can move, bending forward is the manoeuvre most common to our species. People spend their first nine months growing in their mothers' wombs, folded in a forward bend; it's possible that because people instinctively associate this position with the peace and security of their prenatal lives, they often bend forward after strenuous or unfamiliar activities to calm and comfort themselves.

Forward bends are usually a good way to begin any movement routine (unless you're dealing with spinal disc injuries or certain other back problems). Although back bends are the lively extroverts of the *asana* family, forward bends are the retiring introverts; they are always performed with an exhalation – the passive, contracting phase of the breathing cycle.

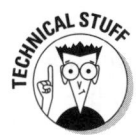

In Sanskrit, the representative sitting forward bend is called *pashcimottanasana* (pronounced *pash-chee-moh-tah-nah-sah-nah*), which translates to the 'extension of the West posture'. In yogic jargon, the West refers to the back, while the East stands for the front. The symbolism refers to both the physical and psychological effects of this posture: It stretches the back of the body, especially the back of the spine and legs, and just as the sun sets in the West, so does the 'light' of our consciousness draw inwards as we fold upon ourselves.

Our constant bending forward *from the waist* tends to put stress on the lower back and neck. Yogic forward bends call for movement *from the hip joints*, which can help you maintain a healthy, stress-free spine as you correct poor forward-bending habits.

Be very careful of all the seated forward bends if you have disc-related back problems.

Book IV

Exploring Yoga and Pilates

Seated forward bend – pashcimottanasana

The seated forward bend intensely stretches the entire back side of the body, including the back of the spine and legs. It also tones the muscles and organs of the abdomen and creates a calming and quietening effect.

1. **Sit on the floor, with your legs at hip width and comfortably stretched out in front of you.**

   Bring your back up nice and tall and place your palms down on the floor near your thighs.

2. **As you inhale, raise your arms forward and up overhead until they are beside your ears (see Figure 5-10a).**

   Keep your arms and legs soft and slightly bent.

3. **As you exhale, bend forward from the hips; bring your hands, chest and head towards your legs.**

   Rest your hands on the floor, your thighs, knees, shins or feet. If your head is not close to your knees, bend your knees more until you feel your back stretching (see Figure 5-10b).

4. **Repeat Steps 2 and 3 three times, then stay folded (Step 3) for 6 to 8 breaths.**

Note: In the classic posture, the inner legs are joined, the knees are straight, and the ankles are extended (the toes point up). Also, the chin rests on the chest, the hands hold the sides of the feet, the back is extended forward and the forehead is pressed against the legs.

If you have a problem sitting upright on the floor in the seated forward bend or in any of the following forward bending postures, raise your hips with folded blankets or firm pillows, as shown in Figure 5-10c.

The Sanskrit word *pashcimottanasana* is composed of the words *pashcima* (pronounced *push-chee-mah)* meaning Western', *uttana* (pronounced *oot-tah-nah*) meaning 'extended', and *asana* or 'posture'.

Head-to-knee posture – janushirshasana

The head-to-knee posture keeps your spine supple, stimulates the abdominal organs, and activates the central channel (*sushumna-nadi*; see Figure 5-11). The central channel is the pathway for the awakened energy of pure consciousness (called *kundalini-shakti*), which leads to ecstasy and spiritual liberation.

1. **Sit on the floor, with your legs stretched out in front of you, bend your left knee and bring your left heel towards the right of your groin.**

2. **Rest the bent left knee on the floor (but do not force it down), and place the sole of your left foot on the inside of your right thigh.**

   The toes of the left foot point towards the right knee.

3. **Bring your back up nice and tall; as you inhale, raise your arms forward and up overhead until they are beside your ears (see Figure 5-11a).**

   Keep your arms and the right leg soft and slightly bent.

4. **As you exhale, bend forward from the hips.**

   Bring your hands, chest and head towards your right leg. Rest your hands on the floor, your thigh, knee, shin or foot. If your head is not close to your right knee, bend your knee more until you feel your back stretching on the right side (see Figure 5-11b).

5. **Repeat Steps 3 and 4 three times; then stay in Step 4 (the final forward bend) for 6 to 8 breaths.**

   Repeat the same sequence on the opposite side.

Keep your back muscles as relaxed as possible, which helps you achieve better extension.

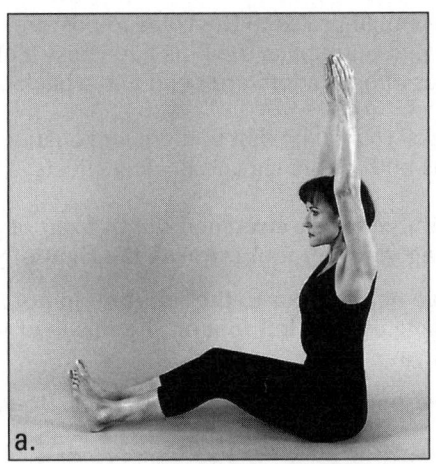

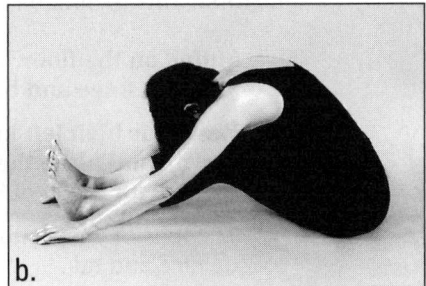

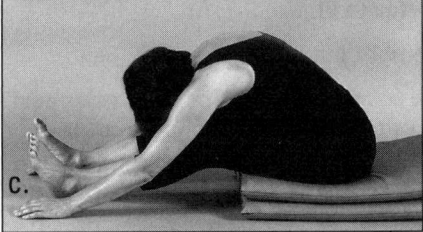

Figure 5-10: If your head is not close to your knees, bend your knees more.

a.

b.

c.

The Sanskrit word *janu* (pronounced *jah-noo*) means 'knee', and *shirsha* (pronounced *sheer-shah*) means 'head'.

Figure 5-11:
This posture
stretches
the back
more on the
side of the
extended
leg.

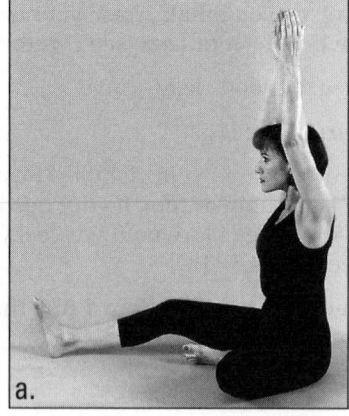
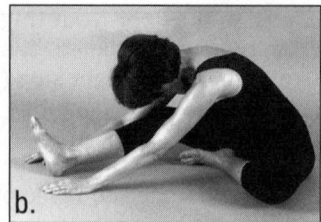

a.　b.

Figure 5-11: This posture stretches the back more on the side of the extended leg.

Volcano – mahamudra

Ancient Hatha Yoga texts give high praise to the volcano posture. It strengthens the back, stretches the legs, and opens the hips and chest. This posture is unique in that has qualities of both a forward bend and a back bend.

When used with special 'locks' (*bandhas*) that contain and channel energy in the torso, this technique has both cleansing and healing effects.

1. **Sitting on the floor, with your legs stretched out in front of you, bend your left knee and bring your left foot towards the right of your groin.**

2. **Rest your bent left knee on the floor to the left (but do not force it down), and place the sole of your left foot on the inside of your right thigh, with the heel in your groin.**

   The toes of your left foot point towards your right knee. Bring your back up nice and tall.

3. **As you inhale, raise your arms forward and up overhead until they are beside your ears (refer to Figure 5-11a).**

   Keep your arms and the right leg soft and slightly bent.

4. **As you exhale, bend forward from the hips, lift your chest forward, and extend your back, but don't let your back round.**

   Place your hands on your right knee, shin or toes and look straight ahead (see Figure 5-12).

5. **Repeat Steps 3 and 4 three times; then stay in Step 4 for 6 to 8 breaths.**

   Repeat the same sequence on the opposite side.

Note: In the classic posture, the front leg and the arms are straight, and the hands are holding the toes of the front leg. The back is extended and the chin is pressed on the chest. The abdominal muscles are pulled up into the abdominal cavity and the anal sphincter is tightened.

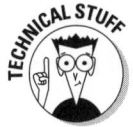

The Sanskrit term *mahamudra* (pronounced *mah-hah-mood-rah*) means literally 'great seal'.

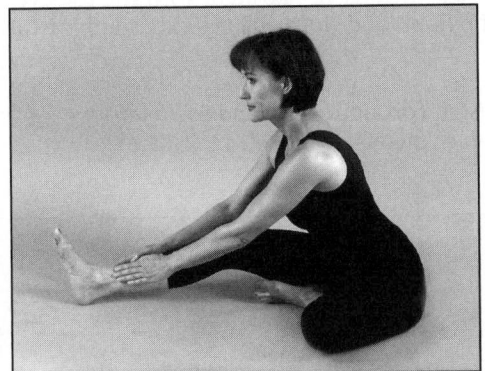

Figure 5-12:
The volcano is a great all-inclusive posture.

Spread-leg forward bend – upavishta konasana

The spread-leg forward bend stretches the backs and insides of the legs (hamstrings and adductors) and increases the flexibility of the spine and hip joints (see Figure 5-13). It improves circulation to the entire pelvic region, tones the abdomen, and has a calming effect on the nervous system.

Note: Muscle density may cause some men to find this posture more difficult.

1. **Sit on the floor with your legs straight and spread wide apart (but not more than 90 degrees).**

   Because this posture is most challenging, give yourself an advantage by pulling the flesh of the buttocks (you may know them as 'cheeks') out from under the sit bones (the ischium) and bending your knees slightly. Alternatively, sit on some folded blankets.

2. **As you inhale, raise your arms forward and up overhead until they are beside your ears.**

   Keep your arms soft and your legs slightly bent. Bring your back up nice and tall (see Figure 5-13a).

3. **As you exhale, bend forward from the hips and bring your hands, chest and head towards the floor.**

   Rest your extended arms and hands, palms down, on the floor. If you have the flexibility, place your forehead on the floor as well (see Figure 5-13b).

4. **Repeat Steps 2 and 3 three times; then stay in Step 3 (the folded position) for 6 to 8 breaths.**

Note: In the classic posture, the legs are straight with the toes vertical, the chin and chest are on the floor, and the arms are extended forward with the palms joined.

The Sanskrit term *upavishta* (pronounced *oopah-vish-tah*) means 'seated' and *kona* (pronounced *koh-nah*) means 'triangle'.

Figure 5-13:
Muscle density may make this posture difficult for some men.

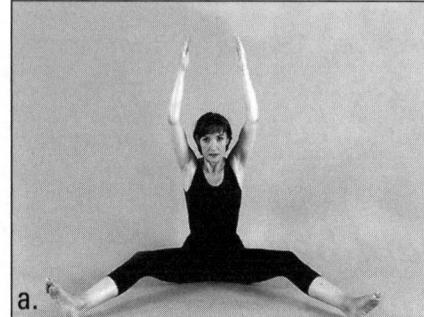 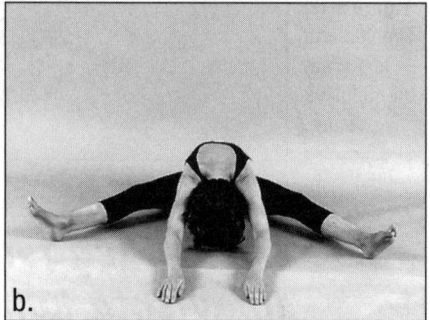

Putting a Positive Spin on Twisting

Approach all twists with caution if you're suffering from disc problems anywhere in your spine. Consult your doctor or work with a reputable Yoga teacher.

Easy chair twist

If you're like most people, you probably sit most of the day. So why, you may wonder, do we ask you to sit on a chair for this exercise? Trust us – this is an excellent way for a beginner to achieve a good twist safely. Your spine will be grateful to you!

1. **Sit sideways on a chair with the chair back to your right, feet flat on the floor and heels directly below your knees.**

2. **Exhale, turn to the right, and hold the sides of the chair back with your hands.**

3. **As you inhale, extend or lift your spine upwards.**

4. **As you exhale, twist your torso and head further to the right (see Figure 5-14).**

5. **Repeat Steps 1 to 4, gradually twisting further with each exhalation for 3 breaths (don't force it); then hold the twist for 6 to 8 breaths.**

   Repeat the same sequence on the opposite side.

If your feet are not comfortably on the floor for the easy chair twist, place a folded blanket or a phone book under your feet for elevation.

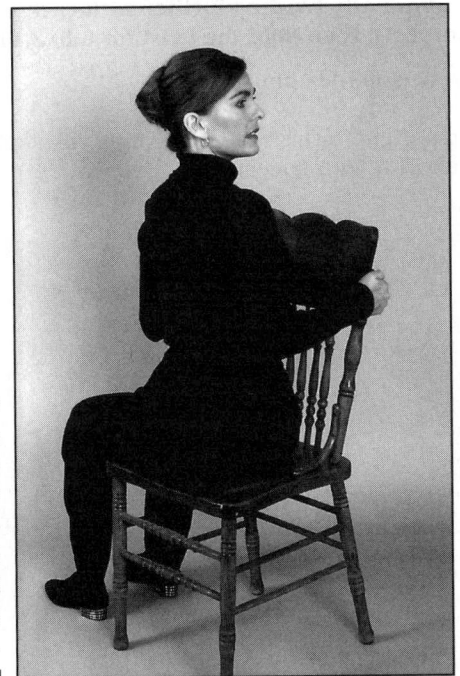

Figure 5-14:
Twist mainly
from your
shoulders —
the head
and neck
come along
for the ride.

Easy sitting twist

Once you can twist comfortably while seated on a chair, you can transfer your newly gained skill to the floor and try the following exercise. Its effect is similar to that of the easy chair twist described in the previous section. The easy sitting twist is usually more convenient during regular Yoga practice because you do most yogic exercises on the floor. Of course, if you're at the office and want to liberate your spine with a yogic twist without drawing too much attention to yourself, you may opt to stay seated instead.

1. **Sit on the floor with your legs in a simple, cross-legged position and extend your spine upwards nice and tall.**

2. **Place your left hand, palm down, on top of your right knee.**

3. **Place your right hand, palm down, on the floor behind your right hip to prop yourself up.**

4. **As you inhale, extend your spine upwards.**

5. **As you exhale, twist your torso and head to the right (see Figure 5-15).**

6. **Repeat Steps 4 and 5, gradually twisting further with each exhalation for 3 breaths (don't force it); then hold the twist for 6 to 8 breaths.**

Repeat the same sequence on the opposite side.

If you have difficulty sitting upright in this seated twist, use blankets or pillows to make your hips even with your knees.

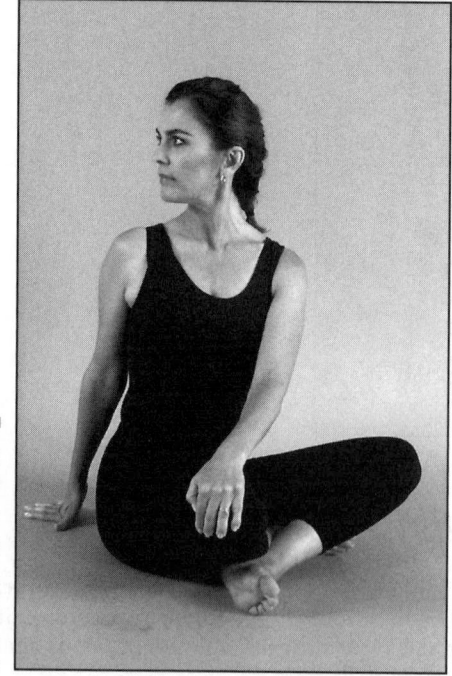

Figure 5-15:
Seated twists usually emphasise the upper back.

The sage twist

The easy chair twist and the easy sitting twist are the simplest yogic twists. By changing the position of your legs, you can alter the level of difficulty and also enhance the overall benefit. The sage twist gives you extra rewards for your investment.

1. **Sit on the floor with both legs extended forward; bend your right knee and place your right foot on the floor just inside your left thigh, with toes facing forward.**

2. **Place your right hand, palm down, on the floor behind you; wrap the palm of your left hand around the side of your right knee.**

3. **As you inhale, extend or lift your spine upwards.**

4. **As you exhale, twist your torso and head to the right (see Figure 5-16).**

5. **Repeat Steps 3 and 4, gradually twisting further with each exhalation for 3 breaths (don't force it), and then hold the twist for 6 to 8 breaths.**

   Repeat the same sequence on the opposite side.

If you have difficulty sitting upright in this seated twist, use blankets or pillows to sit on until your hips are even with your knees.

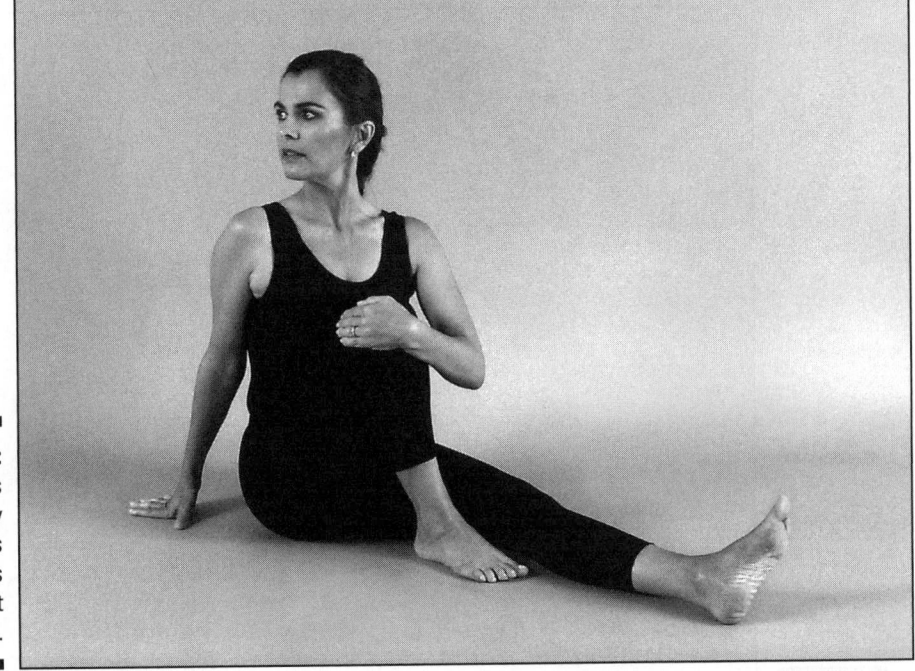

Figure 5-16: Beginners can enjoy benefits from this sage twist variation.

Book IV

Exploring Yoga and Pilates

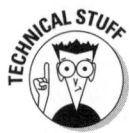

This posture is a variation of the classic posture called *maricyasana*. The Sanskrit word *marici* (pronounced *mah-ree-chee*) means 'ray of light' and is the name of an ancient sage.

Bent leg supine twist

The previously described twists all require you to sit upright. This exercise calls for you to lie down, which sounds easy enough – but there's a twist to this stipulation, literally. And it's in the twist that you harvest all kinds of benefits, including a delicious feeling of energy being released in your spine.

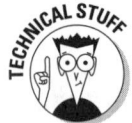

The bent leg supine twist is a variation of the classic posture known as *parivartana*. The Sanskrit word *parivartana* (pronounced *pah-ree-vahr-tah-nah*) means 'turning'.

1. **Lie on your back with your knees bent and feet on the floor at hip width, extend your arms out from your sides like a 'T', palms down, in line with the top of your shoulders.**

2. **As you exhale, slowly lower the bent legs to the right side, while turning your head to the left (see Figure 5-17).**

   Keep your head on the floor.

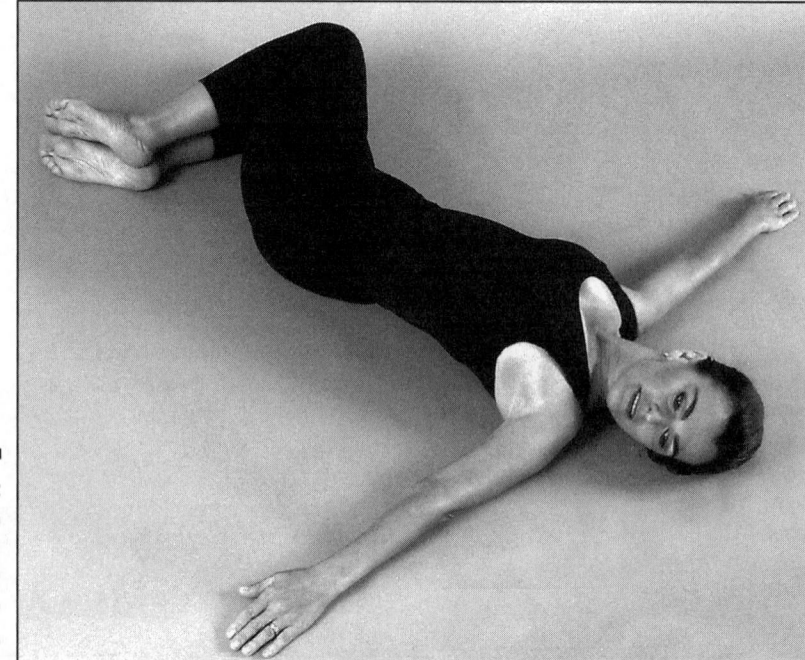

Figure 5-17:
This posture has a calming effect on the lower back.

3. As you inhale, bring your bent knees back to the middle.

4. As you exhale, slowly lower your bent knees to the left while turning your head to the right.

5. Follow Steps 1 to 4 alternating three times slowly on each side, and then hold one last twist on each side for 6 to 8 breaths.

Book IV

Exploring Yoga and Pilates

Chapter 6

Following the Classic Yoga Formula

In This Chapter

▶ Outlining the classic formula

▶ Listing the categories

*H*ow much time you choose to spend on your yoga practice is up to you. Some people like creating their own order of exercises; others prefer guidance to know which exercises to do as part of a routine.

In this chapter we introduce you to a classic Yoga formula which takes you through a range of postures including time for rest and relaxation.

The sequence will help work your mind and body and help you to keep enjoying your yoga practice.

Introducing the Classic Yoga Formula

What we call the Classic Formula consists of the following 12 categories:

1. Attunement (integrating body, mind and breath)

2. Preparation or warm-up (also used between main exercises wherever necessary)

3. Standing postures

4. Balance postures (optional)

5. Abdominals

6. Inversions (optional)

7. Back bends

8. Forward bends

9. Twists

10. Rest (to be inserted between main exercises whenever you feel the need)

11. Compensation (to be inserted after main exercises)

12. Final relaxation

You don't have to use all these categories as long as you follow the proper sequence (from 1 to 9 and always concluding with 12). The categories of *rest, preparation/warm-up* and *compensation* are repeated where appropriate. Balancing postures and inversions are marked *optional,* because their inclusion depends on your available time.

The Classic Formula is optimal for 30- to 60-minute general conditioning programmes, but we also refer to it in the 15- and 5-minute programmes. The beauty of our formula is that, as your Yoga practice grows over the years, you can explore safe postures from any book or system and then insert them into their appropriate slots within our 12-category module.

Attunement

To help you understand *attunement* – your personal connectedness – think of it this way: Attunement is like logging on to the Internet. Your 'password' is the type of breathing you select for your attunement and the rest of your programme. After you log on and establish the conscious link between your body, breath and mind, all the benefits of the Yoga universe are yours. If you forget about the attunement stage, you'll be logged off the cosmic Internet before you have a chance to receive all the benefits of your Hatha Yoga session.

First, for routines of any length, select a style of breathing from Book IV Chapter 2. If you're a beginner, choose something simple like focus breathing or belly breathing. Later you can try either the classic three-part breathing or chest-to-belly breathing, or adopt the *ujjayi* technique.

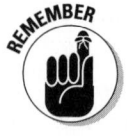

Be sure not to confuse these styles of breathing with the traditional techniques of breath control (*pranayama*) that we also describe in Book IV Chapter 2.

Next, select one of the resting postures from Book IV Chapter 4 or a sitting posture from Book IV Chapter 3, depending on your frame of mind, physical condition or what you have planned for the rest of your routine. The corpse posture (lying flat on your back) is always a good starting point for beginners. With our hectic lifestyles, we usually need to adjust and slow things down before we can begin our postural exercises. Lying flat on your back definitely shifts your mood towards relaxation. However, sitting in the easy posture or standing in the mountain posture also makes a great starting point. Figure 6-1 shows some examples of rest postures that you can use to help achieve attunement.

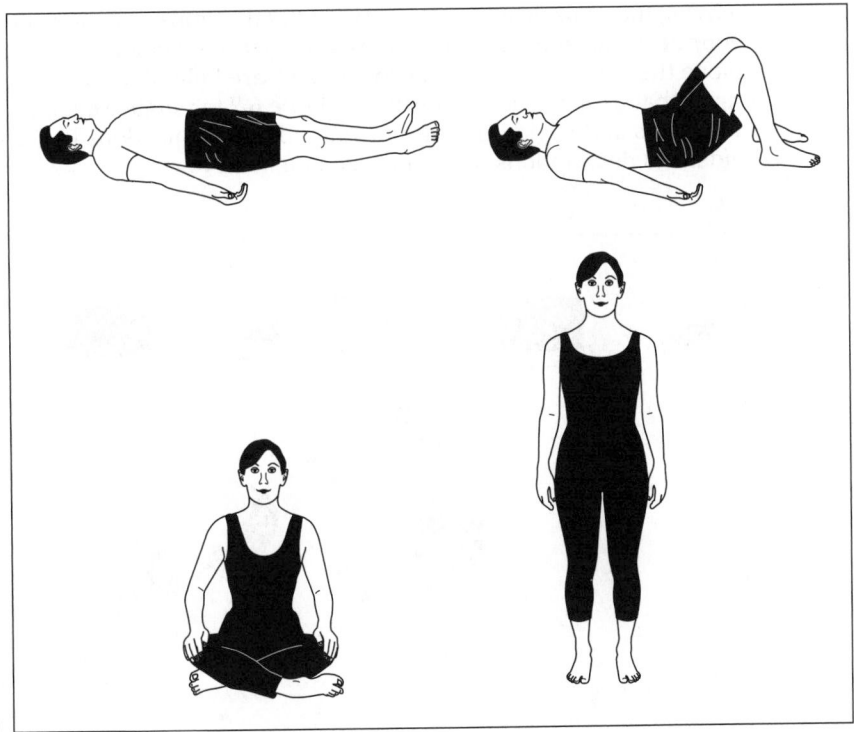

Figure 6-1:
These rest postures are great starting points when working towards attunement.

Use 8 to 12 breaths to achieve attunement. The more you 'remember' (pay attention to) the breath and your attunement, the more benefit you can expect to derive from your programme.

Warm-up

You may notice that almost all the warm-ups in Book IV Chapter 3 are folding and opening motions (flexion and extension). Either motion provides the easiest way for your body to prepare for breath and movement. Select a warm-up posture or sequence from Book IV Chapter 3 that is a *similar* position to your attunement posture.

TIP Make your Yoga practice as smooth as possible. Flow like a gentle river. For example, your attunement and warm-up both can take place on the floor; then you can stand up for all the standing postures. Avoid getting up and down like a yo-yo. Economy of movement is one of the principles of good Hatha Yoga practice.

TIP If you're composing a routine designed for 30 minutes or more, you usually have room for at least two warm-up postures. Because the neck is a frequent site of tension, we often suggest using a warm-up posture that incorporates moving the arms. In addition to stretching the spine, arm movement prepares your neck and shoulders and helps you release tension. Also, warm-ups that move the legs and prepare the lower back are helpful for the standing postures that usually follow. Check out Figure 6-2 for some examples of common warm-ups in the lying, sitting and standing positions. Book IV Chapter 3 provides full descriptions of all our recommended warm-ups.

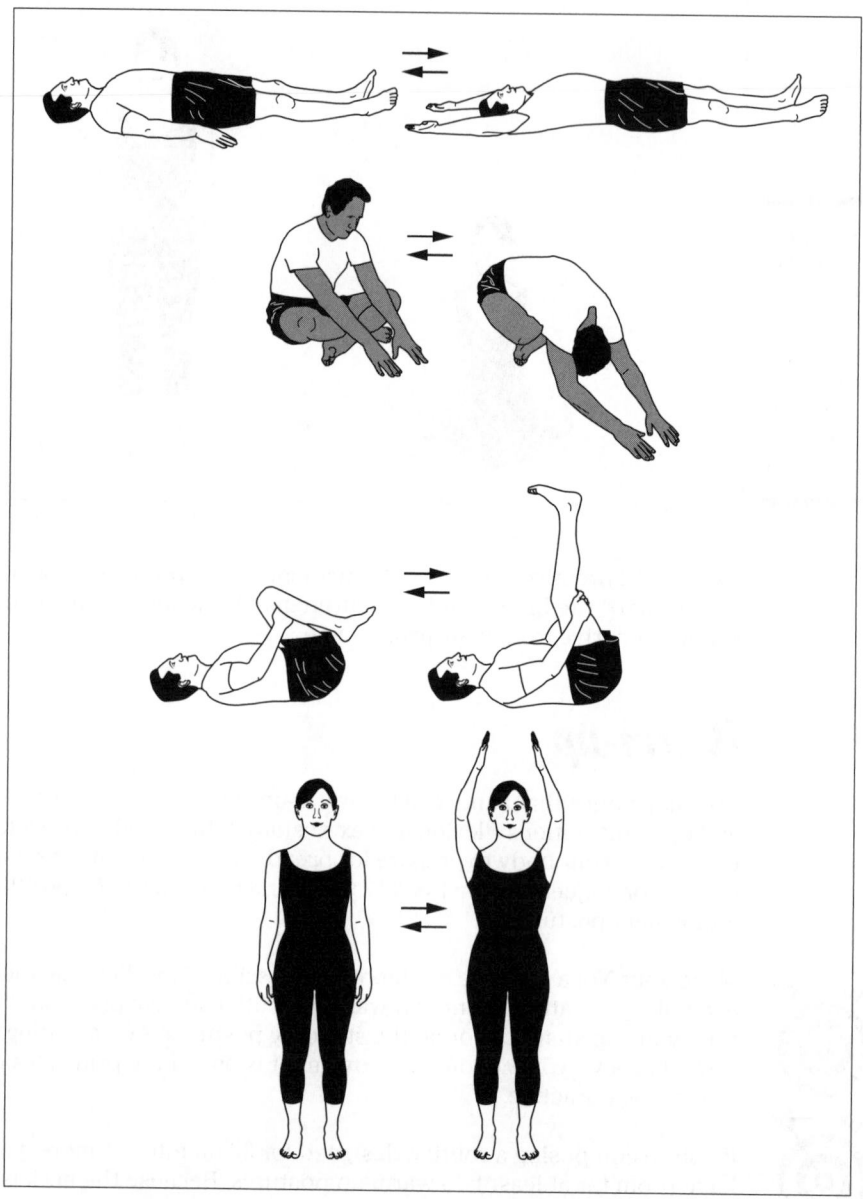

Figure 6-2:
Examples
of warm-up
postures.

Standing postures

The standing postures tend to be the most 'physical' part of a programme. If you're doing a 30-minute routine, you usually have time for three or four standing postures. In a 60-minute programme, you may have as many as six or seven main *asanas*. You can choose any of the standing postures from Book IV Chapter 3 for this portion of your routine.

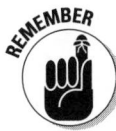

Before you begin picking your postures, run through a simple rule of sequencing: *back bends, twists and side bends are usually followed by forward bends.* Therefore, you want to include standing forward bends after most of the standing postures you choose. Figure 6-3 shows you examples of standing postures for a 30-minute or 60-minute programme. If you want your routine to be more physically challenging, simply do two sets of the standing postures.

The simplest way to expand a 30-minute routine into a 45-minute routine is to do two sets of your chosen standing postures and add one extra posture to the abdominal, back bend and forward bend categories.

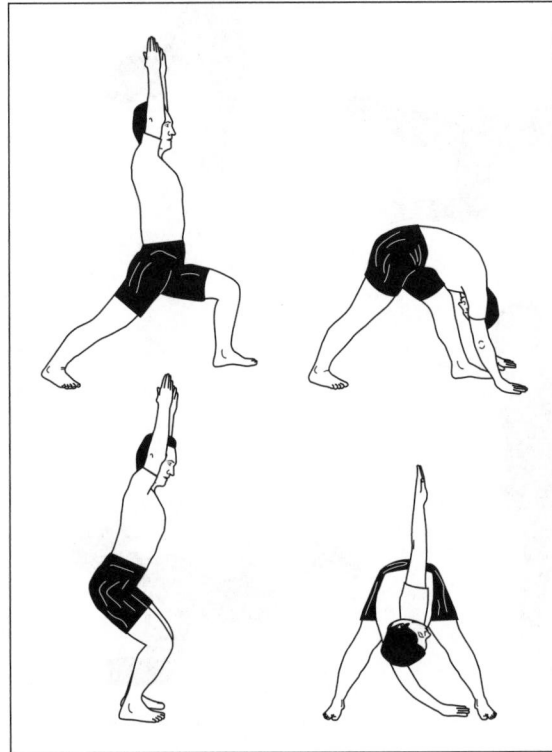

Figure 6-3:
Examples
of common
standing
postures.

Book IV

**Exploring
Yoga and
Pilates**

Balancing postures (optional)

Balancing postures are optional and depend on your time and stamina. They are often the most athletic postures and require overall co-ordination. Balancing postures are very rewarding because you can see your progress immediately. They fit nicely after the standing postures because at this point in your routine, you're fully warmed up. Also, all our recommended balancing postures are either standing or kneeling, which means they fit smoothly into the sequence. Choose one balancing posture from Book IV Chapter 4 for a 30-minute to 60-minute routine (see Figure 6-4).

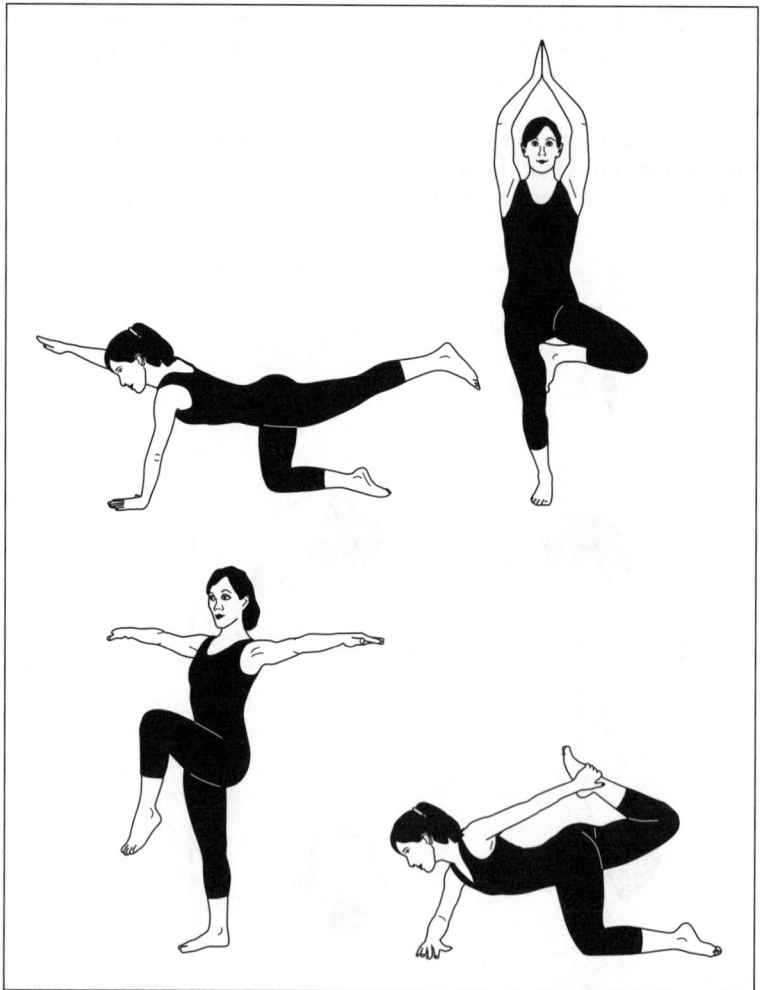

Figure 6-4:
Examples of balancing postures.

Abdominals

We recommend that you include at least one, but not more than two, abdominal postures in any programme lasting 30 minutes or more. Think of your abdomen as 'the front of your back' – a very important place. Choose one of the abdominal postures that we describe in Book IV Chapter 4 for a 30-minute routine or one or two for a 60-minute routine, or check out Figure 6-5.

Compensation and preparation

Take a short rest when you finish the abdominal exercises and then use the dynamic bridge, the dynamic bridge with arm variation, or the lying arm raise 6 to 8 times (see Book IV Chapter 3 and Figure 6-6). The action of the dynamic bridge plays a dual function here, because it *compensates* the abdomen, returning it to neutral. The bridge also warms up or *prepares* the back and the neck, if you choose to include an inversion posture or move on to back bends next.

Note: Compensation and preparation are normally done dynamically (moving).

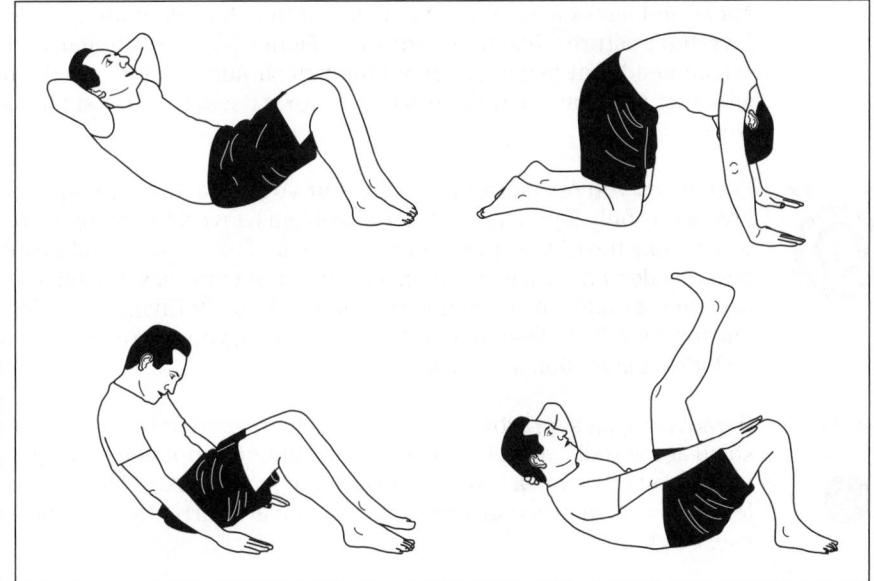

Figure 6-5: Abdominal postures strengthen the front of your back.

Book IV

Exploring Yoga and Pilates

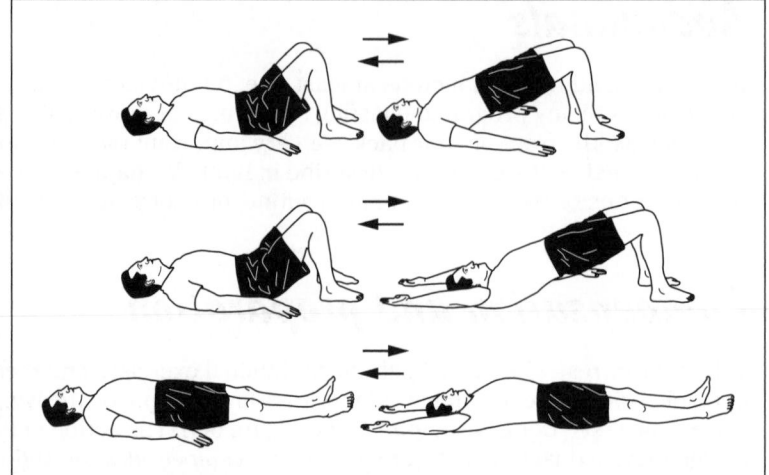

Figure 6-6:
Compen-
sation for
abdominals
can also be
prepara-
tion for
inversions.

Inversion (optional)

Indian Yoga teachers often teach inverted postures near the beginning
or at the end of a class. For Westerners, we prefer inverted postures closer
to the middle of the programme, when they've properly prepared their
backs and necks and they have plenty of time for adequate compensation.
Inverted postures, like those shown in Figure 6-7, are optional, and we
recommend that beginners avoid the half shoulder stand and the half
shoulder stand at the wall until they've practised Yoga for six to eight
weeks.

Even when you're comfortable with your yogic practice, attempt
inversions only if you have no neck problems. Inverted postures are
worthy of a healthy respect rather than fear. They're powerful postures,
but they demand a sense of balance and strong muscles. We offer you
several easy and safe inversion postures in Book IV Chapter 5. Select just
one for your 30- to 60-minute routine, assuming you are ready and want to
include an inversion in your practice.

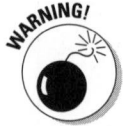

We advise against practising the half shoulder stand or the half shoulder
stand at the wall if any of the following conditions applies to you: glaucoma,
high blood pressure, a history of heart attacks or stroke, hiatal hernia, the first
few days of menstruation, pregnancy, or you are currently 18 or more kilos
overweight.

Compensation for inversions and preparation for back bends

You should rest after the simpler inverted postures, normally in the corpse posture (see Book IV Chapter 4). After the half shoulder stand, rest and then compensate further with any one of the cobra postures (see Book IV Chapter 5). The cobra postures also prepare you for further back bends. Figure 6-8 shows these examples.

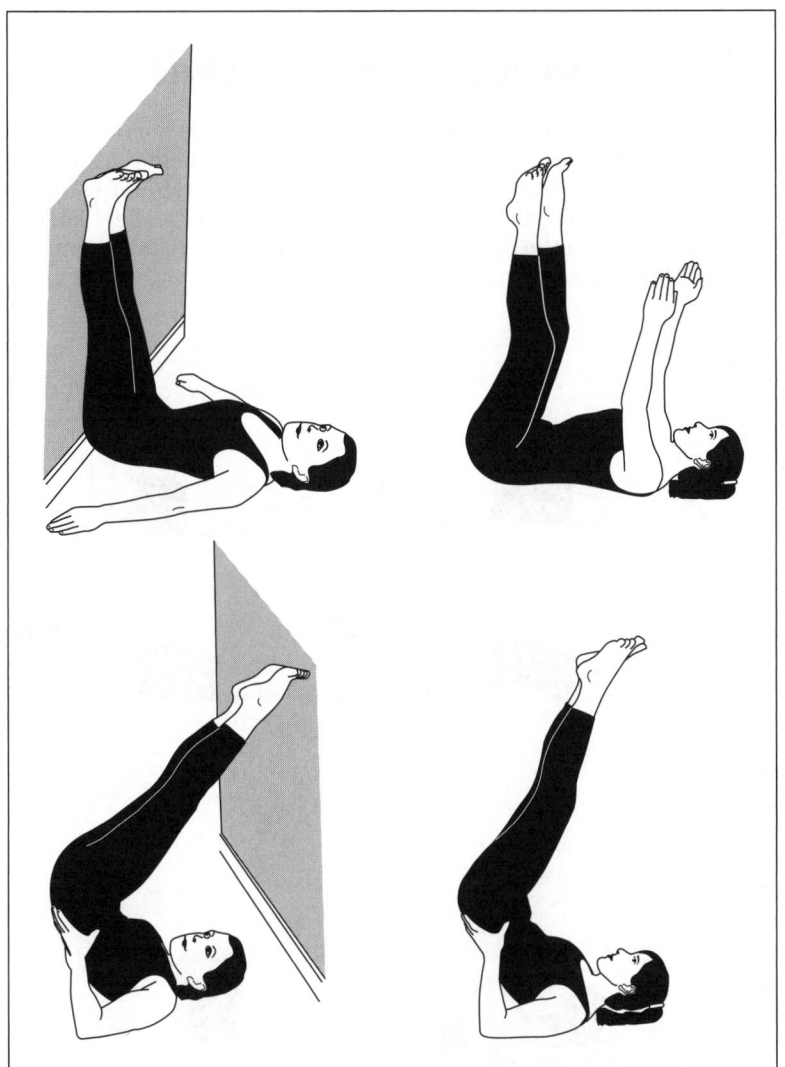

Figure 6-7:
Inversions are powerful postures that deserve respect.

Book IV

Exploring Yoga and Pilates

Back bends

Check for yourself how well back bends work after an inverted posture, and also how the cobra is an excellent compensation for the shoulder stand. The cobra is also a gentle back bend that serves as good preparation for more physical back bends. As Westerners, we bend forward far too much – that fact makes back bends a vital part of your Hatha Yoga practice. Whenever possible in general conditioning Yoga routines, select one back bend from Book IV Chapter 5; in programmes over 30 minutes, select two back bends. Figure 6-9 shows some common back bends you can try.

Compensation for back bends

The compensation for prone back bends is usually some form of a bent knee forward bend (see Figure 6-10). We often recommend the knees-to-chest or the child's posture (see Book IV Chapter 4). After more strenuous back bends, we suggest a short rest followed by one of the bent knee forward bends, and then the dynamic bridge posture as a second compensatory posture. This sequence helps neutralise the upper back and neck.

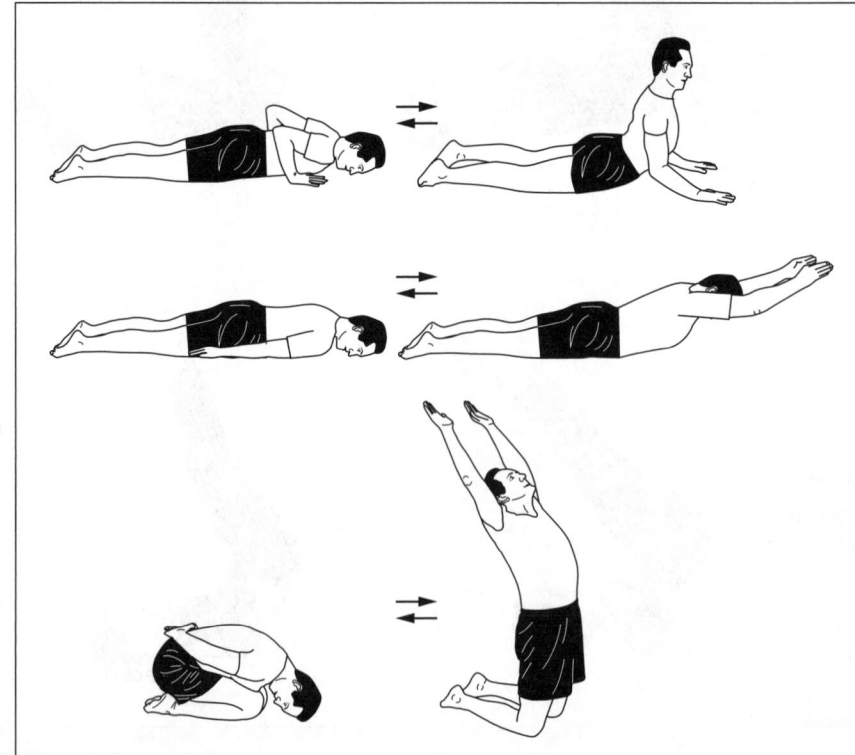

Figure 6-8:
These postures help you either compensate for an inversion or prepare for deeper back bends.

Figure 6-9:
Examples
of two com-
mon back
bends.

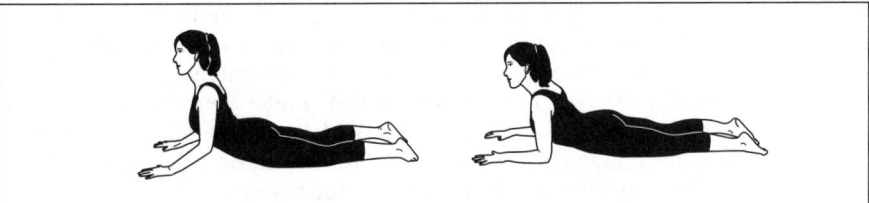

Figure 6-10:
Compen-
sating for
back bends
is an
important
part of your
Yoga
programme.

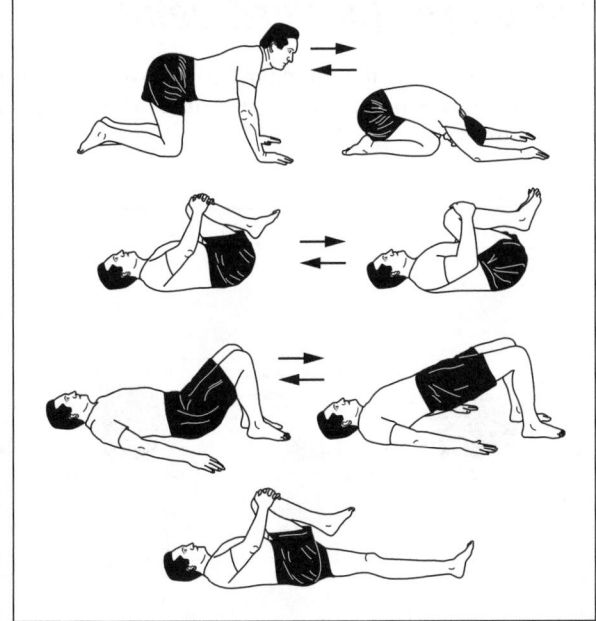

Preparation for forward bends

Preparation is particularly critical in the performance of extended leg forward bends. Stretching the hamstrings or the hips just before any of the recommended seated forward bends (see Book IV Chapter 5) not only improves
the posture but also is safer for your back. Use the hamstring stretch, or the
double leg stretch for a 30-minute routine. See Figure 6-11 for examples of
some of these stretches.

Forward bends

The seated forward bends are normally done towards the end of an exercise
programme because they have a calming effect. Of all the postures described
in this book, the seated extended leg forward bends divide the sexes the most.

Book IV

**Exploring
Yoga and
Pilates**

Men have a higher muscle density, especially in the hip and groin area, and are usually tighter in the hamstrings. Preparation of the hamstrings is particularly important. If you have a hard time with this category, bend your knees more and, if necessary, place some blankets under your hips to give yourself a better angle for the forward bends (see Book IV Chapters 3 and 5). For a 30-minute routine, choose just four forward bend from Book IV Chapter 5. For a 60-minute routine, select two forward bends (see Figure 6-12).

Compensation for forward bends

The forward bends are usually self-compensating. However, sometimes you may want to use a gentle back bend like the dynamic bridge as a counter pose (see Book IV Chapter 4).

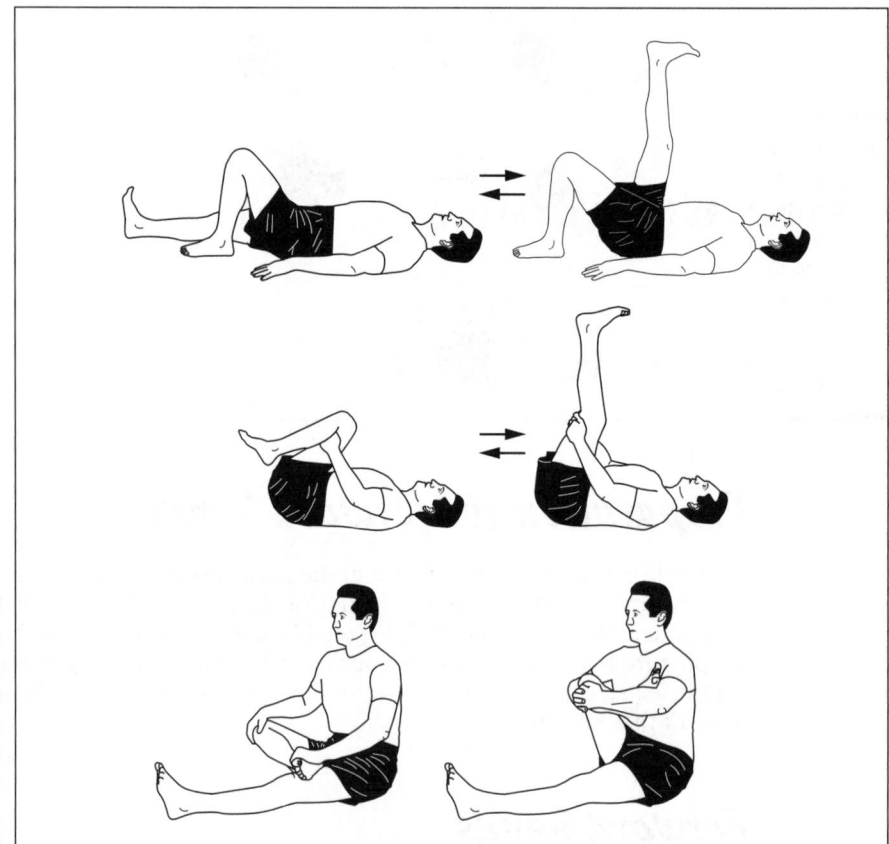

Figure 6-11: These postures help you prepare for forward bends.

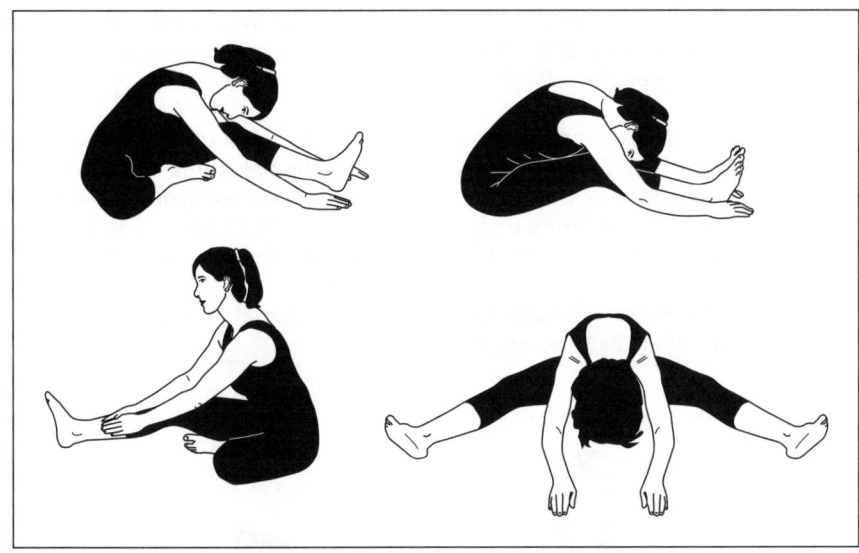

Figure 6-12:
Examples
of forward
bends.

Preparation for twists

The preparation for all twists is a forward bend. So, moving from the category of forward bends to twists is another grouping in the classic schema that flows naturally.

Twists

Twists, like forward bends, have an overall calming effect. The floor twists are the dessert in our programme, because at the end of the routine they just feel so good. Choose one floor twist from Book IV Chapter 5 for a 30-minute routine and one or two for a 60-minute routine. Figure 6-13 shows some common twists.

Relaxation

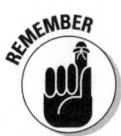

No matter how short your programme, remember to include some form of relaxation. Rest provides a place where 'absorption' can take place: You digest all the marvellous energies unleashed by your Yoga exercises.

Book IV

Exploring Yoga and Pilates

This final category in our classic formula can take several forms: a relaxation technique (see Book IV Chapter 4), yogic breathing called *pranayama* or meditation (see Book IV Chapter 2).

First, choose one of the rest postures or one of the sitting postures from Book IV Chapter 4. Next, select one of the breathing or *pranayama* techniques Book IV Chapter 2, a relaxation technique from Book IV Chapter 4, and/or a meditation technique from Book IV Chapter 2. In a 60-minute routine you may choose both a breathing and a relaxation technique.

Whichever technique you choose, use it for at least 2 to 3 minutes and not more than 15 minutes.

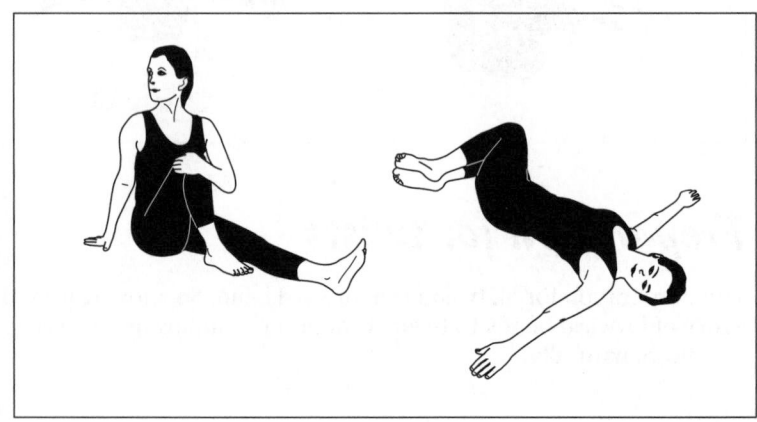

Figure 6-13: Twists are calming postures and they just feel good.

Chapter 7

Seeing What Pilates Can Give You

....

....

*B*efore you get serious about Pilates, this chapter tells you what you need to know so you understand the Pilates principles and concepts. We introduce you to some gentle exercises as a warm-up so you understand the key movements that are at the foundation of all Pilates exercises.

Getting the key principles right at the beginning enhances your Pilates practice and ensures the exercises are performed safely and effectively to benefit your body.

Seeing Is Believing: Some Pilates Images

Pilates isn't like, say, jogging. Many people find jogging relaxing because they can let their mind wander. The body goes on autopilot, and the mind is free to do other things. Not so with Pilates. Pilates – although relaxing in its own way – requires concentration. You have to think about what you're doing.

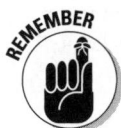

Visual images play an important role in Pilates because they help your body assume the correct position. Keep the following images in mind as you do your Pilates exercises.

> ✔ **Pull the navel towards the spine.** This image reminds people to engage their deep abdominal muscles. This image is the most essential one in Pilates.

✔ **A golden string at the back of the top of your head pulls you up to the sky.** This image helps people lengthen their whole spine when sitting or standing. Sitting up straight and standing with your head aligned with your hips is essential to strengthening the deep muscles of the back. These postural muscles tend to get very weak and overstretched in people who slouch or sit all day at a computer. This weakness is one of the main causes of back pain.

✔ **Keep the shoulders back and down.** This image counteracts the tendency to let the shoulders creep up by the ears when doing exercises, especially difficult ones. People tend to use their upper traps (trapezius) to help perform an exercise for no good reason; it is a tension response that is unnecessary and important to address. By keeping the shoulders back and down, you are engaging your back muscles, which stabilises the shoulders and helps counteract the overworking upper traps.

✔ **Keep your ears growing away from your shoulders and your shoulders dropping down away from your ears.** Another image to help relax the upper traps. This image helps remind people to keep their spine long, especially the neck.

✔ **Lower the ribcage.** Letting your ribcage protrude from your chest when using your upper body is a common response. Remember, however, that keeping the ribcage down or 'knitted' into the abdomen helps to maintain upper torso stability and keeps the upper abdominal muscles engaged.

Getting on a Mat and Learning the Pilates Principles

The mat is the essence of Pilates. A daily mat regimen guarantees you a strong centre and enables you to progress as a Pilates student, whether you continue with the mat work only or decide to try one of the many pieces of Pilates equipment.

Mat work strengthens your deep abdominal, bottom and back muscles; teaches torso stability; increases your overall flexibility; and improves your posture. Mat work, when done at an advanced level, is a full-body workout, and a quite challenging one at that.

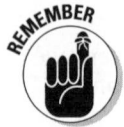

Although it's best to have a firm mat under you, Pilates mat work can be done anywhere you have a soft but supportive surface under your spine. You have no excuse not to do a little mat work every day.

Most mat work focuses on core strength (that is, strength in your stomach, back and bottom), so it trains your middle to be more compressed. You may see definition you never had before in your abdominals, and the whole middle region will begin to tone in a very delightful way. Because Pilates focuses on the deep abdominals, the sides of your torso will become more defined and the superficial bulging muscles of your stomach will disappear.

Women naturally have abdominal fat, which may or may not diminish. Losing abdominal fat is a function of weight loss – not muscular definition – but Pilates can be an important part of your weight-loss plan when it's combined with aerobic exercise.

Deciding Whether Mat Exercises Are Right for You

Pilates exercises address tightness by stretching the body in each exercise. Pilates exercises address weakness by strengthening the body in each exercise. The most important thing to remember is to just do the work regularly. Your body will change in time. As you advance in your levels and get to an exercise that you can't do, just skip over it and come back later. We guarantee that in time everything will come together. Pilates makes sense for everybody – remember that it's magic!

If you have a neck or spinal injury, especially if the injury involves a vertebral disc problem, we recommend seeing an experienced Pilates practitioner trained in rehabilitation before trying Pilates at home. People who have suffered certain kinds of spinal injuries should not do many of the Pilates mat exercises. The mat series is designed for the healthy body, and exercises must be modified by a rehabilitation professional if a spinal injury is present.

Learning Some Pilates Principles

The Pilates Principles are at the core of all the exercises. Understanding the principles right at the beginning will help you as you work your way through the different exercises. Pilates aims to increase your strength, muscle tone and body conditioning. The principles also focus on proper alignment, improving balance and coordination to help prevent injury. Taking time to understand the following principles will benefit your Pilates practice.

Book IV

Exploring Yoga and Pilates

Neutral Spine

Neutral Spine is one of the most subtle yet powerful principles in Pilates. It belongs to the less-is-more approach to movement, like most of the fundamental concepts underlying the Pilates method.

Here's how you can feel Neutral Spine: Lie on your back with your knees bent and your feet flat on the floor. Your spine should have two areas that do not touch the mat underneath you: your neck and your lower back (the cervical spine and lumbar spine, respectively). These natural curves in your back function to absorb shock when you're standing, running, jumping or simply walking around town. When you sit, it's important to maintain the natural curves in your spine to prevent lower back and neck strain. Neutral Spine is basically universal proper posture.

You often work in Neutral Spine when performing stability exercises in Pilates in order to maintain and reinforce these natural curves in the spine. Many people are taught to flatten the curve of their lower back when doing exercises or when standing. This method is no longer thought to be posturally correct; instead, the natural curve is indicated. Figures 7-1a and 7-1b show the back with too much curve and not enough curve, respectively. Figure 7-1c shows true Neutral Spine. Note that Neutral Spine can be called for even when you're not on your back – some of the exercises in Book IV Chapter 9 call for Neutral Spine when you're on all fours, for example.

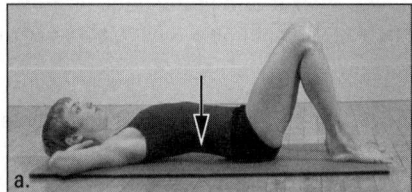

Too much curve (anterior pelvic tilt)…

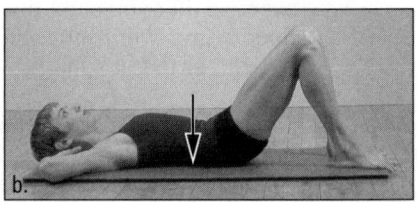

not enough curve (posterior pelvic tilt)…

Figure 7-1:
Finding
Neutral
Spine.

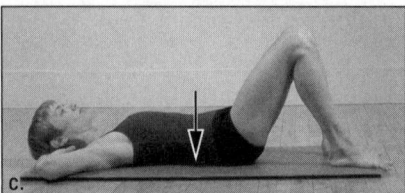

and just right (neutral pelvis).

Abdominal Scoop

You can do the Abdominal Scoop in any position, anywhere, anytime. It is easy and fun to do in your spare time, and it hides your spare tyre! Basically, it's the act of pulling your navel in towards your spine. Imagining that you're pulling in your gut to zip up a tight pair of trousers will do the job.

What you're doing, anatomically, is engaging your deepest abdominal muscle (called your _tranversus abdominis_), which functions to hold your viscera in and, when contracted, decreases the diameter of the abdominal wall. When pulled taut, it works a lot like a drawstring around a pair of tracksuit bottoms. The reason you scoop in Pilates is that your deep abdominals help to stabilise your back and tend to be weak in most people. The superficial abdominal muscle _(rectus abdominis),_ on the other hand, tends to be a workaholic and takes over the work of the deeper layers if you're not careful. So keep reminding your tummy to pull in! Figure 7-2 shows the Abdominal Scoop in action.

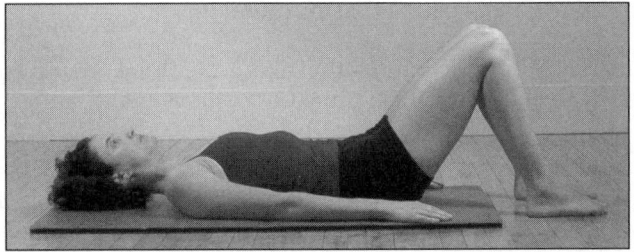

Figure 7-2:
The
Abdominal
Scoop.

Spine Curl

Lie on your back with your knees bent and your feet flat on the floor. Push your hips up as high as you can and hold them there. Take a deep breath in, and as you exhale, squeeze your bottom, drop your ribcage, and pull your navel in towards your spine to make your torso as flat as possible. Your body should make a flat plane, with no bowing of the body up or down. You can maintain this tabletop torso by continuing to squeeze your bottom and knitting your ribcage down into your belly. You'll feel a good burn in the back of your legs _(hamstrings)_ and in your bottom _(gluteus)_. Figure 7-3 shows the position.

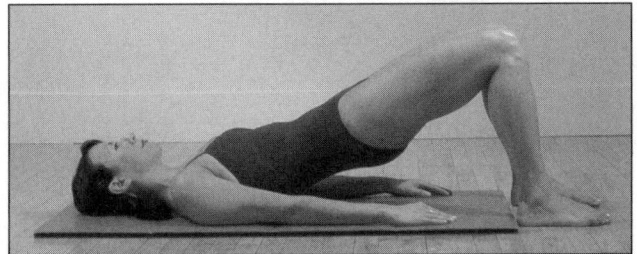

Figure 7-3:
The Spine
Curl
position.

Book IV

**Exploring
Yoga and
Pilates**

C Curve

The classic C Curve is always initiated by the abdominals. Try a C Curve by sitting up tall with your legs slightly bent in front of you. Imagine someone punching you in the lower stomach, and allow your spine to round by scooping in your deep abdominals. Your upper back, neck and head may naturally follow this motion and round forward. So you initiate the C Curve with the lower back (*lumbar spine*), then you add the upper back (*thoracic spine*), and finally you add the head and neck (*cervical spine*). Now your whole spine is making a capital C. This movement should feel like a big stretch for your whole spine and all the muscles that surround it.

Here's a little more specific information about the three natural curves of the spine and how they participate in the C Curve movement.

Lumbar C Curve

The Lumbar C Curve movement is always initiated by your lower abdominals. This is the most difficult spinal movement to initiate because the lumbar spine has thick vertebrae that are meant to stabilise and hold the weight of the body. When you're standing or lying, the natural curve of your lumbar spine is in slight extension (like Neutral Spine), so when performing a Lumbar C Curve, you must pay much attention to pulling in your abdominals from the lowest part of your abdomen and attempting to reverse the natural curve of your low spine. You can accomplish this only by deep and strong low abdominal engagement. Figure 7-4 shows the Lumbar C Curve.

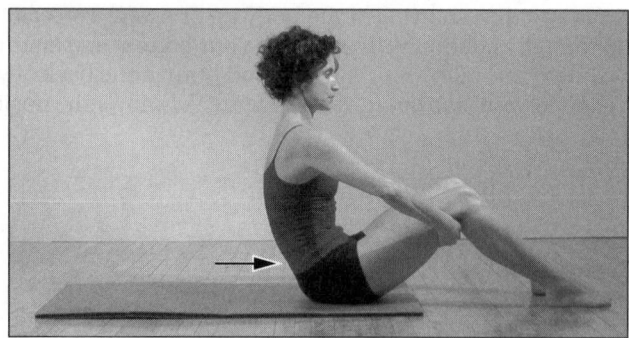

Figure 7-4:
The Lumbar
C Curve.

Thoracic C Curve

The upper back (thoracic region) naturally curves forward in a C shape (at least with most people – longtime dancers and gymnasts can develop a flattened or reverse thoracic curve from years of sticking out their chest). When performing a Thoracic C Curve, think of pulling your ribs in and allowing your shoulders to round forward, as in Figure 7-5. Doing so creates a nice stretch in the upper back.

The Thoracic C Curve naturally follows the Lumbar C Curve, but it is easy to do the Thoracic C Curve without actually starting from the lower back. In other words, it's easy for people to round their upper back because the back naturally rounds in that direction. Initiating the rounding from the lower back is more difficult and takes low abdominal work. The idea in Pilates is generally to try to do more work from the belly and to move the spine starting from the lower back and then adding in the upper back afterwards. Be aware that you may have a tendency to just hunch forward like Quasimodo when doing a C Curve and round only from your upper back, without actually using your low tummy!

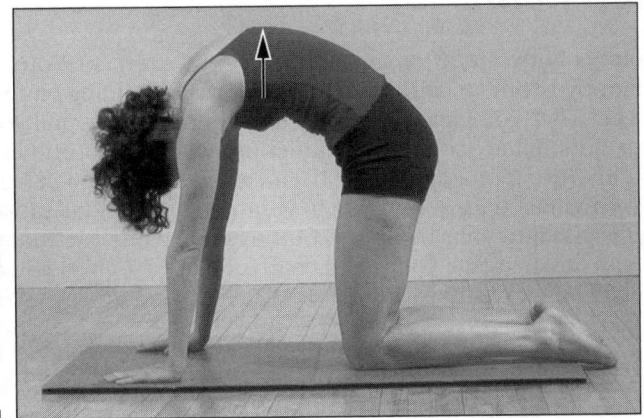

Figure 7-5:
The
Thoracic C
Curve.

Cervical C Curve

One of the most common complaints we get from novice Pilates students after their first mat class is 'My neck bothers me!'. That's why we go into painstaking detail about the correct way to lift your head when doing a sit-up. We use the Cervical C Curve mostly as a way to visualise the correct way to lift your head off the mat during an abdominal exercise. If you know the right way to lift your head up and understand proper neck alignment, you won't overstrain your neck when doing the abdominal-related exercises in Pilates.

Book IV

Exploring
Yoga and
Pilates

Lie on your back with your hands interlaced behind your head to support the neck. Lift your head off the mat by lengthening the back of the neck and by imagining that you're squeezing a tangerine under your chin to bring the head up (kind of like nodding your head 'yes' as you lift it off the mat). Don't lead up with your chin. Once your head is off the mat, you have created your Cervical C Curve; the C shape begins at the top of your head and ends at the base of your sternum (or ribcage). You must lift your head high enough to form the shape of the C. Think of your abdominal muscles lifting up the weight of the head, not the neck muscles. If you're very tight in your neck or very weak in your tummy, you may not be able to make a complete C shape. But if you keep doing the work, you will! Figure 7-6 shows a Cervical C Curve.

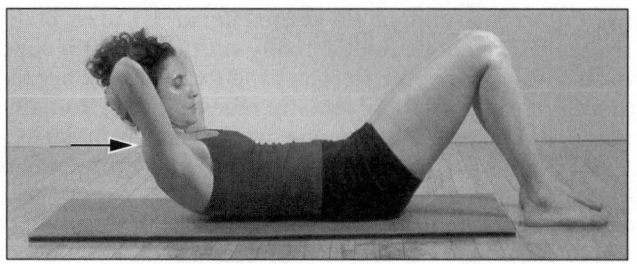

Figure 7-6:
The Cervical
C Curve.

Balance Point

Balance Point is both a position and a fundamental exercise. You can practise Balance Point by sitting up with your knees bent and holding on to the backs of your thighs. Then roll back slightly behind your tailbone, pull your stomach in (your Abdominal Scoop, from earlier in this chapter), and lift your feet off the mat. In order to maintain your balance and stop yourself from rolling backwards, you must engage and pull in your deep abdominal muscles. This position pulls you into your Lumbar C Curve and teaches you that to balance with ease, you must engage your deep centre. Figure 7-7 gives you an idea of what Balance Point looks like.

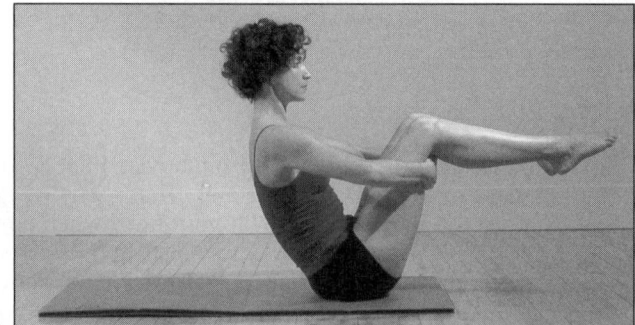

Figure 7-7:
Balance
Point.

Stacking the Spine

Stacking the Spine is a finish to several exercises in the Pilates method. It teaches *articulation* of the spine (full movement throughout all the vertebrae) as well as how to sit up vertically. It's a fluid way to sit up or stand erect from a hunched-over position. Also, Stacking the Spine is a wonderful stretch for your back. Figure 7-8 shows Stacking the Spine in action.

To practise Stacking the Spine, start by sitting cross-legged (or with your knees bent and your feet on the floor) with your back against a wall. If this is a difficult position for you because you're tight in your hips or low back, then sit on a pillow. Allow your whole spine to round forward, letting your head hang heavy. Then begin to Stack the Spine by pulling your navel in towards your spine and trying to press your lower back into the wall. Start at the lowest vertebra possible and keep pressing your spine into the wall, moving up one vertebra at a time and allowing your head to hang heavy until the end. Finally, you're sitting up tall, with your whole spine and head against the wall. You have just Stacked your Spine! You can try again, but this time try reversing the stacking to get to the starting point. In other words, allow your head to initiate the roll down and then peel off the wall one vertebra at a time until you're rounded forward (in a C Curve) and are ready to stack up again.

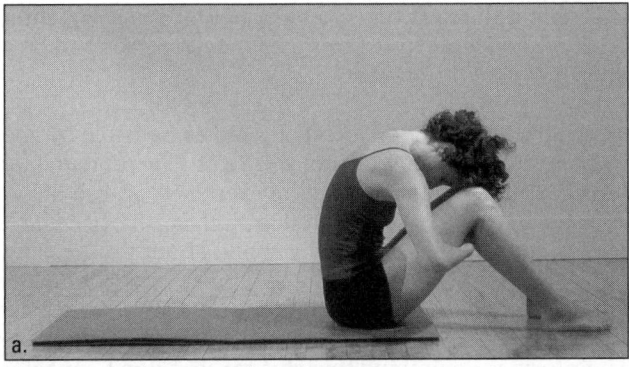

Move your back one vertebra at a time.

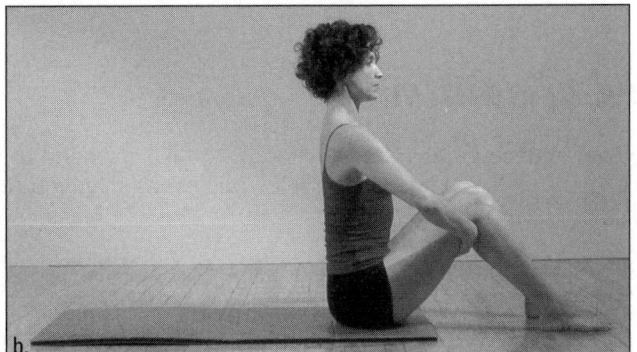

Figure 7-8: Stacking the Spine.

Pre-Pilates: The Fundamentals

The exercises in this section are sometimes called pre-Pilates because they are preparations to get your body ready to do the harder stuff. These are definitely what you should do when you're first introducing yourself to Pilates, and then you can do them in the future as a warm-up for the more advanced exercises. And you can always come back to these basics, no matter how advanced you get, to refresh your form.

Practise this fundamental series until you understand these basic concepts in both your body and your mind, then move on to the beginning series.

We include some of these fundamental exercises in the beginning and intermediate series. We think that the Upper Abdominal Curls and Coccyx Curls are two exercises that are always great to start your workout. Why? Well, Coccyx Curls warm up your lower back and get you connected to your deep abdominals, while the Upper Abdominal Curls warm up your neck and upper back and get you feeling that Pilates Abdominal Position.

When doing this series of exercises, be aware of the sensations in your body. If you really get the concept that the exercise is trying to teach, then you may not need to repeat it the next time you work out. Ultimately, the goal is to incorporate these concepts in the more advanced series and be able to build more complex movement phrases.

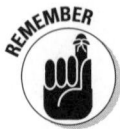

In this book, we try and give you as much help as possible by giving you a set of exercises that match whatever level you're at. The fundamentals are in this chapter, Book IV Chapter 8 has beginning exercises, and so on. Do the exercises in the order that they're presented in each series, because this order makes sense for your body. And don't feel bad about progressing slowly!

One other thing: The models in this book are all experienced Pilates instructors. Don't feel like you need to look like them, exactly, as you perform the exercise. Their form is something to strive for, but don't expect yourself to match it perfectly.

A word of caution

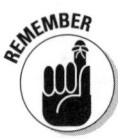

Before you get started doing Pilates, we want to take a second to remind you to please be careful. If you injure yourself while exercising, you're hurting your health, not improving it!

Here are some signs that an exercise isn't right for you:

- ✔ You feel a sharp, shooting or tingling pain while exercising.
- ✔ You feel a muscle pulling while doing an exercise, and the pain doesn't subside in a few minutes.
- ✔ Your neck hurts while doing an exercise.
- ✔ One or more of your joints hurts while doing an exercise.

Your low back may feel sensations when doing Pilates, but that may not be a bad thing. Bad back pain is the kind that doesn't go away after a few minutes but lasts for days afterwards. If you feel your back hurting when doing an abdominal exercise, you must modify it until you don't feel your back anymore. Usually you just need to pull your navel in a lot more! As your abdominal muscles get stronger, your back will stop bothering you.

Breathing in Neutral Spine

Most people don't breathe into the lower portions of their lungs, but only breathe superficially. This exercise focuses on increasing lung capacity, and especially on bringing air into the deeper parts of the lung.

Breathing is something we all do automatically, and yet some people tend to hold their breath when exercising. Holding your breath tenses your muscles and makes your body more rigid. Even though the following exercise may seem unbearably easy, it's actually the fundamental essence that underlies all future Pilates exercises.

Getting set

Lie down on your back with your knees bent, feet flat on the floor about hip distance apart. Relax your back into Neutral Spine (see section in this chapter). Place your hands on either side of your lower ribcage just above your waist, putting your thumbs towards your back and your other fingers towards your breast bone.

The exercise

Inhale: Breathe deeply into your lungs, allowing the ribs to expand laterally in your hands. Think of breathing into your kidney area (your low back) and filling up your lungs to their fullest capacity. Try not to arch your back off the mat at all.

Exhale: Allow all the air to come out of your lungs.

Imagine you are playing an accordion. As you inhale, the squeeze box expands open, as you exhale, it comes back together.

Do's and don'ts

- ✔ Don't arch your back when you inhale. Keep your upper back in contact with the mat.

- ✔ Do continue this exercise until you feel relaxed and grounded and ready to proceed with the next exercise.

Book IV

Exploring Yoga and Pilates

Shoulder Shrugs

Feeling uptight? Tension is a physical as well as an emotional reality. Most people unknowingly hold tension in their neck and shoulders; especially if they work at a computer or have a desk job. Not overusing your upper trapezius muscles (the muscles at the back of your neck and at the top of your shoulders) is almost impossible if you hold your arms in front of you hour after hour. But once you become aware of this holding pattern, it is possible to correct through this simple exercise.

Getting set

To begin, lie down on your back with your knees bent and your feet flat on the floor about hip distance apart, arms straight down by your sides. Relax your back into Neutral Spine (see Figure 7-9a).

The exercise

Inhale: Bring your shoulders up by your ears, contracting your upper trapezius muscles (Figure 7-9b).

Exhale: Relax and release your shoulders, letting them drop down quickly away from your ears.

Complete four repetitions. On the final repetition, slow down and on the exhale let your shoulder blades melt slowly down your back. Try to feel the muscles in your back that keep the shoulder blades down and away from your ears.

Do's and don'ts

- ✔ Do follow the breathing cues in this exercise. Exhaling always helps relax your muscles.

- ✔ Don't hold your breath.

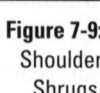

Figure 7-9:
Shoulder
Shrugs.

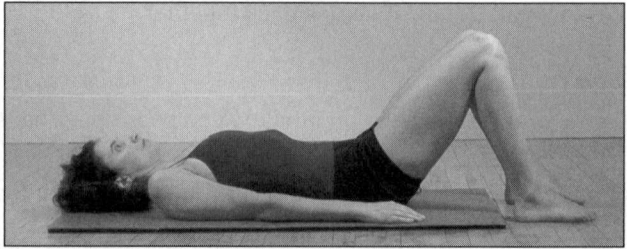

Shrug, then release, your shoulders.

Shoulder Slaps

Shoulder Slaps are another safe and simple way to discover how to relax and release your shoulder muscles as well as a way to discover how to engage the stabilising muscles of your shoulder.

Getting set

Lying on your back with your knees bent and your feet flat on the floor, bring your arms up so that your fingers point towards the ceiling.

The exercise

Inhale: Reach your arms up to the sky, allowing your shoulder blades *(scapulae)* to come off the mat (Figure 7-10a).

Exhale: Keep your arms straight and reaching up as you relax and release your shoulder muscles, letting your scapulae slap back to the mat (Figure 7-10b).

Complete four repetitions.

On the final repetition, allow your shoulder blades to return slowly, imagining your shoulder blades melting back into the mat. Keep pushing your scapulae back into the mat, and feel the muscles that are working – these are your *latissimus dorsi muscles.* It is important to know where the latissimus dorsi is because you use it all the time in Pilates to pull your shoulders down away from your ears, helping to release shoulder tension.

Do's and don'ts

  ✔ Do really release on the exhale, allowing your shoulder blades and arms to truly drop with gravity.

  ✔ Don't bend your arms when you slap your shoulder blades down.

Book IV

Exploring Yoga and Pilates

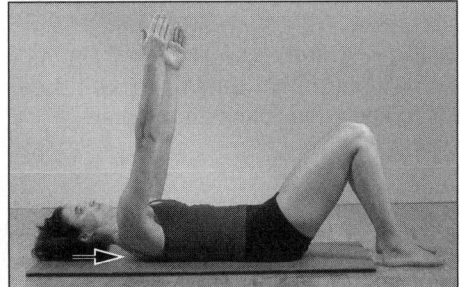

Figure 7-10:
Shoulder
Slaps.

Lift your shoulders off the mat.

Arm Reaches/Arm Circles

This exercise has the dual function of stretching out the chest and back muscles while teaching upper torso stability.

If you are tight and need to stretch, focus on opening your chest when performing this exercise. If you have lots of flexibility in your body, then focus on stabilising your torso (don't let your upper back arch off the mat!).

Getting set

Lie on your back with your knees bent and your feet flat on the floor, approximately hip distance apart, and your back in Neutral Spine, arms down by your sides.

The exercise

Inhale: Reach your arms up to the ceiling at a 90-degree angle to the floor, keeping your arms shoulder distance apart (Figure 7-11a).

Exhale: Drop your ribcage and think of knitting your ribs into your tummy, and reach your arms back towards your ears. (Figure 7-11b). Use your upper abdominals to keep your upper back from arching off the mat. Figure 7-12 shows incorrect posture, with the back arched off the mat.

Inhale: Circle the arms open to a 'T' shape (keeping the arms on the floor, as in Figure 7-11c), then down by your sides, then back to the starting position, reaching up to the sky.

Complete three repetitions and reverse directions.

Do's and don'ts

✔ Do maintain absolute stability in your torso by keeping your ribs down.

✔ Do keep your shoulders down away from your ears as you initiate the exercise.

✔ Don't let your upper back arch off the mat (Figure 7-12). As you raise your arms, your upper back naturally wants to go with them – the whole point of this exercise is to keep your back on the mat.

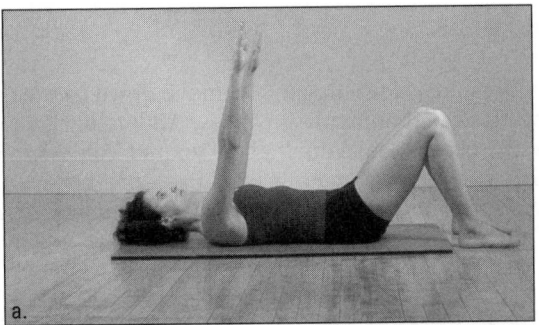

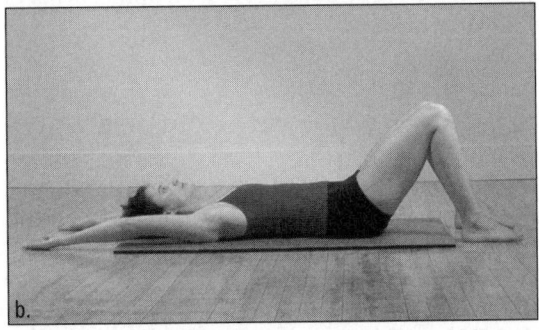

Figure 7-11:
Arm
Reaches/
Arm Circles.

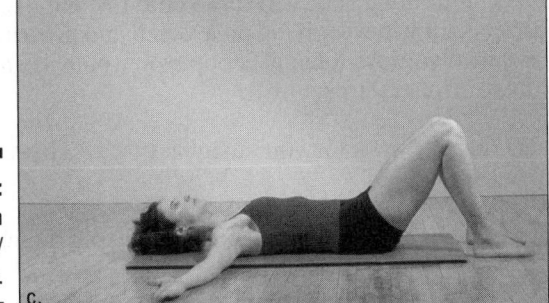

Figure 7-12:
What not to
do when
performing
Arm
Reaches/
Arm Circles.

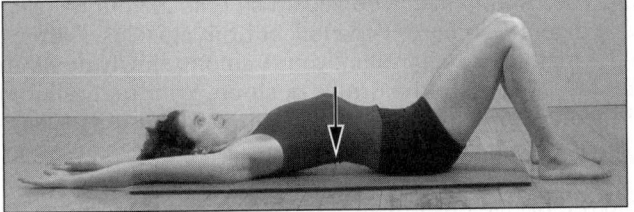

Don't allow your back to arch off the mat.

Coccyx Curls

Now that your shoulders are released, you can move down to the centre of it all. This is your first exercise that involves the low Abdominal Scoop that is so prevalent in Pilates exercises. Please don't allow your shoulders to rise and hold tension now that you've got some release there – just because you're not focusing on the shoulders doesn't mean that you get to go back to bad habits!

Getting set

Lie on your back with your knees bent and your feet flat on the floor, approximately hip distance apart, and your back in Neutral Spine, arms down by your sides (Figure 7-13a).

The exercise

Inhale: Breathe in deeply.

Exhale: Begin the Coccyx Curl by first finding your deep Abdominal Scoop: Pull your navel in towards your spine and gently squeeze your low bottom muscles and flatten your low back onto the mat.

Imagine that your stomach is so pulled in that it's pressing the vertebrae of your low back onto the mat. This is sometimes called imprinting because you're picturing yourself imprinting your vertebrae onto the mat beneath you with your Abdominal Scoop. If you were lying on a beach and pressing your low back onto the sand with your Abdominal Scoop, you would see an imprint of the vertebrae on the sand afterwards.

If the imprinting image doesn't work for you, imagine that you have to zip up a very tight pair of trousers.

If neither of the above get you to scoop, think of scooping out a melon, which is your stomach!

Inhale: Release and go back to a comfortable Neutral Spine.

Exhale: Find your Abdominal Scoop again by pulling your navel in towards your spine and gently squeezing the low bottom muscles. Flatten your low back onto the mat, then keep rolling your tailbone slowly up off the mat to the count of 5. Roll up to the Bridge position. Your body should make a straight line from your shoulders to your knees. Don't press your hips up so high that you can't see your knees.

Inhale: Hold the Bridge position.

Exhale: Roll down one vertebra at a time, again by pulling in your tummy. Return to Neutral Spine at the end.

Why engaged Neutral Spine is so important

If you carry over engaged Neutral Spine to standing up, you will have the beginnings of very good posture. It allows you to keep the natural curves of the spine while still having deep abdominal engagement to support the back. Engaged Neutral Spine on the mat simply means your stomach is pulled in but you have not changed the position of your pelvis on the mat. To make sure you are in Neutral Spine, make sure your tailbone is still making contact with the mat.

Complete three repetitions, each time making the movement smaller and smaller until on the last one you're not even moving out of Neutral Spine, but are pulling the abdominals in as if you were going to initiate a Coccyx Curl but don't. This is called engaged Neutral Spine. See the sidebar 'Why engaged Neutral Spine is so important' for more info.

Do's and don'ts

- Do focus on initiating this movement with the Abdominal Scoop.

- Don't tense your upper body when doing this exercise. Keep your neck long and your shoulders relaxed.

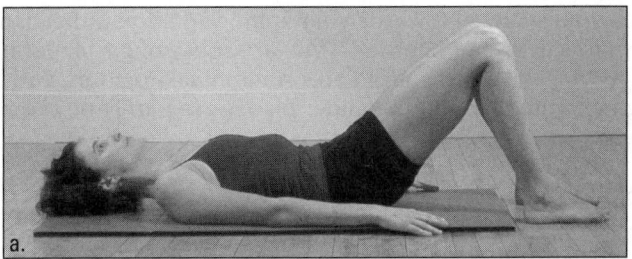

Figure 7-13: Coccyx Curls.

a.

b.

Upper Abdominal Curls

This exercise may be hard for you for two reasons:

- ✔ If you have weak upper abdominal muscles, you will shake when attempting to roll up. Don't worry too much if you cannot come up in this curl; you'd be surprised how many people have a hard time with this exercise at first.

- ✔ If you have a very tight upper back and neck, you may not be able to get into the position. If this is the case, then it will be virtually impossible for you to come up and you may or may not feel any work in your abdominal muscles. You will, however feel a stretch in the back of your neck and upper back.

In either case, keep trying. If you get frustrated, just move on to the next exercise and revisit this one after a few weeks of other Pilates exercises. You'll slowly transform, and may find this one easier at a future date.

Getting set

To begin, lie down on your back with your knees bent, feet flat on the floor about hip distance apart. Relax your back into Neutral Spine. Interlace your fingers and put your hands behind your head (Figure 7-14a).

The exercise

Exhale: Pull your navel in towards your spine and lift your head, pulling your chin in towards your chest as if you are squeezing a tangerine under your chin, as you roll up to your Pilates Abdominal Position. You should roll up just high enough that your shoulder blades are barely off the mat, as in Figure 7-14b).

Inhale: Hold this position.

Exhale: Control the movement back down to the mat.

Complete eight slow repetitions.

Do's and don'ts

- ✔ Do maintain Neutral Spine as you roll up.

- ✔ Don't let your low back flatten; keep your tailbone anchored to the mat.

- ✔ Don't strain your neck. Allow your hands to hold the weight of your head and keep the space of a tangerine between your chin and your neck.

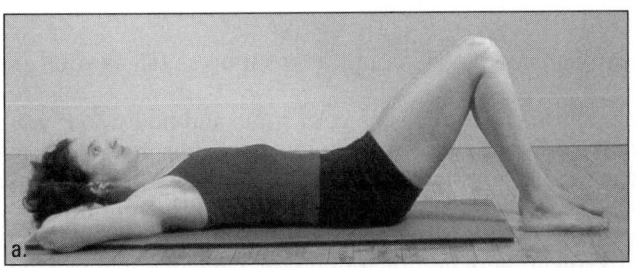

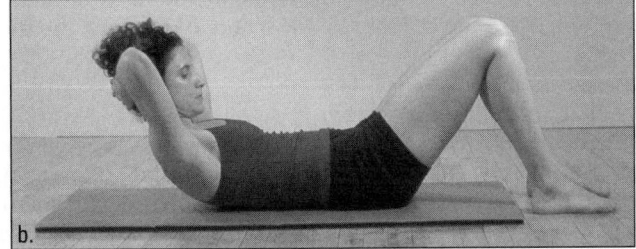

Figure 7-14:
Upper
Abdominal
Curls.

C Curve Roll Down Prep

Now we're getting into the fun stuff. This exercise is a preparation for Roll Down, which is a preparation for Roll Up! You may be strong enough already to do a full Roll Up. If so, you will progress quickly through this series and the next. But, if you have little awareness of your deep abdominals and little strength, plan on taking things slowly, and know that you are in the majority.

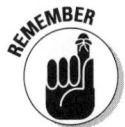

Ultimately, one of the most satisfying things about Pilates is that it is challenging – take up the challenge, and you'll feel great as you slowly conquer more and more difficult exercises.

C Curve Roll Down Prep – the name is pretty self-explanatory. You guide yourself as you become aware of how to feel your C Curve in your low back. You also get some practice with Stacking the Spine.

Getting set

Sitting up, bend your knees and put your feet flat on the floor. Hold the back of your thighs with your hands, wrapping them around the outside of your legs (Figure 7-15a). Sit up as tall as you can by imagining you have a golden string attached to the back of the top of your head that is pulling you up to the sky.

Book IV

Exploring Yoga and Pilates

The exercise

Inhale: Breathe in deeply and continue to sit up as tall as you can.

Exhale: Pull your navel in towards your spine and hollow out your low belly, making a C Curve shape in your low back. Imagine that someone punched you in your low belly. Begin rolling backwards down your spine, allowing your tailbone to roll underneath you. Allow your arms to walk slowly down your thighs as needed, and use them to assist you in the roll down. Try to roll far enough down that you can feel the bones of your lower back pressing onto the mat. Your whole back, including your neck and your head, should look like a big C. Figures 7-15b and 7-15c show the model rolling down.

Inhale: Take in a breath at the bottom.

Exhale: Pull your navel in towards your spine, and think of pressing your lower back into the mat with your abdominal muscles as you slowly roll back up. Again, use your arms to assist you, and allow them to walk back up your thighs. Allow your whole back to stay round in a C Curve and your tummy to stay hollow, and return to sitting on your tailbone. You should be making a C shape with your whole spine (Figure 7-15d).

Inhale: Stack up the Spine, starting from your low back, then your upper back, then your head and neck. Think of keeping your head hanging heavy until the very end.

Exhale: Keep sitting up tall, and allow your shoulders to drop down away from your ears. Feel the back muscles engage, keeping the shoulders down in their proper place (Figure 7-15e).

Complete six repetitions.

Do's and don'ts

✔ Do focus on using the abdominals to perform the exercise.

✔ Do attempt to articulate through the spine on the way down and on the way up.

✔ Do minimise the tension in the upper body; keep the neck long and relaxed.

✔ Don't hold your breath. Use long, slow breathing to assist the movement.

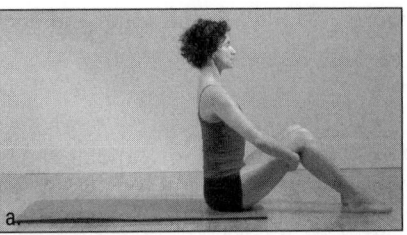
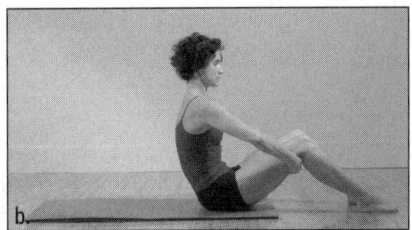
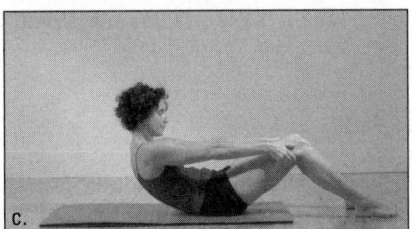
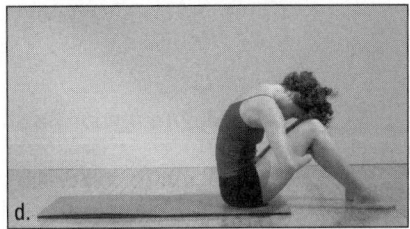
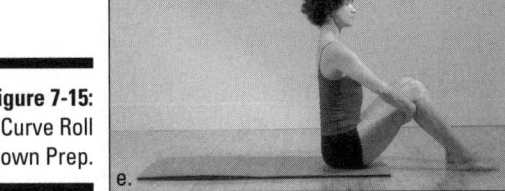

Figure 7-15:
C Curve Roll
Down Prep.

Balance Point/Teaser Prep

Balance Point is basically a C-Curve Roll Down Prep with your feet off the floor. Your feet being off the floor makes it much harder to keep your balance. If you find this exercise too daunting, simply practise the previous exercise until you're ready to progress.

Balance Point is one of the best exercises we know to find your deep abdominal muscles. You can't cheat and use other muscles to help out in this exercise; you are forced to use your deep abdominals because if you don't you'll fall out of position. This exercise really separates the women from the girls and the men from the boys.

In this exercise and in Pilates in general, articulating your spine is important. *Articulating* your spine just means to move your spine one vertebra at a time, instead of moving the spine in chunks of four or five vertebrae. Articulating

Book IV

Exploring
Yoga and
Pilates

one vertebra at a time brings more flexibility to the spine and enables the abdominals to work more.

Getting set

Sit up, bend your knees and lift your feet off the floor, holding the back of your thighs with your hands (right hand wrapping around the outside of the right thigh and left hand around the outside of the left thigh). You should be balanced right behind your tailbone (coccyx), with your low back rounded and your tummy hollowed out (Figure 7-16a). This is the Balance Point position.

The exercise

Inhale: Maintain your Balance Point.

Exhale: Begin to roll down your spine, pushing your thighs away as a counterbalance. Pull your navel in and control the movement from the centre. Only go back as far as where you can control the movement (Figures 7-16b and 7-16c show the model rolling down).

Inhale: Do nothing.

Exhale: Press your legs away and come back to the Balance Point position, using the hollow abdominal muscles to bring you back up.

Complete six repetitions. Attempt to increase the distance you go backwards every time.

Do's and don'ts

- ✔ Do focus on using your abdominals to perform the exercise.
- ✔ Do attempt to articulate through your spine on the way down and on the way up.
- ✔ Do minimise the tension in your upper body; keep your neck long and relaxed.
- ✔ Don't overuse your arm muscles by heaving yourself up with your biceps.

Modifications

If this exercise is too hard for you to do and you keep falling backwards, put your feet on the ground and proceed with the same instructions.

When you get the strength and control, you'll be able to go all the way to the floor and back up to the Balance Point. Once you've mastered that, try letting your arms free and allowing them to come down and open on the way down and come together and forward on the way up.

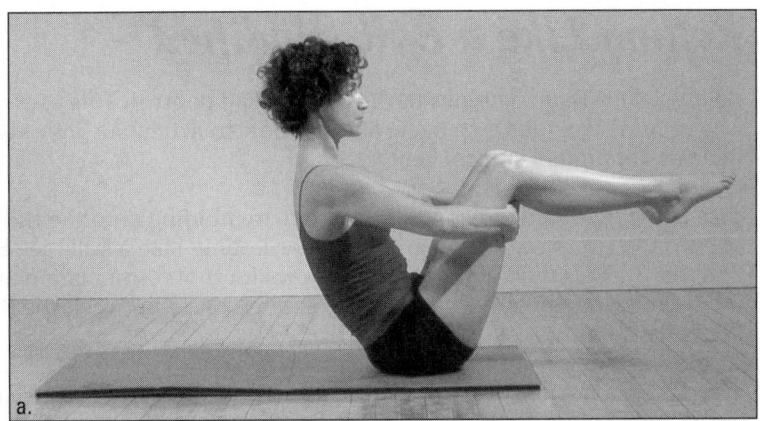

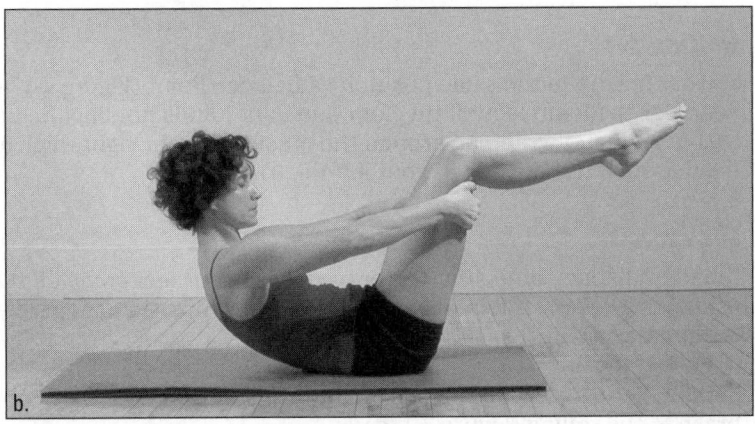

Figure 7-16:
Balance
Point/
Teaser
Prep.

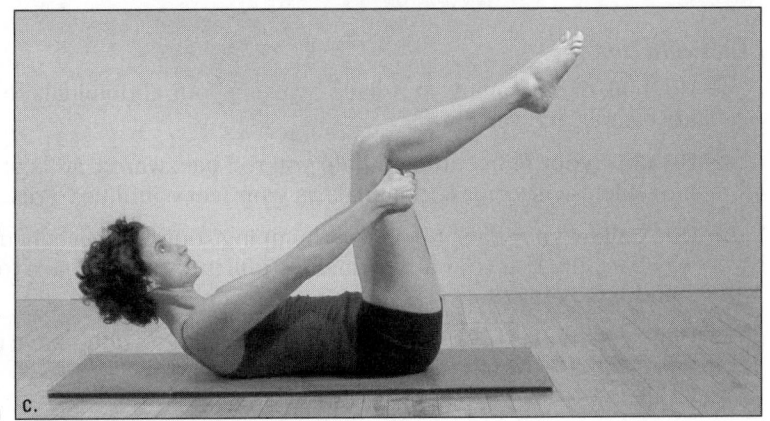

Rolling Like a Ball, Modified

Rolling Like a Ball combines both strength and control. This exercise is a fun way to massage your own back, find out how to articulate your spine, and find the abdominal control centre.

This is the modified version because you are holding onto the thighs instead of onto the shins, as you do in the regular Rolling Like a Ball (see Book IV Chapter 8). This modified handhold allows for more articulation and ease in the rolling movement because it allows more space between the thigh and the body.

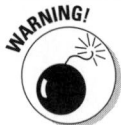

If you have a neck injury, proceed with caution. Skip this exercise if it causes any strain in your neck.

Getting set

Start sitting up in the same position as Balance Point (Figure 7-17a), with your legs bent and feet off the floor and your hands holding the back of your legs (right hand wrapping around the outside of your right thigh and left hand around the outside of your left thigh).

The exercise

Inhale: Roll back onto your upper back until your feet come off the floor, using your lower Abdominal Scoop to lift your hips, and squeeze your bottom to get an extra lift (Figures 7-17b and 7-17 c).

Exhale: Return to your Balance Point, using your Abdominal Scoop as the brake to the rolling (Figure 7-17d).

Do's and don'ts

- ✔ Do think of massaging your back by using your abdominals to help you articulate each vertebrae.

- ✔ Do allow your momentum to help you roll backwards, and control the movement with your abdominals as your feet continue to rise.

- ✔ Don't allow your back to make a thumping sound, especially on the way back up. Use your abdominals to pull into the low back to make a smooth movement.

- ✔ Don't roll too far back onto your neck. Even if you don't have neck problems, you don't want to start having them now.

Modification

Rolling Like a Ball becomes more difficult the smaller the ball you make.
If you hold your hands on the front of your knees, you tighten your 'ball',
making this more of a control and abdominal exercise and less of a massage
and articulation exercise.

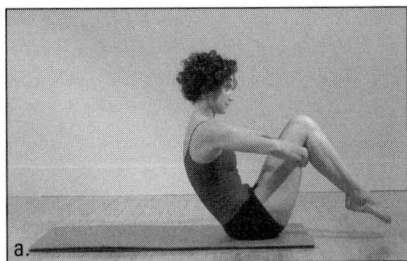
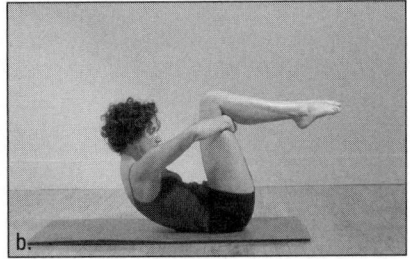

Figure 7-17:
Rolling Like
a Ball,
modified.

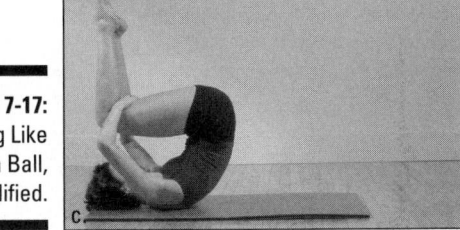
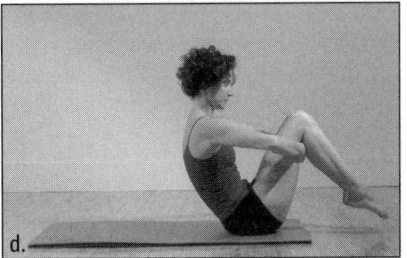

Return to the Balance Point.

Chapter 8

Giving Yourself the All-Body Pilates Workout

*E*ach Pilates exercise helps to tone and strengthen your muscles. The exercises are also designed to teach the muscles how to work together for greater efficiency and movement.

Once you've mastered the key Pilates principles you're ready to push your body a little further. In this chapter we take you through the beginning mat series so you can master some of the basics. We then take you up a level to try some intermediate exercises.

The Beginning Mat Series

If you started your Pilates experience by doing the series in Book IV Chapter 7 (as we recommend), you've mastered what we call pre-Pilates exercises. You understand the fundamentals, both in your body and in your mind, so you're ready for a full-blown Pilates series.

Even the Hundred, which is the first new exercise in this series, requires a huge amount of upper abdominal strength and neck strength – so don't feel bad about having to take it slow and incorporating these exercises into your routine a little at a time. Before you move on, though, you should be able to move through this series fluidly and without much difficulty.

Hundred, Beginning Level

The Hundred got its name because you hold the exercise for 100 beats. It is a great exercise to come early in a series because it gets your whole body warm, possibly even breaking a sweat. It gets your breath going strong and your blood moving. In addition, the Hundred is an excellent exercise for increasing torso stability and abdominal strength. You may have some difficulty keeping your head up for so long. See the 'Do's and don'ts' section for ways to protect your neck.

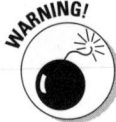

Never continue if your neck feels strained.

Getting set

Lie on your back with your knees bent and up in the air, your knees and hips forming 90-degree angles. Your back should be in Neutral Spine (see Book IV Chapter 7 for an explanation of Neutral Spine). Figure 8-1a shows the starting position. If this position feels like a strain on your lower back, try keeping your feet down on the floor for now.

The exercise

Inhale: Reach your arms straight up to the sky, palms facing forward.

Exhale: As you reach your arms back down to the floor, lift your head (think of squeezing a tangerine under your chin on the way up) and roll up to the Pilates Abdominal Position with your shoulder blades just off the mat. Your palms gently slap the floor in a percussive rhythm (Figure 8-1b).

Inhale: Inhale deeply for 5 beats (keep the rhythm with your arms), using accordion breathing.

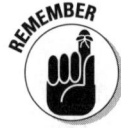

Accordion breathing is *lateral chest breathing.* Imagine that your rib cage is an accordion. On the inhale, the accordion expands laterally, and on the exhale, the accordion squeezes back together.

Exhale: Using percussive breathing, exhale for 5 beats (saying shh, shh, shh, shh, shh).

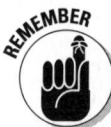

Percussive breathing is forced exhalation using the abdominal muscles; think of forcing the air out in short percussive blows.

Hold the position and continue pulsing your arms for 10 breaths, which is 100 total beats (5 for each inhale and 5 for each exhale).

Do's and don'ts

- ✔ Do remember that this is an abdominal exercise, not a neck exercise. You must be rolled up off the mat high enough to maximise the abdominal workout and minimise neck strain.

- ✔ Do press your lower back into your mat by using your Abdominal Scoop, especially on the exhale, maintaining your pelvis in its neutral position by keeping your tailbone grounded to the mat.

- ✔ Do think of reaching long, away from yourself, with your fingers and try to think of pulsing your arms from your back muscles, keeping your shoulder blades pulling down your back.

- ✔ Don't continue if your neck strains. Instead, change positions. Put one hand behind the head to support the neck, and switch hands at 50 beats.

- ✔ Don't let yourself lose the Pilates Abdominal Position by sinking downwards; accentuate the upper abdominal curl up on every exhale.

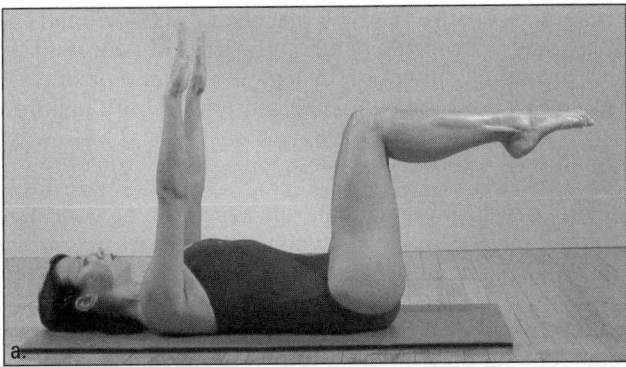

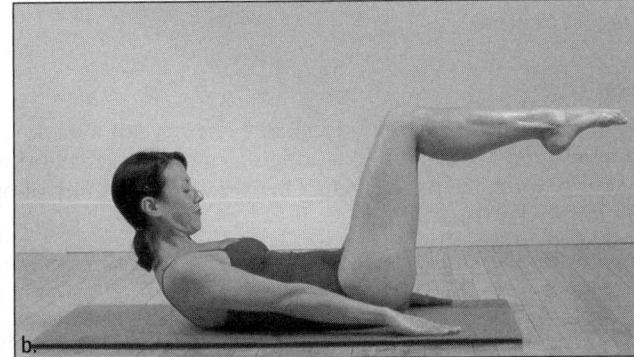

Figure 8-1:
Hundred,
Beginning
Level.

Book IV

Exploring Yoga and Pilates

Single Leg Stretch

This is one of the most basic torso stability exercises in the Pilates method. Because you reach out only one leg at a time, the challenge to stability is not as demanding as it would be if you were reaching out two legs.

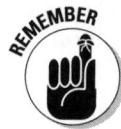

A torso stability exercise is one in which your torso doesn't move while your arms and/or legs are moving to challenge torso stability.

Getting set

To begin, lie down on your back with your knees bent and your feet flat on the floor about hip distance apart. Relax your back into Neutral Spine. Gently lift your head, maintaining Neutral Spine, pull your navel towards your spine and lift one leg at a time off the floor towards your chest. Take both hands by your right knee, right hand by your right calf and left hand by your right knee. Gently straighten your left leg out to about 45 degrees from the floor (the lower the leg, the more challenging the exercise). As you change legs to perform the exercise, ensure that you place your outside hand on the ankle of your bent leg, and your inside hand on the knee of your bent leg (this position maintains proper alignment of the leg). If this hand position is too confusing at first, simply hold the bent knee gently with both hands.

The exercise

Inhale: Switch legs twice on one inhale, always grabbing your bent leg with your outside hand on your ankle and your inside hand on your knee. Figure 8-2 shows the model switching legs.

Exhale: Switch legs twice on one exhale, grabbing onto the other bent leg with your outside hand on your ankle and your inside hand on your knee.

Repeat for eight breaths.

Do's and don'ts

- ✔ Do remember that this is an abdominal exercise, not a neck exercise, so you must hold the head high enough to maximise the abdominal workout and minimise neck strain. On every exhale, think of pulling your navel in to lift your head up.

- ✔ Do keep your navel pulled in to the spine, accentuating this pulling in on every exhale.

- ✔ Don't let yourself lose the Pilates Abdominal Position by sinking downwards; accentuate the upper abdominal curl up on every exhale.

- ✔ Don't continue if your neck strains. Rest your head down when your neck feels strained. Continue after a breath.

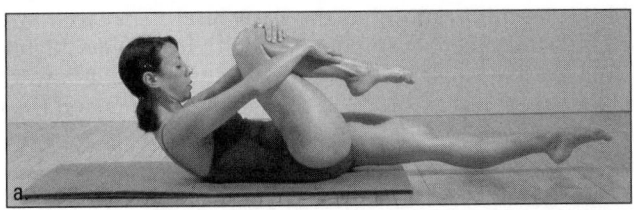

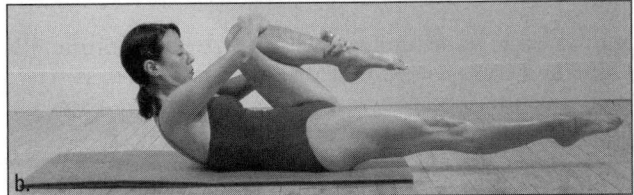

Figure 8-2:
Single Leg
Stretch.

Rising Swan

This is the first and only back extension exercise in this series. This exercise strengthens your neck, back and bottom muscles. Please include this exercise in your daily routine to counteract the negative effects of forward bending on your spine.

Getting set

Lie face down with your forehead flat on the mat, your arms bent with your elbows close to your side, and your palms facing down by your ears. Allow your legs to turn out from the top of your hip (drop your heels towards each other). You can keep a comfortable distance between your legs; if you have slim hips, you can pull your inner thighs together.

Pull your navel up off the mat so that you could slide a piece of paper under your stomach and press your pubic bone down into the mat. Squeeze your bottom to help accomplish this tucking under of your pelvis. This is your powerhouse at work!

The exercise

Inhale: Maintain your position.

Exhale: Scoop your stomach in, squeeze your bottom, and slowly rise up from your upper back, keeping the back of your neck long and gently lifting your head off the mat (Figure 8-3a).

Pretend to see an ant on the floor below your head. Follow the ant as it crawls away from you, raising your upper back and head off the mat as it crawls up the wall in front of you.

Book IV

**Exploring
Yoga and
Pilates**

Inhale: Hold this position, known as the Baby Swan. Test your strength by taking your hands off the mat. You don't need to be up very high to get the benefits of this exercise. Keep lifting your tummy up and in towards the spine and keep squeezing your bottom. Don't let your legs come off the mat!

Exhale: Return to the starting position.

Inhale: Maintain your position.

Exhale: Again scoop in your tummy and squeeze your bottom. Rise up a little higher this time and place your forearms down in front of you to prop you up (Figure 8-3b). You should be positioned like a sphinx. As shown in Figure 8-4, don't let your navel stay on the mat!

Inhale: Hold the sphinx position.

Exhale: Straighten your arms by pressing your hands into the mat. Protect your lower back by again pulling your stomach in and squeezing your bottom (Figure 8-3c).

Inhale: Hold this position, known as the High Swan.

Exhale: Lower yourself down to the mat.

If, when in the High Swan, you feel a lot of compression or discomfort in your lower back, avoid this part of the exercise until you gain more strength in your bottom and abdominals.

Finish by pushing back to the rest position. Sit on your heels with your spine rounded and relaxed forward like a foetus, as shown in Figure 8-5.

Do's and don'ts

- ✔ Do support your head by lifting the top of your head up and away to keep your neck long and strong.

- ✔ Don't allow your lower back to sag; keep your powerhouse working overtime.

Roll Downs

Roll Downs are a beginning variation of the classical Pilates Roll Up. It's always easier to start sitting up and roll down than to start lying down and roll up. This exercise increases abdominal strength and articulation of the spine.

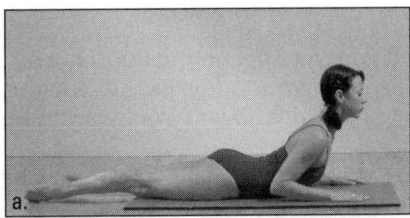
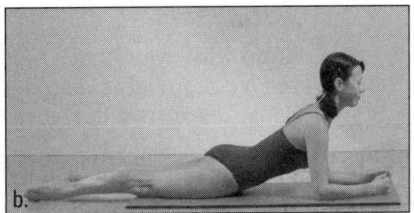

Figure 8-3: Rising Swan.

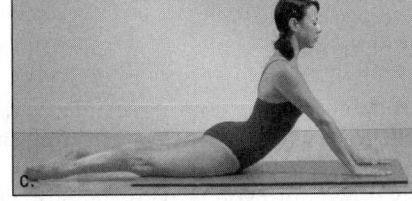

Figure 8-4: The wrong position for Rising Swan.

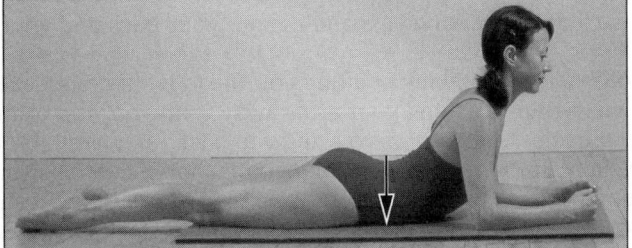

Don't let your navel stay on the mat.

Figure 8-5: Taking a rest in the rest position.

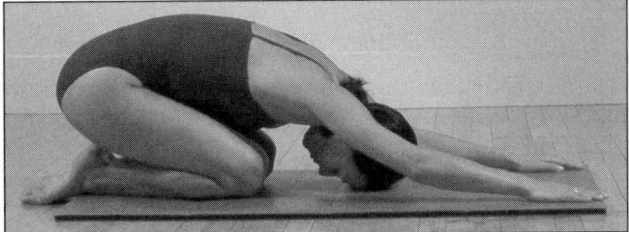

Getting set

Sit up with your knees bent and your feet flat on the floor, hip distance apart, and a comfortable distance away from your body. Extend your arms in front of you, as shown in Figure 8-6a. Think of lifting up from your lower back.

Sit up as tall as you can by imagining that you have a golden string attached to the back of the top of your head pulling you towards the sky.

The exercise

Inhale: Lift up from the base of your spine.

Exhale: Begin to roll down your spine, pulling your navel in, creating a C Curve with your lower back, and controlling the movement from the centre (Figure 8-6b). Think of pressing your spine down onto the mat one vertebra at a time. Roll slowly all the way down until you're lying flat, arms by your sides (Figure 8-6c).

Inhale: Take a deep breath in, expanding into your back and your lungs.

Exhale: Roll back up, thinking of lifting your head by first squeezing a tangerine under your chin, reaching your arms away from you, and using the hollow abdominal muscles in a C Curve to bring you back up (Figures 8-6d and 8-6e). Finish the exercise by Stacking the Spine. You should end up sitting tall, in your starting position, with your arms extended in front of you and your shoulders relaxed and dropped.

Complete six repetitions.

Do's and don'ts

- ✔ Do focus on using your abdominals to perform the exercise.
- ✔ Do attempt to articulate through your spine on the way down and on the way up.
- ✔ Do minimise the tension in your upper body, keeping your neck long and relaxed.
- ✔ Don't hold your breath. Use long, slow breathing to assist the movement.

Modifications

If this exercise is too hard for you to do and you keep falling backward or you can't get up, grab onto your legs and use your arm strength to help you control the movement down and to get yourself up (like the C Curve Roll Down Prep in Book IV Chapter 7).

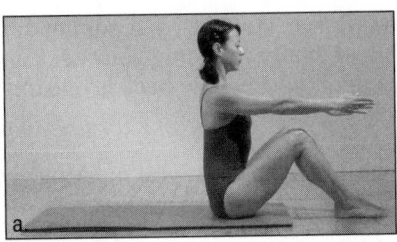
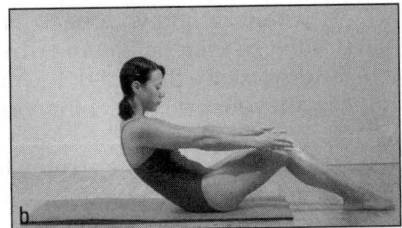

Roll down...

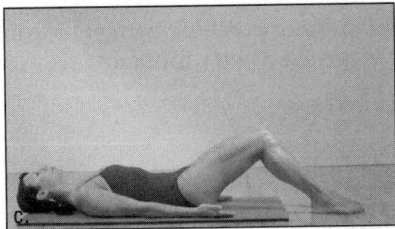
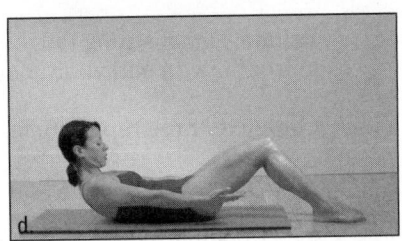

breathe in...   and roll back up.

Figure 8-6:
Roll Down.

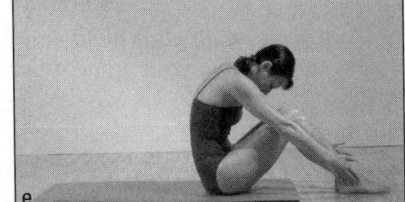
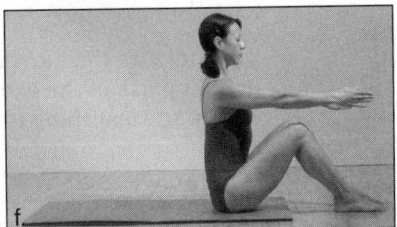

Spine Stretch Forward

Spine Stretch Forward is exactly that: a stretch for the whole spine, especially the neck and upper back.

Getting set

Sit up tall with your legs straight and spread a little wider than the width of your hips. You can bend your legs if it's impossible for you to sit up straight with your legs straight – for example, if you have tight hamstrings.

The exercise

Inhale: Sit up as tall as you can from the base of your spine. Flex your feet and reach through your heels to engage your leg muscles. Your arms should be shoulder width apart and straight ahead, with your palms facing down (Figure 8-7a).

Exhale: Round your back into a C Curve, starting by scooping out your low tummy, then pulling the ribs in, and finally rounding your neck and head forward. By the end of the movement, your whole back is making a C shape, with your arms reaching forward (Figure 8-7b).

As you perform the stretch forward, imagine that you're lifting your spine up and over a barrel.

Inhale: Stack up your spine, bone by bone.

Exhale: Finish sitting tall, in your starting position, with your arms extended in front of you and your shoulders relaxed and dropped.

Complete three repetitions.

Do's and don'ts

- ✔ Do initiate the C Curve with your low tummy.

- ✔ Don't do all the curving from your upper back; try to get your lower back rounded, too.

- ✔ Don't initiate the movement from your head; your head should trail in both parts of the exercise. When stacking your spine, your head is always the last thing to rise.

Modifications

Bend your knees if necessary, or sit on a small pillow if you have tight hamstrings. You can also do this exercise against a wall to practise Stacking the Spine.

Side Kicks

Side Kicks are a nice side-lying stability exercise. It focuses on control from the stomach and strengthens your thighs and your bottom. This exercise is not about how far you can kick your leg; it's about how stable your body can be while you move your legs freely.

Getting set

Lie on your side with your legs slightly in front of your body and slightly turned out in the Pilates First Position. Let your head rest on your bottom hand, propped up on a bent elbow on the floor, while your top arm is bent with the palm down on the mat in front of you for stability (Figure 8-8a).

The exercise

Inhale: Flex your foot as you kick your top leg straight out in front of you, pulsing your leg once to test your stability (Figure 8-8b).

Exhale: Kick your leg behind you, pointing the foot, keeping it the same height as your hip, and pulsing the leg once to test your stability. Squeeze your bottom and pull your navel in for stability. See Figure 8-9 for an example of an advanced hand placement for this exercise.

Complete 10 repetitions on each side.

Do's and don'ts

- ✔ Do press your weight into your front palm on the floor to maintain balance throughout the exercise.
- ✔ Don't wobble around. Maintain stability in your body as your leg moves freely, especially when kicking to the back.
- ✔ Do keep your neck long and relaxed.
- ✔ Do keep your body square, shoulder over shoulder and hip over hip.

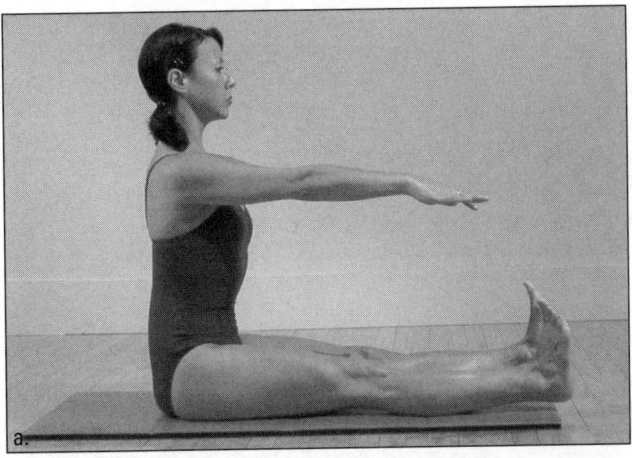

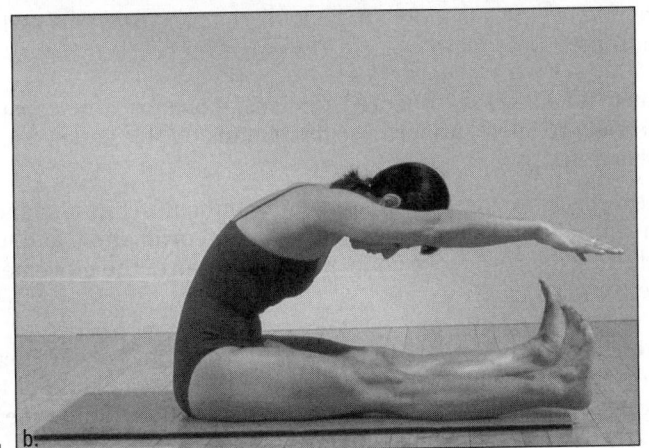

Figure 8-7:
Spine
Stretch
Forward.

Book IV

Exploring Yoga and Pilates

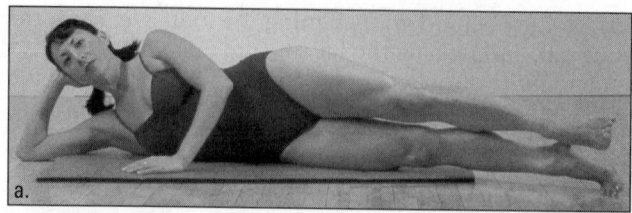

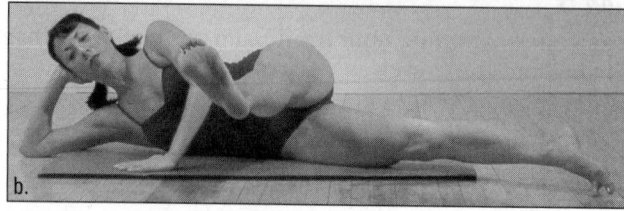

Figure 8-8: Side Kicks.

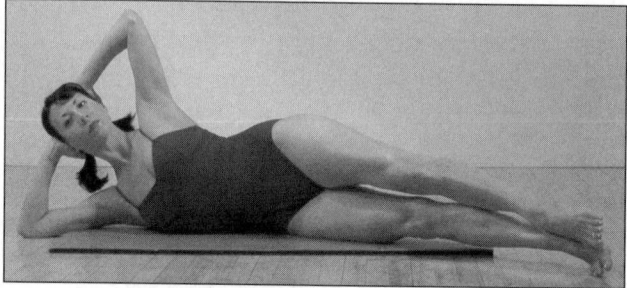

Figure 8-9: The advanced hand placement for Side Kicks.

Feeling Stronger Every Day: Intermediate Mat Exercises

The intermediate series is more challenging than the previous series for a couple reasons:

✔ Because it's longer, with more exercises, it is more time-consuming (you can expect to spend about 25 to 35 minutes on this series once you get familiar with it.)

✔ The exercises themselves are just more difficult. They demand more from your abdominal muscles, from your co-ordination, and from your mind (they demand more concentration because the movements are more complex).

Pilates exercises are not meant to be done in isolation. They're meant to be done in a chain; you fluidly move from one exercise to another in a prescribed series. We present the exercises in this section in the order that you should do them to attain the maximum benefit.

As you progress in the Pilates series, you want to make sure that you are really flowing through the exercises. It's not enough to clunk through the exercises one by one, stopping in between. Instead, begin to try to transition seamlessly from one exercise to the next as you grow more and more independent from this book. Doing so brings a new challenge and makes your workout more aerobic.

Even though they're not officially a part of the intermediate series, try starting your workout with Coccyx Curls and Upper Abdominal Curls. Both of these exercises are described in Book IV Chapter 7, and are familiar to you if you've been doing the series in order. This is an especially good idea if you haven't warmed up at all.

Hundred, Intermediate Level

This exercise is excellent for increasing torso stability and abdominal strength, but you may find it difficult to keep your head up for the hundred counts that give this exercise its name. Never continue if your neck feels strained; see the do's and don'ts for ways to protect your neck. As you get stronger in your neck and your abdominals, you will not notice this strain.

In the intermediate Hundred, your legs are straight. In the beginning version of the Hundred, your knees are bent in the tabletop position. This increases the difficulty of the exercise because the weight of the legs puts a little more load on the torso, forcing the abdominals to work a little harder.

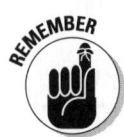

This exercise call for accordion and percussive breathing. For accordion breathing, imagine that your rib cage is an accordion. On the inhale, the accordion expands laterally, and on the exhale, the accordion squeezes back together. Percussive breathing is forced exhalation using the abdominal muscles; think of forcing the air out in short percussive blows.

Getting set

Lie on your back with your knees bent and up in the air. Your knees and hips should be in the table top position, inner thighs squeezing together, knees bent at a 90-degree angle, arms down by your sides.

The exercise

Inhale: Reach your arms straight up with your palms facing forward, as shown in Figure 8-10a.

Exhale: As you reach your arms back down to the floor, lift your head and roll up to the Pilates Abdominal Position with the shoulder blades just off the mat. Simultaneously straighten your legs up to the sky, as shown in Figure 8-10b.

Why do we say *reach* your arms down to the floor instead of *lower* them down? To remind you to keep your arms stretched and long as you drop them.

Book IV

Exploring Yoga and Pilates

As you roll up into your Pilates Abdominal Position, think of squeezing a tangerine under your chin. This image helps you keep space between your chin and your chest so that your neck isn't overstretched.

Keep your legs in the Pilates First Position, slightly turned out from the hip, with your inner thighs pulling together. Your palms gently slap the floor in a quick, percussive rhythm.

Inhale: Inhale deeply for 5 beats (keep the rhythm with your arms), using accordion breathing.

Exhale: Using percussive breathing, exhale for 5 beats (saying 'shh, shh, shh, shh, shh').

Hold the position and continue pulsing your arms for 10 breaths, which is 100 total beats (5 for each inhale and 5 for each exhale).

Lower your head to the mat and bring your knees into your chest to relax your back. Then extend your arms and legs long on the mat to get ready for the Roll Up.

Do's and don'ts

- ✔ Do remember that this is an abdominal exercise, not a neck exercise. You must keep your head high enough to maximise the abdominal workout and minimise neck strain.

- ✔ Do press your low back into the mat by using your Abdominal Scoop, especially on the exhale.

- ✔ Do think of reaching long away from you with your fingers and try to think of pulsing your arms from your back, imagining that the movement of the arms initiates at the shoulder blades.

- ✔ Don't continue in this position if your neck strains. Put one hand behind your head to support the neck; switch hands at 50 beats.

- ✔ Don't let yourself lose the Pilates Abdominal Position by sinking downwards; accentuate the abdominal curl on every exhale.

Modification

To make the Hundred more advanced, lower your legs to a 45-degree angle, making sure to keep your low back flat on the mat by scooping your abs and squeezing your bottom.

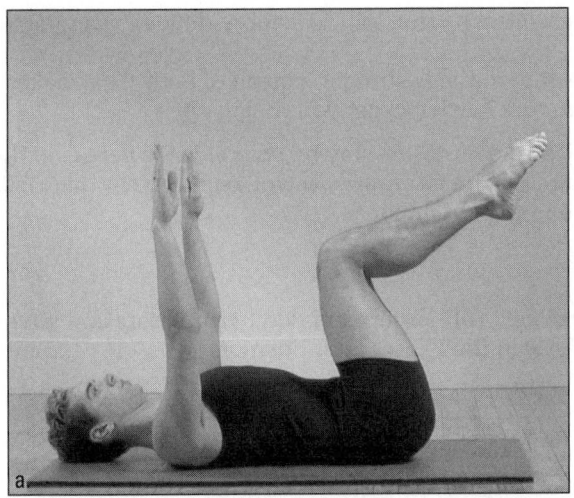

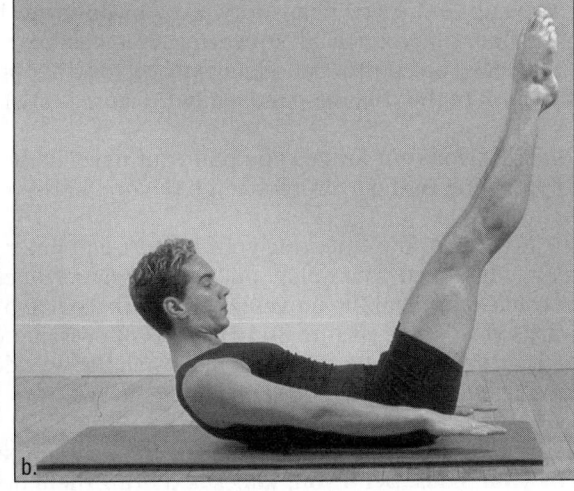

Book IV

Exploring Yoga and Pilates

Figure 8-10: The intermediate level Hundred.

Roll Up

The Roll Up is the more difficult version of the Roll Down. Before doing this exercise, you should be able to do a Roll Down with control and mastery. Like the Roll Down, the Roll Up increases abdominal strength and articulation of the spine.

There are two reasons why the Roll Up is more difficult than the Roll Down:

- You begin with your legs straight instead of bent. This makes your abdominals work harder to get you rolling up.

- In the Roll Down, your arms stay by your sides, whereas in the Roll Up your arms are reaching upwards as you come off the mat. This also puts more load on your abdominals.

Getting set

Lie down on your back with arms extended by your ears and your legs straight on the floor in the Pilates First Position.

The exercise

Inhale: Breathe in deeply. Stretch your arms and legs away from each other like you do when waking up in the morning (Figure 8-11a).

Exhale: Lift your arms up to the sky, palms forward. As your arms become perpendicular to the floor, lift your head, squeezing an imaginary tangerine under your chin. Squeeze your bottom and inner thighs together and scoop your abdominals to initiate the rolling up movement (Figure 8-11b).

Inhale: Stretch forward over your legs as you pull your navel in, hollowing your stomach in opposition to the forward stretch (Figure 8-11c).

Exhale: Initiate the Roll Down by squeezing your bottom and inner thighs together and begin to roll down your spine, pulling your navel in, creating a C Curve with your back. Control the movement from the centre by pulling your navel in towards your spine (Figure 8-11d). Think of pressing your spine down onto the mat one vertebra at a time. Roll slowly all the way down to lying flat, your arms reaching above your ears, and begin again.

Complete six repetitions. Finish the last one by lying flat on your back with your arms down by your sides. Bend your knees and bring them up to your chest, grabbing onto them with your hands. Roll yourself up to sitting to prepare for Rolling Like a Ball.

Do's and don'ts

- Do focus on using your abdominals to perform the exercise.

- Do attempt to articulate through your spine on the way down and on the way up.

- Do minimise the tension in your upper body; keep your neck long and relaxed.

- Don't hold your breath. Use long, slow breathing to assist the movement.

- Don't let your feet or legs lift off the floor as you roll up.

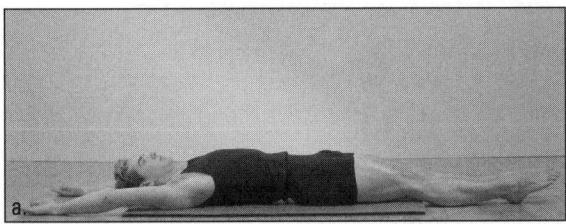

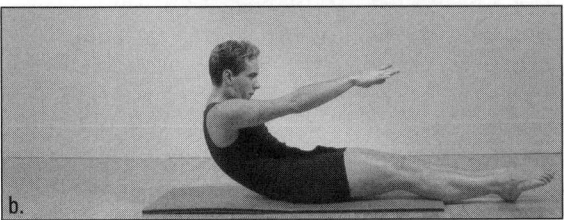

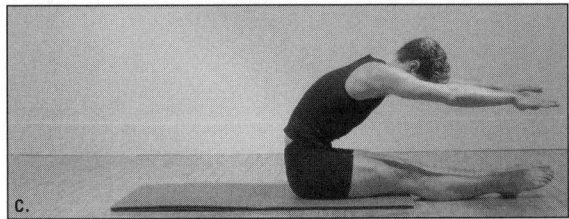

After stretching forward...

Figure 8-11:
Roll Up.

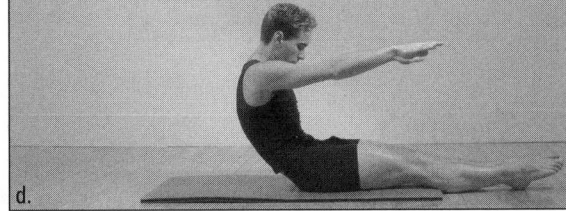

control the movement back down.

Rolling Like a Ball

At this point in the series, do the Rolling Like a Ball exercise that we introduce in the beginning series. See Figure 8-12 for photos. Complete six repetitions, then slowly roll down to your Pilates Abdominal Position, allowing one knee to bend into your chest (outside hand on the ankle, inside hand on the knee) and straightening the other leg as you transition into the Single Leg Stretch.

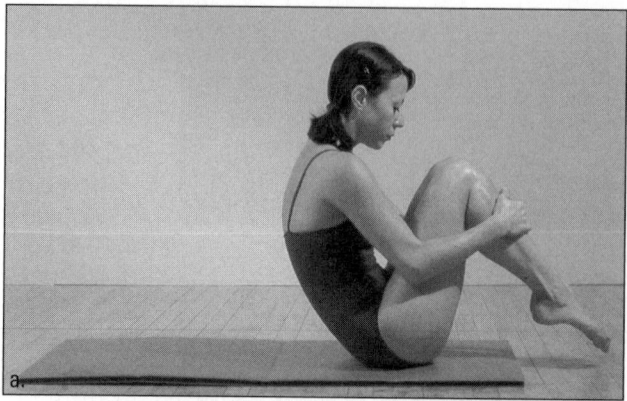

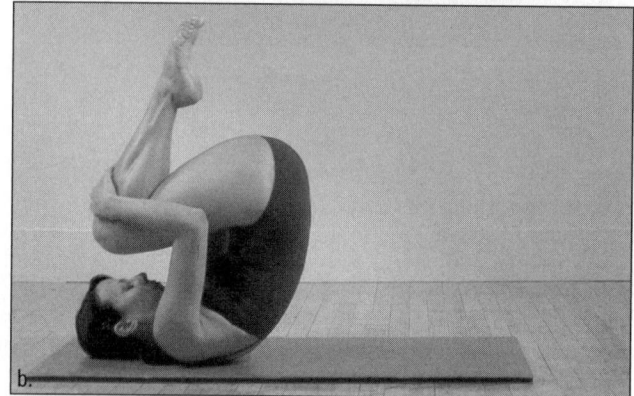

Figure 8-12:
Rolling Like
a Ball.

Single Leg Stretch

After Rolling Like a Ball, do the Single Leg Stretch. See earlier in the chapter for instructions and Figure 8-13 for photos. Complete 20 repetitions, alternating sides. Transition to the Double Leg Stretch by bringing both knees into your chest, holding one knee with each hand.

Double Leg Stretch

The Double Leg Stretch is much more challenging than the Single Leg Stretch. Not only are you supporting two legs rather than one, but the arms are also added to the equation, making torso stability that much more difficult. This exercise requires a huge amount of abdominal strength and requires full-torso stability, meaning both upper and lower torso stability.

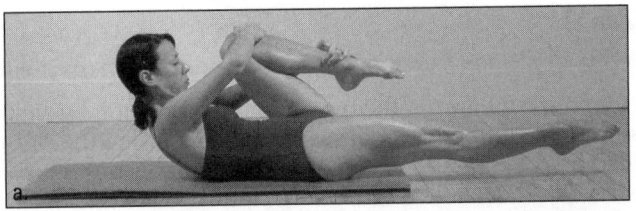

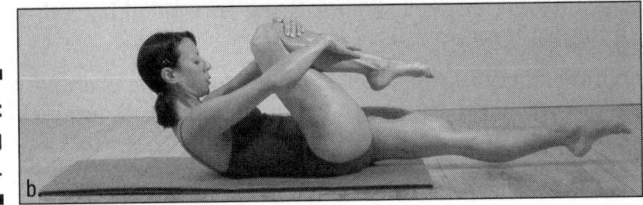

Figure 8-13:
Single Leg
Stretch.

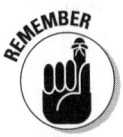

A torso stability exercise is one in which your torso does not move while your arms and/or legs are moving to challenge this stability.

As you perform this exercise, you should reach your legs only as low as you can while still maintaining absolute stability in your torso. Absolute stability means that your back should not arch off the mat at all and your tummy must stay pulled in and scooped. If you feel any discomfort in your lower back, you are dropping your legs too low, meaning your abdominal muscles can't support their weight. This may cause injury to the back, so please bring your legs back up!

Getting set

Lie on your back with your knees on your chest, holding onto one knee with each hand. Roll up into the Pilates Abdominal Position (Figure 8-14a).

The exercise

Inhale: Send your arms and legs out into a 'V', your arms by your ears and your legs at a 45-degree angle to the floor. Keep your lower back in contact with the mat with your Abdominal Scoop and by squeezing your bottom (Figure 8-14b). Hold this position for a second, feeling the stability in your body.

Exhale: Return to the start position, pulling your knees to your chest and hollowing your stomach.

Complete six repetitions. On the last one, hold onto your knees and lower your head down to the mat. Place your hands behind your head to get ready for Crisscross.

Book IV

Exploring Yoga and Pilates

Do's and don'ts

- ✔ Do keep your stomach scooped in when your limbs are extended.

- ✔ Don't let yourself lose the Pilates Abdominal Position by sinking downwards. People tend to let their head drop back when their arms are extended by their ears. To counteract this tendency, keep your focus on your stomach the whole time.

- ✔ Don't continue if your neck strains. Bring your head back down to the mat. Continue after a breath.

- ✔ Don't continue if your lower back strains. Modify the exercise by reaching your legs straight up to the sky until you gain more abdominal strength.

Modification

The lower your legs, the more abdominal work is needed to keep your low back flat on the mat. Lower your legs as low as you can while still maintaining contact with the mat with your lower back.

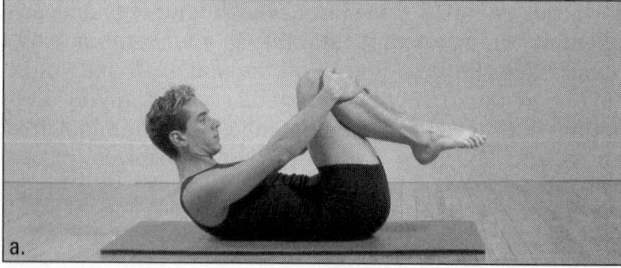

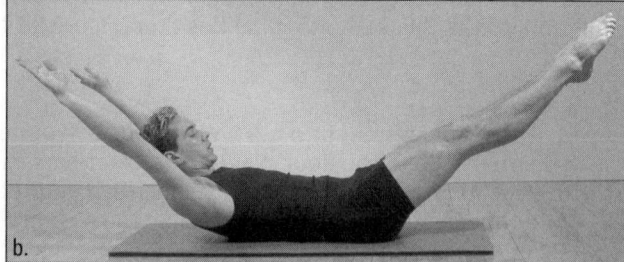

Figure 8-14: Double Leg Stretch.

Crisscross

Crisscross is similar to the Single Leg Stretch, but it adds a twist to the body that strengthens the oblique abdominal muscles. If this exercise is too difficult for you, repeat the Single Leg Stretch from earlier in the series instead.

Getting set

Bring your hands behind your head and roll up into the Pilates Abdominal Position with your knees bent and in the air.

The exercise

Inhale: Reach one elbow to the opposite knee and extend your other leg long in front of you. Then change sides, reaching your other elbow to your other knee. Imagine pulling your shoulder blade off the mat and twisting from your back muscles as you twist your body. Do not drop out of the Pilates Abdominal Position; try to keep your shoulder blades off the mat. Figure 8-15 shows the crisscrossing motion.

Exhale: Continue the crisscrossing motion, making two twists on the exhale.

Do two movements for each inhale and two movements for each exhale. Repeat for eight total breaths (an inhale and an exhale is a breath). Finish by bringing your knees into your chest and lowering your head to the mat. Straighten out your legs and split them apart, leaving one on the mat and the other pointing up to the sky. Grab onto the leg that's pointing up, as high on the leg as you can reach, while rolling up to the Pilates Abdominal Position. This gets you set for Scissors.

Do's and don'ts

- Do keep your navel pulled into your spine, accentuating this pulling in on every exhale.

- Do keep your elbows wide and make sure you're twisting from your centre; move your centre, not just your elbows.

- Don't let yourself lose the Pilates Abdominal Position by sinking downwards; think of rotating the body without touching your shoulder blades to the mat.

Scissors

Scissors is both an abdominal exercise and a hamstring stretch. If straightening your leg to a 90-degree angle is difficult, then you may want to start by stretching out the hamstring first and then proceed to this exercise. See Figure 8-16 for a hamstring stretch.

Getting set

Start on your back with your knees on your chest, one hand on each knee. Roll up into the Pilates Abdominal Position.

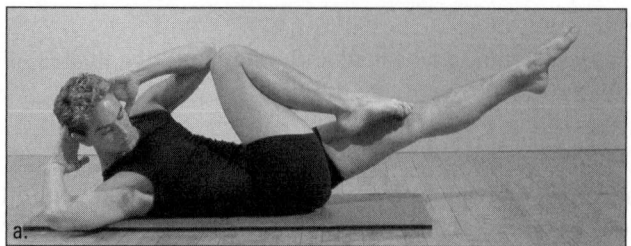

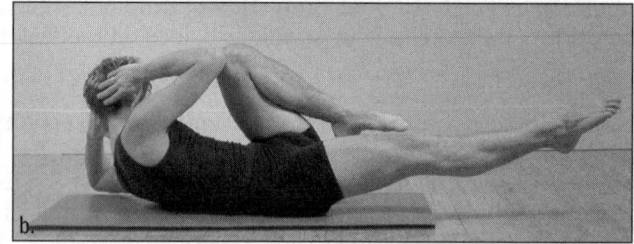

Figure 8-15: Crisscross.

The exercise

Inhale: Extend one leg to the sky and grab it below the ankle. If you have tight hamstrings, simply hold your leg closer to your knee and allow the knee to bend a little. Straighten the other leg in front of you, keeping it slightly above the mat (Figure 8-17a).

Exhale: Switch legs, and as you pull the other leg towards your body pull it twice quickly to make a double pulsing motion (Figure 8-17b).

Complete 10 breath cycles, or 20 total leg pulls.

'Nose to your knee and knee to your nose.' Always think of raising your head a little higher to touch your nose to your knees. Doing so will keep your abs working!

Do's and don'ts

- ✔ Do keep your navel pulled into the spine, accentuating the scoop on every exhale.
- ✔ Do keep your legs as straight as possible.

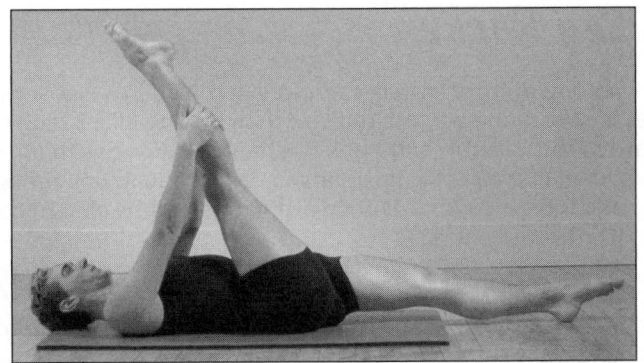

Figure 8-16:
Stretching
the
hamstring.

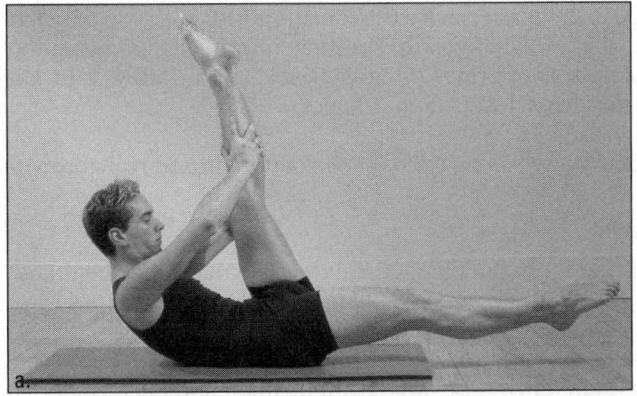

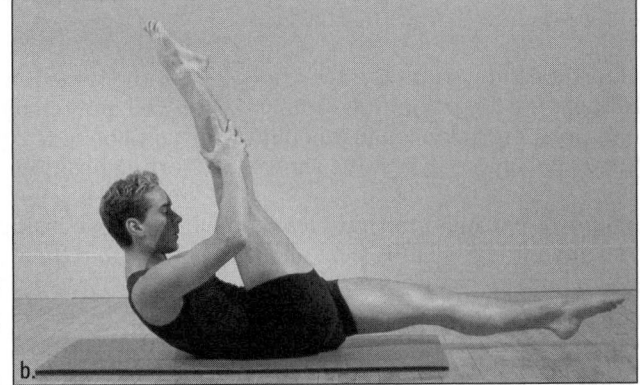

Figure 8-17:
Scissors.

Open Leg Rocker

This is the second of three rolling exercises in the Pilates mat series. Open Leg Rocker is substantially more difficult than Rolling Like a Ball, versions of which are in this chapter and Book IV Chapter 9. For one thing, you must have a good deal of hamstring flexibility in order to maintain proper form. Also, you must have a good deal of co-ordination and be able to control the movement from your centre.

Open Leg Rocker requires both strength and control. The exercise is another fun way to massage your own back, learn how to articulate your spine, and develop abdominal control.

This exercise may seem daunting at first, but there is a sharp learning curve as you repeat the exercise. By the fourth or fifth roll, you may feel a little more sure of yourself. If you find getting into the starting position difficult because of tight hamstrings or a tight back, simply allow your knees to bend and hold your legs closer to your knees.

As when doing any rolling exercise, be careful not to roll onto your neck!

Getting set

Start by sitting up in the Balance Point, with your knees bent and open to the sides, feet off the floor, and your hands holding the outsides of your ankles.

To practise finding your balance, first straighten one leg out to the side in front of you, maintaining your Balance Point position and deep Abdominal Scoop. Bend your knee back in and then repeat with your other leg. Figures 8-18a and 8-18b show you how to find your balance.

Now to find the starting position, extend both legs at the same time into a 'V' shape in front of you. Keep your low stomach hollowed and remain in your Balance Point position, balanced just behind your tailbone to feel your stomach helping you balance. Figure 8-18c shows the starting position.

If you have tight hamstrings (the muscles on the backs of your thighs) or a tight back, keep your legs slightly bent and don't try to hold them near the ankles. Instead, hold on closer to your knees.

The exercise

Inhale: Roll onto your upper back raising your feet off the floor and over your head (Figure 8-18d). Use your lower Abdominal Scoop to lift your hips, and squeeze your bottom to get an extra lift.

Exhale: Return to your Balance Point, using your Abdominal Scoop as a brake to halt the rolling motion.

Complete six repetitions.

Do's and don'ts

- ✔ Do think of massaging your back by using your Abdominal Scoop to help you articulate each vertebra.

- ✔ Do allow your momentum to help you roll backwards, and control the movement with your abdominals as you raise your feet off the floor and over your head.

- ✔ Don't allow your back to make a thumping sound, especially on the way back up. Use your Abdominal Scoop to help you articulate the rolling – especially through your low back – to make a smooth movement.

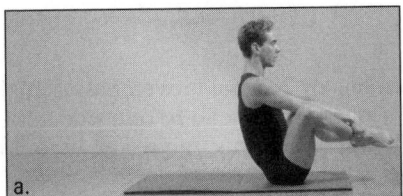 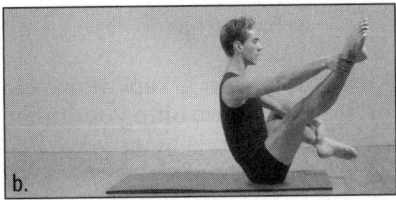
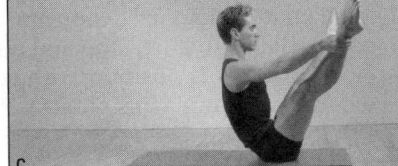 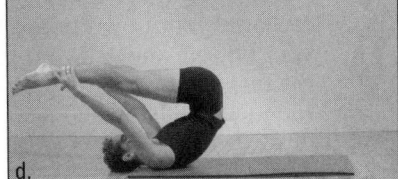

Figure 8-18: Open Leg Rocker.

Single Leg Kick

This exercise strengthens your back muscles, trains your shoulders to drop down your back, and simultaneously stretches the fronts of your legs and hips (the quadriceps muscles) while toning the back of your thighs (the hamstrings) and your bottom (the gluteus muscles).

Getting set

Start by lying on your tummy, and then prop yourself up like a sphinx on your elbows. Figure 8-19a shows the proper position, but it's a little more complicated than the photo may indicate:

✔ Your forearms should be shoulder width apart, with your hands in fists pressing into the mat.

✔ Your inner thighs are together, your navel is up off the mat, and your pubic bone is pressed down into the mat. Squeeze your bottom to accomplish this tucking under of your pelvis. This is your powerhouse at work!

✔ Your elbows are pushed into the mat while your shoulder blades are pulled down your back. Really try to feel the muscles underneath your shoulder blades pulling and maintaining this shoulder position while you do the exercise.

The exercise

Inhale: Kick your right heel to your bottom with a double beat, the first beat with a pointed foot and the second beat with a flexed foot (Figures 8-19b and 8-19c). Point your foot as you straighten your leg to the mat.

Exhale: Change legs.

Complete 10 repetitions on each leg, or 20 total movements. Finish by coming back down onto your tummy, bringing your head to one side, and allowing your hands to interlace behind your back. Now you're ready to flow into the Double Leg Kick.

If you feel yourself sinking in the middle and your low back compressing, recharge your powerhouse by finding your Abdominal Scoop and squeezing your bottom anew. If your low back continues to hurt, stop and push back to the rest position (sitting on your heels in a foetus position, with your back rounded and head and neck relaxed forward, your arms outstretched in front of you).

Do's and don'ts

✔ Do maintain a lifted upper body and absolute stability in your torso during this exercise.

✔ Do support your head by lifting the top of your head up and away to keep your neck long and strong.

✔ Do keep pressing your elbows into the mat to keep your shoulders pulling down your back.

✔ Do keep your inner thighs and knees glued together.

✔ Don't allow your back to sag; keep your powerhouse working overtime.

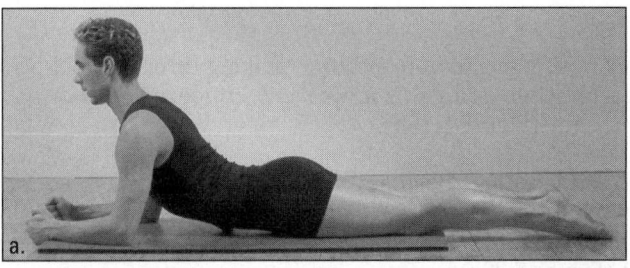

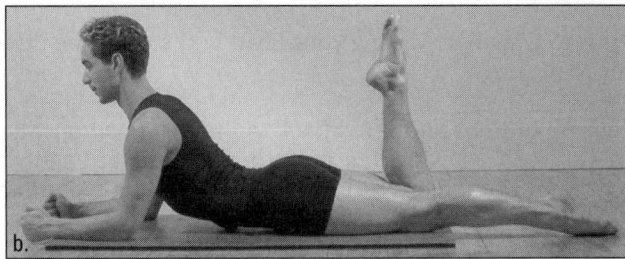

Pointed foot

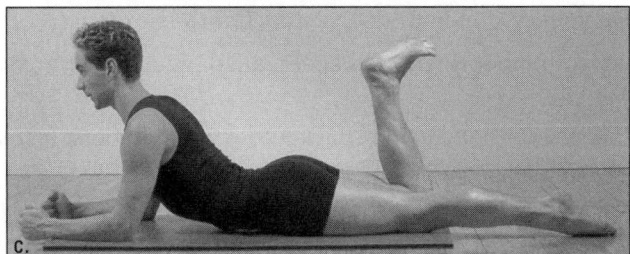

Figure 8-19:
Single Leg
Kick.

Flexed foot

Double Leg Kick

This exercise opens your chest, strengthens your back, and tones the back of your legs and your buttocks.

Getting set

Start by lying on your belly with your head turned to one side. Bend your arms behind your back and interlace your fingers. Place your hands as high on your back as you comfortably can and let your elbows drop down onto the mat (Figure 8-20a).

Book IV

Exploring Yoga and Pilates

The exercise

Inhale: Kick both heels to your bottom, making three beats. Be sure not to let your back arch when doing this movement; squeeze your bottom to counteract this tendency (Figure 8-20b).

Exhale: Extend your legs back down to the floor and reach your arms back as you arch your back up off the mat. Reach your arms long behind you and think of squeezing your shoulder blades together to increase the stretch in your chest (Figure 8-20c).

Inhale: Return to lying flat, turning your head in the opposite direction and again kicking your heels.

Complete four repetitions and press back to the rest position. Sit on your heels in a foetus position, with your back rounded forward and your arms on the floor in front of you (Figure 8-21). After you've rested your back for a few breaths, roll onto your side for the Side Kicks.

Do's and don'ts

- Do keep your Abdominal Scoop throughout the exercise.
- Do keep your inner thighs and knees glued together throughout the exercise.
- Don't allow your head to sink back into your shoulders. Instead, lengthen the back of your neck.
- Don't arch your back off the mat while doing the kicks. Instead, concentrate on pressing your pubic bone down to the floor and lifting your abdominals up off the mat.
- Don't allow your back to sag; keep your powerhouse working overtime.

Side Kicks

After you've been in the rest position, roll over to your side and do Side Kicks. For instructions, see section in this chapter. For photos, see Figure 8-22. Complete 10 repetitions.

For Side Kick variations that give your backside more of a workout, see later in the chapter.

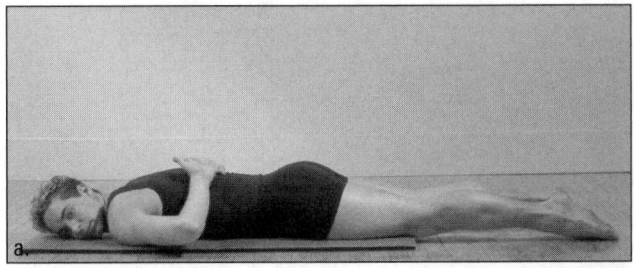

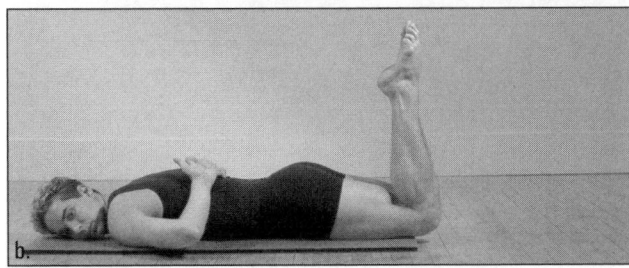

Figure 8-20:
Double Leg
Kick.

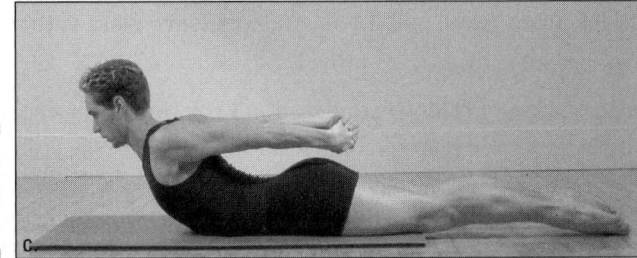

Figure 8-21:
Ahhh . . .
the rest
position.

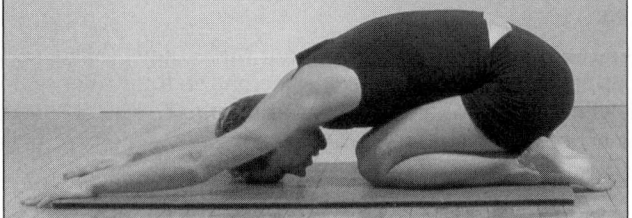

Book IV

**Exploring
Yoga and
Pilates**

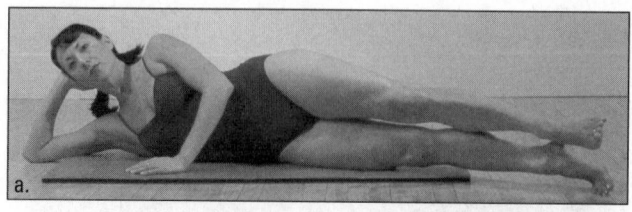

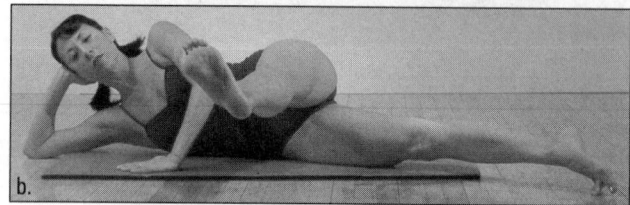

Figure 8-22: Side Kicks.

The Seal

We think the Seal was developed to promote humility. This exercise often concludes a mat class, and it lets students leave class with a smile.

As when performing any rolling exercise, don't roll onto your neck.

Getting set

Start by sitting up in the Balance Point position, with your knees bent and open to the sides, your feet together and slightly off the floor, and your hands grabbing your ankles from the inside (Figure 8-23a).

The exercise

Inhale: Clap the soles of your feet together three times (like a seal), roll back onto your upper back, until your feet come off the floor (Figure 8-23b shows the model rolling back). Use your lower Abdominal Scoop to lift the hips and squeeze your bottom to get an extra lift. Clap your feet again three times at your highest point (Figure 8-23c).

Exhale: Return to your Balance Point, using your Abdominal Scoop as the brake to the momentum. Again, clap your feet three times.

Complete six repetitions . . . and you're done with the intermediate series! Congrats.

The Fives: Five abdominal exercises to do every day

If you want ten minutes of excruciating abs work, the Fives are for you. These exercises, when done regularly, keep your middle taut and prevent injury to the back. You can also use the Fives as a warm-up for doing other exercise forms, because these exercises will awaken your middle and help your form, no matter what you choose to do with your body.

Remember, don't push yourself if you aren't ready for them. If you feel your lower back straining, please modify the exercises by raising your legs higher off the floor. The lower you reach your legs, the more work your abdominal muscles have to do to stabilise the spine. If you see your tummy protrude suddenly when you reach your legs out for one of these exercises, you need to modify by lifting up the legs.

I like to insert Rolling Like a Ball into this series to break up the burn and to give the back a little rest after the Hundred. So you could call these exercises the Sixes, but it just doesn't sound as good.

✔ Hundred

✔ Rolling Like a Ball

✔ Single Leg Stretch

✔ Crisscross

✔ Double Leg Stretch

✔ Scissors

Do's and don'ts

✔ Do think of massaging your back using your abdominals to help you articulate each vertebra.

✔ Do allow your momentum to help you roll backwards, and control the movement with your abdominals as your feet continue to rise.

✔ Don't allow your back to make a thumping sound, especially on the way back up. Use your abdominals to pull into your low back to make a smooth movement.

✔ Don't roll too far back onto your neck. Even if you don't have neck problems, you don't want to start having them now.

Modification

The hardest part of this exercise is maintaining the Balance position long enough to clap three times. So instead, start with one clap on your way back and then add another and another as you gain control.

Book IV

Exploring Yoga and Pilates

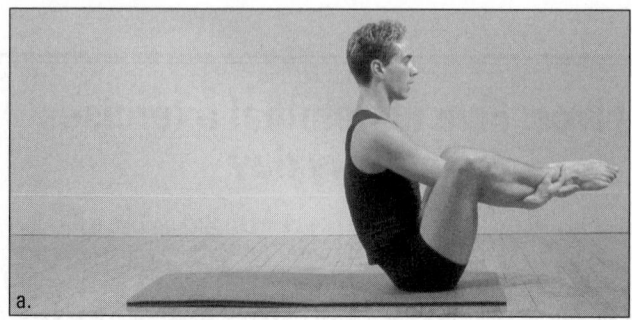

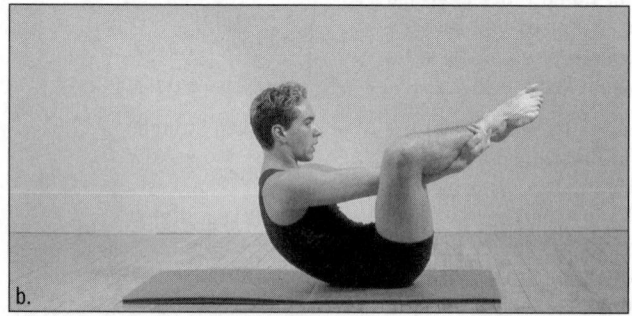

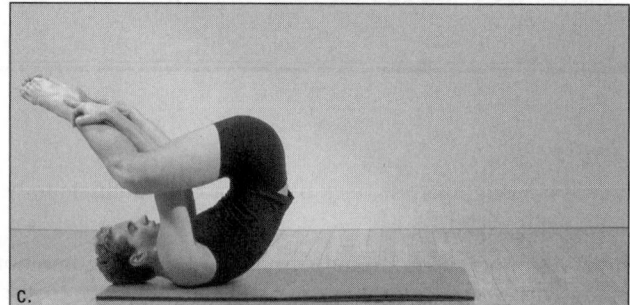

Figure 8-23:
The Seal.

Chapter 9

Challenging Yourself with Advanced Pilates Exercises

- -

In This Chapter

▶ Becoming advanced

▶ Helping your bottom and thighs

▶ Stretching like a cat

▶ Using a foam roller

- -

*T*his chapter includes more exercises to tempt you into challenging your-self further. The exercises in this chapter are more difficult and often have more repetitions to push you a bit harder. They help you strengthen and tone your body even more.

More Than a Washboard: The Advanced Mat Series

Don't try the series we present in this chapter until you can complete the earlier intermediate series with confidence and ease. You need core strength and core stability before you can move on to the advanced exercises. Once you've built up your core, you'll be able to add on the fancy variations that make up the advanced work.

Not only are the exercises more challenging in the advanced series, but the workout gets a lot longer, as you may notice. So part of becoming more advanced is gaining endurance as well as strength – a powerful combination!

I think it's a good idea to warm up with Coccyx Curls and Upper Abdominal Curls before launching into this series, especially if you're not warmed up at all. Both of these exercises are described in full in Book IV Chapter 7.

To carry out a more advanced workout, use the following exercises (all previously described in Book IV Chapter 8) and increase to 10–15 repetitions as you feel able:

- Roll Up
- Rolling Like a Ball
- Single Leg Stretch
- Double Leg Stretch
- Crisscross
- Scissors
- Spine Stretch Forward
- Rising Swan
- Single Leg Kick

Try these additional exercises, which are more challenging:

Hundred, Advanced Version

This exercise is excellent for developing torso stability and abdominal strength. In the advanced version of this exercise, your legs are straight and dropped to at least a 45-degree angle. In order to keep absolute stability in your torso with the weight of your legs dropping down, the abdominals need to work much harder than in the intermediate version (with the legs straight up) or in the beginning version (with the knees bent).

Getting set

Lie on your back with your legs in the tabletop position (your hips and knees bent at 90-degree angles and your inner thighs squeezing together) and your arms by your sides.

The exercise

Inhale: Reach your arms up to the sky, palms facing forward (Figure 9-1a).

Exhale: As you reach your arms back down to the floor, lift your head and roll up to the Pilates Abdominal Position, with your shoulder blades just off the mat. Simultaneously, straighten your legs, stretching them forward in front of you at about a 45-degree angle to the ground. Figure 9-1b shows this position.

Lower your legs only as far as you can while maintaining a scooped-out tummy and flattened lower back. Keep your legs in the Pilates First Position, slightly turned out from your hips, your knees facing away from each other, and your inner thighs pulling together. Gently slap your palms on the floor in a quick, percussive rhythm.

Inhale: Pump your arms up and down for 5 beats, making very small pulses.

Exhale: Keep the rhythm by pumping your arms up and down for 5 more beats. (Say, 'Shh, shh, shh, shh, shh.')

Hold this position and continue the arm pulsing for 10 full breaths (10 beats per breath makes 100 total beats).

If your neck feels strained, put one hand behind your head to support your neck, and switch hands at 50 beats.

Relax your head down to the mat, bring your knees into your chest, and gently circle your knees to relax your back. Rest for 1 or more breaths before continuing in the series. This exercise really works your abdominals and neck muscles, so you may need to rest your head on the mat for a moment before continuing. Once you're ready to move on, lengthen your legs out in front of you and reach your arms above your head to get ready for the Roll Up.

Do's and don'ts

- ✔ Do remember that this is an abdominal exercise, not a neck exercise. You must maintain the head high enough to maximise the abdominal workout and minimise neck strain.

- ✔ Do press your lower back into the mat by using your Abdominal Scoop, and squeeze your bottom to help stabilise your lower back.

- ✔ Do think of reaching long away from yourself with your fingers and try to think of pumping your arms from the back.

- ✔ Do think of squeezing a tangerine under your chin to keep a little space between your chin and your chest so that you don't overstretch the back of your neck.

- ✔ Don't let yourself lose the Pilates Abdominal Position by sinking downwards; accentuate the upper abdominal curl up on every exhale.

Modification

To make the Hundred easier, raise your legs straight up to the sky as you pulse your arms.

The Saw

The Saw is a great twisting stretch for your lower back. It incorporates breathing to clean out the lungs and get out all the old air. The Saw is difficult if you have tight hamstrings.

Book IV

Exploring Yoga and Pilates

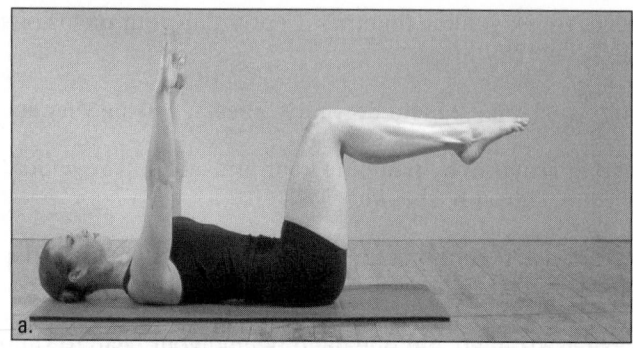

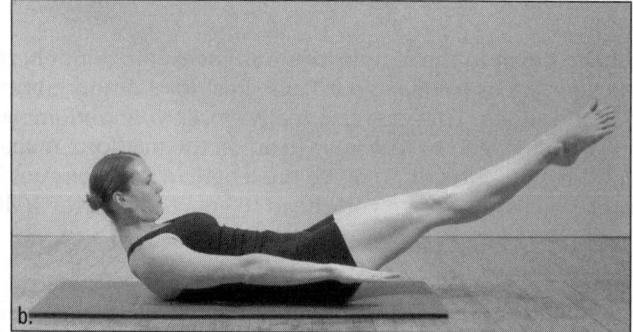

Figure 9-1:
Hundred,
Advanced
Version.

This exercise can be potentially stressful for your lower back. Be careful if you have any serious problems with your back.

Getting set

Sit up tall with your legs straight and a little wider than the width of your hips. You can bend your legs if it's impossible for you to sit up tall with your legs straight – in other words, if you have tight hamstrings. Or you can sit on a pillow to give yourself a little lift. Reach your arms out in a 'T', extending your arms away from each other, palms facing down.

The exercise

Inhale: Sit up as tall as you can from the base of your spine, flex your feet, and reach through your heels to engage your leg muscles. Think of grounding your hips into the mat (Figure 9-2a).

Exhale: Lift up and out of your hips as you scoop out the low stomach and twist from your waist to reach your left arm to your right calf (Figure 9-2b). Hold onto your calf and feel the stretch in your right lower back. Hold for 1 breath.

Inhale: Come back up to the erect spine position.

Exhale: Lift up off your hips and reverse the stretch (Figure 9-1c). Hold again for 1 breath.

Inhale: Come back up to the erect spine position.

Exhale: This time, instead of holding your calf, reach your right arm towards your left leg, stretching past your left foot with your hand, and think of sawing off your left little toe with your right little finger. Keep your right hip grounded onto the mat as a counterbalance.

Inhale: Return to the erect spine position.

Exhale: Twist to the left and stretch your left arm past your right foot, as you imagine that you're sawing off your right little toe with your left little finger.

Inhale: Return to the erect spine position.

Complete three repetitions, alternating sides, for six total sawing motions. Roll onto your front for the Single Leg Kick.

Do's and don'ts

- ✔ Do keep your shoulders relaxed and down in your back.

- ✔ Don't let your hips lift off the mat when twisting. Think of reaching your opposite heel forward and grounding the opposite hip bone when stretching.

- ✔ Don't let your knees roll in as you stretch forward.

Modification

Slightly bend your knees throughout the exercise if necessary, or sit on a small pillow if you have tight hamstrings.

Single Leg Kick

The Single Leg Kick is great for your back and legs. Complete 10 repetitions, alternating legs each time (see Figure 9-3). Finish by coming back down onto your belly, bringing your head to one side, and allowing your hands to interlace behind your back. Now you're ready to flow into the Double Leg Kick.

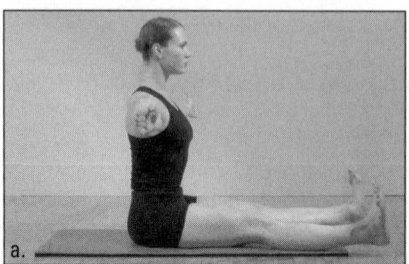
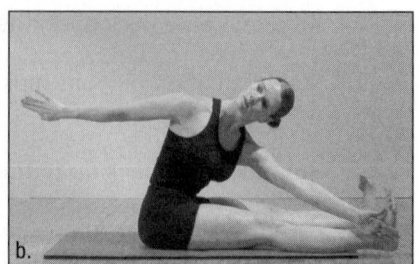
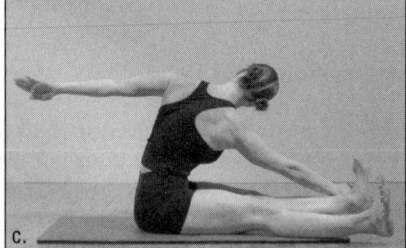

Figure 9-2:
The Saw.

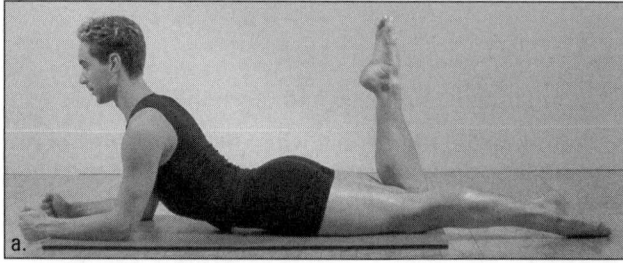

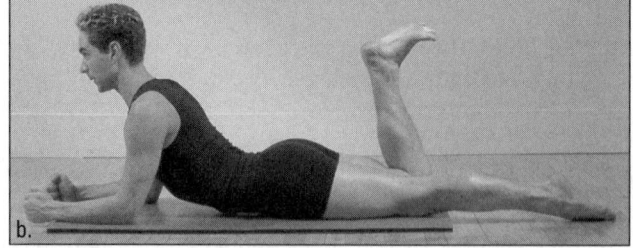

Figure 9-3:
Single Leg
Kick.

Double Leg Kick and Rest

The Double Leg Kick, from Book IV Chapter 8, is shown in Figure 9-4.
Complete four repetitions and press back to the rest position.

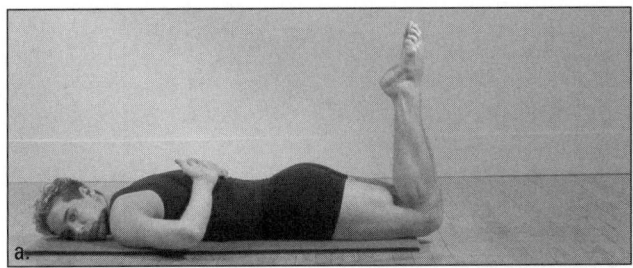

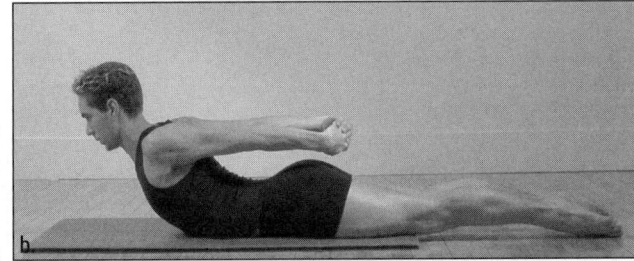

Figure 9-4:
Double Leg
Kick.

The rest position (Figure 9-5) isn't really an exercise, but a position that enables you to relax and release your back.

Sit on your heels and stretch your body forward onto the mat with your arms extended out in front of you. Imagine your lower back lengthening and releasing as your stomach hollows inwards. Breathe into your back. When you feel ready, roll down onto your back to get ready for the Neck Pull.

Hip Flexor Stretch

Lie on your front and bend your left leg, grabbing your left foot with your left hand. Reach your right arm out in front of you on the mat (Figure 9-6a). To increase the intensity of the stretch, try lifting your left thigh as high off the mat as possible by pulling your left foot up with your hand and pressing away with your left foot. Also, pull your navel in towards your spine and squeeze your bottom, trying as hard as you can to tuck your pelvis under. You should feel a deep stretch in the front of your hip. Breathe deeply for 4 or 5 breaths, trying to increase the stretch on every exhale. Switch sides and repeat the stretch (Figure 9-6b). Roll over onto your back, propping yourself up on your elbows for the Hip Circles.

Book IV

**Exploring
Yoga and
Pilates**

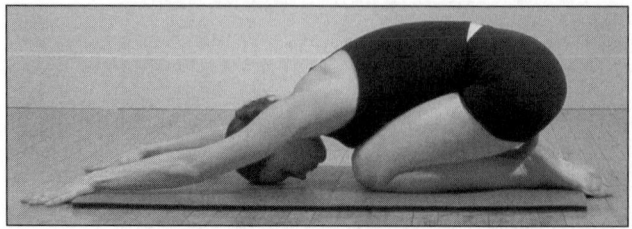

Figure 9-5:
The rest
position.

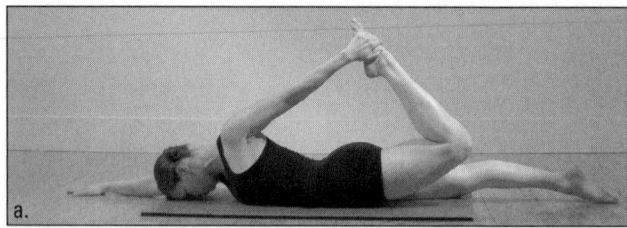

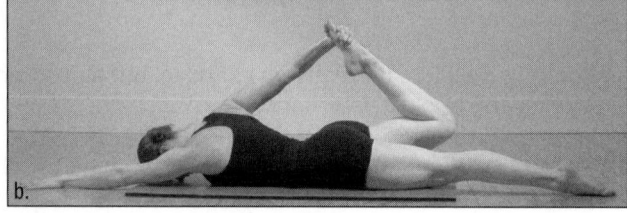

Figure 9-6:
Hip Flexor
Stretch.

Swimming

Whenever you start an exercise by lying on your stomach, you can be pretty sure that you'll be working the muscles of the back. So it's okay to feel the back working, but not straining. Swimming strengthens all the muscles on the back of your body: bottom, thigh and back muscles.

Getting set

Lie flat on your stomach with your arms stretched out in front of you and legs outstretched behind you (Figure 9-7a). Squeeze your inner thighs and heels together, in the Pilates First Position. If this position feels too compressive on your lower back, allow your legs to open slightly but still keep them turned out, with your heels dropped towards each other and your knees facing away from each other.

The exercise

Breathing continuously: Pull your navel up off the mat and raise your upper back and head off the mat slightly as you simultaneously lift your right arm and your left leg off the mat (Figure 9-7b). Squeeze your bottom and try to keep pressing your pubic bone down to the mat.

Switch arms and legs and begin an even rhythm of swimming, alternating arms and legs (Figure 9-7c). Think of reaching your arms and legs long away from yourself, extending your body as much as possible.

Swim continuously, trying to complete 4 swimming beats on the exhale and 4 beats on the inhale, for a total of 24 beats (6 full breaths).

Finish by pressing back to the Rest Position, sitting on your heels to release your back (Figure 9-8). Come up to your plank position (as if you were about to do a push-up) to get ready for Control Front.

Do's and don'ts

- ✔ Do keep stretching your limbs long in opposite directions.

- ✔ Do keep squeezing your bottom and pulling your navel up off the mat to protect your lower back.

- ✔ Don't let your shoulders hunch up by your ears. Instead, keep your shoulder blades pulling down your back. You may need to widen your arm width to accomplish this.

- ✔ Don't crane your head upwards, but think of lengthening the back of your neck.

Modification

To make Swimming easier, don't lift your upper body and head up very high and keep your arms and legs very low and close to the mat. The higher you lift up your limbs and upper body, the more work for your bottom and back muscles.

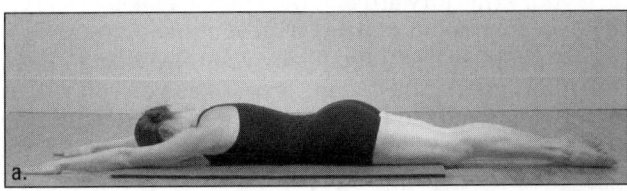

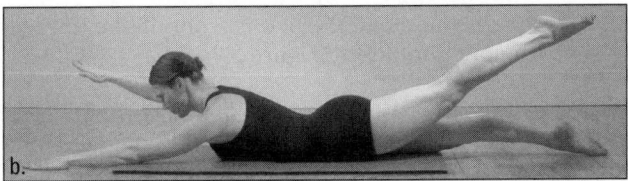

Figure 9-7: Swimming.

Book IV

Exploring Yoga and Pilates

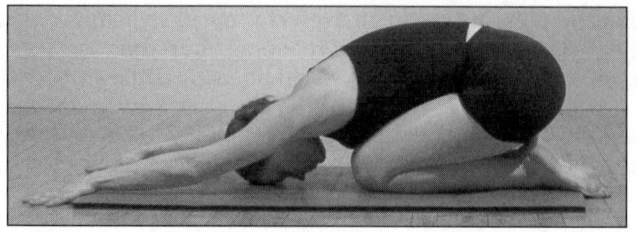

Figure 9-8:
Rest
position.

Pilates Push-Up

The Pilates Push-Up combines a nice stretch and release for the back and hamstrings with a classic push-up. The exercise strengthens your shoulders, back and bottom and increases spinal articulation.

Getting set

Stand up at the back of your mat, with your legs in the Pilates First Position (slightly turned out from the top of your hips, knees facing away from each other, and inner thighs squeezing together) and your arms reaching overhead. (Figure 9-9a).

The exercise

Inhale: Pull your navel in and squeeze your bottom, stretching your arms high overhead like you've just woken up and you're getting your first stretch of the day.

Exhale: Reach your arms forward and then down, making an arc, as you begin to roll down your spine, starting with your head dropping forward, then your neck and upper back, and finally your lower back, and come to a forward bend. Allow your arms to hang forward as you roll. Come all the way down and reach your hands to the mat in front of you (Figure 9-9b). Think of keeping your abdominals lifting up as your back goes down. This exercise is opposition at work and helps protect your back.

Inhale: Walk your hands out along the mat in front of you until your hands are directly beneath your shoulders (Figure 9-9c).

Exhale: Lower your hips and come into a push-up position: Place your hands shoulder distance apart and your legs together, lift your tummy, and squeeze your bottom. Keep your heels together, a position that will help you feel your bottom and your inner thighs working. Make sure that your body is in a straight line, rigid and strong like a wooden plank (Figure 9-9d). If you feel strain in your lower back, think of lifting up your hips slightly and really squeezing your bottom.

Inhale and exhale: Maintaining your plank position, do eight push-ups, trying to keep your elbows by your sides as you go down. Inhale on the way down and exhale on the way up. Try to go slowly and with control. Keep your torso stable by pulling in your stomach, using your Abdominal Scoop, and squeezing your bottom (Figure 9-9e).

Inhale: Walk your hands back towards your feet and hang down in your forward bend stretch, keeping your head hanging heavy. You may need to bend your knees slightly if the stretch is too excruciating.

Exhale: Soften your knees and begin stacking up the spine, lifting your navel up and in towards your spine as if you're being lifted from the middle. Keep your head hanging heavy as you rise, one vertebra at a time. Finish by standing tall, your head being the last thing to rise.

Do's and don'ts

- ✔ Do keep the crown of your head reaching long in front of you.

- ✔ Do keep squeezing your bottom and pulling your navel in by using your Abdominal Scoop throughout the exercise.

- ✔ Don't let your shoulders hunch up by your ears. Instead, keep your shoulder blades pulling down your back.

Modifications

You'll gain upper body and core strength just by holding the plank position. When you can hold the plank for 10 seconds, roll back up to standing.

To make the Pilates Push-Up even harder, once you get out to the plank position, lift one leg off the mat and do the push-up sequence on one leg. You may need to lift your pelvis up a little to maintain balance. Finish the sequence and repeat on the other side.

Book IV

Exploring Yoga and Pilates

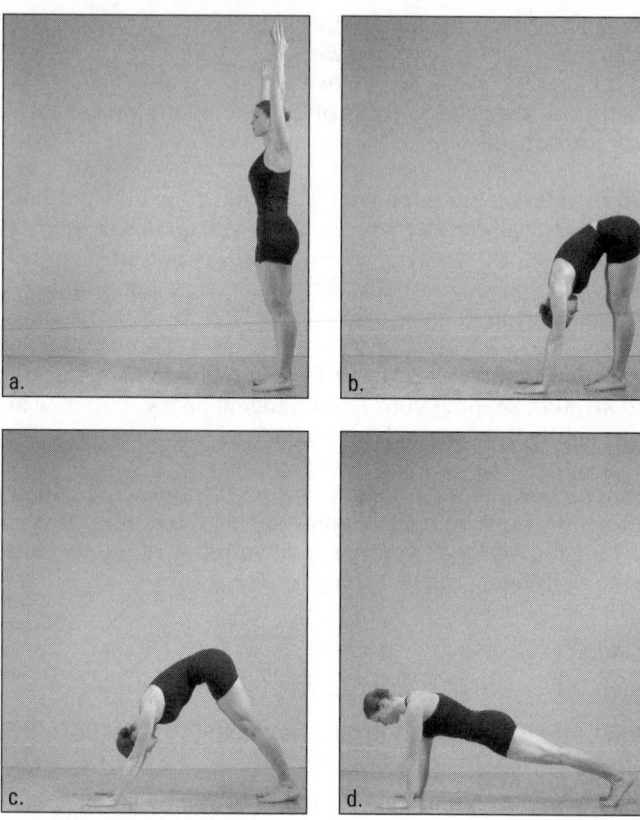

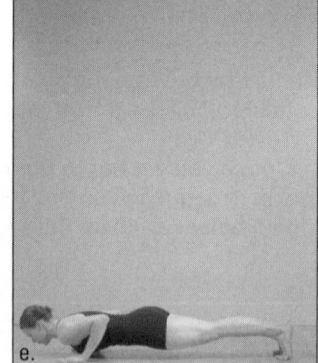

Figure 9-9:
Pilates
Push-Up.

Extra Help for the Bottom and Thighs with the Side Kick series

If you spend ten minutes a day focusing on the exercises in this section, you'll see a difference in the tone and shape of your thighs and bottom.

The bottom is made up of three muscles: the gluteus maximus, the gluteus medius and the gluteus minimus. All three help to stabilise your pelvis when you walk, and when weak, they can cause low back pain or a number of other problems. The gluteus maximus is the main fleshy part of your bottom, the gluteus medius and minimus are both on the side of your bottom, just behind your hip bones.

The exercises that follow comprise the Side Kick series. Try to do all the exercises in a row; they're meant to follow each other. If you can complete the whole series, you'll definitely feel a delicious burn all around your bottom.

Please note that some exercises in the Side Kick series are more advanced than others. If you come to an exercise in this series that feels too advanced for you, skip it and move on to the next one. We state the difficulty of the exercise next to its name.

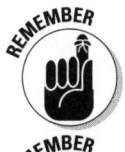

There's a lot of flexing and pointing of the feet in this section, so we thought we'd remind you what the terms mean. You're flexing your foot when you pull your foot up so that it makes an 'L' shape with your shin. You're pointing your foot when it makes a straight line with your leg.

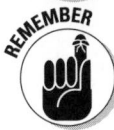

Go through the series on one side, then flip over and do the series lying on your other side.

Side Kicks (Beginning)

It's no surprise that the classic Side Kick series starts with Side Kicks. If you've done the series in Book IV Chapter 8, you've done Side Kicks already. Try doing the advanced variation, where both your hands are behind your head. Figure 9-10 shows Side Kicks, and Figure 9-11 shows the advanced hand position.

Book IV

Exploring Yoga and Pilates

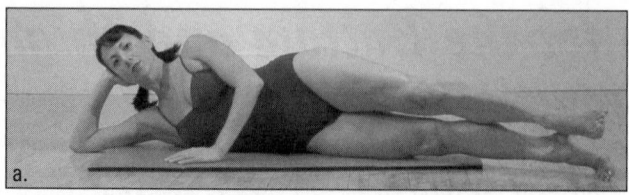

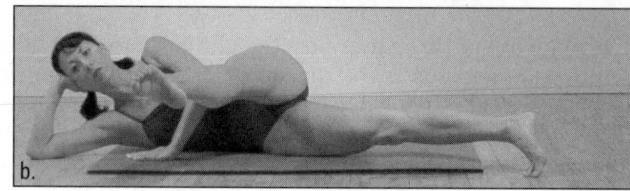

Figure 9-10:
Side Kicks.

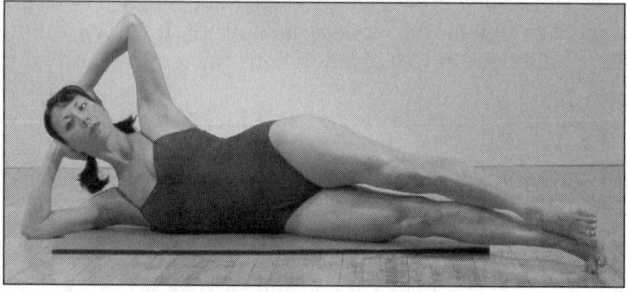

Figure 9-11:
Make Side
Kicks more
difficult by
changing
your hand
position.

Bicycle (Beginning)

In this exercise, you move your legs like you're riding a bike – only you're lying on your side.

Getting set

Lie on your side, propped up on one elbow with your hand supporting your head. Place your other hand behind your head. Your legs should be together and slightly in front of your body. Place your top palm on the mat in front of you for support. Keep your hips square during the exercise. Point your knees straight ahead (as opposed to facing slightly away from each other), in what is known as the parallel position. Point your feet. (Figure 9-12a shows the starting position).

If you're struggling with this exercise, put the palm of your top arm on the mat for support.

The exercise

Breathing continuously: Lift your top leg up slightly so that it's even with your hips. Point your foot and swing your top leg forward as far as you can while still maintaining stability in your torso (Figure 9-12b), then bend the knee as if you're pedalling a bicycle (Figure 9-12c). As you complete your pedalling motion, straighten the leg behind you (Figure 9-12d) and swing it back forward to start the cycling motion again.

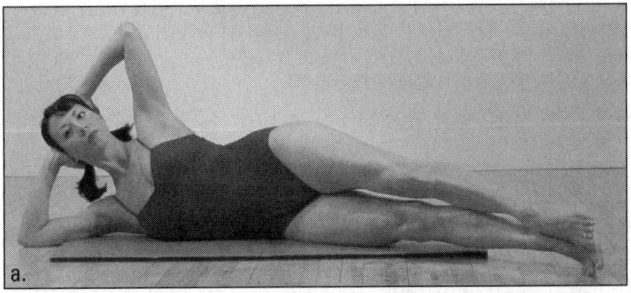

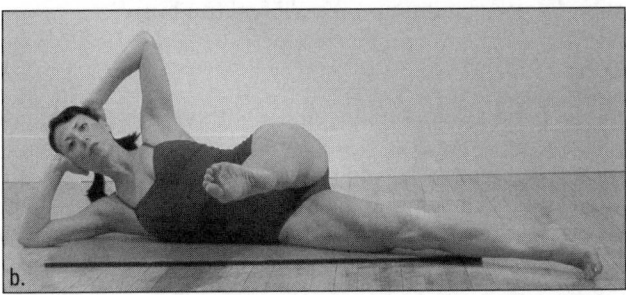

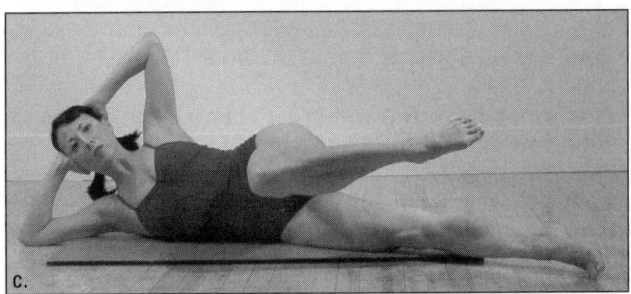

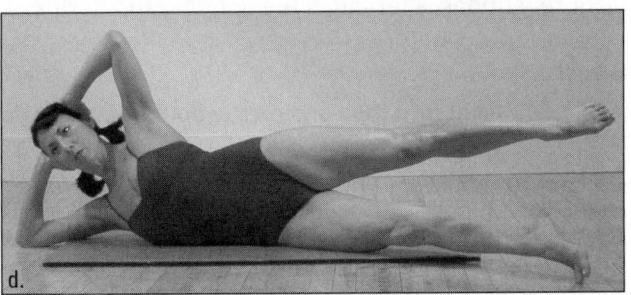

Figure 9-12:
Bicycle.

Book IV

Exploring Yoga and Pilates

After three forward pedals, reverse the pedalling by swinging your top leg back, then bending it while the knee is still behind you, and extending the leg as it comes to the front. Do three backward pedals.

Do's and don'ts

- ✔ Do place your palm on the floor in front of you to help you maintain balance throughout the exercise, if you need to do so.

- ✔ Do keep your neck long and relaxed.

- ✔ Do keep your body square, hip over hip.

Up/Down in Parallel (Beginning)

Up/Down in Parallel strengthens the side of your hips and bottom (the gluteus medius and gluteus minimus). You'll feel the burn!

Getting set

Lie on your side, propped up on one elbow with your hand supporting your head, and place your other arm's palm on the mat in front of you for support. Your legs should be straight and together and slightly in front of your body. Keep your hips square during the exercise. Point your knees straight ahead, in what is known as the parallel position. Point your feet. (Figure 9-13a shows the starting position.)

The exercise

Inhale: Lift your top leg about a foot off the floor (Figure 9-13b).

Exhale: Flex your foot at the top and bring your leg back down to the starting position, pulling your navel in and squeezing your bottom.

Think of pressing down an imaginary spring as you lower your leg, creating resistance in the inner thigh. Imagine reaching your heel long away from you, as if your top leg will reach longer than your lower leg.

Complete eight repetitions, alternating the pointing and flexing of the foot.

Do's and don'ts

- ✔ Do press your weight into the palm on the floor in front of you to maintain balance throughout the exercise.

- ✔ Do keep your neck long and relaxed.

- ✔ Do keep your body square, hip over hip.

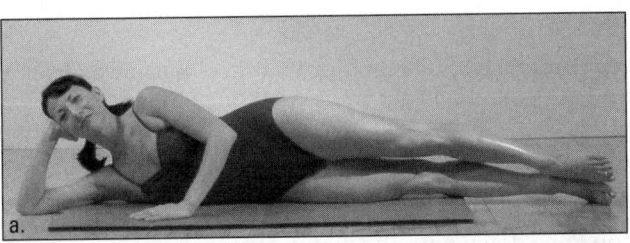

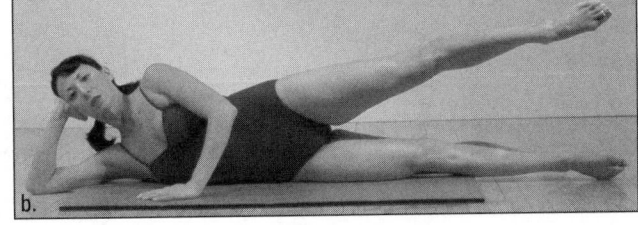

Figure 9-13:
Up/Down in
Parallel.

Bottom Cruncher (Beginning)

Bottom Cruncher addresses the side of the bottom (the gluteus medius muscle). This exercise will make you wince with pain, but it will give you the desired side-of-the-bottom firmness.

Getting set

Lie on your side propped up on one elbow, with your hand supporting your head, and place your other arm's palm on the mat in front of you for support. Fold your knees and hips at 90-degree angles, then straighten your top leg so that it is at a 90-degree angle from your body. If you're tight in your legs, come as close to 90-degrees as you can. You can also bend your knee slightly to make this position more comfortable. Flex your top foot. (Figure 9-14a shows the starting position.)

The exercise

This exercise has two parts: First you pulse, then you circle.

Pulses

Breathing continuously: Think of reaching your heel way away from you as you lift and lower your top leg, making small pulsing movements (Figure 9-14b). Accent the up direction of the movement for eight pulses (think up and up and up and up . . .).

Book IV

Exploring Yoga and Pilates

Circles

Breathing continuously: Still reaching your heel long away from you, make small circles with your heel as if you're painting circles on the wall that's in front of you. Circle eight times in one direction and then eight times in the opposite direction.

Transition by straightening your lower leg, bending your top leg, and dropping your top knee down onto the mat in front of your lower leg. Now you're ready for the Inner Thigh Pulses.

Do's and don'ts

- Do keep your body square, hip over hip.
- Don't let your leg turn in as you repeat the movements. Keep your knee facing straight ahead.

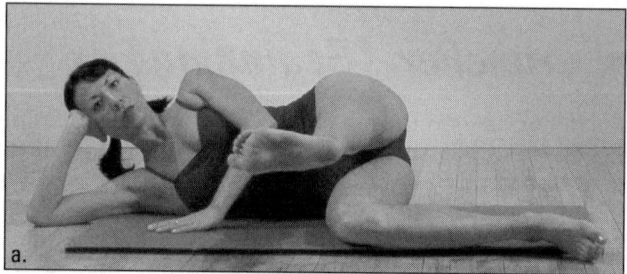

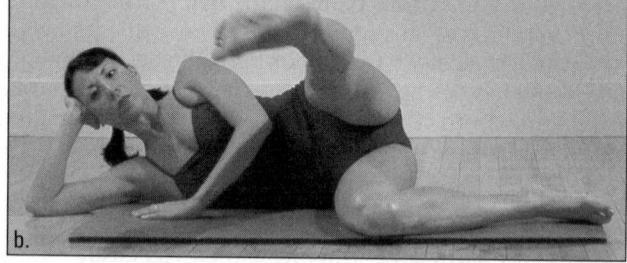

Figure 9-14:
Bottom
Cruncher.

Inner Thigh Pulses (Beginning)

Women are always coming to us wanting to tone their inner thighs. Well, ladies, here's your exercise! Because this exercises works your inner thighs, it gives your bottom a much-needed break.

Getting set

Lie on your side, one arm holding up your head and the other on the mat, and straighten out your lower leg. Bend your top leg and bring it in front of you so that your lower leg has room to move straight up (Figure 9-15a).

The exercise

Inhaling and exhaling: Flex the bottom foot and reach the heel long away from you as you lift and lower the leg, making large pulsing movements (Figure 9-15b). Try to lift the leg as high as you can without losing your control and balance. Think of initiating the movement from your tummy by pulling your navel in towards your spine on every upward pulse.

Accent the up direction for 10 pulses – think up and up and up and up.

Transition to Up/Down in Turnout by straightening both legs and bringing them together, back to the side-lying position. Your legs should be slightly in front of your body. Place your top arm down on the mat for support.

Do's and don'ts

  ✔ Do lift your leg as high as you can, really challenging your inner thigh.

  ✔ Do keep your body square, hip over hip.

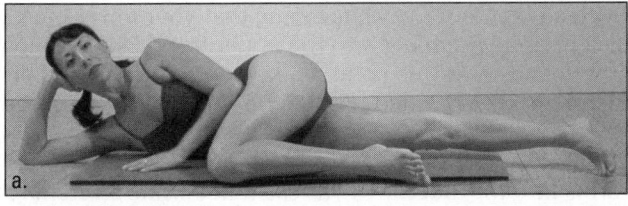

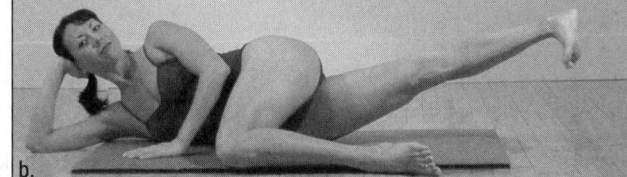

Figure 9-15:
Inner Thigh
Pulses.

Book IV

**Exploring
Yoga and
Pilates**

Meow! Stretching the Spine

If you wake up in the morning with a stiff back or neck, spend a couple minutes doing one of the following stretches.

Basic Cat (Beginning)

The Basic Cat is one of the gentlest and simplest ways to stretch out the back. You see cats making this movement in the morning when they wake, and you can do it too!

Getting set

To begin, get on all fours. Align your hands beneath your shoulders and your knees beneath your hips. Allow your back to assume its natural position, in Neutral Spine (Figure 9-16a).

The exercise

Inhale: Arch your back slightly, allowing your head to rise and your bottom to stick up and out (Figure 9-16b).

Exhale: Pull your navel in towards your spine and squeeze your low bottom. You begin with a Lumbar C Curve, meaning that your lower back is curved like a C, then continue rounding into the upper back. Finally, allow the head to slowly drop forward. At this point, your whole spine should be making a C shape (Figure 9-16c). Your back should be rounded to the greatest extent possible.

Push your arms into the mat for extra resistance while stretching your upper back. Keep your abdominals and ribcage pulled in. Think of using this pulling action to stretch through your whole spine.

Think of pulling your imaginary tail between your legs and rounding your back up as high as you can like a cat arching its back.

Inhale: Return to Neutral Spine, then go further into the arch, sticking your tail and head upwards.

Complete four repetitions.

Do's and don'ts

✔ Do go for the fullest stretch in each direction.

✔ Don't hunch your shoulders. Let them relax down away from your ears.

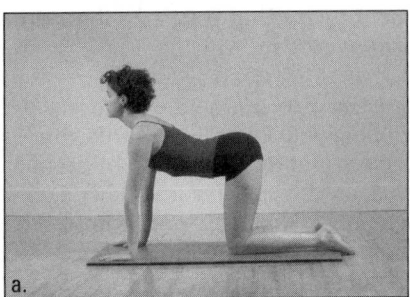
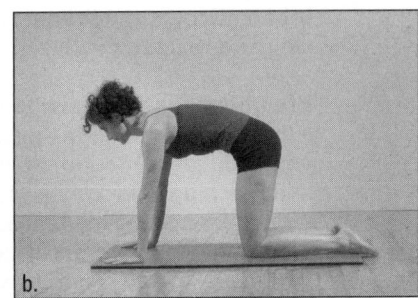
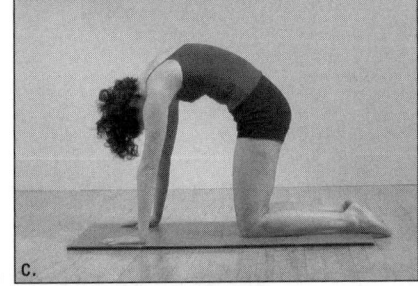

Figure 9-16:
Basic Cat.

The Mermaid (Intermediate)

You can do the Mermaid exercise on the mat and on all the other pieces of Pilates equipment. It is an excellent stretch for the sides of the torso (both the side abdominal and the side back muscles). We recommend it for people with low back tightness and chest tightness. You'll know if you have tightness in these areas once you try this exercise! It feels wonderful.

Getting set

Sit on your left hip, with your knees bent and your legs folded on top of each other, feet facing towards the right and behind you. You can adjust your legs to be either on top of one another or more separate until you find a comfortable position for your hips. You should be sitting like a mermaid, with your tail to one side. Figure 9-17a shows the mermaid position.

You can sit on a pillow if your knees hurt in the initial position.

The exercise

Inhale: Place your left elbow down on the mat beside you. Simultaneously, reach the right arm overhead as far as you can (Figure 9-17b).

Exhale: Reverse the direction of the stretch and reach your left arm overhead, thinking of pulling your navel in towards your spine or using your Abdominal Scoop (Figure 9-17c).

Book IV

Exploring Yoga and Pilates

Inhale: Repeat the first movement by putting your left elbow down by your side and reaching your right arm overhead.

Breathing continuously: Reverse the direction of the stretch and reach your left arm overhead, thinking of pulling your navel in towards your spine or using your Abdominal Scoop. Now add a spiral to this stretch by arching your back and reaching your arm as far back as you can (Figure 9-17d). Continue the stretch by making the biggest circle you can with your arm. As your arm comes in front of you, your back should now round forward (Figure 9-17e). Pulling your navel in and scooping your tummy, complete the circle and come up to sitting tall. Reverse the circle of your arm, rounding your back as you circle forward and arching your back as your arm circles behind you.

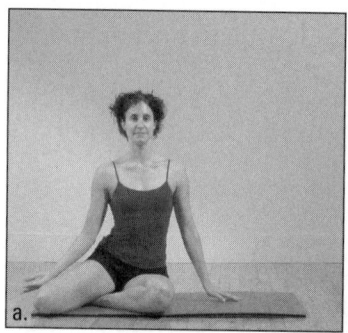
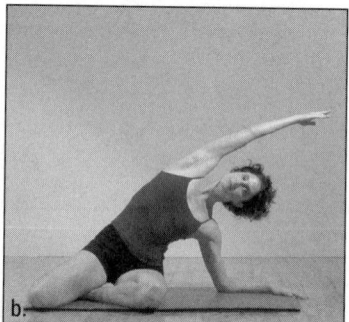
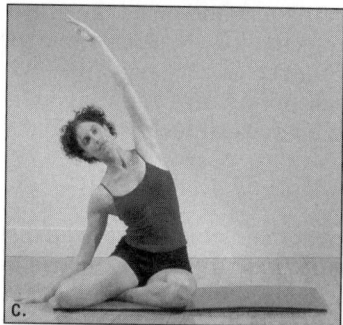
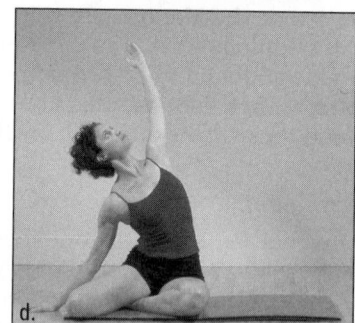
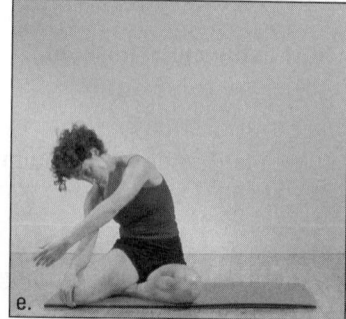

Figure 9-17:
The
Mermaid.

Imagine someone is holding your hand and pulling your arm in the biggest possible circle it can make.

Do only once and repeat the exercise on the other side.

Do's and don'ts

✔ Do allow your arm to reach far back behind your body to open your chest and give you the maximum chest stretch.

✔ Do sit on a pillow if your knees hurt.

Plastic Foam Never Felt So Good: The Roller

The foam roller is a great accessory. It isn't part of classic Pilates but it's a wonderful tool to use in conjunction with Pilates exercises. It helps people better feel the alignment and posture they're striving for.

Shoulder Slaps

We describe how to do Shoulder Slaps as a mat exercise in Book IV Chapter 7. When you do them on the roller, Shoulder Slaps are even more effective at releasing your shoulder muscles and teaching proper shoulder placement.

Getting set

To get into the starting position, sit on the edge of the roller and roll slowly down onto your back, placing your hands on the floor to help you control the movement down. Now you should be lying back with the roller along your spine, your knees bent, your feet flat on the floor approximately hip distance apart, your arms down by your sides, and your palms facing down. Make sure that your head and your whole spine are on the roller; adjust forward or back if you're falling off. The roller is too unstable for you to maintain Neutral Spine; instead, flatten your low back onto the roller by using your Abdominal Scoop.

The exercise

Inhale: Reach your arms up to the sky, allowing your scapulae (shoulder blades) to come off the roller (Figure 9-18a).

Exhale: Keep your arms straight as you completely relax and release the shoulder muscles, letting your scapulae slap back down again (Figure 9-18b).

Book IV

Exploring Yoga and Pilates

Complete four repetitions. On the final repetition, allow your scapulae to come down slowly, imagining your shoulder blades melting down into your back. Keep pushing your scapulae back and feel the muscles that are working. This concept of having 'your shoulders down your back' is very important and is repeated over and over again in Pilates.

Do's and don'ts

✔ Do really release on the exhale, allowing your shoulder blades and arms to truly drop with gravity.

✔ Don't bend your arms when you slap your shoulder blades down.

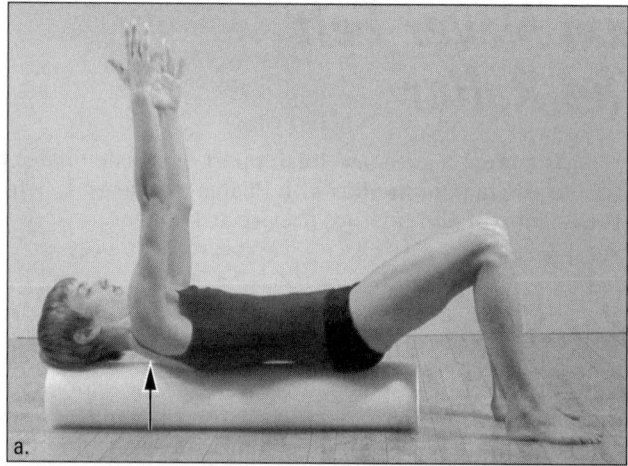

Lift your shoulders off the roller...

Figure 9-18:
Shoulder
Slaps.

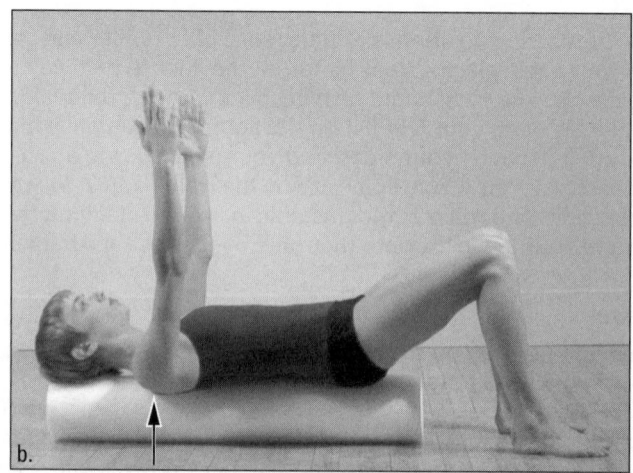

and then let them slap back down.

Arm Reaches/Arm Circles

You can do Arm Reaches/Arm Circles (which we describe in Book IV Chapter 7) on the mat as well as on the roller. Like Shoulder Shrugs, this exercise is even more effective in both its goals – stretching out your chest and back muscles and teaching upper torso stability – when done on the roller. Feel free to hold the stretch if it feels good and if you feel like you need it.

If you're tight and need to stretch, focus on opening your chest when performing this exercise. If you have lots of flexibility in your body, then focus on stabilising your torso (don't let your upper back arch off the roller!).

Getting set

You should already be in the correct position after doing Shoulder Slaps: The roller is along your spine, your knees are bent, your feet are flat on the floor approximately hip distance apart, your arms are down by your sides, and your palms are facing down. Make sure that your head and your whole spine are on the roller; adjust forward or back if you're falling off the edge. The roller is too unstable for you to maintain Neutral Spine; instead, flatten your lower back onto the roller by using your Abdominal Scoop.

The exercise

Inhale: Reach your arms straight up to the ceiling, keeping them shoulder distance apart (Figure 9-19a).

Exhale: First, think of knitting your ribs into your belly, and reach your arms back towards your ears. If you're very tight in your shoulder area, you may not be able to reach all the way back. Just go to the position where you feel a stretch. Feel the contact of your whole back on the roller; use your upper abdominals to keep your upper back from arching off the mat and to keep your ribs from popping up (Figure 9-19b).

Inhale: Bring your arms back to the starting position – reaching straight up to the ceiling.

Complete three repetitions.

On the last reach backwards, allow your arms to reach all the way back to the floor behind you. Allow your back to arch and your chest to expand open. Take a deep breath in and expand into your rib cage and lungs. This movement will transition you into the next exercise, Chicken Wings.

Book IV

Exploring Yoga and Pilates

Do's and don'ts

↳ Do maintain absolute stability in your torso by keeping your ribs down until the very last repetition.

↳ Do keep your shoulders down away from your ears as you initiate the exercise.

↳ Don't let your upper back arch off the mat. This is the whole point of this exercise! As you raise your arms, your upper back naturally wants to go with them. Figure 9-20 shows the back arched off the mat. This is a model of what *not* to do . . . until the last one, when you can go for your stretch.

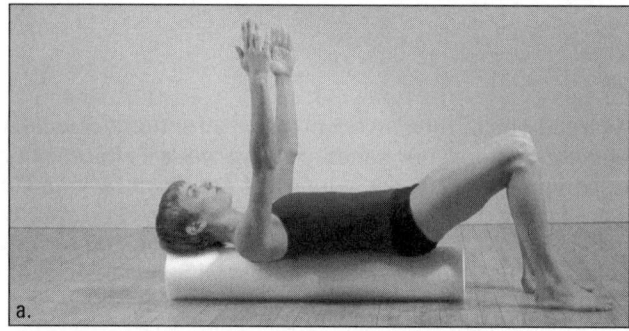

Figure 9-19:
Arm
Reaches/
Arm Circles.

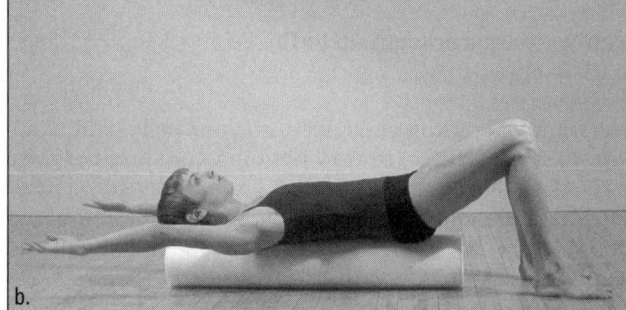

Keep your back on the roller.

Figure 9-20:
How *not*
to do Arm
Reaches/
Arm Circles.

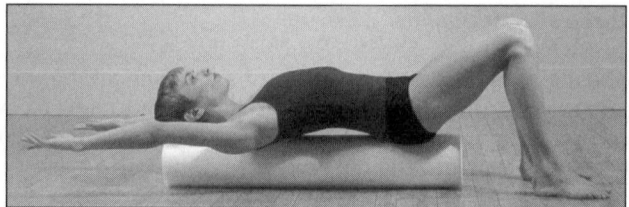

Don't allow your back to arch off the roller.

Chicken Wings

Chicken Wings is a delicious stretch for your chest and shoulder muscles. If you're extremely tight and the stretch is too intense for whatever reason, roll off the roller onto the floor and try the exercise on the mat instead. As your muscles begin to open up, try it again on the roller.

Getting set

You should already be in the correct position after doing Arm Reaches: The roller is along your spine, your knees are bent, your feet are flat on the floor approximately hip distance apart, your arms are down by your sides, and your palms are facing down. Make sure that your head and your whole spine are on the roller; adjust forward or back if you're falling off the edge. The roller is too unstable for you to maintain Neutral Spine; instead, flatten your lower back onto the roller by using your Abdominal Scoop.

Inhale: Reach your arms back by your ears, toward the wall behind you (Figure 9-21a). Expand into your chest and allow your back to arch off the mat a little.

Exhale: Start to slowly bend your elbows, trying to let them touch the floor as you pull them down, as if aiming them for your back pockets (Figure 9-21b). If you're very tight, your elbows won't touch the floor, so just let them drop back as far as feels comfortable. Try to keep your upper arm and lower arm at about a 90-degree angle to each other as you do the exercise. Imagine pulling your shoulder blades down your back with your back muscles. Once you've pulled your elbows down as far as you can, let your arms straighten and come down by your sides.

Inhale: Turn your palms up to the sky and go right into Angels in the Snow.

Complete three repetitions.

Do's and don'ts

- ✔ Do allow your arms to drop down to the mat to get your best stretch.
- ✔ Do allow your back to arch off the roller to get a better stretch in your chest.
- ✔ Do inhale deeply and hold any part of the movement that feels like a particularly great stretch.

Angels in the Snow

Angels in the Snow is a great exercise for teaching the proper shoulder alignment while stretching out the chest (the pectoral muscles).

Book IV

Exploring Yoga and Pilates

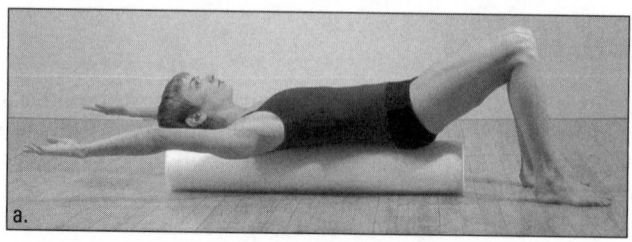

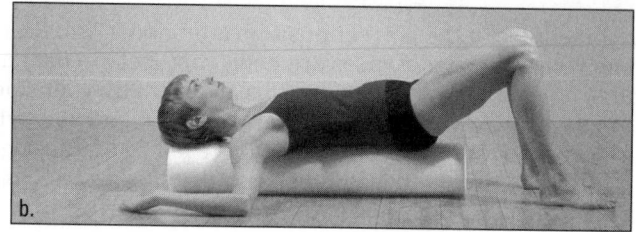

Figure 9-21: Chicken Wings.

Getting set

You should already be in the correct position after doing Chicken Wings: The roller is along your spine, your knees are bent, your feet are flat on the floor approximately hip distance apart, your arms are down by your sides, and your palms are facing up. Make sure that your head and your whole spine are on the roller; adjust forward or back if you're falling off the edge. The roller is too unstable for you to maintain Neutral Spine; instead, flatten your lower back onto the roller by using your Abdominal Scoop.

The exercise

Exhale: Pull your shoulder blades down your back as you begin to drag your arms slowly along the floor, opening them to a 'T' shape with your body (Figure 9-22a).

You're making angels in the snow with your arms. Imagine that you're lying in the snow and pushing up the snow with your arms by using your back muscles and allowing your chest to open and release.

Inhale: Keep your arms heavy on the floor to get a wonderful stretch in your chest as you allow your arms to keep moving, completing a semicircle that ends with your arms up by your ears (Figure 9-22b).

Exhale: Move your arms back down with the Chicken Wings motion from the previous exercise: Slowly bend your elbows, trying to let them touch the floor as you pull them down, as if aiming them for your back pockets. If you're very tight, your elbows won't touch the floor, so just let them drop back as far as feels comfortable. Try to keep your upper arm and lower arm at about a 90-degree angle to each other as you do the exercise. Imagine pulling your shoulder blades down your back with your back muscles. Once you've pulled your elbows down as far as you can, let your arms straighten and come down by your sides.

Alternate Angels in the Snow (going up with your arms) and Chicken Wings (coming down with your arms).

Complete three repetitions.

Do's and don'ts

- ✔ Do allow your arms to stay heavy on the floor, and try to drag them only from the back muscles.

- ✔ Do inhale deeply and hold any part of the movement that feels like a particularly great stretch.

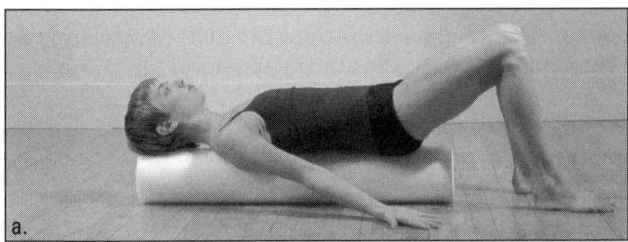

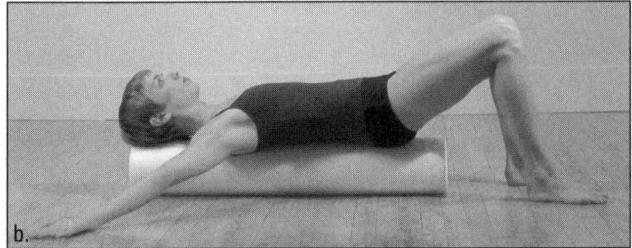

Figure 9-22:
Angels in
the Snow.

Book IV

Exploring Yoga and Pilates

Tiny Steps

Any mat stability exercise becomes more challenging when you do it on the roller, and Tiny Steps is no exception. The roller likes to wobble from side to side; that's what round things like to do. To keep the roller from rolling, you must engage even deeper into your core muscles which makes it a much more challenging exercise.

Tiny Steps is a stability exercise that tests the strength and stability of your lower abdominals. The point of this exercise is to not move your hips or lower back while moving your legs up and down. It looks simple, but it actually takes quite a bit of inner strength. You're going for absolute stability here!

TIP

Feel free to use your arms, pressing on the floor to help you stabilise yourself during this exercise, and make sure that your whole back makes contact with the roller (Figure 9-23a).

Getting set

You should already be in the correct position after doing Angels in the Snow. The roller is along your spine, your knees are bent, your feet are flat on the floor approximately hip distance apart, your arms are down by your sides, and your palms are facing down. Make sure that your head and your whole spine are on the roller; adjust forward or back if you're falling off the edge. The roller is too unstable for you to maintain Neutral Spine; instead, flatten your low back onto the roller by using your Abdominal Scoop.

Exhale: Pull your navel in towards your spine and lift your right knee up to your chest (Figure 9-23b).

Inhale: Bring your right leg back down to the mat, controlling the movement from the centre, and return to the starting position.

Change sides and repeat eight times.

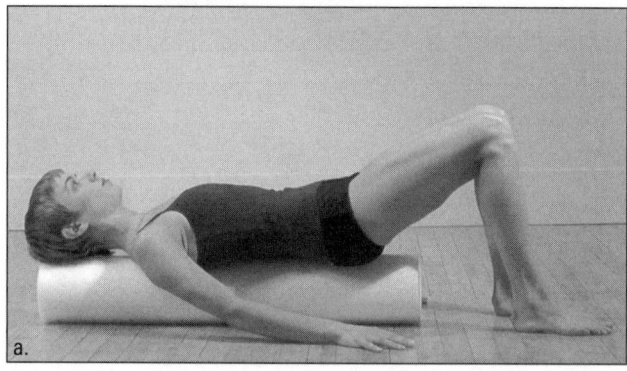

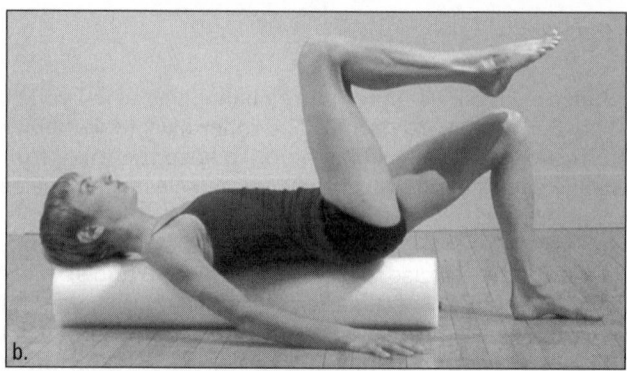

Figure 9-23:
Tiny Steps.

Do's and don'ts

✔ Don't let your lower back arch or your hips rock from side to side.

✔ Don't tense your upper body when doing this exercise. Keep your neck long and your shoulders relaxed.

Pilates exercises can be enhanced even further by using some equipment within a Pilates studio, and small equipment and accessories including foam rollers, magic circles, balls, bands and weights you can use at home – for more information please refer to *Pilates For Dummies*.

Book V
Mental Health

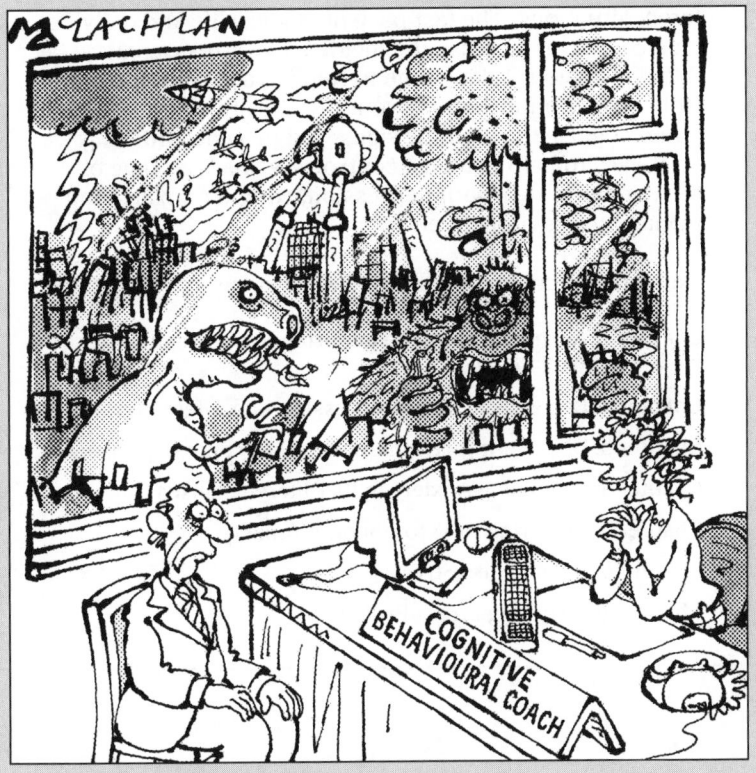

'Now for a start, we have to get rid of your negative
patterns of thought about the world.'

In this book . . .

Mental health relates to your personal well-being, how you think and feel, and how you manage different situations. The fast pace of modern life and daily challenges can increase the incidence of stress, anxiety and depression. Taking time to think about your personal well-being is important for your own health. Book V helps you recognise the warning signs, and provides thinking strategies to help you take control. We share a range of techniques to deal with depression, conquer anxiety and manage stress proactively.

Here are the contents of Book V at a glance:

Chapter 1

Acknowledging the Importance of Personal Well-Being

• •

In This Chapter

▶ Measuring your well-being

▶ Linking stress and health

▶ Eating well to avoid stress

▶ Exercising for health

▶ Helping yourself get quality sleep

• •

*F*eeling healthy and happy has a positive effect on your life in general. Your personal well-being can be affected by eating, exercise and sleep, so this chapter helps you assess your own well-being and in particular the effect of happiness and stress. We also consider the impact of certain foods on stress, describe some exercises to calm your mind and take time to help you think about how you sleep at night.

Understanding Your Level of Well-Being

Assessing your own well-being is a helpful starting point. The following questionnaire developed by Professor Stephen Joseph and his colleagues helps to measure life satisfaction and well-being. Take a few minutes to complete the questionnaire if you wish to understand your level of well-being.

A number of statements that people have made to describe how they feel are given in Table 1-1. Please read each one and tick the box which best describes how frequently you felt that way in the past seven days, including today. Some statements describe positive feelings and some describe negative feelings. You may have experienced both positive and negative feelings at different times during the past seven days.

Table 1-1:	Level of Well-Being			
	Never	*Rarely*	*Sometimes*	*Often*
1. I felt dissatisfied with my life.				
2. I felt happy.				
3. I felt cheerless.				
4. I felt pleased with the way I am.				
5. I felt that life was enjoyable.				
6. I felt that life was meaningless.				

To work out your score, use the following scoring key to turn your answers into numbers.

> ✔ **For items 2, 4, and 5:** Never = 0, rarely = 1, sometimes = 2, often = 3.

> ✔ **For items 1, 3, and 6:** Never = 3, rarely = 2, sometimes = 1, often = 0.

Now, using the scoring key above, add scores on all 6 items to give a total score, with a possible range of 0 to 18. Most people score between 11 and 13. Higher scores indicate greater happiness. As scores decrease, however, happiness fades into unhappiness, which fades into depression. Research estimates that scores below nine are increasingly indicative of depressive states. If you scored very low on the questionnaire, it is possible that you are suffering from what psychologists call clinical depression. Of course, one short questionnaire can't give us all the answers – that would take a full assessment from a psychologist – but it may be useful in giving you a sense of where you lie on the spectrum of well-being.

Making the Case for Being Happy

Perhaps you feel that you don't deserve to be happy. If so, you're probably someone who often experiences guilt and self-blame. You may need to do further work on certain core change-blocking beliefs or habitual ways of thinking before starting down the path towards authentic happiness.

Perhaps you feel you deserve happiness as much as anyone else, but you think happiness is an overrated idea? This perspective can spring from the messages you got from your parents when you were a child. Some children

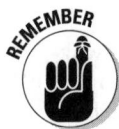

are told that work is the one and only valuable activity in life, and that anything else is merely a diversion from what's really important.

A growing body of studies increasingly highlights and confirms the value of happiness. Today we now know that happy people:

- ✔ Live longer
- ✔ Are more creative
- ✔ Have lower blood pressure
- ✔ Have more active immune systems
- ✔ Have more empathy with others
- ✔ Are more successful financially
- ✔ Are more productive

So, if work is your main concern in life, it seems that happiness means you're going to work more efficiently and productively. Happiness is also good for your health and well-being, and it also means you're likely to live longer. Now those are pretty convincing arguments.

Stress and Health

If we perceive events to be a threat to our normal functioning, well-being, or self-esteem, we experience the negative thoughts and emotions we all associate with stress. However, the effects of stress are not limited to what goes on within our brains – they permeate our whole body and, if sustained, can have powerful and harmful effects on our physical health. It's the link between what we think or feel and the activity in the rest of our body that's mediated (at least in part) by the stress hormone *cortisol*. The more stressful we perceive life to be, the more cortisol is released into the bloodstream. Although cortisol is an essential hormone that performs a wide range of vital functions (see 'Understanding how cortisol works' later in this chapter), producing too much at the wrong times of day can put our health at risk.

The reason why the links between stress and health are so difficult to prove is because stress, and stress alone, does not cause a specific disease. Rather, a sustained period of stress can increase our chances of succumbing to a range of illnesses, depending on individual susceptibilities in terms of genetic predisposition and lifestyle. Potentially, stress can also worsen some existing conditions. Although it can be difficult to tease out all the factors that may lead to illness, research continues to find clear evidence that stress is an issue we should all take seriously: Stress not only threatens the quality of our lives but also the state of our health.

Understanding how cortisol works

Healthy levels of cortisol rise sharply within the first 30 minutes after awakening in the morning and then decline throughout the rest of the day to reach their lowest levels before going to bed and in the early stages of sleep. This pattern is important as a 24-hour signal to the rest of the body, maintaining a healthy balance between the different organ systems during the course of the day. If too much stress is superimposed upon this normal, healthy pattern then the rest of the body doesn't know whether it's night or day, and this can cause a problem for efficient functioning.

In addition, body organs detect stress-related increases in cortisol and respond in a variety of ways – for example, by increasing blood pressure, altering the balance of our immune systems, and increasing blood glucose levels for use as energy. Over-activity in any of these departments may increase the risk of cardiovascular problems, infection, and/or allergic disorders, as well as diabetes.

Preparing for fight or flight

Your body responds to threats by preparing for action in three different ways: physically, mentally, and behaviourally. When danger presents itself, you reflexively prepare to stand and fight or run like you've never run before. Your body mobilises to respond to danger in complex and fantastic ways.

Figure 1-1 gives you the picture.

First, the brain sends signals through your nervous system for your body to go on high alert. Production and release of the stress hormone, cortisol, increases. The brain tells the adrenal glands to rev up production of adrenaline and noradrenaline. These hormones stimulate the body in various ways. Your heart pounds faster and faster, and you start breathing more rapidly, sending increased oxygen to your lungs, which is transferred to the blood that flows to the large muscles, preparing them to fight or flee from danger.

Digestion slows to preserve energy for meeting the challenge, and pupils dilate to improve vision. Blood flow decreases to hands and feet in order to prevent blood loss if injured and keep up the blood supply to the large muscles. Sweating increases in order to keep the body cool, and it makes you slippery, so aggressors can't grab hold of you. All your muscles tense to spring into action.

Mentally, you automatically scan your surroundings intensely. Your attention focuses on the threat and nothing else. In fact, you can't attend to much of anything else.

Behaviourally, you're now ready to flee or fight. You need that preparation in the face of danger. When you have to take on a bear, a lion, or a warrior, you'd better have all systems on high alert.

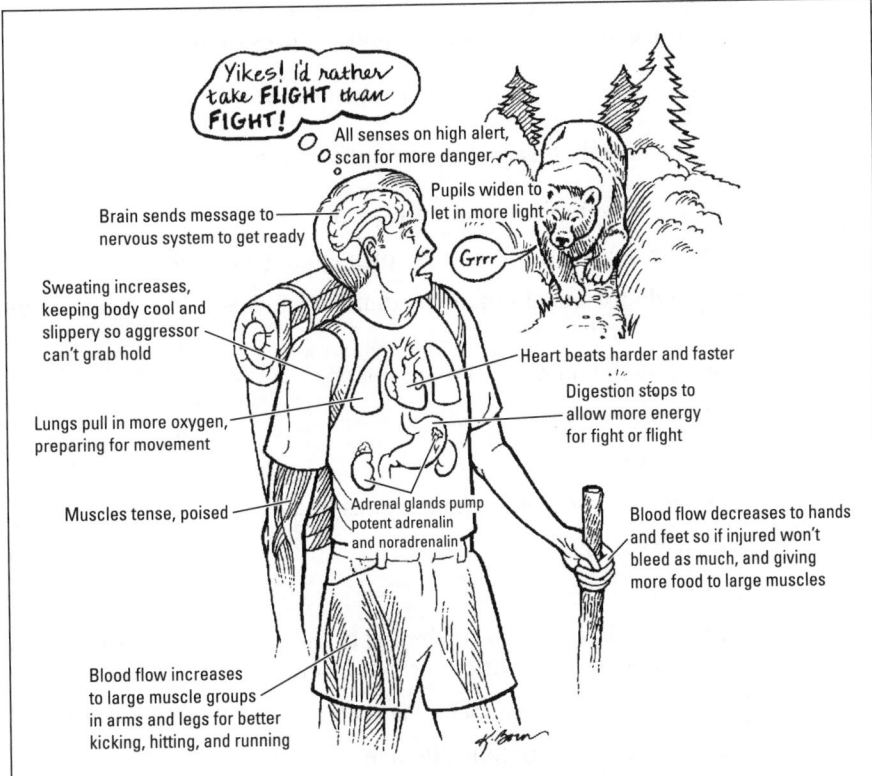

Figure 1-1:
Choices,
choices!

Just one problem – in today's world, most people don't encounter lions and bears. Unfortunately, your body doesn't know this and automatically reacts with the same preparation for facing dangers, even though these are fighting traffic, meeting deadlines, speaking in public, and other everyday worries.

When human beings have nothing to fight or run from, all that energy has to get out somehow. So you may feel the urge to fidget by moving your feet and hands. You feel on edge – like jumping out of your skin. You may be highly irritable with those around you.

Homing in on anxiety-related disorders

Most experts believe that if you experience these physical effects of anxiety on a frequent, chronic basis, it can't be doing you any good. Various studies have suggested the possibility that chronic anxiety and stress may conceivably contribute to a variety of physical problems, such as abnormal heart rhythms, high blood pressure, irritable bowel syndrome, asthma, ulcers, stomach upsets (diarrhoea, constipation, cramping, bloating, and excessive production of digestive acids in the stomach, which may cause a painful burning sensation), chronic muscle spasms, tremors, chronic back pain, tension, headaches (which may only start some time after the event), and a depressed immune system.

Figure 1-2 illustrates the toll of chronic anxiety on the body.

Chronic anxiety has also been implicated in:

- ✔ The development of depression.
- ✔ The development of full-blown anxiety disorder.
- ✔ Reduced quality of life by diminishing feelings of pleasure and accomplishment.
- ✔ Potential damage to relationships.
- ✔ Heart disease.
- ✔ Stroke.
- ✔ Effects on the inflammatory response.
- ✔ Weight gain or loss.
- ✔ Diabetes.
- ✔ Sleep disturbances, including both insomnia and/or waking up in the middle of the night or early morning.
- ✔ Diminished sexual desire and an inability to achieve orgasm in women.
- ✔ Temporary impotence in men.
- ✔ Negative effects on both fertility and pregnancy.
- ✔ Memory, concentration, and learning disorders.
- ✔ Allergies
    - eczema and other rashes
    - headaches
    - asthma
    - sinus problems
- ✔ Skin conditions, including
    - hives
    - psoriasis
    - acne
    - rosacea
    - eczema
    - unexplained itching

✔ Unexplained hair loss (*Alopecia areata*): where hair is lost in discrete patches. The cause is unknown, but stress is suspected as a player in this condition. For example, hair loss often occurs during periods of intense stress, such as grieving after a death.

✔ Gum disease leading to tooth loss.

If stress becomes chronic, sufferers often experience loss of concentration at work and at home, and they may become inefficient and accident-prone. In children, the physiological responses to chronic stress can make learning difficult. Chronic stress in older people may also play an even more important role in memory loss than the aging process.

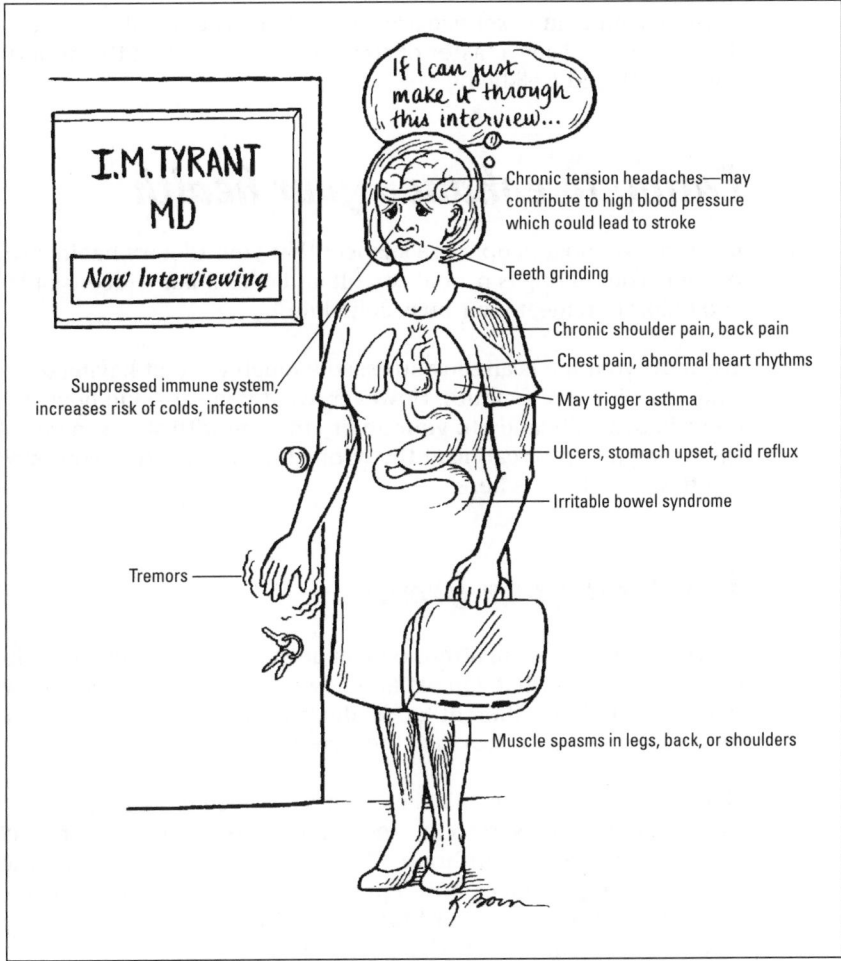

Figure 1-2:
The chronic effects of anxiety.

However, before you get too anxious about your anxiety, please realise that hard, definitive evidence doesn't exist yet to show that anxiety is a *major* cause of most of these problems. Nevertheless, enough studies have suggested that it can make these disorders worse and that you should probably take chronic anxiety seriously. In other words, be concerned, but DON'T PANIC!

Using Eating, Exercise and Sleep to Enhance Your Well-Being

Food, nutrition and exercise are covered in more detail in Book II and Book III. Here you will see a taster of some ideas to highlight the importance to your health and well-being.

Eating to enhance your health

If you're like most people, we suspect that your dietary habits are less than perfect. Your eating is probably a hit-and-miss affair – inconsistent, rushed and tailored to meet your busy schedule.

We know your life is already stressed enough without having to worry about what goes into your mouth. However, what you eat – and how you eat it – can contribute significantly to your ability to cope with stress in your life. Eating the wrong things or eating at the wrong times can add to your stress level. Not to worry. Help is here.

Feeding your brain

In recent years, a lot of attention has been paid to the relationship between food and mood – what you eat and how you feel. Researchers now have a better idea of how different foods affect your psychological states and how food can increase or decrease the stress in your life.

One of the major biochemical elements involved in your stress experience is something called serotonin. Serotonin is a naturally occurring chemical neurotransmitter in your brain. Changing serotonin levels can dramatically change the way you feel. Antidepressant drugs like Prozac can alter the amount of serotonin in your brain, which can alter your mood and affect the ways in which you cope with a potential stress.

The foods you eat can also change the serotonin levels in your brain. Your diet is an important way of regulating your serotonin levels. Putting the right stuff on your plate means you have a better chance of giving your brain what it needs.

Choosing low-stress foods

The following are some specific food guidelines that can help you choose foods to lower your stress as well as help your body cope with all the stress in your life:

- ✔ **Include some complex carbohydrates in every meal.** Complex carbohydrates, such as pasta, cereals, potatoes and brown rice, can enhance your performance when under stress. Foods rich in carbohydrates can increase the levels of serotonin in the brain, making you feel better. Too many complex carbohydrates, however, are not the best thing for you. Remember: Moderation.

- ✔ **Reduce your intake of simple carbohydrates.** Sweetened, sugary foods – simple carbohydrates – like carbonated drinks and sweets can make you feel better in the short run, but feel worse in the long run.

- ✔ **Eat adequate amounts of protein.** This means eating more fish, chicken and other lean meats. Foods high in protein enhance mental functioning and supply essential amino acids that can help repair damage to your body's cells.

- ✔ **Eat your vegetables.** Beans, peppers, carrots, squash and dark-green leafy vegetables, whether cooked or raw, provide your body with the vitamins and nutrients it needs to resist the negative effects of stress.

- ✔ **Get plenty of potassium.** Milk (especially the low-fat variety), whole grains, wheat germ and nuts can all provide your body with potassium, a mineral that can help your muscles relax. Bananas, a personal favourite, are also a good source of potassium.

Stop feeding your stress

Are you an *emotional eater*? If so, you may eat whenever you are anxious, upset, nervous or depressed. Although emotional eaters can still put it away when they're happy, delighted, non-anxious and non-depressed (and yes, during those rare times when they're actually hungry), most emotional eaters eat when they feel they need to feed their stress.

When you feed your stress, a destructive cycle begins. You feel stressed, so your food choices are not always the best. For some reason of cruel fate, foods that tend to make you feel good are usually the foods that are not so good for your body. Chocolate, ice cream, pizza, cake, doughnuts and biscuits may make you feel terrific – but, unfortunately, only for about 17 seconds. Then, of course, your stress returns (plus a ton of guilt) and you feel the need for another bout of eating. The cycle then repeats itself.

The first step in breaking the cycle is becoming aware of exactly when you are distressed and identifying your feelings. When you feel the urge to open the refrigerator door, you need to realise that you are experiencing some form of discomfort. It could be hunger; but more likely, it is stress.

Before you put any food in your mouth, stop and take stock of your emotional state. Ask yourself, 'Am I really hungry or am I feeling emotionally distressed?' If it is truly hunger, eat. Otherwise label your feelings (for example, 'I'm upset', 'I'm nervous' or 'I'm a wreck!'). Simply breaking the stress-eating connection for even a moment can give you a different perspective and an increased level of motivation that can sustain you – until you find something a little more redeeming than filling your mouth.

The following are some other tips that you can use to improve your relationship with food when you're stressed:

Distract yourself

One of the better things you can do is involve yourself in some activity you enjoy that will take your mind off eating. Do something. Anything. Some eating substitutes that will keep you away from the kitchen include the following:

- ✔ **Get out of the house.** Often, simply changing your environment can rid you of the old eating cues. Go for a walk. Do an errand. Visit a friend.

- ✔ **Get some exercise.** Hit the exercise bike or treadmill, or simply do some floor exercises like sit-ups or even just stretching.

- ✔ **Read a good book.** Or watch an interesting television programme.

- ✔ **Cook something.** This may seem like asking for trouble, but often the process of cooking can serve as a substitute for your eating. A hint: Don't make biscuits or cakes. Try something like a soup or a casserole, something that is filling, takes time to cook and prepare, and is not immediately ready to eat.

Substitute relaxation for food

Whenever you are about to open the refrigerator to calm your frayed nerves, consider substituting a relaxation break. Simple deep breathing, some rapid relaxation, or some relaxation imagery can induce a feeling of emotional calm that can reduce your desire to eat. That's all you may need to ease you past a difficult moment.

Work with a stress cue

Sometimes a little reminding goes a long way. Create a stress-eating reminder that you could put on your fridge or on the cabinet where you keep delicious snacks. One of our patients came up with what we thought was a beauty: She put a not terribly attractive picture of her in her heavier days in a small magnetic frame that she stuck on her fridge.

You may decide to be less brutal and opt for something more neutral. One friend has the question, 'Are you really hungry?' taped to her kitchen door. Even more innocuous is a simple little coloured circle of paper you can affix at strategic places in your kitchen. It reminds you that you shouldn't open the door unless you are hungry. Only you know what it represents and why it's there.

Eat your breakfast

Again, your mother was right! Research shows that eating a nutritious (low-fat, high-carbohydrate) breakfast makes you more alert, more focused, and in a much better mood than if you have a high-fat, high-carbohydrate breakfast; have a moderate-fat, moderate-carbohydrate breakfast; or have no breakfast at all.

Skipping breakfast can lower your body's ability to cope with the stress that lies in wait for you later in the day. Starting the day on the right nutritional foot is important. When you wake up in the morning, as many as 11 or 12 hours have passed since you last ate. You need to refuel.

And don't forget lunch

Lunchtime tends to be one of the busier times of your day. With a lot to do, eating lunch may be low on your list of priorities, but don't skip lunch. Your body functions best when it gets fed regularly. Missing lunch can leave you feeling tense and edgy.

When you do have lunch, don't overdo it. A big lunch can leave you lethargic and dreaming of a mid-afternoon siesta, a practice frowned upon by many businesses.

Eat like a cow

Eating a big meal can result in your feeling lethargic soon after eating. To digest that heavy meal, your body needs a greater supply of blood. This blood has to come from other places in your body like your brain, depriving it of some of the oxygen it needs to keep you alert. The solution? Graze like a cow.

Spread out your eating fairly evenly throughout the day. Avoid those huge meals that load you down with calories and leave you feeling ready for a nap. Instead consider smaller, lighter meals at your regular mealtime. Supplement them with healthy snacks. Have a mid-morning snack, and then a light lunch, another snack later in the afternoon (a piece of fruit is good), and a *moderate* dinner. A snack later in the evening (try some air-popped popcorn) should avert any hunger pangs. It seems to work for cows, doesn't it?

Drink like a camel

Most people do not get enough liquids into their bodies during the course of the day. The notion of drinking the recommended eight glasses of water, for most of us, is a joke. If you're like most people, you usually wait until you're thirsty before heading for the kitchen. Unfortunately, by then it's a little late. Your body needs the liquid *before* you feel that thirst. Coffee and tea can act as diuretics and therefore should not be considered as part of your 'daily 8s'.

Load up earlier in the day

For most people, the simplest way to lose weight is to eat more in the first half of the day than they do in the last half. Then they have time to burn off many of those earlier calories. Recall that old bit of nutritional wisdom, 'Eat like a king in the morning, a prince at noon, and a pauper at night.'

Simply supplement

If you think that you may not be getting enough of your needed vitamins and/ or minerals, consider taking a daily multiple vitamin and mineral supplement. If your daily diet gives you all the nutritional good stuff you need, this may not be necessary. However, you may be one of the many whose diet is not nutritionally praiseworthy and could benefit from some supplemental help.

Mastering the art of anti-stress snacking

Feeling anxious, nervous, stressed out? Need a quick food-fix? Snacking, when done right, is an art. Anyone can down a chocolate bar or a bag of crisps and a fizzy drink. The real skill is coming up with a snack that not only doesn't add to your stress level but helps you reduce the stress you already have. Here are some guidelines:

- ✔ Avoid highly sugared treats. They'll give you a boost in the short run but let you down in the long run. You'll crash.

- ✔ Stick with snacks that have high-energy proteins and are high in complex carbohydrates. They'll give you a longer-lasting sustained pick-me-up.

Here are some specific suggestions of quick bites and snacks that can boost your mood and help alleviate some of your stress:

- ✔ A piece of fruit: an orange, peach, apple or banana – just about any fruit is fine.

- ✔ A handful of mixed nuts. (Until only recently, nuts were considered low on the health-food hierarchy. These days they're are on the okay list.)

✔ A bowl of wholegrain cereal with a sliced banana.

✔ A spinach salad.

✔ A bowl of fruit salad.

✔ Air-popped popcorn.

✔ A muffin. (Go easy on the butter or margarine.)

✔ A container of low-fat yoghurt.

✔ A piece of chocolate (but just a piece!).

Exercise and Activity to Boost Your Health

Exercise is one of the better ways of helping you cope with the stress in your life. Exercise and sustained activity – in whatever form – can decrease your blood pressure, lower your heart rate, and slow your breathing – all signs of reduced arousal and stress. Exercise is a natural and effective way of slowing and even reversing your body's fight-or-flight response. This section shows you how you can make exercise and activity your allies in winning the battle against stress.

Calming your brain naturally

When you exercise, you feel different; your mood changes for the better. This difference is not only a psychological response to the fact that you are doing something good for your body. It is physiological as well.

When you exercise, you produce *endorphins* (literally, natural morphine from within your body), which can produce feelings of well-being and calming relaxation. This positive feeling helps you cope more effectively with stress and its effects.

Think activity, rather than exercise

You may think of exercise as something falling outside the range of your normal day-to-day activities. However, a better way of thinking about the goal of staying fit is to replace the word *exercise* with the term *activity*.

We all recognise that after a hard day of work, or taking care of the kids, the chances of your putting on a tracksuit and lifting weights or completing a 6-kilometre run are slim. The good news is, you don't have to. The trick is to find naturally existing outlets for activity that are readily available and easily integrated into your lifestyle and work style.

Exercise, cleverly camouflaged as daily physical activity, is all around you. The hard part is knowing it when you see it.

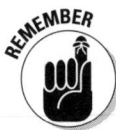

The following are some simple ways in which you can introduce small bits of activity into your day:

- ✔ **Park your car a little farther from your office and walk the rest of the way.**

- ✔ **Use your TV time effectively.** While you are watching television, do some sit-ups, push-ups or stretches.

- ✔ **Walk away from your stress.** As an exercise, walking has always had wimp status. But if done consistently and for a sustained period of time, it can be a terrific way of staying in shape. The nice thing about walking is that it can be pleasantly camouflaged as strolling or sightseeing – both painless activities. And if you crank up the pace and distance a bit, you have a wonderfully simple form of aerobic exercise that can enhance your feeling of well-being, mentally and physically. Walking is a great way to clear your head and calm your mind.

  And remember to take a mini walk or two during your day. Your walks can be as short as down the street to the corner shop or a lap around your office or house.

- ✔ **Do something you like.** Jake was on the swimming team in school, and although he was pretty good he really disliked it and dreaded the early-morning dips in the overly chlorinated pool. As soon as he could, he dropped out. The moral here is, if you don't like the exercise or activity you're doing, the chances of you sustaining it are small. Find something you really enjoy, like one of the following:

  - • **A favourite sport.** Golf, tennis, cricket, basketball, squash – whatever.

  - • **A favourite activity.** Horse-riding, dancing, trampolining, swimming, ice-skating or abseiling – anything that gets your body moving.

  - • **Gardening.** Yes, if done for a sustained period, gardening can be considered a form of exercise.

  - • **Cycling.** Find a place where you can bike safely and enjoyably. If you don't know where those places are, contact your local council. Or ask friends or people you see on bikes what they suggest.

✔ **Become a member of a sports team.** One of the better ways of staying in shape is playing at something you like. Every big city has just about every conceivable kind of sports team; everything from minor league to friendly games in the park on a Saturday or Sunday morning. You don't even have to be especially proficient at a sport to get on board. Check with your local gym or community centre for teams forming, and ask at work if teams already exist.

Getting a Good Night's Sleep

Most people do not get enough quality sleep. Unfortunately, when you're tired, your emotional threshold is lowered. You are more vulnerable to all the other stresses around you. Stress breeds even more stress. Breaking the cycle and getting a good night's sleep becomes very important. Most people need about seven or eight hours of sleep a night.

No fixed rules will tell you how much sleep you need. So take the simple sleep quiz in the nearby sidebar to help see whether you're getting enough sleep at night.

To get the most benefit from your sleep, try the following:

✔ **Hit the sheets earlier.** We recognise that for many, getting to bed earlier is easy to suggest, but much harder to do. Face it, staying up at night is when you do the things you need to do (laundry, house cleaning, paying bills). Or, if you're lucky, late nights are when you do the things you want to do, whether that's vegging out in front of the television or turning the pages of the latest bestseller. You may try to burn the candle at both ends – stay up later and get up early. Often, this strategy just doesn't work, and you're tired the next day. An important element in helping you get the sleep you need is realising that you have to get to bed earlier. It's as simple as that.

✔ **Try the 20-minute approach.** If you determine that you are, in fact, not getting enough sleep at night, try getting to bed 20 minutes earlier and see if the quality of your day is improved.

To get to bed just a few minutes earlier, turn off the TV at a more reasonable hour.

Getting quality sleep

Okay, you may get to bed earlier, but you either aren't falling asleep as you'd like or the quality of your sleep is somehow disturbed. Here are some suggestions and direction that can help you attain that night of restful bliss:

Need more sleep?

Here are some of the more important signs and symptoms of someone who probably isn't getting enough sleep at night. Answer true or false, depending on whether the following statements apply to you.

1. I notice a major dip in my energy level early in the afternoon.

2. I need an alarm clock to wake up in the morning.

3. On the weekends, when I don't have to get up, I end up sleeping much later.

4. I fall asleep very quickly at night (in about 5 minutes).

5. On most days, I feel tired and feel as though I could use a nap.

Answering 'That's me' to any of the above suggests that you may want to re-evaluate how much sleep you're getting and how much sleep you truly need. Try experimenting by getting a bit more sleep at night and see if you notice any changes in your stress levels.

Develop a sleep routine

The best sleep comes from having a regular sleep pattern. Your body's internal clock becomes stabilised with routine. This means getting to bed at the same time and getting up at the same time.

Getting up at the same time may be controllable, but hitting the mattress at the same time every night is not that easy. We often get a second wind later at night and develop an unexplainable urge to work on some project that needs far more time than is reasonable. Burning the candle at both ends usually spells stress. Get to bed at about the same time each night. Save the parties for the weekend.

Bed = Sleep

Ideally, you want to establish a set of reminders and habits that promote an effective sleep routine. The relationship in your mind should be that lying down in bed means that you are going to sleep.

That's the ideal. However, if you live in a small house or flat, you may not have the luxury of keeping a whole room dedicated to just one or two activities. You may be one of the many who uses the bedroom for just about everything. This is understandable, but unfortunately, it's less than ideal for the purposes of optimising your sleep patterns.

Create a sleep ritual

If you can't make your bedroom a room devoted only to sleeping, you may find that creating a bedtime ritual is more realistic. At a certain hour, make the bedroom a place where you wind down and relax. This means no upsetting discussions, no work taken home from the office, no bill-paying, no arguments with the kids, no unpleasant phone calls, or anything else that may trigger worry, anxiety or upset. You can read, watch some relaxing TV, or whatever else it is that calms your body and quietens your mind. We would advise against watching the local news. Hearing about today's robbery, fire, or general mayhem is not the last thing you want to hear before your head hits the pillow.

Don't exercise within three hours of your bedtime

Exercising is great, but doing it too close to your bedtime can rev you up and keep you awake.

Turn the noise down

You may have trouble sleeping soundly because of noise. This is especially the case if you live in a place where wailing car alarms or party-loving neighbours interrupt even the pleasantest of dreams. Worse yet, you may be a very light sleeper, and vulnerable to a host of far less dramatic noises.

Watch the pills and the booze

The quality of your sleep is as important as the number of hours you sleep. A nightcap does little harm, but greater amounts of alcohol (even though they may help you fall asleep) can disturb the quality of your sleep and leave you waking up feeling tired. Sleeping pills have their place, and when used appropriately, they can be very useful. However, routine use of medication for sleeping can quickly become psychologically addictive and often impair sleep itself.

Dealing with bedtime worries

Sometimes distractions are external – noise from the street outside or voices in another room of your house. Sometimes, the noises are internal – racing in your mind. You're worried, upset, angry or otherwise distressed, and this keeps you revved up and awake. You can try several techniques to help you stop this pattern of worry:

- ✔ **Jot it down.** Keep a small pad and pencil near your bed. Jot down the worrisome problem or thought on a piece of paper and decide to yourself that you will work on the problem the next day. This strategy will give you some closure and allow you to leave that little bit of business alone.

- ✔ **Just stop it!** Try something called the *Stop Technique*. Whenever you catch yourself obsessing or ruminatively worrying about something, visualise a large red and white Stop sign. At the same time as you're visualising the Stop sign, silently yell the word stop to yourself. What you'll find is that this temporarily interrupts your worrying. Then replace the worry with a welcome and pleasant thought or image. Keep repeating this process until you have sufficiently broken the worry cycle or have fallen asleep. This technique takes a bit of practice, but it really works.

Sleep tight!

Chapter 2

Recognising How Depression Can Affect You

*W*orldwide research shows that the number of people suffering from depression is increasing alarmingly. Depression is now so common that one in five people suffer from it at some point in their lives. Yet depression's still stigmatised, with sufferers often afraid to tell families and friends, let alone their employer.

Everyone gets overwhelmed sometimes, but when you descend into depression, the level of misery can feel unprecedented. It can take an inordinate effort to admit to the problem and accept help.

In this chapter, we help you recognise the signs of depression and highlight the damaging effect on health. We explore the main types of depression that can affect people at different stages of their life. We also consider how certain drugs and medications can precipitate depression.

Understanding and Overcoming Depression

Depression can feel like being locked away in a prison. Feeling frightened, alone, miserable and powerless, you can find yourself withdrawing into a shell. Hope, faith, relationships, work, play and creative pursuits – the very paths to recovery all seem meaningless and impossible. Like a cruel punishment, depression imprisons the body, mind and soul.

Though depression may feel isolating and inescapable, we have a set of keys for unlocking the prison door. You may find that the first key you try works, but usually the door is double locked and opening it needs a combination of keys. We're here to help, and have a pretty impressive bunch of keys for you to try out, taking you from darkness into the light.

Feeling blue, or depressed?

'For better, for worse; for richer, for poorer; in sickness and in health, 'til death do us part . . .' You may recognise these words from a certain ceremony, dating way back in time. They sum up the inevitability of life's ups and downs, and it's ultimately inescapable end. Even if nothing goes seriously wrong, everyone, sooner or later, is going to die. Expecting to live a life without times of sadness, despair or grief is unrealistic. But experiencing sorrow makes you truly appreciate life's blessings.

Misfortune and loss can cause sadness and grief, but they don't have to lead to depression. The difference is that sadness and grief lessen in intensity as time passes, while depression often does not. Misfortune and loss may feel pretty overwhelming at the time they occur. But time does eventually heal.

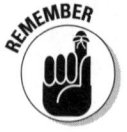

Unlike periods of sadness, depression involves deep despair, misery, guilt and loss of self-esteem. People suffering from depression feel hopeless, helpless, and blame themselves not only for this, but also for just about everything else that goes wrong. Depression disrupts the body's rhythms, often disturbing sleep, appetite, concentration, energy, sexual activity and enjoyment. The net result is that depression seriously reduces your ability to love, laugh, work and play.

Depression is a mood disorder making you feel profoundly sad, without joy, despondent and unable to experience pleasure. Depression appears in a variety of forms, with varying symptoms.

The many faces of depression

Depression can affect anyone regardless of race, social class or status. Symptoms include deep sadness, loss of energy, loss of interests, low self-esteem, feelings of guilt and changes in appetite and sleep. These symptoms are experienced by both men and women, young and old. However, the symptoms of a depressed toddler may be different to those of a depressed 80-year-old.

Here, we show you how to identify depression in different people at different life stages.

Young and depressed

Depression can affect children of any age, from preschool through to young adulthood. Experts agree that the rates of depression in young people have gone up enormously. The rates are probably underreported because children aren't usually able to identify that they're suffering from depression, and parents and professionals often fail to recognise the problem. Parents are sometimes reluctant to accept that their children are depressed. Children can often be unaware of their feelings, or not have the words to describe what they are experiencing. They rarely spontaneously tell others what is happening to them. Instead, they may show changes in their behaviour, appetite and sleep.

When children are depressed they lose interest in activities that they previously enjoyed. If you ask them if they're sad, they may not be able to put their feelings into words. However, children may show signs of depression, such as low energy or motivation, sleep problems, appetite changes, irritability, low self-esteem and self-criticism. They may feel unloved, pessimistic or even hopeless about the future. In fact, depressed children experience more anxiety and physical symptoms than do depressed adults.

Grandparents: Grumpy or depressed?

Some people view old age as inevitably depressing. They assume that the older you get, the greater the deterioration in quality of life. Of course it's true that the longer you live, the more opportunity you have of experiencing negative as well as positive events. And certain illnesses, aches, pains and disabilities do become more likely with increasing age, as do losses of family, friends and social support. Therefore, *some* sadness is to be expected.

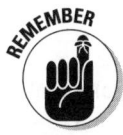

Nonetheless, depression is absolutely *not* an inevitable consequence of old age. Most symptoms of depression in the elderly are identical to those in people of all ages. However, the elderly are more likely to focus on the physical and talk about their aches and pains rather than their feelings of despair. Furthermore, elderly people commonly express regret and remorse about past events in their lives.

Depression interferes with memory. If you notice increased memory problems in Grandpa or Grandma, you likely suspect the worst-case scenario – Alzheimer's disease, otherwise known as dementia. However, these memory problems can often be the result of depression.

And depression in the elderly increases the chances of death. Yet, if you ask elderly people whether they are feeling depressed, they may not recognise their feelings, or may even ridicule the idea. But by denying depression, the older person may not receive the treatment he or she needs.

Men don't do depression, or do they?

Most studies show that men are half as likely as women to report that they get depressed. Men tend to cover up and hide their depression; they feel far more reluctant to talk about what they see as weaknesses and vulnerabilities than women do. Why?

Many men have been taught that admitting to any form of psychological or emotional problem is unmanly. From early childhood experiences, men get to know how to hide such feelings.

Francis looks forward to retirement from his job as a marketing executive. He can't wait to start travelling and having time for all those hobbies he's wanted to take up for ages. Three months into retirement, his wife of 20 years asks for a divorce. Shocked, yet showing little emotion, Francis makes light of his situation to friends and family, saying, 'Oh well! Life goes on.'

But gradually Francis starts drinking more heavily than usual. He becomes interested in extreme sports. He pushes his abilities to the limit in rock climbing, hang-gliding and skiing in remote areas. Francis distances himself from family and friends. His normally even temperament turns sour. Yet Francis denies the depression, so obvious to those who know him well.

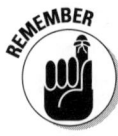

Rather than admit to disturbing feelings, men commonly turn to drugs or alcohol in an attempt to cope. Some depressed men express anger and irritation rather than sadness. Others report the physical signs of depression, such as lack of energy, body aches, changes in sleep and in appetite, but strongly deny feeling depressed. The cost of not expressing feelings and not getting help may account for the four-fold rate of suicide among depressed men compared to women.

Women and depression

Why are women around twice as likely as men to report depression? Biological factors, including those related to reproduction, may play a role. The rates of depression during pregnancy, after childbirth and before the menopause are higher than at any other times in women's lives. Research on women in 2002 found that women who had given birth had a 27 per cent higher rate of depression or anxiety compared to men. For women who had not given birth, 19 per cent were more likely than men to suffer from anxiety and depression.

Cultural and social factors are likely contribute to women's depression. For example, women are more likely than men to have been sexually or physically abused, and such abuse increases the likelihood of depression. Likewise, risk factors such as low income, stress and multiple responsibilities like juggling housework, childcare and a career, occur more frequently in women than men.

Janine gently lays her baby down in the cot. Finally, the little one falls asleep. Exhausted after a tough day at work, Janine desperately longs to go to bed herself. But the washing's piling up, she's got to pay those red bills, and the house is a total tip. Six months ago, her husband changed jobs and became a long-distance lorry driver, and life hasn't been the same since his lengthy absences started. Janine realises her overwhelming fatigue and loss of appetite are quite possibly because she's starting to suffer from depression.

Getting to the root of depression

There are lots of theories about what causes depression. Some experts suggest that depression is caused by imbalances in brain chemistry, while others believe that the chemical imbalances are due to genetics. Others experts are convinced that the cause of depression goes back to childhood. Still others say that depression is a result of negative thinking. There are also those who suggest that depression is caused by impoverished environments and/or cultural experiences. Unwanted patterns of behaviour are also seen as a cause of depression. Finally, some experts have identified relationship problems as the major contributor.

Yet the field of mental health does have both knowledge and ideas about how depression develops. There is strong evidence supporting the theory that education, thinking, biology, genetics, childhood and the environment all play important roles in the development, maintenance and potential treatment of depression. All these factors interact in amazing ways.

For example, a growing body of studies shows that medication alters the physical symptoms of depression such as loss of appetite and energy. And antidepressant medication also improves the negative, pessimistic thinking that accompanies most forms of depression. Perhaps that's not too surprising.

Similarly, studies show that psychotherapy alone decreases negative, pessimistic thinking, much like medication does. Some medical practitioners are shocked to find studies showing that certain psychotherapies, even if carried out without antidepressant medication, also alter brain chemistry.

Overall, recent studies on the roots of depression fail to support any theory that puts forward one specific cause of depression. Rather, they support the idea that a variety of physical and psychological factors interact with each other.

The brain's brew

Your brain contains around 100 billion *neurons* (nerve cells), give or take a few. Busy neurons take in information about the state of the world outside and inside the body. These 100 billion nerve cells don't touch each other. They send information back and forth by releasing tiny molecules which the next nerve picks up. This communication process involves chemical messengers, called *neurotransmitters* that move through and between the neurons.

Depressed people do show changes in the balance of brain chemicals. Several theories have been offered to explain the relationship between depression and the chemical messengers. Many researchers believe that neurotransmitters such as norepinephrine,

serotonin and dopamine play important, interactive roles in mood regulation. Furthermore, these neurotransmitters may interact with other brain chemicals in as yet unknown ways.

What researchers do know is that for some people with depression, the chemical 'soup' may need a different balance of 'spices' or medication. So one person's brain requires a dash of salt (one medication), and for another, pepper (a different medication) may be necessary to lift the depression. But that doesn't necessarily mean that the depression was caused by a lack of pepper or salt, that is, a particular chemical! Experts haven't yet reached agreement on how all this works.

Personal costs of depression

The profound suffering caused by depression affects both the sufferer and the carer. These include:

- ✔ The anguish of a family suffering from the loss of a loved one to suicide.
- ✔ The excruciating pain experienced by someone with depression.
- ✔ The diminished quality of relationships suffered by people with depression and those who care for and about them.
- ✔ The loss of purpose and sense of worth suffered by those with depression.
- ✔ The loss of joy.

The composer, Berlioz, wrote about his fits of depression:

> *The fit fell upon me with appalling force. I suffered agonies and lay groaning on the ground, stretching out abandoned arms, convulsively tearing up handfuls of grass and wide-eyed innocent daisies, struggling against the crushing sense of absence, against a mortal isolation. Yet such an attack is not to be compared with the tortures that I have known since then in ever-increasing measure.*

Detailing depression's physical toll

Depression's destructive effects go beyond personal and economic costs – depression can damage the body itself. Research provides a constant flow of new information about the intricate relationship between mood and health. Today, we know that depression affects:

- ✔ **Your immune system:** Your body has a complex system for warding off infections and diseases. Studies show that depression changes the way the immune system responds to attack. Depression exhausts the immune system and makes people more susceptible to disease.

- ✔ **Your skeletal system:** Untreated depression increases your chances of getting osteoporosis, though it's unclear exactly how depression may lead to this problem.

- ✔ **Your heart:** The relationship between depression and cardiovascular disease is powerful. Johns Hopkins University studied healthy doctors and found that among those doctors who developed depression, their risk of heart disease increased two-fold. This risk is comparable to the risk posed by smoking. Likewise for those with heart problems, having depression doubled the chance of having another heart attack.

- ✔ **Your mind:** Although depression can mimic dementia in terms of causing poor memory and concentration, depression also increases the risk for dementia. We're not sure why, but scientists have discovered that an area in the brain thought to govern memory is smaller in those with chronic depression. If left untreated, depression can disrupt and possibly damage connections in your brain and may lead to the degeneration and death of brain cells.

- ✔ **Your experience of pain:** Depression contributes to the experience of physical pain. Thus, if you have some type of chronic pain, such as arthritis or back pain, depression may increase the amount of pain you feel. Scientists aren't entirely sure how depression and pain interact, but the effect may be due to disruption of neurotransmitters involved in pain perception. Many people with depression fail to realise they're depressed and only complain about a variety of physical symptoms such as pain.

Depression seems to affect everything about the way the whole body functions. For example, altered appetite may lead to obesity, or to under nourishment and serious weight loss. Also, depression is associated with disrupted hormonal levels and various other subtle physiological changes.

Examining the Six Types of Depression

In this section, we turn our attention to the six major types of depression to look out for:

- ✔ Major depressive disorder
- ✔ Dysthymic disorder
- ✔ Adjustment disorder with depressed mood
- ✔ Bipolar disorder
- ✔ Seasonal affective disorder
- ✔ Depression related to hormones

Major depressive disorder: Can't even get out of bed

Major depressive disorders include a seriously low mood or a notable drop in pleasures and interests lasting for two weeks or more. Sometimes depressed people deny these low feelings and any loss of interest – on purpose, or without being aware of it. However, despite the denial people who know the depressed person well can usually spot the difference.

As well as low mood and lack of pleasure, to qualify as experiencing a major depressive disorder, you usually have a wide variety of other symptoms, such as:

- ✔ Clear signs of increased agitation or slowed functioning
- ✔ Extreme fatigue
- ✔ Inability to concentrate or make decisions
- ✔ Intense feelings of guilt and self-blame
- ✔ Major changes in sleep patterns
- ✔ Repetitive thoughts of suicide
- ✔ Striking changes in appetite or weight (an increase or decrease)
- ✔ Very low sense of personal worth

With major depressive disorders, these symptoms occur almost every day over a period of at least two weeks or more. Major depressive disorders vary greatly in terms of severity. However, even mild cases of major depressive disorder need treatment.

If you're suffering from an episode of severe major depressive disorder, just how low you feel is difficult for someone who has never had the same experience to imagine. A severe, major episode of depression takes over a person's life and slowly destroys all pleasure. But it does far more than wipe out joy; severe depression can make you feel that you are at the bottom of an unscalable pit of utter, unrelenting despair that stops you from showing and even feeling love. People caught in such a pit of depression lose the ability to care for themselves, others and even life itself.

If you suffer from such a severe case of depression, there's definitely good reason for hope. Many effective treatments work even with severe depression. So no matter how low and hopeless you feel – do get help.

Major depressive disorders can significantly reduce your ability to function at work or deal with other people. Such disorders deprive you of the very resources you need for recovery. That's why getting help is so important. If you allow the major depressive disorder to continue, it may result in death from suicide. If you or someone you know *even suspects* the presence of a major depressive disorder, you need to seek help promptly.

Dysthymic disorder: Chronic, low-level depression

Dysthymic disorder, or *dysthymia*, is similar to major depressive disorder (see the previous section). However, dysthymic disorder is less severe, tends to be chronic, and persists for longer periods of time. With dysthymic disorder, the symptoms occur for at least two years (though often for far longer), with the depressed mood obvious on most days for the majority of each day. However, you only need to display two of the following chronic symptoms, as well as a depressed mood, in order for your condition to qualify as a dysthymic disorder:

- ✔ Guilty feelings
- ✔ Low sense of personal worth
- ✔ Poor concentration
- ✔ Problems making decisions
- ✔ Thoughts of death or suicide

Compared with major depressive disorder, dysthymic disorder displays fewer physical symptoms such as problems with appetite, weight, sleep and agitation.

Dysthymic disorder frequently begins in childhood, adolescence or young adulthood and can easily continue for many years if left untreated. Also, people with dysthymic disorder are at an increased risk of developing a major depressive disorder at some point in their lives.

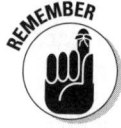

Although someone with dysthymic disorder generally isn't as devastatingly despondent as a person with a major depressive disorder, they are frequently lacking in energy and the joy of living. A person suffering from dysthymic disorder isn't always easy to identify, but they are noticeable for being pessimistic, cynical and grouchy a good deal of the time.

People with dysthymic disorder often see their problems as merely 'just the way they are', and so don't look for treatment. If you suspect that you or someone you care about has dysthymic disorder, get help. You have the right to feel better than you do, and the long-lasting nature of the problem means that it isn't likely to go away on its own. Besides, you certainly don't want to risk developing a major depressive disorder, which is even more debilitating.

Adjustment disorder with depressed mood: Reactive depression

Life's road isn't always easy. You have to expect the rough with the smooth. Most of the time, people handle their problems without extreme emotional upset. At other times, they don't.

Adjustment disorders are reactions to one or more difficult issues, such as marital problems, financial setbacks, conflict with colleagues, and traumatic events including natural disasters. When a stressful event occurs and your reaction lessens your ability to work or participate effectively with others, in combination with symptoms such as a low mood, crying spells and feelings of worthlessness or hopelessness, you may be experiencing an adjustment disorder with a depressed mood. Adjustment disorder is a much milder problem than a major depressive disorder, but it can still disrupt your life.

People suffering from an adjustment disorder with depressed mood quite often don't seek treatment. They assume if they wait long enough, the problem will just go away by itself. However, if you suspect that you or someone you care about has this problem, do get help. Otherwise you may still have difficulties long after the original triggering problem is resolved, and these can become a major problem for you and those around you.

Bipolar disorder: Ups and downs

Bipolar disorder is a mood disorder, just like other forms of depression. However, bipolar disorder is quite different from other types of depression because people with a bipolar disorder can experience episodes of irrational 'highs', called *mania*.

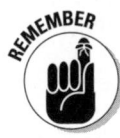

In bipolar disorder, moods fluctuate between extreme highs and lows. This makes the treatment of bipolar disorder different from other types of depression. We want you to be familiar with the symptoms so that you can seek professional help if you experience manic episodes within your depression. Self-help isn't sufficient for the treatment of bipolar disorder.

Although individuals with mania may seem quite cheerful and happy, the people who know them can tell that their good mood is a little too good to be true. During manic episodes, people feel they need less sleep, may show signs of unusual creativity, and have loads more energy and enthusiasm. Sounds pretty good, doesn't it? Who wouldn't want to feel wonderful and totally on top of the world? Well, just hold your horses . . .

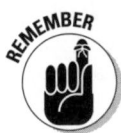

The problem with manic episodes related to bipolar disorder is that the 'highs' increase to a level where the person loses touch with reality. During manic episodes, sound judgement goes out the window. People who have bipolar disorder disorder often:

- ✔ Engage in risky sexual escapades
- ✔ Gamble excessively
- ✔ Make foolish business decisions
- ✔ Spend too much money, and get into serious debt
- ✔ Talk fast and furiously
- ✔ Think that they have super-special talents or abilities

Manic episodes can involve mildly unwise decisions and excesses, or reach extremes. People in manic states can cause ruin for themselves or their families. Their behaviour can get so out of control that they may seek hospital treatment and a period of inpatient care. Alternatively, they may be sectioned – detained in hospital under certain sections of the Mental Health Act at the request of the authorities, or their closest relative.

Most people with bipolar disorder also go through cycles of mild to severe depression. They go from feeling great to gruesome, sometimes during the same day. The depression that follows a manic episode can be unexpected and devastating. The contrast from the high to the low is particularly painful. People with untreated bipolar disorder typically feel out of control, hopeless and helpless. Not surprisingly, the risk of suicide is higher for bipolar disorder than for any of the other type of depression.

Bipolar disorder is generally *chronic* (lasts for a long time), but if you're diagnosed as having bipolar disorder, don't despair. The condition can be successfully managed. Medication and psychotherapy, usually in combination, can ease a lot of the most debilitating symptoms. Research is also finding new treatments and medication.

Bipolar disorder is a complicated and serious illness. The condition has many subtle variations. If you suspect that you or someone you know has any signs of bipolar disorder, seek professional help at once.

Seasonal affective disorder: Dark depression

Some depressions come and go with the seasons, as regularly as clockwork. People who repeatedly experience depression during autumn or winter may have *seasonal affective disorder* (SAD). They may also experience a few unusual symptoms, such as:

- A sense of heaviness in the arms and legs
- Carbohydrate cravings
- Increased appetite
- Increased desire for sleep
- Irritability

What does a bear do to get ready for winter? Bears energetically forage for food, get as fat as they can, and then hibernate in a cosy cave. Perhaps it's not a coincidence that people with SAD typically gain weight, crave carbohydrates, have reduced energy, and feel like staying snuggled in bed for the winter.

SAD is increasingly being recognised, and a variety of treatments are available, some with more scientific backing and evidence than others. Research is also finding new treatments and medication. Taking a walk outside to experience more natural light may be helpful – and certainly can't hurt.

Premenstrual dysphoric disorder and postnatal depression: Horrible hormones?

Occasional, minor premenstrual changes in mood occur in a majority of women. A smaller percentage of women experience significant and disturbing symptoms known as *premenstrual dysphoric disorder* (PDD). PDD is a more extreme form of the more widely known premenstrual syndrome (PMS) or premenstrual tension (PMT).

Although hormones probably play a significant role in PDD, research hasn't yet explained the causes. Women suffering from full-blown PDD experience some of the following symptoms almost every month, during the week before their period. (These same symptoms can also occur – probably because of hormonal fluctuations – in the years leading up to, during and following menopause.)

✔ Anger

✔ Anxiety

✔ Bloating

✔ Fatigue

✔ Food cravings

✔ Guilt and self-blame

✔ Irritability

✔ Sadness

✔ Tearfulness

✔ Withdrawal

Postnatal depression is another type of serious mood disorder that's widely thought to be related to hormonal fluctuations, although no one knows for sure how and why the hormones profoundly affect the moods of some women and not others. This depression occurs within days or weeks after giving birth. The symptoms appear quite similar to those of major depressive disorder. (For a complete discussion of these symptoms, see 'Major depressive disorder: Can't even get out of bed', earlier in this chapter.)

Faith had tried unsuccessfully to conceive for the past eight years. She and her husband Sean are overwhelmed with joy when at last the home pregnancy test registers positive. Their cheerful, cosy nursery looks like a picture in a baby magazine, only better, because it's theirs.

Faith and Sean weep with happiness at the sight of their newborn. Faith feels exhausted, but Sean assumes that's normal. He takes charge the first day home so that she can rest. Faith feels the same way the next day, so Sean continues to take over the responsibilities of caring for the baby. Sean becomes alarmed when Faith shows no interest in holding the baby. In fact, she seems irritated by the baby's crying and mentions that maybe she shouldn't have become a mother. At the end of the second week, Faith tells Sean that he can't go back to work because she doesn't think that she can take care of the baby. Faith is suffering from postnatal depression.

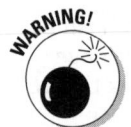

Most women feel a bit low shortly after delivery – it's called the 'baby blues'. The down feelings aren't usually severe and they tend to go within two weeks. However, if you begin to feel like Faith, you need to get professional help immediately.

Linking Drugs, Diseases and Depression

The interaction of depression with illness and disease can form a vicious cycle. Illness and disease (and related medications) can hasten the onset or intensify the effects of depression. And depression can further complicate the various diseases. Depression can suppress the immune system, release stress hormones, and affect your body and mind's capacity to cope. Depression may increase whatever pain you have and further diminish your crucial resources. In this section, we focus on the role of medication and illness in the development and worsening of depression.

Drugs with depressive side effects

Dealing with an illness is hard enough without having the medication make you feel even worse. Some medication can actually appear to cause depression. Of course, recognising whether it's merely the experience of the illness, or if it's the drug that's causing the depression is difficult. However, in a number of cases, medication does appear to contribute directly to depression.

If you notice inexplicable feelings of sadness shortly after starting a new prescription, tell your doctor. The medication could be causing your feelings, and an alternative treatment that won't affect you in this way may be available. Table 2-1 lists the most common medications that have potential depressive side effects.

Table 2-1	Potentially Depressing Drugs
Medication	*Condition Typically Prescribed For*
Antabuse	Alcohol addiction
Anticonvulsants	Seizures
Barbiturates	Seizures and (rarely) anxiety
Benzodiazepines	Anxiety and insomnia
Beta blockers	High blood pressure and heart problems
Calcium channel blockers	High blood pressure and heart problems
Corticosteroids	Inflammation and chronic lung diseases
Hormones	Birth control and menopausal symptoms
Interferon	Hepatitis and certain cancers
Levodopa, amantadine	Parkinson's disease
Statins	High cholesterol
Zovirax	Herpes or shingles

Depression-inducing illnesses

Chronic illnesses interfere with life. Some chronic illnesses require lifestyle adjustments, frequent GP and hospital appointments, and time off work. These illnesses disrupt relationships, and cause physical pain. Feeling upset by such things is normal. But these problems may trigger depression, especially in vulnerable people.

Also, some illnesses can disrupt the nervous system in ways that cause depression. If you suffer from one of these diseases, talk to your doctor, especially if you find your mood begins to deteriorate. Diseases that are thought to directly influence depression include:

- AIDS
- Asthma
- Cancer
- Chronic fatigue syndrome
- Coronary artery disease and heart attacks
- Diabetes

- ✔ Hepatitis
- ✔ Lupus
- ✔ Multiple sclerosis
- ✔ Parkinson's disease
- ✔ Stroke
- ✔ Ulcerative colitis

Discovering the Distorting Perceptions Behind Depression

Everyone views the world from different perspectives, which we call *life-lenses*. As you look at your world through your life-lenses, they filter what you see. The correct lenses can make your view clearer, but others distort what you see. Lenses can be clear, grey, cloudy, rose-tinted, cracked, dirty, or distorted.

Introducing the problematic life-lenses

Most people don't realise that they look at their world through life-lenses, and they're usually quite unaware of precisely which ones their minds use.

The potential list of possible life-lenses is long. But working with people suffering from depression we have found that there are 12 life-lenses which cause particular problems. Our list covers most of the problematic issues dealt with by mental health professionals.

- ✔ **Entitled:** A perspective that you always deserve the best and you feel outraged when your needs go unmet
- ✔ **Guilty:** A pervasive sense that you inevitably, usually unwittingly, do the wrong thing, and you deserve punishment for this
- ✔ **Inadequate:** A sense that you lack important skills, abilities, or other vital qualities
- ✔ **Inferior:** Viewing yourself as insignificant and less important than others

✔ **Intimacy avoidant:** You don't like getting close to people

✔ **Invulnerable:** No recognition of the need to take special care because you believe you can come to no harm

✔ **Without conscience:** Shameless disregard for ethics and morality

✔ **Perfectionistic:** A belief that you can and *should* do everything perfectly

✔ **Scared of abandonment:** Worry that people you care about plan to leave you

✔ **Superior:** The view that you are far better than others

✔ **Unworthy:** A sense that you don't deserve good things, or to have good things happening to you

✔ **Vulnerable:** A belief that the world is a dangerous place, and you are at imminent risk of coming to harm

Seeing the world through cracked life-lenses

Now, to show you precisely how these lenses operate, here's an example of how viewing the *exact same event* through different lenses leads to totally contrasting thoughts and feelings.

Imagine you're giving a presentation to a group of colleagues. You feel slightly nervous at the start, but quickly relax and gain confidence as you get your point across. After the talk, a colleague comments, 'I noticed you were a little nervous up there.'

Depending on your particular life-lens or perspective, your reaction to the comment may lead to very different thoughts and feelings. Table 2-2 illustrates how these lenses work.

In Table 2-2, you may notice that the final lens, 'good enough,' wasn't on the list of problematic lenses listed earlier. If so, you observed correctly. That's because some lenses are not distorted, or 'cracked' and do give a clear view of yourself and the world. We discuss clear lenses in the section on 'Seeing clearly: Replacing the distorting lenses' later in this chapter.

Table 2-2	How Life-Lenses Lead to Contrasting Thoughts and Feelings	

Event: You give a talk, and a friend says that you looked a little nervous.

Life-Lens: Definition	Thoughts (or Interpretations)	Resulting Feelings
Inadequate: I'm not very bright or good at anything.	I'm never going to be a good speaker. I shouldn't even try. Everyone thinks I'm a twit and an idiot. How stupid can I be?	Shame Despair
Scared of abandonment: I really worry about whether people like and approve of me. Eventually, everyone leaves.	My friend won't want to associate with me any more. No one else is going to, either.	Worry Anxiety Isolation
Superior: I'm better than others and therefore I look down on them.	My so-called friend is trying to undermine me! Who is he to say something like that? As if he could do any better. I never thought much of him anyway.	Anger Rage
Good enough: I know and accept that I have both strengths and weaknesses. I like to do well, but I can learn from mistakes too.	My friend is right; I did feel nervous, and it probably did show a bit. I don't particularly like looking nervous, but I'm sure I can improve my performance with practice.	Mild, Short-lived Distress Optimism

Same event, different perspectives. When viewing life through various lenses, people can't help but see starkly contrasting pictures. This process explains why people have such conflicting thoughts and feelings when facing the same situations.

For example, Lionel's life-lens, of seeing himself as inferior, causes him to have a multitude of thoughts, which in practice actually do him a disservice in a variety of different situations. At parties, he has thoughts about how poorly others regard him, so he tries to blend into the background. At work, he fails to put himself forward for promotion because he doesn't rate his own abilities, and also thinks that others at his level are loads better than him. At the neighbourhood association meetings, he's loath to participate, because he assumes that no one is going to take him, or his ideas, seriously. Though his thoughts in each situation are different, they all relate to his one lens, the perspective that he's inferior to others.

Finding self-forgiveness

Finding self-forgiveness is a crucial step that ultimately leads to removing and replacing your distorted life-lenses. All too often, people beat themselves up for having distorted perspectives. Punishing yourself merely drains you of much needed energy for making difficult changes. It's like running a race and hitting yourself on the head with a hammer at the same time because you haven't yet reached the finishing line.

Focus on what you can do about future changes rather than beating yourself up over a past that you can't change.

Separating then from now

Your life-lenses are largely shaped by emotionally intense events in child-hood. As an adult, when you look at current life experiences, the lens makes you see occurrences from the perspective of childhood events, as if they are now happening all over again. You may find it useful to compare and contrast the events triggering your problematic life-lens with how you viewed the world in your childhood. When you do, take into account that your reaction probably has more to do with events from long ago than with what's happening now.

Carrying out a cost/benefit analysis

Many people would be willing to change their problematic lenses sooner than they do, but are held back because they believe the lenses protect or benefit them in some way. At first sight, you may think that idea sounds unlikely. For example, why is someone going to think that feeling unworthy is in any way beneficial?

One of the reasons life-lenses feel beneficial is that people believe in the view, and they fear the consequences which may arise if they discard the lens.

Here are a few of illustrations of how such concerns play out for several different lenses:

> ✔ **Entitled:** Someone with this lens fears that if they give up feeling entitled to everything they want and need, this means that they're not going to get what they want.

- ✔ **Inadequate:** If a person with this lens decides that he is in no way inadequate, but is the equal of others, he may start taking risks, such as volunteering to lead a project at work. But he doesn't do so because he's absolutely convinced that his inadequacy lens is true, and if he does volunteer, that he's going to fail miserably if he tries to discard the view of inadequacy.

- ✔ **Superior:** A person who feels that he stands far above others fears that letting go of this lens is going to cause him to be seen as the opposite – totally inferior to others.

- ✔ **Unworthy:** If a woman with this lens decides to discard it and believe that she's truly worthy of good things, she's likely to fear that others may see her as outrageously greedy and self-centred because, she believes that others really do know that she doesn't deserve those things.

We suggest that you carry out a careful cost/benefit analysis of each problematic life-lens that distresses you.

Seeing clearly: Replacing the distorting lenses

If you've reached the point where you know that your old, distorted lenses aren't doing you much good, then now's the time to try out some new ones. When you look for new lenses, giving them a new name – one that's more flexible and balanced – is helpful. For example, instead of *inferior* or *superior,* you can design a lens you call 'equal to others.' Or instead of *invulnerable* or *vulnerable,* you may come up with a lens you call 'reasonably cautious.'

Hold on to the fact that the process of removing and replacing old lenses isn't quick or easy. The good news is that you can succeed with patience and hard work.

You need to proceed with care and attention because acting against the distorted perspective you've been seeing through your lenses is like being in a foreign country where you are driving on the opposite side of the road. The ingrained, habitual side of your mind says to drive on the left, and the clear-headed, adaptive side says to drive on the right. Preventing the old habit from automatically taking back control means keeping your mind on the task – no doubt you or some one you know has had experience of driving in Europe!

We have four separate strategies that are likely to help you remember which side of the road to stay on. Remember to drive slowly and watch the road signs. You may find that one of these strategies works for you, or you may find it helpful to use two, three, or even all four.

Chapter 3

Discovering Techniques to Overcome Depression

Depression affects people in different ways. It can drain your energy and distort your thinking, causing you to have a pessimistic, bleak outlook. In this chapter we help you on your journey to feeling good again by helping to untangle your thinking by monitoring your thoughts and feelings. We consider techniques to combat lapses in memory, help you see the benefits of taking exercise and alter any negative thoughts to reduce the risk of relapse.

Feeling Good Again

Depression is treatable. With good diagnosis and the right help, most people can expect to recover. If you feel a loss of pleasure, reduced energy, a diminished sense of your worth, or unexplained aches and pains, you may be depressed (see Book V Chapter 2 for more information about the symptoms of depression).

Many types of help exist for depression. This book is one of them and falls under the category of self-help. Self-help does work for many people. However, self-directed efforts may not be enough for everyone. In the following sections, we briefly outline the different kinds of help that you may find useful.

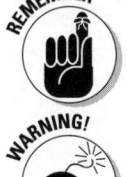

You don't have to choose just one option. You may need or want to combine a number of these strategies. For example, many people with depression find the combination of medication and psychotherapy helpful. And using more than one type of psychotherapy, usually completing one type before starting the next, can prove useful as well.

If your depression doesn't start to lift or if you have severe symptoms such as thoughts of suicide, please seek professional help.

Seeing Things More Clearly: Cognitive Therapy

Cognitive therapy, and the later development of cognitive behavioural therapy, are by far the most widely researched psychological treatments for depression. Studies repeatedly show that cognitive therapy lifts depression and reduces relapse.

Cognitive therapy is one of the psychological therapies. All psychological therapies involve working on your own, or with a therapist using psychological techniques to reduce emotional problems. Cognitive therapy primarily uses techniques designed to change your way of thinking, making you feel better.

A major idea underpinning cognitive therapy is the interconnected nature of feelings (which we also refer to as emotions) and thoughts. Thoughts strongly influence feelings, and vice versa. Both play an important role in the development and maintenance of depression.

But the story doesn't end there. Physical factors can also play a role in depression. Factors such as fatigue, illness, and changes in blood chemistry can lower your mood, which, in turn, prepares the ground for the development of depressing thoughts.

For example, Colin tosses and turns through a third night. He's not sure what's causing his recent bout of insomnia, but every time he feels he's about to fall asleep, another part of his body itches, or his position becomes uncomfortable. Colin's day begins with a long rush-hour drive; irritability overtakes his usual calm acceptance. His tiredness worsens his growing worry. He starts to think, 'What's wrong with me? I'm not going to be able to get through another day. I feel awful. I can't focus. I'm going to lose my job.'

Colin's thoughts have begun to spiral downwards. Why? Too many consecutive nights of poor sleep bring on fatigue and accompanying negative thoughts. One good night of sleep just may allow Colin to return to normal.

Or not. Sometimes, a physical event can start a train of negative thoughts and feelings that may then hang around for quite a while.

No one knows how to determine which of the three ingredients (feelings, thoughts, or physical factors) triggers depression for any particular person. But the good news is that you can interrupt the cycle of depression in various ways, using cognitive therapy, no matter what started the downward spiral. The goal of cognitive therapy is to help you be fully aware of your negative thinking when it occurs, and then to actively reframe those thoughts into more realistic terms. After you've done so over a period of time, your depression is likely to lift.

Monitoring thoughts and feelings, and relating them to life events

A core element of cognitive therapy involves increasing your awareness of the links between thoughts, feelings, and events in your life. In this section, we show you how to become aware of your feelings about events and to examine the thoughts that go with them.

Some people genuinely are hardly aware of their feelings. Others have difficulty detecting their thoughts. We help you to recognise and identify feelings, and we explain how to work out what you're thinking. You may think that you already know what your feelings and thoughts are, but they aren't always that obvious. After you've got the hang of clearly identifying feelings and thoughts, you can then see the links between your thoughts, feelings, and the events that lead to them, plus keep track of them using a 'Thought Catcher'.

Designing your Thought Catcher

You can use the Thought Catcher when you experience troubling feelings. It can help you follow through and understand the connections between your thoughts, feelings, and the events that trigger them. Also, the Thought Catcher can help you become more aware of the types of events that bother you and prepare you to confront and overcome any problematic thoughts.

Start a new page in your notebook, and divide it into three columns. In each column, fill in the following information (see Table 3-1 for a sample):

✔ **Feelings:** Use this first column to write down negative feelings (not thoughts) and rate them on a 1 (very mild) to 100 (extremely severe) scale. People often notice their feelings before anything else, even though thoughts have usually preceded the feelings, so focus first on what you're feeling. Sometimes you notice yourself experiencing more than one feeling. Record all the unpleasant feelings - they are the key to what depression is all about.

✔ **Events:** Use the second column to write down the event that preceded or triggered the feeling. Such events are usually things that happen to a person, but sometimes they involve a daydream or image that floats into the mind. If you notice the event before you become aware of the feeling, feel free to fill out the event first. But events do precede feelings. So if you become aware of any feelings, stop and ask yourself what happened just before. Only occasionally is the feeling going to emerge more than half an hour after the event. In most cases, the feeling arises almost immediately.

When writing down the event, try to be as specific as possible: Include where you were, who was there, and what happened.

✔ **Negative Automatic Thoughts (NATS):** Use the third column to record the thoughts or interpretations you have about the event – , your understanding of what happened. These thoughts generally occur automatically without careful, conscious reflection, and are usually negative in some way, which is why they are called Negative Automatic Thoughts. Be sure to take time and reflect on the whole range of reactions and interpretations you have.

Sometimes you'll have slightly different thoughts relating to different feelings, but which all stem from the same event. Look at the thoughts you have that relate to each feeling. For example, if you recently got promoted and your new boss asks you to immediately complete and deliver the report you've been painstakingly working on, you may have feelings of both anxiety and despair. The anxiety-related thoughts may centre on concerns of being told off if you don't finish on time, and despair-related thoughts may focus on the belief that you're overwhelmingly inadequate to handle the new promotion.

Here's an example of how the Thought Catcher works. Gita is a software engineer. She's a bit of a perfectionist, which adds further stress to her already highly demanding job. When one of the computer programs she's working on repeatedly crashes, Gita too crashes. She can't sleep; she can't eat; and thoughts of suicide enter her mind. Gita confides her despair to a close friend who strongly urges her to see a therapist. Gita protests at first, but her friend insists.

Her therapist suggests that Gita constructs a Thought Catcher, allowing her to catch her thoughts whenever she finds herself feeling down. Take a look at Table 3-1 to see what Gita comes up with.

Table 3-1	Gita's Thought Catcher	
Feelings (0 to 100)	**Events**	**Negative Automatic Thoughts (or Interpretations)**
Despair (80)	The computer program I'm working on crashed again.	My boss is going to find out that I don't know what I'm doing and fire me.
Helplessness (95)		I'm never going to be able to solve this.

You can see how Gita's thoughts contribute to her low feelings and overall depression. We suggest you fill out a Thought Catcher for about a week. Try to catch in your net at least one or two problematic events each day. After finishing this task, you're ready to tackle the thoughts that lead to your depression.

Catching negative thoughts

It's important to capture any suspiciously negative thought, before you can put it on trial. Think of a time when you felt strong negative feelings such as sadness, despair, guilt, or shame. Where did these feelings begin? A Thought Catcher can tell you by uncovering the links between events, thoughts, and feelings. A Thought Catcher shows you that most of the time, your unpleasant emotions come from the thoughts or interpretations you make in response to events that have happened to you.

To understand the relationship between thoughts, feelings, and events, you need to record your thoughts, plus the events that occurred before them, and also the feelings that followed. Rating the intensity of those feelings in order to find out just how much your thoughts are disturbing you is also a good idea.

Unearthing distortions in thinking

Cognitive therapy uses the well-established idea that certain thoughts you have in response to events lead to depressed feelings (see the previous section 'Monitoring Thoughts and Feelings, and Relating Them to Life Events'). Now we show you that those thoughts are almost always distorted. By *distorted*, we mean that these thoughts don't accurately reflect, predict, or describe events. In this section, we help you analyse your thoughts in order to identify these distortions. In doing so, you can start clearing your vision and see your world in more accurate terms.

By asking you to examine your thoughts and to look for various types of distortions, we are *not* trying to get you to rationalise away everything bad that happens to you. The goal of cognitive therapy is to show you how to identify, reflect upon, and weigh up your distorted thoughts in order to later rework them in such a way that they match reality. When reality is really awful, we don't expect or want you to deny that fact. Rather, we want you to cope when events turn out contrary to your hopes.

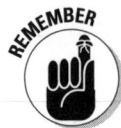

You may find it helpful to know that people with depression aren't the only ones to have distorted thinking. Every person has, at times, significantly distorted thoughts. Depression merely makes these distortions more frequent and intense. Even those who aren't especially depressed can probably benefit from using our strategies for reducing such distortions. And if you're depressed, discovering new ways of thinking may lead to a far happier life.

The mind's seven misleading misperceptions

Everyone distorts reality from time to time. Depressed people just do it more often and to a greater depth, and they find the distortions more credible. In the following list, we review common ways in which your mind can distort reality. See if you can recognise any of the following tricks your mind has tried to play on you.

- **Maximising and minimising:** Your mind uses this distortion to *catastrophise*, or magnify, the importance or 'awfulness' of unpleasant events. This distortion of maximising is also known as *catastrophising*. In a similar fashion, the mind minimises the value and importance of anything positive about yourself, your world, or your future.

- **Filtering:** The depressed mind typically focuses on any dismal, dark data while screening out more positive information. The not-too-surprising result? Both the world, and even you, appear miserable and hopeless.

- **Seeing in black and white, all-or-nothing terms:** This distortion puts everything – you, other people, and even events – into stark terms, with no shades of grey. Thus, a single poor performance is taken to mean complete and utter inadequacy. The problem with polarised thinking is that it sets you up for inevitably experiencing a sense of total failure, disappointment, and self-criticism. All-or-none thinking imposes standards that absolutely no one can ever achieve.

- **Dismissing evidence:** This distortion looks at evidence that may contradict the mind's negative thoughts and dismisses that evidence as not allowable and/or completely irrelevant. For example, suppose you have the thought that you're a failure. Then your boss says that you've earned a promotion for your performance. Your mind may quickly decide that the promotion was both undeserved and meaningless, and that your failure runs much deeper than mere job performance. This misperception is rather like being accused of a crime, and then having the judge throw out as irrelevant every single piece of evidence that proves your innocence. Bet you can guess the verdict. In this case, it's your own mind that throws out the evidence and determines the verdict.

✔ **Discarding positives:** Similar to dismissing evidence, minimising the positive is a distortion the mind uses to trivialise successes, good outcomes, and positive personal attributes and achievements. So if you're successful in your audition for the lead in a play, you decide that this has to be because the drama group is so desperate and of such a poor standard that they welcome with open arms anyone with minimal talent!

✔ **Overgeneralising:** This involves looking at a single, unpleasant occurrence and deciding it represents the way things are, and are always going to be. Thus, if you drop your fork on the floor, your mind tells you that you're a clumsy clot who's *always* dropping things. Words like *always* and *never* are tip-offs to this reality distortion.

✔ **Mind-reading:** Mind-reading occurs whenever you assume, often with unshakable conviction, that you *know* what others are thinking, without checking it out. Thus, someone may not ask out a new acquaintance because, 'I just know she wouldn't go out with someone like me.'

Amending Your Memory

When you're depressed you can feel awful. Your sleep may be disturbed, your appetite practically non-existant, and nothing seems like fun any more. You may also find that your memory is impaired; you may not be able to remember names, dates or shopping lists.

Depression and memory impairment often go hand in hand, but the good news is that when your depression lifts, your memory is likely to improve. In the meantime, there are a number of techniques for making your memory perform better, which may in turn lift your spirits. In this section we show you the ways depression can wear you down and disrupt your memory. We also give you some strategies for dealing with memory problems and boosting your memory skills.

Depressing disruptions

Depression fills you with sadness. Your ability to think clearly can be clouded by feelings of hopelessness, helplessness, guilt, and low self-esteem. But depression also affects your ability to think clearly by having a negative influence on all aspects of your memory. In the following list, we describe the ways that depression affects each aspect of memory.

✔ **Immediate memory:** Depression decreases your ability to pay attention to what's going on around you; you may not even notice important information. Things that you normally pay attention to may just slip by.

✔ **Working memory:** Depression disrupts your ability to concentrate and hold onto information. Your problem-solving ability sharply declines.

✔ **Long-term memory:** Depression makes acquiring new information much harder. Tasks such as studying for an exam can become extremely difficult. Concentrating is more difficult, and the information just doesn't seem to stick. Information refuses to be properly filed into the memory's retrieval storage system – your long-term memory.

✔ **Retrieval:** Depression makes recalling information like dates or doing the shopping without making a list more difficult. Previously known names, faces, and facts are harder to remember. Happy events are particularly difficult to recall. When you're depressed, you're more likely to come up with sad and depressing memories, because depression floods your brain with negative memories. You may actually have trouble remembering whole periods in your life when you were happy.

Forgiving forgetfulness

When you experience memory problems as a result of depression, worrying about these problems may deepen your depression, adding to your forgetfulness. If you're depressed, don't be too surprised if you forget where you parked your car, can't remember a specific word or someone's name, or if you misplace everyday items. Getting upset about minor memory problems can easily make you even more depressed.

Assisting your ailing memory

If you're depressed, you probably don't have lots of enthusiasm for any strenuous exercise that can help improve your memory. So here are some quick, simple tips and techniques to help you cope until your depression lifts and your memory improves.

Putting pen to paper

Acknowledging that you have a problem with your memory, and then taking steps to work on it is a great start. Keep a daily planner next to you at all times, and make sure that you use it. Write down everything you need to remember. List your appointments, what you need from the shops, names of people you recently met, and things you want to get done. Check your daily planner often.

Developing routines

Picture the scene: You finally managed to force yourself to do some shopping, and now you're absolutely shattered. You push your shopping trolley out of the supermarket exit and, suddenly, you can't remember where you parked. You feel such a fool, and are ready to burst into tears. This situation can happen to anyone. But when you're depressed absentmindedness becomes more of a problem, making you feel even more awful, and it can give you yet another reason for feeling bad about yourself.

Try this way of getting round this type of situation. Every time you go shopping, try to park regularly at the end of the row, to either the right or left of the entrance. Alternatively, always choose a particular place on the top floor of the car park, which is usually the least crowded. If you have a favourite shopping centre or supermarket, take some time to select a rarely used space. Park there, even when other spaces nearer the entrance are free. Parking in the same spot increases your chance of remembering where you left the car. It also has the additional benefit of making you walk a little further, by choosing a spot some way from the entrance (see the later section 'Exercising to Lift Depression' for information about the benefits of exercise for depression).

Smelling (and touching and seeing) the roses

Most people experience the world through sight, sound, touch, smell, and taste. Memory experts have discovered that when you use more than one sense, your ability to remember something improves. For example, when you listen to several instructions, you're more likely to remember them if you also see them in writing and then write them down yourself.

When you need to remember something, try to experience it with as many senses as possible. For example, if you want to remember the address '10 Greene Street', picture ten people mowing grass beside a residential road. Using both the image and the smell of the green grass helps plant the address in your memory.

You can also use a familiar melody to help you remember information – just like children do when learning the alphabet. Just change the lyrics of a song to include the information you want remember. But don't forget, one of the very best ways to remember something is to write it down. Writing and singing involve using more than one of your senses.

Remembering names

Are you having difficulty in remembering names? Do you forget someone's name only seconds after being introduced? If so, try this: next time you're introduced to someone, use their name at least three times when you have another conversation with the person. 'Hi, Ryan, nice to meet you, Ryan. So, do you live locally, Ryan?'

Try looking directly at the person and taking a mental photograph. As you make eye contact, use the person's name again in conversation. When you turn away, picture the person's name, face, and anything interesting you discovered about them. Repeat the name to yourself several more times, and then go and write it down on the daily planner or key it into your personal organiser (see the earlier section 'Putting pen to paper').

Biting off no more than you can chew

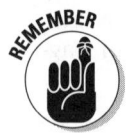

Chunking involves grouping or organising large amounts of information into small units. Doing so greatly helps your memory. Here's an example of how chunking works.

First, read the following numbers and then close your eyes and try to remember them.

632895745

You may find this exercise is difficult. An excellent technique for remembering strings of unrelated numbers is to put them together in shorter units or chunks. Now read the following numbers and then close your eyes and repeat them.

554–759–823

Did you do a little better this time? Your brain, and immediate memory in particular, finds it easier to hold onto greater quantities of small parcels of information than storing one large amount of information.

Decreasing multitasking

Do you ever talk on the phone at the same time as answering your email? Do you sometimes listen to the news while you're reading the newspaper? The modern world encourages, and sometimes demands, multitasking. However, when you're depressed, your ability to pay attention is put under pressure. And multitasking makes heavy demands on your attention.

Understand that, during a time of depression, your concentration may not be as good as usual. If you need to remember something or figure out something new, do so in a quiet setting. Make sure that you concentrate on only one thing at a time.

Following through

Do you have several uncompleted projects hanging over you? The stress of knowing that you have unfinished business may increase your negative mood. When you're having problems with your memory, chasing up progress on several different fronts becomes especially difficult.

Whatever you start, make sure that you finish it. Don't begin another project until you've finished the one you've already begun. Alternatively, you can finish a portion of your project and then plan ahead for a later time, place, and space to tackle the rest. For example, with something as time-consuming as your tax return, you may want to break it down into logical pieces, rather than doing it all at once. And finally, make sure that you plan far enough ahead, so that within your plan you are giving yourself enough time for your project.

Letting it go and reviving recall

One of the most annoying memory problems can be forgetting a word or name in the middle of a conversation. You know that you're going to remember it tomorrow, or in a couple of minutes, but it's on the tip of your tongue and yet won't come out of your mouth! You feel so silly, and the more you try to remember it, the more infuriated you get with yourself.

Stop, take a deep breath, and relax. Tell yourself that it happens to us all, and that remembering the word isn't really that important. Let yourself start thinking about something else. Then, a little later, take some time to think about any associations you may have with that name or word. Most likely, you're then going to find that you remember it. And, whatever else you forget, don't forget to remind yourself that depression

Exercising to Lift Depression

Exercise can substantially improve your feelings, your physical health, and even your quality of life. Exercise helps to drive out depression. However, often depression tries to tell you that you can't even get started. Consider the following ideas to overcome your lethargy and help you choose the type of exercise that's just right for you and your lifestyle.

Introducing endorphins into your life

Who doesn't want to feel good? There are so many ways of feeling great: laughter, a delicious meal, making love, dancing, or perhaps a walk in the great outdoors are just a few examples. But what is it about these activities that actually makes people feel good?

The answer lies, in part, in the brain. The brain has special receptors that receive *opiates*, drugs such as heroin and cocaine that relieve pain and bring about a heightened sense of well-being. The human body produces its own natural substances, called *endorphins* that function like opiates in the brain. Endorphins produce a similar 'high' to that produced by heroin and cocaine: except endorphins are legal substances – and safe! You can generate endorphins through exercise and doing activities you enjoy. Endorphins bring about a feeling of pleasure and well-being that may well hinder depression.

Regular exercise stimulates endorphin production and also tones up your whole body. Exercise improves your cardiovascular system, reduces the risk of various cancers, decreases the risk of diabetes, and balances your cholesterol ratio. As well, exercise gets rid of excessive adrenaline that can cause anxiety and other problems. It's a fact: The right sort of exercise makes you healthier.

Research suggests that exercise can help in easing depression. As yet, it isn't clear if one particular type of exercise works better for lessening your depression (or if all types of exercise work equally well). Although we don't recommend exercise as the only answer to dealing with major depression, you're likely to benefit enormously from *regular* exercise.

Always check with your doctor before beginning an exercise programme – especially if you're overweight, over the age of 40, or have health problems. You also need to see your doctor if you experience serious pain, dizziness, nausea, or other troubling symptoms after exercising, because these symptoms aren't generally normal after moderate exercise.

Easing into exercise

With any luck, you can convince yourself that it may well be easy to start exercising. But that doesn't mean that exercising itself is going to be easy. Depression really does sap your body's energy, so we suggest that you start your exercise programme gently and ever so slowly.

Most exercise gurus preach the importance of exercising for at least 20 minutes, three to five times a week. You may have read recent guidelines recommending that you exercise for at least one hour each day. We don't know about you, but we certainly don't have a spare hour a day. Research shows that doing *any* exercise is far better than none, so even ten minutes, three or four times a week, can help. And you can ease your way into the world of exercise with activities that barely seem like exercise at all:

- ✔ Park a little farther from your workplace.
- ✔ Choose the space in the car park furthest from where you want to go.
- ✔ Take the stairs rather than the lift or escalator.

✔ Do a few brief exercises during work breaks.

✔ If you use a cordless or mobile phone, walk while you talk.

✔ The next time you go shopping, walk a bit further through the shopping centre.

Walking a little farther, taking the stairs, and moving around more all make a good start for your exercise programme. Then, if you want, you can add a little more activity to your daily routine. To get the maximum benefit from exercise, work your body a little harder each day.

The following list shows you three decisions you have to make when designing your exercise programme. For each, start small and build up slowly. And remember that you're not competing with anyone, so don't compare yourself to others if you go to the gym.

✔ **Frequency:** 'How often am I going to work exercise into my life?' As a start, consider planning to exercise twice a week.

✔ **Intensity:** 'How fast and how far am I going to walk, or run? How heavy are the weights I'm going to use?' At first, we suggest the answer be 'not very' to all of these questions.

✔ **Time:** 'How long do I want to exercise each time?' Try starting with just ten minutes.

What type of exercise is going to work best for you? We can honestly say that we have no idea. And you may not know either. So we recommend that you review the various exercise options and pick one that looks the most appealing at first sight (or even just the one that looks the least horrible!).

In this section, we look at strength training, aerobic exercise, and yoga – three of the most popular exercise options. If you want even more info on all the possibilities that are out there, check out at your local health club or sports centre, or pick up a copy of *Fitness For Dummies* by Suzanne Schlosberg and Liz Neporent (Wiley).

Whatever type of exercise you go for, try it out for at least two weeks. If you find that type of exercise isn't for you, choose another. You may have to experiment a little, but you're likely to find an exercise soon that works well for you.

Refer to Book III for more information on exercise options.

Handling Life's Headaches

Depression has a nasty way of slowing down and clogging up your brain's problem-solving machinery. When you're depressed, your problems can quickly grow from molehills to mountains, paralysing you and filling you with hopelessness. This then increases your depression, clouding your ability to find a way out of what's troubling you.

Identifying activities you enjoy

When you're depressed, you may not even be able to remember what fun and pleasure feel like. And coming up with a list of possible pleasurable activities may seem unimaginably difficult. Don't worry – this section helps you get started.

If you're feeling depressed, take a look at the fun things we list in this section. Obviously, not all of these activities are going to appeal. However, we suggest that you circle each of the items that you currently or *used to* find enjoyable. You can rank the activities: from the ones that appeal the most down to the absolutely unthinkable. Then think about which activities are possible for you. For example, if you currently don't have a partner, making love may not be at the top of the list this time round!

The Associates for Research into the Science of Enjoyment (www.arise. org) carried out a survey of adults from all over the world and what gave them the most pleasure. It seems that simple pleasures provide the most enjoyment. These activities include:

- ✔ Drinking a glass of wine
- ✔ Eating chocolate
- ✔ Entertaining friends
- ✔ Exercising
- ✔ Going out for a meal
- ✔ Having a cup of tea or coffee
- ✔ Making love
- ✔ Playing with children
- ✔ Reading
- ✔ Shopping

✔ Spending time with family

✔ Taking a hot bath or shower

✔ Watching TV

If you've ever been to France and gone into a bread shop, it probably won't surprise you to discover that the French have a particular fondness for indulging in pastries. Italians rank sex high on their list of pleasures. And Brits apparently really enjoy a nice cup of tea and drinking alcohol (No! You don't say!).

If nothing on the previous list captures your imagination think about choosing from the good things in life that appeal to the senses, such as:

✔ Eating spicy foods

✔ Having a massage

✔ Listening to music

✔ Looking at beauty in nature or art

✔ Smelling fresh flowers

✔ Spending time in a sauna or steam room

✔ Strolling through the great outdoors

Possibilities for enjoyable activities include experiencing the great outdoors, while indoor activities can be equally great! Here are some suggestions:

✔ Camping

✔ Cinema/video/DVD

✔ Dancing

✔ Hiking

✔ Theatre, concerts, musicals

✔ Reading groups

✔ Participating in sports

✔ Playing games

✔ Playing with pets

✔ Spectator sports

✔ Travel and holidays

Devising life's problem-solving game plan – CRICKET

In recent years, the problem-solving approach to fighting depression has gained wider popularity owing to research showing its effectiveness. The aims of the problem-solving approach, when applied to depression, are to:

✔ Uncover life problems that may be contributing to depression

✔ Figure out how depression lessens chances of finding solutions

✔ Develop effective problem-solving techniques

✔ Prevent relapse by improving coping skills

To make our problem-solving plan easy to remember, we give it the acronym CRICKET. The CRICKET game plan guides you through a series of steps. These steps help you to find effective solutions to your problems and then try them out.

✔ **C** stands for the central *core*, or the problem itself. The core includes how you see the problem and its cause(s), your feelings about the problem, and your beliefs about trying to solve it. For example, you may believe that the problem simply can't be overcome. That belief is part of the core of the problem.

✔ **R** stands for running through the *routes* – these are all the available routes or options you can take to approach the problem creatively.

✔ **I** is for *investigating* the outcomes that carrying out each option creates.

✔ **C** involves committing to a *choice* about which option you want to try.

✔ **K** refers to not *kidding* yourself by saying you 'can't decide'. Remember that no decision is still a decision – you're deciding not to change.

✔ **E** stands for your *emotional plan* for carrying out your option, because some choices may need courage.

✔ **T** stands for the *test* match – testing out your option. You carry out your plan, review the outcome check if it produced the desired result, and work out what to do next, if your plan proved unsuccessful.

Selecting the Best Weapons to Fight Depression

The greater part of this book provides techniques you can use to improve your mood and defeat depression. Most of these are from the fields of cognitive behavioural therapy. We want to encourage you to adopt healthy thinking and behaviour as your first line of defence in your battle against the blues. But no way is psychological therapy the only tool!

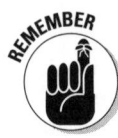

A huge body of studies is available comparing prescribed medication with psychological therapy, mainly cognitive behavioural therapy (CBT), for the treatment of depression. Most studies agree that both types of therapy are equally effective for the treatment of depression. And several studies suggest that a combination of the two brings even better results

Combining medication with therapy appears to give a slight edge over using only the one form of treatment, allowing a person taking antidepressant medication to make better use of psychological therapy.

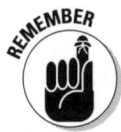

Whatever path you choose, don't forget that depression is an illness that can be treated successfully. If the initial solution you've gone for doesn't work, don't give up hope. Be patient, get help, and try something different.

For more information on medication refer to *Overcoming Depression For Dummies* (Wiley).

Reducing the Risk of Relapse

After successfully getting to grips with your depression, it's very important to keep up your new-found improvement. This book suggests many techniques for helping you conquer your depression and maintaining your well-being. However, if after putting in a lot of personal effort your depression still hasn't improved much, seek professional help. Or, if you're worried that your improvement is slipping and that you're in danger of falling into a relapse, keep on reading this chapter.

Getting the lowdown on relapse rates

So, just how high is the risk of your relapsing? Well, research shows that up to 50 per cent of people who have recovered from one episode of depression find themselves experiencing another bout within the next year or two, and if you've had more than two episodes, there's an 80 per cent chance you're going to have another. In part, your likelihood of relapse depends on whether your depression was treated with medication or psychological therapy.

Combining medication with the therapies we talk about in this book is a very effective way of reducing your risk of relapse.

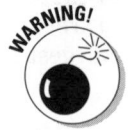

Although there are many treatments available to help reduce the likelihood of relapse, your risk of relapse is much greater if you stop treatment before your symptoms of depression disappear. Don't stop your treatment until you have six months or more of normal energy, appetite, sleep, and you're back enjoying your interests and activities.

Equipping yourself to prevent relapse

If you completely ignore the real possibility of your depression returning, relapse may very well lurk just around the corner, ready to jump out and pounce on you. But you can do a lot to minimise the danger. We're now going to look at strategies for preventing relapse.

Sustaining success

When depression finally goes away, most people feel like stopping treatment. And we don't blame them for feeling that way. All treatments for depression (including self-help) require time, energy, and at least some money.

Given the demands made by treatment, why work harder and longer than you have to – especially when you're feeling good again? The reason is that the risk of relapse is much higher if you stop your treatment too soon, especially when you consider the debilitating nature of depression.

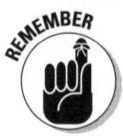

Most professionals believe in treating depression until the symptoms completely subside, not just until they're partially resolved. Also, therapists typically recommend continuing treatment for at least a few months after being free of depression – and a return to normal energy, concentration, appetite, sleep, and enjoyment of life's activities.

The suggestion to continue treatment is based on the idea that adopting new skills, behaviours, and ways of thinking is the best approach. These newly acquired, fledgling skills won't survive in the face of the inevitable adversities of life. You need to repeatedly practise the skills you acquire.

The more skills you acquire and master for handling depression, the less likely you're going to experience relapse in the future. Continuing with psychological therapy or self-help for some months after your depression has gone away helps prevent relapse.

If you choose to treat your depression by using medication alone,, we suggest that you continue taking the medication for at least 6 to 12 months after overcoming your depression. Doing so helps to reduce your chances of relapse, although we highly recommend trying psychological therapy, such as cognitive therapy, as well as medication. Alternatively, some people with a history of recurrent depression find that continuing with lifetime antidepressant medication provides them with reasonable protection against relapse.

Monitoring the signs

Carry out a weekly Depression Review. Choose a convenient time to schedule this activity into your calendar. We recommend continuing doing this review for at least a year after the depression lifts and ask yourself the following questions:

- Have I been having negative or unhappy thoughts?

- Have I started avoiding people or situations that make me feel uncomfortable?

- What is my mood on a 1 to 100 point scale (extremely depressed to completely happy)? Has my mood dropped from its usual rating by more than 10 points and stayed lower for more than a day or two?

If you answer yes to one or more of the questions above, beware! This list contains the early warning signs of possible depression. Of course, anyone can experience a few low thoughts, a little guilt, and difficulty concentrating but still not go on to develop full-blown depression. And we certainly don't expect you to feel 100 per cent fulfilled every week of your life. But, if you're having a lot of negative thoughts they can be warning signs of depression. Pay the signs serious attention, and start some form of treatment, including self-help, if your symptoms are mild, or life feels unsatisfactory.

Preparing a Prevention Plan

No one knows when or where a fire is going to break out. That's why the law requires public buildings such as hospitals, shops, offices, schools to have a regular programme of fire safety drills. Having a fire prevention plan in place makes sure that you're ready and know what to do in the event of fire. The result? Effective damage limitation.

A Prevention Plan for limiting the effects of depression does the same thing. In your Prevention Plan you vividly imagine potentially challenging times and events, and then explore how you *could* cope with them. Finally, you imagine yourself *actually coping*, and doing so in a productive manner.

None of us can predict what the future holds, which is perhaps a good thing, on the whole! However, you probably know what types of events have been difficult for you to handle in the past, and also have an inkling about what you fear about the future. Rather than pretend that your life is going to be a bed of roses, we suggest that you make a list of potentially distressing events that could happen to you at any time and that you fear could overwhelm your capacity for coping.

Here are a few possibilities:

- Humiliation
- Failing to meet a deadline
- Financial reversals
- Illness
- Injury
- Losing a loved one
- Rejection

Next, choose just one item from your list. Imagine that event happening and finding a way of coping. When you make your Prevention Plan, use the questions in this list to help you come up with ideas on how you're going to cope:

- How would someone else handle this situation?
- Have I dealt with something like this in the past? How did I do it?
- How much effect is this event going to have on my life a year from now?
- Is this event as awful as I'm making it out to be?
- What creative ways can I find to deal with this challenge?

Overcoming Depression with Mindfulness

Being aware of the present moment is the goal of mindfulness. In a mindful state, you're aware, engaged, connected, and non-judgemental. Mindfulness is a central aspect of Buddhist teachings, but you don't need to be a practising Buddhist to benefit from mindfulness.

Getting playful

A useful strategy for dealing with negative, self-critical thinking is to treat it playfully. Yes, really. Play with it. Surprisingly, you can change the meaning of your thoughts and your response to them if you start getting playful.

Write down the negative thoughts that are running through your head. Sing those thoughts to yourself over and over again. Then use the negative thoughts as lyrics to a popular tune, or make up your own melody. You find your negative thoughts becoming trivial, even amusing when you give them a tune. Alternatively, experiment with saying them out loud, but in a highly distorted voice. Try a Donald Duck, or Inspector Clouseau voice, or any other exaggerated stereotype. Buying into negative chatter is a lot harder when you hear it coming from Donald Duck!

Letting go of negative thoughts

Here's another suggestion for dealing with your negative thoughts. When you notice yourself having negative thoughts, try picturing them balancing on a giant leaf and see yourself watching the leaf gently float down stream. Practise playing with your negative thoughts as being something outside yourself. Observe them. Watch them float away into the distance. See how they swirl and dance as they go by. Visualising your negative thoughts being washed away is a form of meditation. Try it out for 10 to 20 minutes each day. Simply sit and relax. Watching each thought float away.

You may prefer to visualise your negative thoughts as a swirling mass of clouds. Watch the clouds drift past you in front of your eyes, seeing them gradually dissolving into nothingness. Or, if visualisation doesn't work for you, write your negative thoughts down on a piece of paper. Take the paper outside, put it in an incinerator, and set your negative thoughts alight. Watch them going up in smoke right in front of you. Try backing away and putting some distance between you and your negative thoughts. From a distance quietly observe your negative thoughts (although of course if your negative thought is signalling danger, you need to act there and then). At most, consider your thoughts as possibilities, rather than statements of fact.

Connecting with experience: Life's no spectator sport

Do you know the saying 'the past is history, the future is a mystery, but the here and now is a gift, which is why we call it the present!' This saying nicely sums up what cognitive therapy and mindfulness are about.

Here's the story of two Buddhist monks on a journey. Reaching a stream, they see a small, frail woman. She asks to be carried across – the water's too wide and the current too strong for her. Despite the prohibition of touching a woman, the first monk picks her up, carries her across, and the two monks continue on their way. After two hour's silence, the second monk bursts out 'I can't get over it! You carried that woman! Across the river!' The second smilingly says 'Yes. But I put her down hours ago. You're still carrying her.'

As you bring acceptance into your life (see the earlier 'Acquiring acceptance' section) you're preparing to experience life grounded in the present. The idea of being connected with present-moment experience is rather strange for many people. Staying connected with 'now' takes practice. However, even small steps towards acceptance can lead to some respite and peace in your life.

When you find yourself dwelling on past regrets or future worries, try the Connecting with the Present exercise. This exercise shows you how to observe your thoughts *mindfully*. We suggest you practise 10 or 15 minutes each day, for a few weeks. Try not to let yourself get upset if troubling or distracting thoughts interfere while you're doing the exercise. Remember, that's just what the mind does. If such thoughts come into your mind, merely notice them, rather than judging whether you're doing the exercise correctly.

1. **Focus on each moment that you're experiencing.** Notice all the sensations in your body, including touch, sights, sounds, smell, and taste.

2. **You're probably finding thoughts coming into your mind. Pay attention to them.** Make a note of whether they're about the future, or the past. Just notice them, then return your attention to your body's sensations.

3. **Focus on your breathing, feeling the air as it goes in your nose, into your lungs, and out again.** Notice the rhythm of your breathing.

4. **More thoughts are going to start coming into your mind.** Remember, *thoughts are just thoughts*.

5. **Return to your breathing.** Notice how good the air feels.

6. **If you have sad or anxious feelings, notice *where* you're feeling them in your body.** Is your chest tight, or your stomach churning? Stay with those sensations. Give your sensations your full attention.

7. **If you have thoughts about your feelings, notice how interesting it is that the mind is taking stock of everything that is going on.** Watch those thoughts and let them drift past, like leaves floating down stream, and the clouds drifting across the sky. Return to the present moment and the sensations in your body.

8. **If more thoughts come, notice the *you* observing those thoughts in the present moment.** If dozens of thoughts flood your mind, try imagining them as a torrent, rushing down a waterfall, while you stand watching behind the waterfall.

9. **Return to your breathing.** Pay attention to how nice and rhythmic it feels.

10. **If you hear sounds, try not to judge them.** For example, if you hear loud music outside, just notice the sounds as sounds. Not good or bad. Pick out the rhythm or the notes and let yourself hear them. If the phone rings, be aware of the sound, but don't answer it right now.

11. **Notice what you see at the back of your eyelids when you close your eyes.** See the interesting patterns and forms that come and go.

12. **Once again experience the sensation of your whole body breathing.**

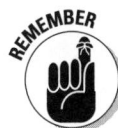

The more you resist what is, the more you're going to build up negative feelings and tension.

Try approaching life's tasks mindfully. At first, dozens of thoughts concerning past regrets, present irritations, and future worries are going to interrupt and disrupt your attempts at connecting with what is. With practice, you're going to become aware of them, let them drift by, and recognise that they really are no more than just passing thoughts. After getting the hang of doing things mindfully you're going to find you're no longer as irritated by or keen to avoid so many everyday tasks. You can even apply this strategy to your home exercise programme for helping you ease depression.

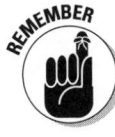

Thoughts are just thoughts . . .

Chapter 4

Examining Anxiety in Its Different Guises

Anxiety comes in many different shapes and sizes. It can cause emotional pain and distress and affect physical health and family relationships. Left untreated, anxiety can cause long-term health problems.

Taking time to consider the symptoms and types of anxiety, as we do in this chapter, can help you start to unearth the roots of anxiety and take control again.

Understanding the Symptoms of Anxiety

The physical symptoms of anxiety can be a part of normal, everyday experience. But sometimes they signal something more serious. Think about yourself. Have you ever thought that you were suffering a nervous breakdown or worried that you were going crazy? Perhaps you felt you were having a heart attack?

To demonstrate the difference between an actual anxiety disorder and a normal reaction, read the following description and imagine ten minutes in the life of Sandy.

At first, Sandy feels restless and slightly bored. Standing, she shifts her weight from foot to foot. Walking forward a little, she notices a slight tightening of her chest. Her breathing quickens. She feels an odd mixture of excitement and mounting tension. She sits down and does her best to relax, but the anxiety continues to intensify. Her body suddenly jerks forward; she grips the sides of her seat and clenches her teeth to choke back a scream. Her stomach feels like it's rising up into her throat. Then it settles down. She feels her heart race and her face flush. Once more her stomach seems to rise up into her throat. Sandy's emotions run wild. Dizziness, fear and a rushing sensation overtake her. It all comes in waves, one after the other.

You may wonder what's wrong with poor Sandy. Perhaps she has an anxiety disorder. Or could she be having a nervous breakdown – and maybe even be going crazy?

But Sandy's just spent those last ten minutes, plus many more, at an amusement park. First, she queued to buy a ticket and felt bored. Then she handed her ticket to the attendant and strapped herself into a roller coaster. After that, well, no doubt you now understand the rest of her experience. Sandy has no anxiety disorder, she isn't suffering a nervous breakdown, and she isn't going mad. As her story illustrates, the symptoms of anxiety can be a normal reaction to life events.

Sorting out what's normal from what's not

Anxiety is good for you! It prepares you to take action. It mobilises your body for emergencies. It warns you about potential problems. Be glad you have some anxiety. Your anxiety helps you stay out of trouble.

Anxiety only poses a problem for you when:

- ✔ Anxiety lasts uncomfortably long or occurs too often.
- ✔ It interferes with doing what you want to do.
- ✔ Anxiety greatly exceeds the level of actual danger or risk. For example, when your body and mind feel like an avalanche is about to bury you, but all you have to do is take a test at school, your anxiety has gone too far.
- ✔ You struggle to control your worries, but they keep disturbing you and never let up.

Anxiety appears in different forms for different people. You may find that anxiety affects your thoughts, behaviours, and feelings. Some of the more common symptoms are listed as follows.

You're *thinking* anxiously if you're:

- ✔ Making dire predictions about the future.
- ✔ Thinking you can't cope.
- ✔ Frequently worrying about pleasing people.
- ✔ Thinking that you need to be perfect.
- ✔ Have excessive concerns about not being in control.
- ✔ Having difficulty concentrating.

You're *behaving* anxiously if you're:

- ✔ Avoiding many social events.
- ✔ Leaving situations that make you anxious.
- ✔ Never taking reasonable risks.
- ✔ Staying away from feared objects or events, such as flying or spiders.

You're *feeling* anxious if you have:

- ✔ Butterflies in your stomach.
- ✔ Dizziness.
- ✔ Muscle tension.
- ✔ A racing heart.
- ✔ A shaky feeling.
- ✔ Sweaty palms.

 The physical symptoms of anxiety may result from medical problems. If you have a number of these symptoms, see a doctor for a quick checkup.

Matching symptoms and therapies

Anxiety symptoms appear in three different spheres:

- ✔ **Thinking symptoms:** The thoughts that run through your mind.
- ✔ **Behaving symptoms:** The things you do in response to anxiety.
- ✔ **Feeling symptoms:** How your body reacts to anxiety.

You may well experience symptoms from all these groups but find one more powerful and disturbing than the others.

The following sections address treatment for these three kinds of symptom.

Thinking therapies

One of the most effective treatments for a wide range of emotional problems, known as *cognitive therapy,* deals with the way you think about, perceive and interpret everything that's important to you including:

- ✔ Your views about yourself
- ✔ The events that happen to you in life
- ✔ Your future

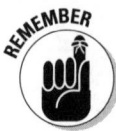

When people feel unusually anxious and worried, they almost inevitably distort the way they think about things, especially those things that are important to them. That distortion actually causes much of their anxiety.

Behaving therapies

Another highly effective type of therapy is known as *behaviour therapy.* As the name suggests, this approach deals with actions you can take and behaviours you can incorporate to alleviate your anxiety. Some actions are fairly straightforward:

- ✔ Simplify your life
- ✔ Get more exercise
- ✔ Get more sleep

On the other hand, one type of behaviour therapy that is likely to be very effective, but which can feel a little scary, is *graded exposure* – breaking your fears down into small steps and facing them one at a time. Exposure, however, is a bit more complicated and does involve a little more than this statement indicates, so turn to Book V Chapter 5 for more about exposure.

Feeling therapies

Anxiety sets off a whirlwind of distressing physical symptoms, such as a racing heartbeat, upset stomach, muscle tension, sweating, dizziness, and so on. We have a variety of suggestions for helping to quell these symptoms.

Presenting the Seven Main Types of Anxiety

Anxiety comes in various forms. The word *anxious* is derived from the Latin word *angere*, meaning to press tightly, strangle or choke. A sense of choking or tightening in the throat or chest is a common symptom of anxiety. However, anxiety also involves other symptoms, such as sweating, trembling, nausea, and a racing heartbeat. Anxiety may also involve fears – fear of losing control and fear of illness or of dying. In addition, people with excessive anxiety avoid various situations, people, animals or objects to an unnecessary degree. Psychologists and psychiatrists have compiled a list of seven major categories of anxiety disorders as follows:

- Generalised anxiety disorder (GAD)
- Social phobia
- Panic disorder
- Agoraphobia
- Specific phobia
- Post-traumatic stress disorder (PTSD)
- Obsessive-compulsive disorder (OCD)

Although we provide the major signs and symptoms of each type of anxiety so that you can get a general idea of which category your anxiety may fall into, to really understand where your particular anxiety fits, you need to see a professional. If you do seek professional help, the ideas in this book can still assist you in alleviating your problems with anxiety.

Generalised anxiety disorder: The common cold of anxiety

Some people refer to *generalised anxiety disorder* as the common cold of anxiety disorders. Generalised anxiety disorder, also known as GAD, afflicts more people throughout the world than any other anxiety disorder. So if you or a loved one has it, you're in good company. GAD involves a long-lasting, almost constant state of tension and worry. Realistic worries don't mean you have GAD. For example, if you worry about money and you've just lost your job, that's not GAD – it's a real-life problem. But if you constantly worry about money and your name is Bill Gates, you just may have GAD!

You may have GAD if you've experienced anxiety almost daily for the last six months. You try to stop worrying but you just can't. *And* you frequently experience a number of the following problems:

- ✔ You feel restless; often irritable, on edge, fidgety or keyed up.
- ✔ You get tired easily.
- ✔ Your muscles feel tense, especially in your back, neck or shoulders.
- ✔ You have difficulty concentrating, falling asleep or staying asleep.

Not everyone experiences anxiety in exactly the same way. That's why only a professional can actually make a diagnosis. Some people complain about other problems, such as twitching, trembling, shortness of breath, sweating, dry mouth, stomach upset, feeling shaky, being easily startled, and having difficulty swallowing. They fail to realise that they actually suffer from GAD.

The following profile offers an example of what GAD is all about.

On the Underground train, Brian taps his foot nervously. He arches his back to stretch his tight shoulder muscles and checks his watch, worrying that he may be three or four minutes late for work. He hates coming in late. He didn't sleep much last night because thoughts about the presentation of his latest project repeatedly invaded his sleep. One preoccupation or another usually disturbs Brian's sleep. Struggling to concentrate on the newspaper that he's holding, he realises that he can't remember what he's just read.

When Brian gets to work, he snaps at his new assistant. After he loses his temper with her, he feels immediate remorse and angrily tells himself off, increasing his anxiety further. His colleagues often tell him to keep cool. His performance has always exceeded his employer's expectations, so he objectively has no reason to worry about his job. Nevertheless, worry he does. Brian suffers from GAD.

Social phobia – avoiding people

Those with *social phobia* fear exposure to public scrutiny. They frequently dread interviews, performing, speaking in groups or even one to one, going to parties, meeting new people, entering groups, using the telephone, writing a cheque in front of others, eating in public, and/or interacting with those in authority. They see these situations as painful, because they expect to receive humiliating or shameful judgements from others. Social phobics often believe that they're somehow defective and inadequate; thus, they assume that they'll mess things up, for instance muff their lines, spill their drinks, shake hands with clammy palms, or commit any of a number of social *faux pas* and thus embarrass themselves.

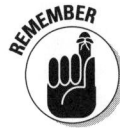

We all feel uncomfortable or nervous from time to time, especially in new situations. So if you've been experiencing social fears for less than six months, you may well not have social phobia. A short-term fear of socialising may be a temporary reaction to a new stress – moving to a new area or starting a new job. However, you may have social phobia if you experience the following symptoms for a prolonged period of time:

✔ You fear being in situations with unfamiliar people or where you may be observed or evaluated in some way.

✔ When forced into an uncomfortable social situation, your physical symptoms and scary thoughts can feel overwhelming. For example, if you fear public speaking, your voice shakes and your knees tremble the moment that you start your talk, and you are convinced that everyone thinks you are stupid.

Feeling panicky

Of course, everyone feels some panic from time to time. People often say that they're panicking about a looming deadline or a presentation, or about planning a party. You're likely to hear the term used to describe concerns about rather mundane events such as these.

But people who suffer with panic disorders are talking about different phenomena entirely. They have periods of horrendously intense fear and anxiety. If you've never had a panic attack, you're lucky. The attacks usually last about ten minutes, and many people who have them really believe that they will die during the attack. Not exactly the best ten minutes of their lives. Panic attacks normally include a range of attention-grabbing symptoms, such as:

✔ Irregular, rapid or pounding heartbeat.

✔ Perspiring.

✔ A sense of choking, suffocation or shortness of breath.

✔ Vertigo or light-headedness.

✔ Pain or other discomfort in your chest.

✔ Feeling that events are unreal or a sense of detachment from yourself.

✔ Numbness or tingling.

✔ Hot or cold flashes.

✔ Feeling that you will faint, have a heart attack or a brain haemorrhage.

✔ Fearing that you will die, though without basis in fact.

✔ Stomach nausea or upset, or feeling that you will vomit.

✔ Jitteriness or trembling.

✔ Thoughts of going insane or completely losing control, or of making a fool of yourself.

✔ Feeling that you will lose control of your bladder or bowels, or both.

Professionals generally agree that in order to have full-blown panic disorder, panic attacks must occur more than once. People with panic disorder worry about when they'll experience the next attack and whether they'll lose control and/or embarrass themselves. Finally, they usually start changing their lives by avoiding certain places or activities.

Panic attacks often begin with an event, such as physical exertion or normal variations in the body's reactions, that triggers some kind of sensation. This triggering event induces responses in the body, such as increased levels of adrenaline. No problem so far.

But the otherwise-normal process goes awry at the next step – when the person who suffers from panic attacks then misinterprets the meaning of the physical symptoms. Rather than viewing the symptoms as normal, the person with panic disorder sees them as a signal that something dangerous is happening, such as a heart attack, brain haemorrhage or a stroke. That interpretation causes escalating fear and thus more physical arousal. In other words, it becomes a vicious cycle. Fortunately, the body sustains such heightened physical responses only for a while, and it eventually calms down.

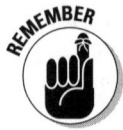

The good news: Many people have a single panic attack and never have another one. So don't panic if you have a panic attack.

Maria's story is a good example of a one-off panic attack.

Maria leaves the hospital after visiting her next-door neighbour. She still can't believe that he had a heart attack at the age of 42. Maria, never one to worry about her health, ponders the fact that she just reached her 46th birthday. She resolves to lose that extra stone or so and to start exercising.

On her third visit to the gym, frustrated with her slow progress, she sets the treadmill to level 6. Almost immediately, her heart rate accelerates rapidly. Alarmed, she decreases the level to 3. She starts taking rapid, shallow breaths but feels she can't get enough air. Reducing the level further doesn't seem to help. She stops the treadmill and goes to the changing room. Sweating profusely and feeling nauseous, she finds an empty cubicle. She sits down and thinks that maybe she just overdid the treadmill a little. But the symptoms intensify and her chest tightens. She wants to scream but feels she can't get enough air. She's sure that she'll pass out and hopes someone will find her before she dies. She hears someone pass by and weakly calls for help. An ambulance whisks her to the nearest casualty department while she prays that she'll live through her heart attack.

In casualty, Maria's symptoms subside, and the doctor comes in to explain the results of her examination. He says that she's apparently experienced a panic attack and enquires about what may have triggered it. She explains that she was exercising due to concerns about her weight and health, and she mentions her neighbour's heart attack.

'Ah ha!' says the doctor reassuringly. 'Your health worries made you hypersensitive to any bodily symptom. When your heart rate naturally increased on the treadmill, you became frightened. That fear caused your body to produce more adrenaline, which in turn created more symptoms, including an increase in heart rate. The more symptoms you had, the more your fear and adrenaline increased. If you understand this, hopefully, in the future, your body's normal physical variations won't frighten you. Your heart's in great shape. I recommend that you go back to exercising but just increase it slowly over time without sudden jumps in intensity. Also, you may try some simple relaxation techniques; I'll ask the nurse to come in and tell you about those. I have every reason to believe that you won't have another episode like this one. Finally, you may want to read *Overcoming Anxiety For Dummies* by Elaine Iljon Foreman, Charles Elliott and Laura Smith (Wiley); it's a great book!'

Maria doesn't have a diagnosis of panic disorder because she hasn't experienced more than one attack and she may never have another panic attack again. If she believes the doctor and takes his advice, the next time that her heart races, she probably won't get so scared. She may even use the relaxation techniques that the nurse explained to her – or even the others she picked up from the book!

The panic companion – agoraphobia

Around half of those with panic disorder have an accompanying problem: *agoraphobia*. The word comes from the Greek *agora,* meaning marketplace, and *phobia* – well you know that one by now. Any open space, whether a beach, a field or a sports stadium, can leave the person paralysed with terror. However, agoraphobia is not just a fear of open spaces; the real underlying fear is more complex, encompassing several aspects of daily life that are closely interlinked. The phobias or fears in agoraphobia involve activities such as leaving home, entering public places or travelling alone. In these situations the person feels especially vulnerable and exposed, with nowhere to escape to or hide if things go wrong. Agoraphobia therefore often includes fear of visiting supermarkets or going to the theatre or cinema.

Unlike most fears or phobias, this disorder usually begins in adulthood. Individuals with agoraphobia live in terror of feeling overwhelmed by panic. In addition, they worry about what will happen to them if they have a panic attack. They desperately avoid situations from which they can't readily escape, and they also fear places where help may not be readily forthcoming should they need it. The agoraphobic may start with one fear, such as being in a crowd, but in many cases the feared situations multiply to the point that the person fears even leaving home. And the last straw for some people is that they then start to worry 'What if I have one of my "funny turns" when I'm at home alone, with no one to help me?' So even home is no longer a sanctuary.

Patricia's story, which follows, demonstrates the overwhelming anxiety that often traps agoraphobics.

Patricia celebrates her 40th birthday without having experienced significant emotional problems. She's gone through the usual bumps in the road of life like losing a parent, her child having a learning disability, and a divorce ten years earlier. She prides herself on being able to cope with whatever cards life deals her.

Lately, she notices that she feels stressed when she goes shopping. She needs to pick up a birthday present and doesn't want to go because the shopping centre is especially crowded at weekends. She finally makes herself go to the shopping centre and finds a parking spot at the very end of a row. As she enters the shopping centre, heart pounding, her sweaty hands leave a smudge on the revolving glass door. She feels as though the crowds of shoppers are crushing her, and Patricia feels trapped. She's so scared that she can't bring herself to buy the present and flees the shopping centre.

Over the next few months, Patricia's fears spread. Although it started in the shopping centre, fear and anxiety now overwhelm her in any busy shop. Later, Patricia feels she can no longer cope when she's simply driving in traffic. Patricia is now suffering from agoraphobia. If not treated, Patricia may end up housebound.

Many times, panic, agoraphobia and anxiety strike people who are otherwise devoid of serious, deep-seated emotional problems. So if you suffer from anxiety, it doesn't necessarily mean you'll need years of psychotherapy. You may not like the anxiety, but you certainly don't have to put up with it!

Top ten fears

Various polls and surveys collect information about what people fear most. In the following list, we compile the most common fears. Do you have any of these?

10 Dogs

9 Being alone at night

8 Thunder and lightning

7 Spiders and insects

6 Being trapped in a small space

5 Flying

4 Rodents

3 Heights

2 Giving a speech

And finally, the number one fear: Snakes

Specific phobias – spiders, snakes, lightning, planes and other scary things

Many fears appear to be almost hard-wired into the human brain, they're so common. Cavemen and women had good reasons to fear snakes, strangers, heights, darkness, open spaces and the sight of blood: Snakes could be poisonous, strangers could be enemies, a person could fall from a height, darkness could harbour unknown hazards, open spaces could leave a primitive tribe vulnerable to attack from all sides, and the sight of blood could signal a crisis, even potential death. Throwing up could be a warning to stop eating immediately – were those mushrooms edible or poisonous? Fear inspired caution and avoidance of harm. Those with these fears had a better chance of survival than the naively brave.

That's why many of the most common fears today reflect the dangers of the world thousands of years ago. Even today, it makes sense to cautiously identify a spider before you pick it up. However, sometimes fears rise to a disabling level. You may have a specific phobia if:

✔ You have an exaggerated fear of a specific situation or object.

✔ When you're in fearful situations, you experience excessive anxiety immediately. Your anxiety may include sweating, rapid heartbeat, a desire to flee, tightness in the chest or throat, or images of something awful happening.

✔ You know that the fear is unreasonable. However, a child with a specific phobia doesn't always know that the phobia is unreasonable. For example, the child may really think that *all* dogs bite.

✔ You avoid your feared object or situation as much as you possibly can.

✔ Because your fear is so intense, you go so far as to change your day-to-day behaviour at work, at home or in relationships. Thus, your fear inconveniences you and perhaps others, and it restricts your life.

Post-traumatic stress disorder: Feeling the aftermath

Tragically, war, rape, terror, serious accidents, brutality, torture and natural disasters can be a part of life. You or someone you know may have experienced one of life's traumas. No one knows why for sure, but some people seem to recover from these events without disabling symptoms. However, many others suffer considerably after their tragedies, sometimes for a lifetime.

More often than not, trauma causes at least a few uncomfortable emotional and/or physical reactions for a while. These responses can show up immediately after the disaster, or sometimes they emerge years later. These symptoms are the way that the body and mind deal with and process what happened. If an extremely unfortunate event occurs, it's normal to react strongly.

You may have PTSD if you personally experienced or witnessed an event that you perceived as potentially life threatening or causing serious injury, or you discovered that someone close to you experienced such an event. If your response to such an event includes terror, horror or helplessness, you may develop PTSD, and you may also experience the following three types of problems:

✔ You *relive* the event in one or more of the ways shown in the following examples:

- Having unwanted memories or flashbacks during the day or in your dreams
- Feeling the trauma is happening again
- Experiencing physical or emotional reactions when reminded of the event

✔ You *avoid* anything that reminds you of the trauma and try to suppress or numb your feelings in several ways. These include:

- Trying to block out thinking or talking about the event because you get upset when you remember what happened
- Staying away from people or places that remind you of the trauma

  - Losing interest in life or feeling distant from people

  - Sensing somehow that you don't have a long future

  - Feeling numb or detached

✔ You feel *on guard and stirred up* in several ways. Examples of this are:

  - Becoming startled more easily

  - Losing your temper quickly and feeling irritable

  - Failing to concentrate as well as before

  - Sleeping fitfully

What's it like to live with PTSD? For Charles, it's a constant struggle.

Charles is in the army. Since the first Gulf War, things have been a struggle for Charles. He sleeps poorly and has frequent nightmares; he loses his temper easily, and he feels detached from life.

Charles assumes his problems all stem from issues relating to the army: his work hours, frequent separations from his family, and numerous transfers, which mean moving house frequently, all the while with the intense pressure for promotion. He looks forward to retirement and a less stressful lifestyle. He promises his wife and children that his first goal on retirement is to spend more time with them.

But when Charles takes early retirement at 50, he finds it less rewarding than he'd hoped. He continues to have trouble sleeping. He tries to fulfil his promise to his family but just can't muster any enthusiasm for their activities. He doesn't find anything to look forward to, and his distance from his family grows. He continues to feel irritable and jumpy. After six months of retirement, Charles's wife insists they go for marital counselling.

In taking their history, the psychologist asks Charles about his Gulf War experience. Charles replies shortly that he doesn't want to talk about it – that's how he handles the disturbing memories of the war. That unwillingness to discuss it, together with Charles' other problems, suggests to the psychologist that Charles may have PTSD.

Obsessive-compulsive disorder – over and over and over again

Obsessive-compulsive disorder (OCD) wreaks incredible havoc on people's lives, because OCD frequently frustrates and confuses not only the people afflicted with it, but also their families and loved ones. If untreated, OCD is likely to last a lifetime. Even with treatment, symptoms often recur. That's the bad news. Thankfully, effective treatments are available. So even if the problem comes back, which it may on more than one occasion, you have the skills to deal with it.

A person with OCD may exhibit behaviours that include obsessional thoughts or compulsions, or both. So what are obsessions versus compulsions?

Obsessions are unwelcome repetitive images, impulses or thoughts that come into your mind. People find these thoughts and images disturbing and can't get rid of them. For example, a religious man may have a thought that he will start shouting obscenities during a church service, or a caring mother may have intrusive thoughts of causing harm to her baby. While the vast majority of people don't carry out these imagined actions, the obsessions still haunt them.

Compulsions are undesired repetitive actions or mental strategies carried out to temporarily reduce anxiety. From time to time, an obsessional thought triggers the anxiety; at other times, the anxiety may be triggered by an obsessional thought or a feared event or situation.

The OCD cycle

A pattern frequently develops in which obsessional thoughts create anxiety, which causes the person to engage in a compulsive act in order to reduce the anxiety and obtain relief. That temporary relief powerfully encourages the person to believe that the compulsive act helps. Unfortunately, the cycle begins again, because the obsessional thoughts return. Table 4-1 shows common thoughts and the behaviours which often follow.

Table 4-1	The Most Common Obsessions and Compulsions
Obsessions	**Compulsions**
Worry about contamination, such as from dirt, germs, radiation and chemicals.	Excessive hand-washing or cleaning due to the obsessive fear of contamination.
Doubts about having remembered to turn the cooker and the lights off, lock the doors, close the windows, and so on.	Checking and rechecking to see that the cooker is off, doors and windows are locked, and so on. Even returning home after leaving to re-check.
Sexual imagery about which you feel ashamed.	Repeating certain words or phrases to stop yourself acting on disturbing thoughts – though you never have acted them out.
Thoughts that would violate your own personal codes of behaviour in some shameful way.	Arranging items in a rigid, precise way. Often, you feel compelled to start again if it doesn't come out perfectly.

Obsessions	Compulsions
Thoughts urging you to behave in a socially strange and unacceptable way.	Preventative behaviours such as counting stairs, ceiling tiles, steps walked, and so on. Can include repeating actions such as walking back and forth through a doorway until 'good thoughts' accompany you through the doorway.
Unwanted thoughts of harming someone you love.	Repeating rituals over and over again, with a belief that this will somehow prevent something bad from happening. The belief is that the ritual must be carried out correctly for it to be effective.
Fears of harming others.	Avoiding using knives even when cooking. Not holding or playing with young children. Repeatedly driving back over your route to check you haven't run someone over. (And then having to drive the route again to check out that journey.) Moving stones and objects off footpaths to stop others tripping – and then worrying that the new placement will cause an accident.

Unearthing the Roots of Anxiety

The three major causes of anxiety are:

- ✔ **Genetics:** Your biological inheritance
- ✔ **Parenting:** The way that you were brought up
- ✔ **Trauma:** The horrifying events that can happen in life

Studies show that when people experience an unanticipated trauma, only a minority end up with severe anxiety. That's because anxiety usually stems from a combination of causes – perhaps genes and trauma, or trauma and parenting, or sometimes all three combine to induce anxiety. At the same time, just one factor, if formidable enough, can possibly cause the entire problem.

For example, Gloria grows up on a tough estate, where gangs and violence are commonplace, without developing terribly distressing symptoms. Even when she is mugged for her new mobile phone, she shows surprising resilience during her recovery. Surely she must have some robust, anti-anxiety genes and perhaps some pretty good parents as well in order to successfully endure such an experience. She moves away from the estate and thinks she has left the past behind her. However, she is then on a train going to work, and a gang come steaming through the train, robbing and threatening the passengers, Following this experience, Gloria develops serious problems with anxiety. She has sustained one trauma too many.

Thus you can never ascertain the exact cause of anyone's anxiety with absolute certainty. However, if you examine someone's childhood relationship with his or her parents, family history, and the various events in his or her life (such as accidents, war, disease, and so on), you can generally come up with some pretty good ideas as to why anxiety now causes problems. If you have anxiety, consider reviewing these possible causes of distress and think about which ones may have given you the most trouble.

But what difference does it make where your anxiety comes from? Overcoming anxiety doesn't absolutely require knowledge of where it originated. The remedies change little whether you were born with anxiety or acquired it much later in your life.

However, more quickly identifying the source of your anxiety can help you to realise that your anxiety isn't something that you brought on yourself. Anxiety develops for a number of good, solid reasons. The blame doesn't belong with the person who has anxiety.

Guilt and self-blame can only sap your energy. They drain resources and keep your focus away from the effort required for challenging your anxiety. By contrast, self-forgiveness and self-acceptance invigorate and vitalise your efforts.

Separating nature from nurture

If you suffer from excessive worries and tension, look around at the rest of your family. Of those who have an anxiety disorder, typically about a quarter of their relatives suffer with them. So your Uncle Ralph may not struggle with anxiety, though Aunt Belinda or your sister Charlotte just may.

But you may argue that Uncle Ralph, Aunt Belinda and your sister Charlotte all had to live with Nan, who'd make anyone anxious. In other words, they lived in an anxiety-inducing environment. Maybe it has nothing to do with their genes.

Various researchers have studied siblings and twins who live together to verify that genes do play an important role in how people experience and cope with anxiety. As predicted, identical twins were far more similar to each other in terms of anxiety than non-identical twins or other siblings. But even if you're born with a genetic predisposition towards anxiety, other factors such as environment, peers, and how your parents raised you enter into the mix.

It's my parents' fault!

Parent-bashing is in. Blaming parents for almost anything that ails you is easy. Parents usually do the best they can. Raising children poses a formidable task. So in most cases, parents don't deserve to be vilified. However, they do hold some responsibility for the way in which you were brought up and so may indeed have contributed to your woes.

Three parenting styles appear to foster anxiety in children:

- ✔ **Over-protective:** These parents shield their kids from every imaginable stress or harm. If their kids stumble, they try to swoop them up before they even hit the ground. When their kids get upset, they fix the problem. Not surprisingly, their kids fail to find out how to tolerate fear, anxiety or frustration.

- ✔ **Over-controlling:** These parents micro-manage all their children's activities. They direct every detail from how they should play to what they should wear to how they solve arithmetical problems. They discourage independence and feed dependency and anxiety.

- ✔ **Inconsistent:** The parents in this group provide their kids with erratic rules and limits. One day, they respond with understanding when their kids have trouble with their homework; the next day, they explode when asked for help. These kids fail to discover the connection between their own efforts and a predictable outcome. Therefore, they feel that they have little control over what happens in life. It's no wonder they feel anxious.

It's the world's fault!

The world today moves at a faster pace than ever, and for many of us, the working week has got longer. Modern life is rife with both complexity and danger. Perhaps that's why mental health workers see so many people with anxiety-related problems. Four specific types of disturbing events can trigger a problem with anxiety even in someone who has never suffered from it much before:

✔ **Unanticipated threats:** Predictability and stability counteract anxiety, and the opposite fuels it. For example, Ahmed works long hours to make a decent living. Nevertheless, he just about manages from month to month, with little left for savings. An accidental slip on an icy pavement leaves him out of action for six weeks, and as he is self-employed, no money comes in. He now worries incessantly over his ability to pay bills. Even when he returns to work, he worries more than ever about the next financial disaster that awaits him.

✔ **Escalating demands:** Nothing is better than a promotion. At least that's what Jake thinks when his supervisor gives him a once-in-a-lifetime opportunity to direct the new high-risk research and development division at work. Jake never expected such a lofty position this early in his career, or the doubling of his salary. Of course, new duties, expectations, and responsibilities are part of the deal. Jake now begins to fret and worry. What if he fails to meet the challenge? Anxiety starts taking over his life.

✔ **Confidence killers:** Tricia is on top of the world. She has a good job and feels ecstatic about her forthcoming wedding. However, she is devastated when her fiancé breaks off the engagement. Now, she worries incessantly that something is wrong with her; perhaps she'll never have the life she envisioned for herself.

✔ **Terrorising trauma:** No one ever wants to experience a horrifying or life-threatening experience. Unfortunately, these events do happen. Physical abuse, horrific accidents, battlefield injuries and rape have occurred for centuries, and we suspect that they always will. When they do, severe problems with anxiety often emerge.

Distinguishing Thoughts from Feelings

People often confuse how they feel about a situation with how they think about the events surrounding it. Taking time to consider the difference between thoughts and feelings is helpful. Some people find describing their feelings and emotions hard. Emotions can hurt, but also society doesn't encourage expressing feelings openly, so feelings are avoided or brushed under the carpet, causing low level stress to build up over time.

Getting in touch with your feelings

Noticing your emotions can help you gain insight and discover how to cope more effectively. If you don't know what your feelings are, when they occur, or what brings them on, you can't do much about changing them.

We realise that some people are aware of their feelings and know all too well when they're feeling the slightest amount of anxiety or worry. If you're one of those, feel free to skip or skim the rest of this section.

Take some time right now to assess your mood. First, notice your breathing. Is it rapid and shallow or slow and deep? Notice your posture. Are you relaxed or is some part of your body in an uncomfortable position? Check out all your physical sensations. Look for sensations of tension, queasiness, tightness, dizziness or heaviness. No matter what you find, just study it and sit with the sensations for a while. Then you may ask yourself what *feeling* captures the essence of those sensations. Of course, at this moment you may not have any strong feelings. If so, your breathing is rhythmic and your posture relaxed. Even if that's the case, notice what it feels like to be calm. At other times, notice your stronger sensations.

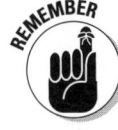

Feeling words describe your physical and mental reactions to events.

Here's a vocabulary list for describing anxious feelings. The next time you can't find the right words to describe how you feel, one of the words that follows may get you started.

Afraid	Panicked
Anxious	Petrified
Agitated	Self-conscious
Apprehensive	Shaky
Disturbed	Tense
Fearful	Terrified
Frightened	Timid
Insecure	Uneasy
Nervous	Uptight
Obsessed	Worried

We're sure that we've missed a few dozen possibilities on the word list, and maybe you have a favourite way to describe your anxiety. That's fine. What we encourage you to do is to start paying attention to your feelings and bodily sensations. You may want to look over this list a number of times and ask whether you've felt any of these emotions recently. Try not to make judgements about your feelings. They may be trying to tell you something useful.

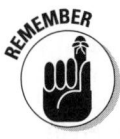

Anxiety and fear also have a positive function: they ready your mind and body for danger. Bad feelings only cause problems when you feel bad repeatedly over a long period of time in the absence of a clear threat.

Negative emotions have an adaptive role to play. They alert you to danger and prepare you to respond. For example, if King Kong knocks on your door, adrenaline floods your body and mobilises you to fight him or run like hell! That's good for situations like that. But if you feel like King Kong is knocking on your door on a regular basis, and he's not even in the area, your anxious feelings cause you more harm than good.

Whether King Kong is knocking at your door or not, identifying anxious, fearful or worried feelings can help you deal with them far more effectively than if you avoid them. When you can see what's going on, you can focus on what to do about your predicament more easily than you can sitting in the dark.

Getting in touch with your thoughts

Just as some people don't have much idea about what they're feeling, others have trouble knowing what they're thinking when they're anxious, worried or stressed. Because thoughts have a powerful influence on feelings, psychologists like to ask their clients what they were thinking when they started to feel upset. Sometimes clients describe feelings rather than thoughts. For example, Dr Baker had the following dialogue with Susan, a client who has severe anxiety:

> **Dr Baker:** So when your supervisor told you off, you said you felt panicked. What thoughts went through your mind?
>
> **Susan:** Well, I just felt horrible. I couldn't stand it.
>
> **Dr Baker:** I know; it must have felt really awful. But I'm curious about what thoughts went through your mind. What did you say to yourself about your supervisor's comments?
>
> **Susan:** I felt my heart pounding in my chest. I don't think I really had any thoughts actually.
>
> **Dr Baker:** That's possible. Sometimes our thoughts escape us for a while. But I wonder, if you think about it now, what did those comments mean to you? What did you think would happen?
>
> **Susan:** I'm shaking right now just thinking about it.

As this example illustrates, people don't always know what's going on in their heads when they feel anxious. Sometimes you may not have clear, identifiable thoughts when you feel worried or stressed. That's perfectly normal.

The challenge is to find out what the stressful event *means* to you. That will tell you what your thoughts are. Consider the example you've just read about. Susan may have felt panicked because she feared losing her job, or she may have thought her boss's criticism meant that she was incompetent.

The reprimand may have also triggered memories of her abusive father. Knowing what thoughts stand behind the feelings can help both Dr Baker and Susan plan the next step.

Tapping into your triggers

If you're like Susan, you don't always know what's going on in your mind when you feel anxious. To figure it out, you need to first identify the *situation* that preceded your upset. Focus on what happened moments before your troublesome feelings. Perhaps you:

- Opened your mail and found that your credit card debt had skyrocketed.
- Heard someone say something that bothered you.
- Read a poor end of term report from your child's school.
- Are wondering why your partner is so late coming home.
- Just got off the scales, having seen a number that you didn't like.
- Noticed that your chest feels tight and your heart is racing for no good reason.

On the other hand, sometimes your anxiety-triggering event hasn't even happened yet. You may be just sitting around and *wham* – an avalanche of anxiety crashes around you. Other people wake up at 4 a.m. with worries marching through their minds. What's the trigger then? Well, it can be an image or a fear of some future event. See the following examples of anxiety-triggering thoughts and images:

- I'll never have enough money for retirement.
- Did I turn off the cooker before I left the house?
- We'll never meet the publication deadline!
- No one is going to like my speech tomorrow.
- What if I'm made redundant tomorrow?
- What if my partner leaves me?

Veronica searches for her anxiety-triggering event.

Veronica works in the university admissions office. The university offers her free tuition for two classes per term. One day, Veronica's manager suggests that she consider taking a course in business administration to increase her chances of getting a promotion in the department. Later, she finds herself feeling unusually anxious. She doesn't know why.

However, after she thinks about it for a while, Veronica realises that the trigger for her anxiety is the thought of studying and having to sit through exams. She has always hated tests. Veronica never considered going to university because she's so anxious about taking tests. Veronica's anxiety trigger is the image of a future event – the idea of taking a test.

Thought-catching

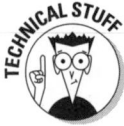

If you know your feelings and the triggers for those feelings, you're ready to become a thought detective. Thoughts powerfully influence emotions. The event may serve as the trigger, but it isn't what directly leads to your anxiety. The meaning that the event holds for you causes the anxiety, and your thoughts reflect that meaning.

For example, suppose your spouse is 45 minutes late coming home from work. You could think *anxious* thoughts:

- ✔ Maybe she's had an accident.
- ✔ She's probably having an affair.

Or you may have different thoughts that don't cause so much anxiety:

- ✔ I love having time alone with the kids.
- ✔ I like having time alone to work on house projects.
- ✔ The traffic must be really bad tonight.

Some thoughts create anxiety; others feel good; still others don't stir up much feeling at all. Capturing your thoughts and seeing how they trigger anxiety and connect to your feelings is important. If you're not sure what thoughts are in your head when you're anxious, you can do something to find them.

First, focus on the anxiety trigger. Think about it for a while; don't rush it. Then ask yourself some questions about the trigger. The following list of what we call *minding-your-mind questions* can help you identify your thoughts or the meaning that the event holds for you:

- ✔ Specifically, what about this event do I find upsetting?
- ✔ What's the worst that could happen?
- ✔ How may this event affect my life?
- ✔ How may this event affect the way others see me?

✔ Does this remind me of anything in my past that bothered me?

✔ What would my parents say about this event?

✔ How may this event affect the way I see myself?

Veronica (you remember her name from earlier in this chapter) suffers from test anxiety. Look at her answers to a few of the following questions from the minding-your-mind list. Her answers indicate what thoughts she has about exams.

✔ **What's the worst that could happen?**

I could fail the test and my boss would find out.

✔ **How may this event affect the way others see me?**

My boss and my colleagues will know how stupid I am.

✔ **How may this event affect the way I see myself?**

I'll finally know for sure that I'm the loser I've always thought I may be.

Even though earlier, Veronica couldn't explain why tests made her so anxious, answering these questions brings her hidden thoughts about exams to light. No wonder she feels so anxious. Perhaps you'll discover some hidden thoughts of your own if you ask yourself these questions about your anxiety triggers.

Here's Andrew's story:

Andrew loves his work. He designs computer systems for a living and relishes creating complex systems to meet his clients' needs. The management appreciates Andrew's expertise and rewards him with a promotion and the opportunity to design a major system for a national laboratory. Andrew can't wait to begin, at least until he realises that part of the project involves giving a number of talks to groups of managers and scientists. Andrew's heart races and he perspires profusely at the mere thought of speaking in front of a group. Andrew has been terrified of speaking in front of an audience since junior school, but he has no idea why.

Andrew has a rather common fear – the fear of speaking in public. He answers a few of the minding-your-mind questions:

✔ **Specifically, what about this event do I find upsetting?**

I'll look silly and forget what I wanted to say.

✔ **How may this event affect my life?**

They'll think I'm incapable of putting this system together, and I'll lose the sale.

✔ **How may this event affect the way others see me?**

They'll know how scared I am and think I'm a fool. Those scientists know more than I do.

When you work with the minding-your-mind questions, use your imagination. Brainstorm and take your time. Even though our examples don't answer all the questions, you may find it useful to build on these ideas.

Tackling your thoughts: Thought therapy

We have three simple strategies for tackling your anxious thoughts:

✔ **Thought court:** Take your thoughts to court and sift through the evidence.

✔ **Rethink risk:** Recalculate the odds of your anxious thoughts coming true – most people overestimate the odds.

✔ **Worst-case scenarios:** Re-examine your ability to cope even if the worst does occur. Most people underestimate their coping resources.

We met Veronica in the section 'Tapping into your triggers', earlier in this chapter. She tracks her anxious thoughts about sitting exams. But she never questions them. She remains anxious and convinced that if she undertakes the course, she will surely fail. And everyone will realise how stupid she is. Veronica needs more than monitoring to deal with her anxious thoughts. She must go to thought court to review the evidence for and against her habitual way of thinking.

Weighing the evidence: Anxiety on trial

The thoughts that lead to your anxious feelings have most likely been around a long time. Most people consider their thoughts to be true. They don't question them. You may be surprised to discover that many of your thoughts don't hold up under scrutiny. If you carefully gather and weigh the evidence, you just may find that your thoughts rest on a foundation made of sand.

Keep in mind that gathering evidence to challenge your thoughts when you're feeling really anxious isn't always easy to do. At those times, it's hard to consider that your thoughts may be inaccurate. When that's the case, you'll be better off waiting until you calm down before hunting for the evidence. At other times, if your anxiety isn't too out of control, you may be able to find evidence. You may find it useful to consider the following *evidence-gathering questions* when judging the accuracy of your anxious thoughts.

✔ Have I had thoughts like these at other times in my life? Have my dire predictions ever come true?

✔ Do I have experiences that would contradict my thoughts in any way?

✔ Is this situation really as awful as I'm making it out to be?

✔ A year from now, how much concern will I have with this issue?

✔ Am I thinking this will happen just because I'm feeling anxious and worried? Am I basing my conclusion mostly on my feelings or on the true evidence?

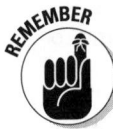

Feelings are always valid in the sense that you feel what you feel. But they are not evidence for supporting anxious predictions. For example, if you feel extremely anxious about taking an exam, the anxiety is not evidence of how you will perform.

Rethinking risk

Another important way to challenge your anxious thoughts is to look at how you assess probabilities. When you feel anxious, like many people, you may *overestimate the odds* of unwanted events actually occurring. It's easy to do. For example, when's the last time you heard a news bulletin reporting that no one got bitten by a snake today, or that half a million planes took off and landed today and not a single one crashed? No wonder people overestimate disaster. Because dramatic events grab our attention, we focus on these events rather than routine ones. That's why it's useful to think about the real, objective odds of your predicted catastrophe happening.

Thoughts are just thoughts. Subject them to a reality test.

Mary from Manchester fears flying. Her father-in-law, who lived in Italy, dies unexpectedly. Mary drives across Europe to the funeral rather than join her husband who chooses to fly. Not only is Mary less available to help her family with arrangements, she misses several extra days of work. Her choice is ironic because, by driving, she greatly increases her odds of being hurt or even dying. Flying is still the safest form of travel available.

Len enjoys walking his dog. Unfortunately, Len also worries that he may have forgotten to lock the door when he leaves the house. More often than not, after he turns the first corner, he goes back to check the lock. Some days, he checks the doorknob four or five times. He feels almost panicked at the idea of someone breaking into his house. Len doesn't realise that he's overestimating two risks. First, although his *thoughts* tell him he probably left the door unlocked, *reality* says that he has never done that. Secondly, only a few break-ins have occurred in his neighbourhood in the past several years. The odds of a burglar plotting to rob Len's home during his 30-minute foray with the dogs are astronomically small.

Both Len and Mary spend too much time and effort avoiding facing their fears, and what they fear is unlikely to occur. Subject your fears to a reality test. Weigh the odds carefully.

Whenever possible, look up the statistical evidence relating to your fears. Unfortunately, you can't always find statistics that help you.

Worst-case scenarios

Some peoples' fears involve issues that go way beyond social embarrassment or temporary financial loss. Severe illness, death, terror, natural disasters, disfigurement, major disabilities, and loss of a loved one are worst-case scenarios. How would you possibly cope with one of these? We're not going to tell you it would be easy, because it wouldn't be.

When you have anxiety about something dreadful happening, it's important to stop avoiding the end of the story. Go there. The more you avoid contemplating the worst, the bigger the fear gets. In our work, we repeatedly find that our clients come up with coping strategies for the worst-case scenario, even the big stuff. When people avoid grappling with their fears instead of becoming copers, they turn into victims.

George, for example, fears flying. He recalculates the risks of flying and realises they're low. He says, 'I know it's relatively safe and that helps a little, but it still scares me.' Recently, George got a promotion. Unfortunately for George, the new position requires considerable travel. George's worst nightmare is that the plane will crash. George asks himself our coping questions and answers them as follows:

✔ **Have I ever dealt with anything like this in the past?**

No, obviously I've never been in a plane crash before.

✔ **How much will this affect my life a year from now?**

Not much, I'd probably be dead!

✔ **Do I know anyone who has coped with something like this, and how did they do it?**

No. None of my friends, relatives or acquaintances has ever been in a plane crash.

✔ **Do I know anyone to whom I could turn for help or support?**

Obviously not. I mean, what could they do?

✔ **Can I think of a creative new possibility that could result from this challenge?**

How? In the few minutes I'd have on the way down, it's doubtful that many creative possibilities would occur to me.

Hmmm. George didn't seem to get much out of our coping questions did he? These questions don't do much good for a small number of worst-case scenarios. For those situations, we have the *ultimate coping questions:*

1. What is it about this eventuality that makes you think you absolutely could not cope and could not possibly stand it?

2. Is it possible that you really could deal with it?

George answers:

1. Okay, I can imagine two different plane crashes. In one, the plane would explode and I probably wouldn't even know what happened. In the other, something would happen to the engine, and I'd experience several minutes of absolute terror. That's what I really fear.

2. Could I deal with that? I suppose I've never thought of that before; it seemed too scary to contemplate. If I really put myself in the plane, I'd probably be gripping the seat, maybe even screaming, but I guess it wouldn't last for long. I suppose I could stand almost anything for a short while. At least if I went down in a plane, I know that my family would be well taken care of. When I really think about it, as unpleasant as it seems, I guess I could deal with it. I'd have to.

Most people fear dying to some extent – even those with strong religious convictions (which can help) rarely welcome the thought. Nevertheless, death is a universal experience. Although most people would prefer a painless, quick exit during sleep, many deaths aren't as easy.

If you have a particular way of dying that frightens you, actively contemplating it works better than trying to block it out of your mind. If you face your fear, you're likely to discover that, like George, you can deal with and accept almost any eventuality.

If you find yourself getting exceptionally anxious or upset by such contemplation, professional help may be useful.

Chapter 5

Exploring How to Conquer Anxiety

· ·

· ·

To help explore anxiety you need to be aware how powerfully your thoughts influence your emotions and perceptions. Taking time to become a thought detective can help you uncover the thoughts that contribute to anxious feelings so you can start to make positive changes.

In this chapter we help you identify your anxious thoughts and give you some strategies to calm your thinking and deal with worry and fear. We also highlight some solutions to simplify your life including relaxation and using all your senses to get back in control again.

Cultivating Calm Thinking

Anxious thoughts capture your attention. They hold your reasonable mind hostage. They demand all your calmness and serenity as ransom. Thus, when you have anxious thoughts, it helps to pursue and destroy them by weighing the evidence, recalculating the odds, and reviewing your true ability to cope.

Another option is to overwhelm your anxious thoughts with calm thoughts. You can accomplish this by using one of two techniques. First, you can try what we call the friend perspective, or you can construct new, calm thoughts to replace your old, anxious thoughts.

Being your own best friend

Sometimes, simple strategies work wonders. This can be one of them. When your anxious thoughts hold most of your reasonable mind hostage, you still have a friend in reserve. Where? Within yourself.

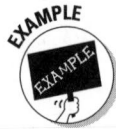

Pick a worry. Any worry. Listen to that worry and everything outrageous it has to say to you. For example, Roger worries about his bills. He has a credit card balance of a few thousand pounds. His car insurance is coming up in a couple of weeks, and he doesn't have the money to pay for it. When Roger contemplates his worry, he thinks that maybe he'll be made bankrupt, his car will be repossessed, and that eventually, he'll lose his house. He feels he has no options and that his situation is hopeless. Roger loses sleep because of his worry. Anxiety shuts down his ability to reason and analyse his dilemma.

Now we ask Roger to help an old friend. We tell him to imagine that James, a friend of his, is sitting in a chair across from him. His friend is in a bit of a mess financially and needs advice on what to do. James fears he will lose everything if he can't come up with the money to pay his car insurance. We ask Roger to come up with some ideas for James.

Surprising to Roger, but not to us, Roger comes up with a whole host of good ideas. He tells James, 'Talk to your car insurers about monthly rather than annual payments. Also, you can possibly increase your limit on your credit card as a short-term solution. Isn't there also a chance of doing some overtime at work? Talk to a debt adviser. Can a friend or relative help out with a short-term loan? In the long run, you need to chip away at that credit-card debt and pull back a little on your spending.'

Another way in which you can use the best friend technique is a development of *cognitive therapy*, the therapy on which this book is based, called 'compassionate mind training'. Using this method, you learn to catch those critical voices and to identify the unpleasant and upsetting things others have said to you and that you now say to yourself.

Compassionate mind training involves providing counter-arguments to those critical thoughts you have about yourself. In the same way that hearing the horrible things others say about you makes you feel bad, saying positive, supportive, encouraging things to yourself, about yourself, can make you feel far better about yourself. You learn to say the helpful things to yourself with the full expression, emotion and compassion that someone special and encouraging would use. You will usually find this has an even more powerful effect than just listing the counter-arguments against your negative thoughts. The arguments are so much more powerful, convincing and meaningful if you can hear them caringly spoken in your imagination. Using this technique, rather than requiring the support to come from others, you can learn to be your own best friend.

Try this technique when you're all alone – alone, that is, except for your friend within.

Truly imagine that your good friend is sitting across from you and talk out loud. Take your time and really try to help. Brainstorm with your friend. You don't have to come up with instant or perfect solutions. Seek out any and every idea you can, even if it sounds foolish at first – it just may lead you to a creative solution.

This approach works because it helps you pull back from the overwhelming emotions that block good, reasonable thinking. Don't dismiss this strategy just because of its simplicity!

Creating calm

Another way to create calm thoughts is to simply look at your anxious thoughts and develop an alternative, more reasonable perspective. The key to this approach is to put your reasonable thoughts on paper. This exercise can have the same effect as chemical medication, but writing your reasonable thoughts down, rather than just thinking of them in your head, is like taking a stronger dose of the medicine and increasing its effectiveness.

Using CBT to Overcome Anxiety

Cognitive behavioural therapy (CBT) techniques have been developed from extensive research, and studies indicate that treatments based on CBT principles lead to the greatest long-term success. The principles underlying all the exercises in this book have come from the development of CBT.

CBT works on the principle that people's behaviour and emotions depend to a large degree on their perception of what they understand is happening. What we think and anticipate can greatly affect our reaction to events and people. Having understood what you're thinking and how to deal with your thoughts, it is possible to train yourself in a different way. This new behaviour can then lead to a potentially more satisfying way of life and become part of your normal lifestyle.

A helpful way to think about understanding and using CBT to overcome anxiety is that the crux of CBT is as straightforward as ABC.

- ✔ **A** refers to the *Antecedent*, or the trigger that sets you off in a direction you didn't want to go in.
- ✔ **B** is for the *Beliefs* that you then apply to the situation.
- ✔ **C** is for the *Consequences* – the outcome.

Learning your ABC goes like this:

1. **First, identify the trigger thought or feeling and call it A – the antecedent event.**

2. **Identify B – your belief about the antecedent.**

3. **Finally, identify C – the consequence of your belief. How did you act and emotionally or physically feel about the situation?**

As you've seen, it's beliefs that largely cause the stressful consequences, not necessarily the actual antecedent event itself. This explains why many people aren't stressed about meeting important deadlines, giving a presentation, or meeting new people – they believe they will cope well and don't predict any awful consequences.

A key part in the process of challenging beliefs is to question the demands that say you must, ought, should or have to achieve a particular outcome. Ask yourself:

✔ Who says you have to believe certain things?

✔ Is it just you in your head or do others make these demands too?

✔ Are others necessarily infallible?

✔ What would happen if you did fail?

✔ Would it really be that unbearably awful?

✔ Are you exaggerating the outcome?

Think of how you could bear it, reminding yourself you don't have to like it. Challenge those over-generalisations – how does not meeting one target make you a total failure in everything? Isn't that a bit unfair on you – and would you judge others in this way?

The aim, having identified A, the antecedent, and challenged B, your beliefs about the antecedent, is to enable you to make your beliefs more realistic and flexible and less demanding, and no longer so absolute. When beliefs are modified, you find that you usually feel emotionally and physically different, and this enables you to evict catastrophising and its companion, procrastination, and get on with the task in hand.

It's very important to tell yourself that like any new skill, learning your ABC takes a while before you know it by rote and incorporate it automatically into your daily routine.

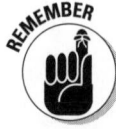

Think of learning your ABC as a daily mental workout – the gym for your mind, where you practise challenging unhelpful, anxiety-inducing thinking. Your workout strengthens you as you develop new stress-reducing, life-improving beliefs.

See Book IV Chapter 3 for more information on Cognitive Behavioural Therapy.

Watching Out for Worry Words

I'll never get this right . . . I always stumble over my words . . . I should really lose some weight . . . Nothing suits me . . . I look an utter mess . . . How can I be so stupid? . . . It will be terrible if I don't get that pay rise . . . I must get this finished, or I'll be in big trouble . . . What if I fail? . . . I'm totally useless at sport.

Imagine inner conversations like these. How would you feel talking to yourself like this? Probably not very good. This section explains how words alone can stir up a whirlwind of anxiety. We help you discover worry words to look out for. They come in several forms and categories, and you'll see how to track them down. Then we give you alternative words and phrases to calm your anxiety.

Getting to grips with worry words

'Sticks and stones may break my bones, but words will never hurt me.' Perhaps you heard this saying as a child. Parents often try to make their children feel better by teaching them this retort to use when others have said nasty things to them. But it usually doesn't work, because words do have power. Words can frighten, judge and hurt.

If those words only came from other people, that would hurt enough. But the words that you use to describe yourself, your world, your actions and your future may have an even greater impact on you than what you hear from others.

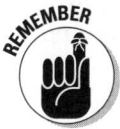

Worry words are words that provoke and increase anxiety. The worry words that you use when you think and talk to yourself easily inflame anxiety and are rarely supported by evidence or reality. Using them unwittingly becomes a bad habit. However, we have good news: Like any habit, the anxiety-arousing word habit can be broken.

Worry words come in four major categories. We go through each of them with you in a moment:

✔ **Extremist:** Words that exaggerate or predict a catastrophe (*catastrophise*).

✔ **All-or-none:** Polar opposites with nothing in between.

> ✔ **Judging, commanding and labelling:** Harsh evaluations and name calling.
>
> ✔ **Victim:** Words that underestimate your ability to cope.

Extremist words

It's amazing how selecting certain words to describe events can make mountains out of molehills. Extremist words grossly magnify troubling situations. In doing so, they aggravate negative emotions.

All-or-none, black-or-white words

Pick up a black-and-white photograph. Any photo will do. Look carefully and you'll see many shades of grey that tend to dominate the picture. Most photos contain very little pure black or white at all. Calling a photo black and white oversimplifies matters and fails to capture the complexity and richness of the images. Just as calling a photograph black and white ignores much of the detail, describing an event in black-and-white terms ignores the full range of human experience. Like a photograph, very little in life is pure black or white.

Nevertheless, people easily slip into language that oversimplifies. Like extremist language, only using words that are opposites – black and white words – rather than the ones in between, intensifies negative feelings.

Judging words

Judging words come in the following three varieties, and we show you examples in Table 5-1:

✔ **Judgements:** These are harsh judgements about yourself or what you do. For example, when you make an all-too-human mistake and call it an utter failure, you're judging your actions rather than merely describing them.

✔ **Commandments:** This category contains words that dictate absolute, unyielding rules about your behaviour or feelings. If you tell yourself that you *should* have taken or *must* take a particular action, you're listening to an internal drill sergeant. This zealous drill sergeant tolerates no deviation from a dogmatic code of conduct.

✔ **Labels:** Finally, self-degrading labels put the icing on the cake. Steve's accounting mistake, for example, leads to all three types of condemnations: He judges his error as *stupid,* he *shouldn't* have allowed it to happen, and he declares himself an *idiot.* It's no wonder that Steve feels anxious when he works on his accounts. Ironically, the increased anxiety makes further mistakes more likely.

Table 5-1	The Three Categories of Judging Words	
Judgements	*Commandments*	*Labels*
Bad	Have to	Fool
Despicable	Must	Imbecile
Failure	Ought	Idiot
Inadequate	Should	Twit
Pathetic	Or else!	A nothing
Stupid	Got to	A nobody
Undeserving	It's imperative	Pig
Feeble	It's vital	Greedy guts
Wrong	Now!	Wimp

Victim words

You may remember the story *The Little Engine That Could* by Watty Piper about the train that needed to climb a steep hill. The author of the book wisely chose not to have the engine say, 'I think I *can't;* I'll never do it; this hill's impossible.'

The world feels a much scarier place when you habitually think of yourself as a victim of circumstance. Certain words can serve as a flag for that kind of thinking, such as the list of victimising words that follows:

✔ Can't

✔ Defenceless

✔ Frail

✔ Helpless

✔ Impossible

✔ Impotent

✔ Incapacitated

✔ Overwhelmed

✔ Powerless

✔ Shattered

✔ Too much

✔ Vulnerable

✔ Worn out

Nadia, suffering from severe generalised anxiety, jumps whenever she hears loud noises. Married for 20 years to a husband who's been repeatedly unfaithful, Nadia doesn't consider leaving him, because she worries that she *can't* survive on her own. She feels *helpless* to deal with the demands of life on her own and believes that it would be *impossible* for her to handle working and caring for her two teenage kids. Even now, she feels *overwhelmed* by housework.

Victim words demoralise. They offer no hope. With no hope, there's little reason for positive action. When victims believe themselves to be defenceless, they feel vulnerable and afraid.

People who describe themselves as victims often don't feel compelled to even try to do much about whatever predicaments they face. Some people express sympathy for them, and others may offer to take care of them. Whether this constitutes much in the way of an advantage or compensation, we leave you to decide.

Refuting and replacing your worry words

Ask yourself how you truly want to feel. Few people like feeling anxious, worried and stressed. Who would choose those feelings? So perhaps you agree that you prefer to feel calm and serene rather than wound up. Set that as your goal.

A good way to start on your journey towards feeling better is to change your worry words. However, you aren't likely to stop using worry words just because we told you that they create anxiety. That's because you still may think that these words accurately describe yourself and/or your world. Many people go through life without questioning their self-talk, simply assuming that words equate with reality.

In order to refute the accuracy of your internal self-talk, consider a small change in philosophy. This shift entails questioning the idea that thoughts, language and words automatically capture truth. Substitute that idea with a new one, using logic and evidence-gathering to structure your reality. At the same time, keep in mind that your goal is to experience greater calm.

Disputing all-or-none words

People use all-or-none words, such as *never, always, absolute, forever, unceasing* and *constant,* because they're quick, easy, and they add emotional punch. But these terms have insidious downsides: They push your thinking to extremes, and your emotions tag along for the ride. Furthermore, all-or-none words detract from coping and problem solving.

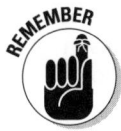

Rarely does careful gathering of evidence support the use of all-or-none words. Many people use all-or-none words to predict the future or to describe the past. But look carefully and you'll see that people often talk about the past in the present tense; for example, 'You *always* criticise me' or 'I *never* get promoted.' This then states, in black and white terms, that this is the reality of the past, the present, and by implication the future as well. You're saying that that's what happened to you in the past and it's happening now, and you're predicting that it will always happen in the future – it's just the way it is! Whether you're talking to yourself or someone else, these words hardly facilitate calmness, nor do they describe what really happened or what's likely to happen in the future. So try to stay in the present and also to drop evidence-gathering words that keep you *in the present without exaggeration.*

Book V

Mental Health

Judging the judging words

Words that judge, command or label, such as *should, must, failure, fool, undeserving* and *twit,* inflict unnecessary pain and shame on their recipients. You may hear these words from others or from your own critic within.

Like the other types of worry words, commandments don't inspire motivation and seldom improve performance. Yet people use these words for those very purposes. They think that saying I *must* or I *should* will help them, but it's more likely that those words will cause them to feel guilty or anxious. Self-scolding merely increases guilt and anxiety, and guilt and anxiety inevitably decrease both motivation and performance.

Try replacing your judging, commanding and labelling words with more reasonable, accurate and supportable alternatives:

- ✔ **Judging:** I got pathetic results for my end-of-term exams. I must be stupid.

  Reasonable alternative: It wasn't the result that I wanted, but I can study more and do better next term. Given how little work I actually did, the results were pretty reasonable.

- ✔ **Commanding:** I must have a happy marriage. I should have what it takes to keep it happy, so it must be all my fault if problems arise.

  Reasonable alternative: Much as I'd like to have a happy marriage, I was okay before I met my wife, and I can learn to be okay again if I have to. Being happily married is just my strong preference, and I don't have complete control over the outcome; it does take two, after all.

In the earlier section 'Judging words', Steve made an error in his accounts. He promptly condemned himself by calling himself a fool and telling himself he should never make an error like that again. After Steve tackles this bad habit, he changes his views. Like most people, Steve makes another mistake in his cheque book three months later. This time he realises the world will not end and that he is not stupid. He stops and reflects. Reflection allows him to see that most of his mistakes happen when he tries to do two or three tasks at once. He decides to slow down a little. Using less harsh judgements allows Steve to learn from his mistakes rather than berate himself.

Vanquishing victim words

Victim words, such as *powerless, helpless, vulnerable, overwhelmed* and *defenceless,* put you in a deep hole and fill you with a sense of vulnerability and fear. They make you feel as though finding a way out is impossible and that hope remains out of reach. Yet, as with other worry words, only rarely do they convey unmitigated truth. It is worth remembering the old adage that when you find yourself in a hole, it's best to stop digging.

Victim words can become what are known as self-fulfilling prophecies. If you *think* that a goal is impossible, you're not likely to achieve it, and there will be little point in attempting it at all. If you *think* that you're powerless, you won't draw upon your coping resources. Instead, you're likely to remain stuck in your adversity. As an alternative, consider the logic of your victim words. Is there anything at all that you can do to remedy or at least improve your problem?

Gather evidence for refuting victim words that appear in your self-talk. Ask yourself whether you've ever managed to cope with a similar situation before. Think about a friend, an acquaintance, or anyone at all who has successfully dealt with a burden like yours.

Facing Fear One Step at a Time

This section explains how you can get back in control and overcome your fears in manageable steps. We discuss how to face fears in your imagination. That prepares you for the next step of tackling your fears by facing them head on, but in small steps.

Exposure: Coming to grips with your fears

No single strategy discussed in this book works more effectively in the fight against anxiety than exposure. Simply put, exposure involves putting yourself in direct contact with whatever it is that makes you anxious. Well now, that may just sound a little ridiculous to you.

After all, it probably makes you feel pretty anxious to even think about staring your fears in the face. We understand that reaction, but please realise that if you're terrified of heights, exposure doesn't ask you to go on the London Eye tomorrow or climb Ben Nevis. Or if you worry about having a panic attack in crowds, you don't have to sit in the stands of the new Wembley Stadium as your first step.

Graded exposure – taking one step at a time

Exposure involves a systematic, gradual set of steps that you can tackle one at a time. You don't move from the first step until you master it. Then, when you're comfortable with the first one, you move to the second. While it's true that each new step brings on anxiety, you'll find it's not an overwhelming amount.

Don't try exposure if your anxiety is severe. You'll need professional guidance. If any step raises your anxiety to an extreme level, stop any further self-help attempts unless you get professional help as well. Also, don't attempt exposure if you're in the midst of a crisis or have a current problem with alcohol or substance abuse.

Getting ready

Why practise relaxing? Exposure makes you anxious. No way around that. Working out how to relax can help you feel more confident about dealing with that anxiety. Relaxation can help keep the inevitable anxiety within tolerable limits.

We suggest a breathing strategy:

1. **Inhale slowly, deeply and fully through your nose.**

2. **Hold your breath for a slow count of six.**

3. **Slowly breathe out through your mouth to a count of eight, while making a slight hissing or sighing sound as you do. That sound can be ever so soft.**

4. **Repeat this type of breath ten times.**

Building blocks

Breaking down the exposure process into manageable steps is important. To start the process:

1. **Pick one and only one of your worries – perhaps there's one within the following list of examples:**

   • Enclosed spaces

   • Financial ruin

   • Flying

   • Having a panic attack (a fear of a fear)

   • People

2. **Think about every conceivable aspect of your fear or worry.**

   What triggers your fear? Include all the activities surrounding your fear. For example, if you're afraid of flying, perhaps you fear driving to the airport or packing your luggage. Or if you're afraid of dogs, you avoid walking near them, and you probably don't visit people who have dogs in their homes. Whenever the fear occurs, take some notes on it. Think about all the anticipated and feared outcomes. Include all the details, such as other people's reactions and the setting.

Imagining the worst

Many times, the best way to begin exposure is in your imagination. That's because imagining your fears usually elicits less anxiety than actually confronting them directly. In addition, you can use your imagination when it would be impossible to replicate your real fear. For example, if you fear getting a disease, such as hepatitis C, actually exposing yourself to the virus wouldn't be a good idea.

You may think that viewing your fears through your mind's eye wouldn't make you anxious. However, most people find that when they picture their fears in rich detail, their bodies react. As they gradually master their fears in their minds, generally the fears reduce when confronting the real-life version.

Facing your fears (gulp)

Although we usually recommend starting exposure in your imagination, the most effective type of exposure happens in real life. The strategy works in much the same way as imaginary exposure; you break your fears down into small steps and stack them into a tower of fear from the least problematic to the most intensely feared. Now, it's time to face your fears head on. Gulp.

1. **Start with a brief relaxation procedure, such as the one of those described earlier in this chapter.**

2. **Select a fear or a group of worries with a similar theme, such as fear of rejection or risk of personal injury.**

3. **Next, break the fear into a number of sequential steps, each step being slightly more difficult than the prior step.**

4. **Finally, take one step at a time.** If your anxiety starts to rise to an unmanageable level, try using one of the brief relaxation techniques. Keep working on each step until your anxiety drops, generally by at least half.

See the following hints to help you get through the exposure process:

✔ Get help from your partner or a friend, but only if that person is someone you really trust. This person can give you encouragement and support.

✔ If you must, take a small step back. Don't make a complete retreat unless you absolutely feel out of control.

✔ Your mind will tell you, 'Stop! You can't do this. It won't work anyway.' Don't listen to this chatter. Simply study your body's reactions and realise that they will not harm you.

✔ Find a way to reward yourself for each successful step that you take. Perhaps indulge in some desired purchase or treat yourself in some other way.

✔ Use a little positive self-talk to help quell rising anxiety, if you need to.

✔ Understand that at times you will feel uncomfortable. View that discomfort as progress; it is part of how you overcome your fears.

✔ Practise, practise, and practise.

✔ Don't forget to practise a brief relaxation procedure before and during the exposure.

✔ Remember to stay with each step until your anxiety drops. Realise that your body can't maintain anxiety forever. It will calm down if you give it sufficient time.

✔ Expect exposure to take time. Go at a reasonable pace. Keep moving forwards, but remember that you don't have to conquer your fear in a few days. Even with daily practice, self-exposure can take a number of months.

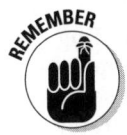

Remember to choose realistic goals. For example, let's say you're afraid of spiders, so much so that you can't enter a room without an exhaustive search for hidden horrors. You don't have to get to the point where you let tarantulas crawl up and down your arms. Let yourself feel satisfied with the ability to enter rooms without unnecessary checking. And if you do see a spider, either to be able to ignore it until it goes away or use a glass and a piece of cardboard to pick it up and deposit it outside.

Simply Simplifying Your Life

Simply by simplifying your life you can have a positive effect on reducing your anxiety. Consider the following tips and ideas.

Delegating tasks to free up extra time

Many people with anxiety feel they must take all the responsibility for their jobs, the care of their families, and their homes. Unless they have a role in everything, they worry things may not get done. And if someone else takes over a task, they fear the result will fall short of their standards.

Grace works many long hours and still feels the need to cook, clean, transport her kids, and do most of the household errands. Sometimes her husband offers to do the washing or cooking, but she turns him down, thinking that he'll only mess it up. But when Grace makes the decision to reorganise her life, she knows that she'll have to start delegating. She ponders what, how, who and when. Talking to some close friends, she discovers they're as stuck and dissatisfied as her. Remembering some brainstorming techniques learned at a business seminar, she invites a couple of her friends over with their partners and suggests they all work together on the ideas. They come up with tasks that can be delegated, to share out the onerous workload. See the following list to find out what they came up with:

- ✔ **Take the risk of letting husband do some laundry and cooking.** If he makes a mess of it, Grace can show him how to improve next time.

- ✔ **Employ a cleaner to do the ironing and the more time-consuming domestic chores.** While it may cost a bit, Grace's long working hours earn her more than enough money to cover it.

- ✔ **Buy good quality pre-prepared foods, with minimal or preferably no additives, that just need to be placed in the oven to cook.**

- ✔ **The whole family can spend one hour a week in a concentrated, joint cleaning effort.** Her husband suggests that if everyone does the cleaning at the same time, with specific delegated tasks, it may even be fun.

- ✔ **Grace's secretary will take on some more responsibilities, including dealing with some client phone calls and scheduling Grace's appointments.** Grace realises that because she so seldom delegates, her secretary has quite a bit of free time. Grace also discovers that her secretary is much happier with the additional responsibility and challenges.

- ✔ **Employ someone to come in monthly and do the heavy, time-consuming work in the garden.** Grace's husband says that he doesn't mind doing some of the work, but employing someone would give them more time together.

- ✔ **Read *Time Management For Dummies* by Clare Evans (Wiley).** It's got some great tips on how to save time and effort and get organised. When you're organised, tasks go more smoothly and faster.

We realise a number of these ideas cost money. Not always as much as you may think, but still they do cost something. Partly it's a matter of how highly you rate money on your priority list. Balance money against time for the things that you value.

However, not all families can consider such options. While not all these options have financial implications, why not get creative? Ask your friends, colleagues, and family for ideas on how to delegate. It may change your life.

Come up with two tasks that you can delegate to someone else. They don't need to cost money, just relieve one or more of your burdens in a way that can save you time and give you more energy to spend on what you enjoy.

Just saying no

We have one more idea. Say no. If you're anxious, you may have trouble standing up for your rights. Anxiety often prevents people from expressing their feelings and needs. When that happens, resentment joins anxiety and leads to frustration and anger. Furthermore, if you can't say no, other people can purposefully or inadvertently take advantage of you. You no longer own your time and your life.

Grace agrees to do nearly all that anyone asks of her. When her boss asks her to work late at the last minute, she always agrees. Even if working late impinges on important plans, she rarely expresses unwillingness. She also finds it difficult to hang up on annoying cold-call telephone sales people. She gives a few pounds to every charity request, even if she's never heard of the organisation. She drives other people's children more than any of the other parents who are in the lift-sharing scheme. When her children need last-minute help on homework projects because of their own procrastination, she pitches in despite her own fatigue and better judgement.

If you're a little like Grace, we have some suggestions for learning how to say no. Realise it will take you some time to incorporate this new habit. You've probably been agreeing to fulfil everyone's requests for many years, so it will take a while to do something different.

First, notice the situations in which you find yourself agreeing when you don't really want to. Does it happen mostly at work, with family, with friends, or with strangers? When people ask you to do something, try the following:

- ✔ **Validate the person's request or desire.** For example, if someone asks you if you would mind dropping off something at the post office on your way home from work, say, 'I know it's more convenient for you if I drop it off . . .' This will give you more time to consider whether you really want to do it.

- ✔ **After you make up your mind, look the person who's making the request in the eye.** You don't need to rush your response.

- ✔ **Give a brief explanation, especially if it's a friend or family member.** However, remember that you really don't owe anyone an explanation; it's only good manners. You can say that you'd like to help out, but it just isn't possible, or you can even simply state that you really would rather not.

✔ **Be explicit that you if are choosing to do what you've been asked, this does not mean you're setting a precedent that you will always follow.** You can always add 'I can't do this regularly, though.'

✔ **Be clear that you cannot or will not do what you've been asked.** It's a fundamental human right to say no.

✔ **If you do fall into the old habit of saying yes, contact the person the next day and explain that having thought about it, you realise it just isn't feasible.** Allow yourself a second bite at the cherry, rather than telling yourself that now you've agreed, you're saddled with that decision.

Grace answers the phone and a double-glazing salesperson cheerfully begins his spiel. He talks so quickly that Grace can't speak without interrupting him. Then she realises that she has the right to interrupt. After all, he's interrupting her dinner. So she musters up her courage and declares, 'Thank you for calling. I'm just not interested.' The salesperson goes right on and says, 'Can I ask you why not?' She responds 'No!' and hangs up the phone. Her husband and children look on in amazement.

When you say no to bosses, colleagues, friends, or family members, they may be temporarily unhappy with you. If you find yourself overreacting to their displeasure, it may be due to an anxiety-provoking assumption.

Sleep, Sweet Sleep

Have you ever experienced early morning worry? As if falling asleep isn't hard enough, many people wake up before they want to, driven into high alert with anxious thoughts racing through their consciousness. In this section, you can find out how to get the best rest possible. Also, we show that what you do in the hours before going to bed can either help or hinder your sleep. Finally, you will see how to get rid of those recurrent nightmares once and for all.

The tendency towards early morning wakening with an inability to get back to sleep can be a sign of depression as well as anxiety. If your appetite changes, your energy decreases, your mood drops, your ability to concentrate diminishes, and you've lost interest in activities that you once found pleasurable, you may be clinically depressed. You should check with a mental health practitioner or a doctor to find out whether this is the case.

The ABC of getting your Zs

Your sleep environment matters. Of course, some rare birds can sleep almost anywhere – on the couch, in a chair, on the floor, in the car, or even at their desks at work. On the other hand, most of us require the comfort of a bed and the right conditions. Sleep experts report that for a restful sleep, you should sleep in a room that's:

- ✔ **Dark:** You have a clock in your brain that tells you when it's time to sleep. Darkness helps set the clock by causing the brain to release melatonin, a hormone that helps to induce sleep. Consider putting up curtains that block out most of the sun if you find yourself awakened by the early morning light or if you need to sleep during the day. Some people even wear an eye mask to keep light out.

- ✔ **Cool:** People sleep better in a cool room. If you feel cold, adding blankets is usually preferable to a warm room.

- ✔ **Quiet:** If you live near a busy street or have loud neighbours, consider getting a fan or white-noise generator to block out nuisance noises. The worst kind of noise is intermittent and unpredictable. The various kinds of sporadic noise that can be blocked out by the consistent noise of a simple electric fan may amaze you.

- ✔ **Complete with a comfortable bed:** Mattresses matter. If you share your bed with another person or a pet, ensure that there's enough room for all of you.

In other words, make your bedroom a retreat that looks inviting and cosy. Spoil yourself with quality sheets and pillowcases. You may want to try aromatherapy. Many people claim that the fragrance of lavender helps them sleep, although no-one knows for sure whether it works.

Following a few relaxing routines

Sleep revitalises your physical and mental resources. Studies show that sleep deprivation causes people to drive as if they're under the influence of alcohol. Without sufficient sleep over long periods, people are likely to make more errors. Sleep deprivation makes you irritable, crabby, anxious and despondent.

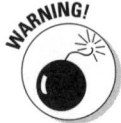

You need to schedule a reasonable amount of time for sleep – at least seven or eight hours. Don't burn the candle at both ends. We don't care how much work you have on your plate; depriving yourself of sleep can only make you less productive and less pleasant to be around.

So, first and foremost, allow sufficient time for sleep. But that's not enough if you have trouble with sleep, so we suggest that you look at the ideas in the subsections that follow to improve the quality of your sleep.

Associating sleep with your bed

One of the most important principles of sleep is to teach your brain to associate sleep with your bed. That means that when you get into bed, don't bring work along with you. Some people find that reading in bed relaxes them, and others like to watch a little TV before bed. That's fine if it works for you, but if those activities don't relax you, avoid doing them in bed.

If you go to bed and lie there for more than 20 or 30 minutes, unable to fall asleep, get up. Again, the point is to train your brain to link your bed to sleep. You can train your brain to dislike getting up by doing some unpleasant (though fairly passive, even boring) chore while you're awake. If you do this a number of times, your brain will find it easier to start feeling drowsy when you're in bed.

Just before hitting the sack

Some people find that taking a warm bath with fragrant oils or bath salts about an hour before hitting the hay is soothing. You may discover that soaking in a scented bath, in a dimly lit bathroom, while listening to relaxing music before going to bed is just the right ticket to solid slumber. Studies show that relaxation can improve sleep.

Whenever possible, go to bed at close to the same time every night. Many people like to stay up late at weekends, and that's fine if you're not having sleep problems. But if you are, we recommend sticking to the same schedule as during the week. You need a regular routine and passive activities before bed.

Don't do strenuous physical or mental exercise within the few hours before going to sleep. Almost any stimulating activity can interfere with sleep.

Watching what you eat and drink

Obviously, you don't want to drink quantities of caffeinated drinks in the couple of hours before you go to bed. Don't forget that many sources other than coffee – colas, certain teas, chocolate, and certain pain relievers – contain caffeine. Of course, some people seem impervious to the effects of caffeine, while others are better off not consuming any after lunchtime. Even if you weren't bothered by caffeine in the past, you can develop sensitivity to it as you age. Consider caffeine's effects on you if you're having trouble sleeping.

Nicotine is also a stimulant. Try to avoid smoking just prior to bedtime. Obviously, it's preferable to quit smoking entirely, but if you haven't been able to stop yet, at least control how much you smoke before bedtime.

Alcohol relaxes the body and should be a great way of aiding sleep, but it isn't. That's because alcohol disrupts your sleep cycles. You don't get as much of the important REM sleep, and you may find yourself waking during the night or up early in the morning, unable to get back to sleep. However, some people find that drinking a glass or two of wine in the evening is relaxing. That's fine, but watch the amount.

Heavy meals prior to going to bed aren't such a great idea either; many people find that eating too much before bed causes mild discomfort. In addition, you may want to avoid highly spiced and/or fatty foods prior to bed. However, going to bed hungry is also not a good idea; the key is balance.

So what should you eat or drink before bed? Herbal teas, such as chamomile or valerian, have many advocates. We don't have much data on how well they work, but herbal teas are quite unlikely to interfere with sleep, and they're pleasant to drink. Some evidence supports eating a small carbohydrate snack before bedtime to help induce sleep.

Medication options

Some people try treating their sleep problems with over-the-counter medications, many of which contain antihistamines that do help, but can lead to drowsiness the next day. Occasional use of these medications is relatively safe for most. Herbal formulas, such those containing valerian, may also help.

If sleep problems are chronic, you should consult your doctor. A medication that you're already taking may possibly be interfering with your sleep. Your doctor may prescribe medication to help induce sleep. Many sleep medications become less effective over time, and some carry the risk of addiction. These potentially addictive medications are only used for a short period. On the other hand, a few sleep medications work for a longer time as an aid to sleep without danger of addiction. Talk about your sleep problem with your doctor for more information and help.

Relaxation: The Five-Minute Solution

In this section, the relaxation procedures fall into two major categories: breathing techniques and ways for relaxing the body. Some of them can take a little longer to become good at, but they can all be done in five minutes when you get the hang of them. The key is daily practice. Like every other skill, the more you practise, the easier and faster it gets.

Blowing anxiety away

Breathing is something you've practised more than anything else in your life. In waking moments, you don't normally even think about your breathing. And it's a safe bet to say that most of us aren't aware of thinking about breathing while we are asleep either. Yet, of all our biological functions, breathing is the most critical to life. Without oxygen, we die! You can go weeks without food, and a couple of days without water, but only minutes without breathing at all. You need oxygen to purify the bloodstream, burn up waste products, and rejuvenate every part of the body and mind. If you're not getting enough oxygen, then your:

- ✔ Thinking becomes sluggish
- ✔ Blood pressure goes up
- ✔ Heart rate increases

You'll also get dizzy, shaky and depressed.

Many people react to stress with rapid, shallow breathing that messes up the optimum ratio of oxygen to carbon dioxide in the blood. This phenomenon is called *hyperventilation,* and it causes a variety of distressing symptoms:

- ✔ Blurred vision
- ✔ Disorientation
- ✔ Jitteriness
- ✔ Loss of consciousness
- ✔ Muscle cramps
- ✔ Poor concentration
- ✔ Rapid pulse
- ✔ Tingling sensations in the extremities or face

Anxiety and relaxation: A recipe for incompatibility

Have you ever known two people who couldn't be in the same room at the same time? If they show up at the same party, there's bound to be trouble. They're like oil and water – they just don't mix.

Anxiety and relaxation are a little like that. Think about it. How can you be anxious at the same time that you're relaxed? Not an easy accomplishment. Psychologists have a term for this phenomenon – *reciprocal inhibition.* Many psychologists believe that the techniques described in this chapter work because relaxation inhibits anxiety and anxiety inhibits relaxation. Training yourself in the use of relaxation skills should therefore help you inhibit your anxiety.

Hyperventilation frequently accompanies panic attacks as well as chronic anxiety. Many of the symptoms of over-breathing feel like symptoms of anxiety, and many people with anxiety disorders tend to hyperventilate. Therefore, finding out how to breathe properly is considered to be an effective antidote to anxiety.

When you came into the world, unless you had a physical problem with your lungs, you probably had no problems breathing – in fact, after you started, you just didn't stop. Look at most babies. Unless they're in distress from hunger, thirst, pain, or cold, they need no instruction on how to breathe in a slow, even, regular way, or in how to relax. Their little tummies rise and fall with each breath in a rhythmic, natural way. The stresses of everyday life, however, can mess up your inborn, natural breathing response.

Under stress, breathing often becomes shallow and fast. People sometimes hold their breath when they feel stressed and aren't even aware of doing it. Try noticing your breathing when you feel stressed and see whether you're a breath-holder or a rapid, shallow breather.

You can also see what your breathing is like when you're not stressed:

1. **Lie down on your back.**
2. **Put one hand on your stomach and the other on your chest.**
3. **Notice the movements of your hands as you breathe.**

   If you're breathing correctly, the hand on your stomach rises as you inhale and lowers as you exhale. The hand on your chest doesn't move so much, and to the extent that it does, it should do so in tandem with the other hand.

The odds are that if you have a problem with anxiety, your breathing probably needs some attention. That's especially so if you have trouble with panic attacks. Breathing practice can start you on the way towards feeling calmer.

The benefits of controlled breathing

Just in case you think that improving the way you breathe sounds like a rather unimaginative, simplistic way to reduce anxiety, you may want to consider the healthy effects. Studies show that training in breathing can contribute to the reduction of panic attacks within a matter of a few weeks. Other studies have indicated that as well as calming worry, controlled breathing can slightly reduce blood pressure, improve the heart's rhythm, reduce certain types of epileptic seizures, sharpen mental performance, increase blood circulation, and possibly even improve the outcome of cardiac rehabilitation efforts following a heart attack. Not a bad list of benefits for such a simple skill.

Abdominal breathing for only five minutes a day

Figure out how to breathe with your *diaphragm*. This is the muscle that lies between your abdominal cavity and your lung cavity. Try this exercise to start breathing like a baby again. You may want to lie down, or you can do this while sitting if you have a large comfortable chair in which you can stretch out.

1. **Check your body for tension. Notice whether certain muscles feel tight or whether your breathing is shallow and rapid. See whether you're clenching your teeth or whether you have other distressing feelings.**

   You may rate your tension on a scale from 1 to 10, with 1 representing complete relaxation and 10 meaning total tension.

2. **Place a hand on your stomach.**

3. **Breathe in slowly through your nose and fill the lower part of your lungs.**

   You'll know you're doing this correctly if your hand rises from your abdomen.

4. **Pause and hold your breath for a moment.**

5. **Exhale slowly.**

   As the air goes out, imagine that your entire body is deflating like a balloon and let it go limp.

6. **Pause briefly again.**

7. **Inhale the same way slowly through your nose to a slow count of four.**

   Check to see that your hand rises from your abdomen. Your chest should move only slightly and in tandem with your stomach.

8. **Pause and hold your breath briefly.**

9. **Exhale to a slow count of six.**

   At first, if you find that hard to do, use a count of four. Later, you'll find that slowing down to a count of six is easier.

10. **Continue breathing in and out in this fashion for five minutes.**

11. **Check your body again for tension and rate that tension on a scale of 1 to 10.**

We recommend that you do this exercise once a day for five minutes. You'll find it relaxing, and it won't add stress to your day by taking up much of your valuable time. Try it for five minutes for ten days in a row. After you do that, try noticing your breathing at various times during your regular routine. You'll quickly see whether you're breathing through the diaphragm, or through the upper chest like so many people do. Slowly but surely, abdominal breathing can become a new habit that decreases your stress.

Panic breathing

Occasionally you may need a faster, more powerful technique. Perhaps you're at a shopping centre and feel trapped, or maybe you're on your way to a job interview and feel overwhelmed. Whatever the situation, when stress hits you and it feels like an unexpected punch in the stomach, try our panic-breathing technique.

1. **Inhale deeply and slowly through your nose.**

2. **Hold your breath for a slow count of six.**

3. **Slowly breathe out through your lips to a count of eight, making a slight hissing sound as you do.**

   That sound can be so soft that only you can hear it. You don't have to worry about what anyone around you may think.

4. **Repeat the above between five to ten times.**

You may think that panic breathing will be difficult to do when stress suddenly strikes like a lightning bolt. We won't deny it takes some practice. However, children have successfully discovered how to use this technique when they face painful medical procedures. When the children used the panic-breathing technique, they felt a little calmer and reported feeling less distress and pain. The key is the slight hissing sound, which gives you a much easier way to slow down your breath.

If panic breathing doesn't help, and you feel like you may be having a full-blown panic attack that won't go away, try breathing in and out of a paper bag. If you're hyperventilating, as people often do during a panic attack, the air that you breathe out is very rich in carbon dioxide, and so the level of carbon dioxide in the blood drops lower and lower. As the level of carbon dioxide decreases and the amount of oxygen in the blood increases, your body releases a variety of chemicals that put you in a state of high alert. You feel a whole host of the physical symptoms of anxiety (racing heart, sweating, and so on), and it's pretty uncomfortable. Breathing into the bag lets you re-inhale some of the carbon-dioxide-rich air that you have just exhaled and so rebalances the ratio of oxygen to carbon dioxide, which should cut the panic attack short.

The gentle inhale/exhale technique

You're likely to find that the gentle inhale/exhale breathing technique is the simplest of all the exercises. It takes just a few minutes and requires only a small amount of attention.

1. **Find a comfortable place to sit down.**

2. **Notice your breathing.** Feel the air as it flows through your nostrils and into your lungs. Feel your muscles pull the air in and push it out.

3. **Let your breathing flow rhythmically, evenly and smoothly.**

4. **Imagine that you're holding a flower with dainty, delicate petals up to your nose.** Allow your breath to soften so that the petals remain undisturbed.

5. **Rhythmically breathe in and out with an even flow.**

6. **Continue to notice the air as it passes through your airways.**

7. **Notice how focusing on nothing but your breathing gently relaxes your mind and body.**

8. **Allow the air to refresh you.**

9. **Continue your gentle breathing and just focus solely on all the sensations of smooth, even breathing.**

Work on the gentle inhale/exhale technique for five minutes a day for ten days. You may then find that you want to continue with one or more of our breathing techniques each day of your life. After all, you have to breathe anyway, so you may as well do it in a relaxing, anxiety-reducing manner.

Relaxing by tightening: Progressive muscle relaxation

Over half a century ago, Edmund Jacobsen developed what came to be the most widely used relaxation technique, *progressive muscle relaxation*. You can find a wide variety of similar techniques, all described as progressive muscle relaxation, in various books and journals. Each of them may use slightly different muscle groups or go through the muscle groups in a different order, but they all do essentially the same thing.

Progressive muscle relaxation involves going through various muscle groups in the body and tensing each one for a little while, followed by a quick letting go of the tension. You then pay close attention to the sensation of release, noticing how the limp muscles feel in contrast to their previous tense state.

Getting ready to mellow

You'll find it useful to look for the right place in which to do your progressive muscle relaxation. You probably don't have a soundproof room, but find the quietest place that you can. Consider unplugging the phone and turning off your mobile.

Choose some comfortable clothing or loosen any clothing you're wearing that's tight and constricting. Take off your shoes, belt, or anything that's uncomfortable.

Realise that when you begin tensing each muscle group, you shouldn't over-exert; don't tighten using more than about two-thirds of your strongest effort. You want firm tension, but you're not body building. When you tense, hold the tension for six to ten seconds and notice how it feels. Then let go of the tension all at once, as though a string holding the muscles up has been cut.

After you release the muscles, focus on the relaxed feeling and allow it to deepen for 10 to 15 seconds. If you don't achieve the desired state of relaxation for that muscle group, you can try once or twice more if you want.

Be aware that you can't *force* relaxation to happen. You *allow* it to happen. Perfectionists struggle with this idea. Don't force it and do try and banish the idea that you *must* do this exercise *perfectly*. Remember it's a skill that you'll acquire slowly over time.

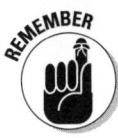

When you tighten one muscle group, try to keep all the other muscles in your body relaxed. Doing this takes a little practice, but you can figure out how to tense one body area at a time. Try and make sure you keep your face relaxed when you're tensing any area other than your face. Yoga instructors often say, 'Soften your eyes.' Though it's unclear exactly what that means, this instruction has often been found helpful – whatever it is that you're actually doing to achieve it.

Occasionally, relaxation training makes people feel surprisingly uncomfortable. If this happens to you, simply stop. If it continues to occur with repeated practice, you may want to seek professional help. Also, don't tighten any part of your body that makes you feel uncomfortable. Avoid tightening any area that's suffered injury or has given you frequent trouble, such as your lower back.

Discovering the progressive muscle technique

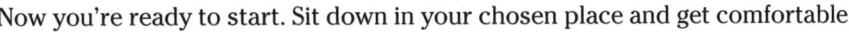

Now you're ready to start. Sit down in your chosen place and get comfortable.

1. **Take a deep breath, hold it, concentrate on the feelings, and then let the tension go.**

   Pulling the air in from your abdomen, breathe deeply. (See the section 'Abdominal breathing for only five minutes a day', earlier in this chapter, if you're unclear about this.) Hold your breath for three or four seconds and slowly let the air out. Imagine your whole body is a balloon losing air as you exhale and let tension go out with the air. Take three more such breaths and feel your entire body getting more and more limp with each breath.

2. Squeeze your hands tight and then relax.

Squeeze your fingers into a fist. Feel the tension and hold it for six to ten seconds. Then, all at once, release your hands and let them go limp. Allow the tension in your hands to flow out. Let the relaxation deepen for 10 to 15 seconds.

3. Tighten your arms and then relax.

Bend your lower arms up so your hands are against your shoulders, and tighten all the arm muscles. Make sure you tense the muscles on the inside and outside of both the upper and lower arms. If you're not sure whether you're doing that, use one hand to do a tension check on the other arm. Hold the tension a little while and then drop your arms as though you've cut the string holding them up. Let the tension flow out and the relaxation flow in.

4. Raise up your shoulders, tighten, and then relax.

Raise your shoulders up to your ears, as though you were a turtle trying to get its head back into its shell. Hold the tension and then let your shoulders drop. Feel the relaxation deepen for 10 to 15 seconds.

5. Tighten and relax the muscles in your upper back.

Pull your shoulders back and bring your shoulder blades closer together. Hold that tension a little while . . . and let it go.

6. Scrunch up your entire face and then relax.

Squeeze your forehead down, screw up your eyes, and furrow your eyebrows. Clench your jaws together and contract your tongue and lips. Let the tension grow and hold it . . . then relax and let go.

7. Tighten and relax the back of your neck.

Avoid causing yourself pain. Gently let your head tip backwards towards your back and feel the muscles tighten in the back of your neck. Notice that tension and hold it; let go and relax. Feel relaxation deepening.

8. Contract the front neck muscles and then loosen them.

Gently lower your chin towards your chest. Tighten your neck muscles and let the tension increase and maintain it; then relax. Feel the tension melting away like candle wax.

9. Tighten the muscles in your stomach and chest and maintain the tension. Then let it go.

Concentrate on noticing the difference between when the muscles are tense and when they're relaxed. Allow yourself to enjoy the sensations when your muscles relax.

10. **Arch your back, hang on to the contraction, and then relax.**

    Be gentle with your lower back and skip this exercise entirely if you've ever had trouble with this part of your body. Tighten these muscles by arching your lower back, pressing your shoulders back against the chair, or tensing the muscles any way you want. Gently increase and maintain the tension, but not too much. Now relax and allow the waves of relaxation to roll in.

11. **Contract and relax the muscles in your buttocks.**

    Tighten your buttocks to gently lift yourself up in your chair. Hold the tension. Then let tension melt and relaxation grow.

12. **Squeeze and relax your thigh muscles.**

    Tighten and hold these muscles. Then relax and feel the tension draining out; let the calm deepen and spread.

13. **Contract and relax your calves.**

    Tighten the muscles in your calves by lifting the balls of your feet upwards while keeping your heels on the floor. Pull your toes upwards. Take care; if you ever get muscle cramps, don't overdo this exercise. Hold the tension . . . then let go. Let tension drain into the floor.

14. **Gently curl your toes downwards, maintain the tension, and then relax.**

    Again, focus on the differences you can feel. Let both of your feet go limp and floppy.

15. **Take a little time to scan your entire body.**

    Notice whether you feel different to when you began. If you find any areas of tension, allow the relaxed areas around them to come in and replace the tension with relaxation. If that doesn't work, repeat the tense-and-relax procedure for the tense area.

16. **Spend a few minutes enjoying the relaxed feelings.**

    Let relaxation spread and penetrate every muscle fibre in your body. Notice any feelings you have. You may feel warmth, or you may feel a floating sensation. Perhaps you'll feel a sense of sinking down. Whatever it is, allow it to happen. When you feel ready, you can open your eyes and carry on with your day, perhaps feeling like you just returned from a short holiday.

Some people like to make a recording of the progressive muscle relaxation instructions to make it easier to go through the exercises without referring to a book. If you do, be sure to record your instructions to yourself using a slow, calming tone of voice.

In the beginning, take a little longer than five minutes to go through the steps of progressive muscle relaxation. You'll find it most effective if you take 20 or 30 minutes to go through the exercises when you first start learning the technique. The more you practise, the more quickly you'll find that you can slide into serenity. So even if you listen to a recording, consider shortening the procedure on your own after a while. For example, you can tense all the muscles in your lower body at once, followed by all your upper body muscles. At other times, you may want to simply tense and relax a few body areas that carry most of your tension. Most frequently these are your neck, shoulder, and back muscles. Some people say that they eventually discover how to relax in just one minute when they've become proficient.

Creating Calm in Your Imagination

People who have vivid imaginations (perhaps people like you) can think themselves into all kinds of anxious situations. Just give them a moment to play with an idea, and they're off on another anxiety trip.

But the good news is that you can also backtrack and rewind to a calmer place if you know how to apply *guided imagery*.

Letting your imagination roam

Some people, thinking of themselves as rather unimaginative, struggle to create pictures in their minds. These people generally feel uncomfortable with their drawing skills and have a hard time recalling the details of events that they've witnessed. Perhaps you're one of them. If so, using your imagination to relax and reduce your anxiety may not be the approach for you.

On the other hand, it just may be. Just remember that the vividness of the images does not predict the depth of relaxation that you can achieve. Guided imagery encompasses more than the visual sense; it includes smell, taste, touch and sound. We can help you sharpen your ability to use all these senses.

We encourage you to give these exercises a go, but people all have different strengths and weaknesses, and you may find that one or more of these exercises just don't work for you. If you discover that guided imagery isn't for you, that's fine. This book discusses many other ways to relax.

To work with each of your senses, follow the three steps below before going through the guided imagery exercises:

1. **Find a comfortable place to sit or lie down.**

2. **Make sure that you loosen any tight garments and shoes.**

3. **Close your eyes and take a few slow, deep breaths.**

Imagining touch

Imagery exercises work best if they incorporate more than one sense. Imagining bodily sensations enhances the overall experience of relaxing by using guided imagery. Try the following steps to see how this works:

1. **Imagine a huge, sunken bath.**

   What colour would you like it to be? How about the shape? Think about the lighting – candlelight, subtle spotlights, or would you prefer something else?

2. **Picture yourself turning on the tap and feeling the water coming out.**

   You can feel that the water is cold and wet as it pours over your hand. Gradually, the temperature increases to what is just perfect for you.

3. **The bath fills, and you can mentally see yourself pouring bath oil in and swirling it around.**

   You can feel how silky the water becomes.

4. **You imagine putting your foot in the water.**

   The water feels just a bit too hot at first, but you find that the warmth soothes you after you slowly lower your whole body into the bath.

5. **You lie back and luxuriate in the silky, smooth, warm water.**

   You can feel it envelop you as the warmth loosens all your muscles.

Were you able to feel the sensations: the wetness and the silky warmth? If not, don't despair. You can heighten the power of your imagination by spending just five minutes a day actively participating in a real experience and then concentrating on storing that experience in your memory. Try one or more of the following exercises each day for five days in a row. You can also experiment with other exercises. Just be sure to focus on touch.

Recalling sounds

You don't have to be a musician to appreciate music or to recreate it in your mind. Guided imagery often asks you to create the sounds of nature in your mind to enhance relaxation. Take the following steps to conjure up what an ocean beach sounds like:

1. **Imagine that you're lying on a beach.**

   You can hear the ocean waves rolling in one after the other. In and out. The soft roar soothes and relaxes. In and out.

2. **In your mind, you hear each wave rolling in. The sound rises to a crescendo and then the wave breaks gently onto the beach.**

   A brief moment of quiet follows as the next wave prepares to roll in. A few seagulls cry out as they fly overhead.

Were you able to hear the sea and the gulls? You can improve your ability to recreate sounds in your mind by actively experiencing the real thing beforehand.

Conjuring up smells

Dogs have a far better sense of smell than we do. They seem to know exactly which bush on their walk needs remarking. We're pretty sure that they know exactly which rival dog did what to which bush. Perhaps it's a good thing that our sense of smell isn't as good as theirs!

But smell has a powerful influence on people as well as dogs. Certain smells alert us to danger – such as the smell of smoke or burning food. Others, such as the aroma of your favourite baked delight or the perfumed scent of a loved one, conjure up pleasant memories and feelings. See whether this description brings a smell wafting into your mind:

1. **Imagine that you're walking across a field of newly mown grass.**

   It's late spring and the first time you've smelled cut grass this year.

2. **You can smell the sweet fragrance of the freshly cut grass.**

   The smell evokes memories of warm, carefree summer days.

3. **You stretch and breathe deeply.**

   A pleasant, refreshing feeling engulfs you.

How does this scene smell in your mind? Smell is often not as easy to consciously reproduce with your imagination as other senses. That may be because a description of smell is more difficult to put into words. However, with practice, you're likely to improve.

Remembering tastes

Which foods do you associate with comfort and relaxation? Many people think of chicken soup or herbal tea. Do you pile the butter and jam on your toast when you're really stressed or occasionally indulge in ice cream – especially the one with chocolate and caramel swirls threaded through rich vanilla? Perhaps you're a chocoholic. Are you salivating yet? If not, try playing out this imaginary scene:

1. **Imagine an exquisite chocolate truffle.**

   You're not sure what's inside, but you look forward to finding out.

2. **In your mind, you take the truffle to your lips and slowly bite off a little piece.**

   The rich, sweet chocolate coats your tongue.

3. **You can imagine taking another bite and detect a creamy, fruity centre.**

   You never tasted anything so rich and delectable, yet not overpowering. The sweet but slightly tangy cherry flavour fills your body with satisfaction.

Could you taste the truffle in your imagination? Perhaps you found the taste easier to imagine than the smell. Either way, you can improve your ability to recall tastes with practice.

Painting pictures in your mind

Many of our clients report that scenes of anticipated disasters and doom enter unbidden into their imaginations. These scenes cause them more anxiety than actual disastrous events usually do. Visual imagery can fuel your anxiety or, alternatively, you can harness your visual imagination to help you quench the fires of anxiety. Try painting this picture in your mind:

Imagine you're at a mountain resort in late spring. The building's made of wood. Nestling into the hillside, it's surrounded by wonderful tall trees. Grey-blue smoke rises lazily from a chimney and curls away into nothingness.

Imagine you spent the day trekking through a forest. Now you're relaxing on the deck overlooking a valley lake ringed by mountain peaks.

The water in the lake is still; the dark blue surface reflects surprisingly clear images of the trees and mountains. The sun sinks behind a mountain peak, painting the clouds above in brilliant hues of red, orange and pink. The mountains are still capped with winter snow. Dark green fir trees stand proudly on a carpet of pine cones and needles.

How did this scene look in your mind? If you practise sharpening your visual imagery, you'll become an expert eyewitness. Wherever you are, take a minute to inspect the view in front of you. It doesn't matter what it is. Scrutinise the image from every angle. Notice colours, textures, shapes, proportions and positions. Then close your eyes. Try to recollect the images in your mind. Focus on every detail. You can practise this anywhere and at any time. It just takes a few minutes. Each day, delay your image retrieval a little longer after turning away from the scene that you just studied.

A selection of herbs and dietary supplements have been beneficial in reducing anxiety for some people. For more information please refer to *Overcoming Anxiety For Dummies*.

Imagining a positive outcome

Athletes commonly use images to reduce their performance anxiety. In addition, many of them create images of success. For example, a gymnast may envision himself making a perfect dismount off the balance beam, over and over. Or a runner may see herself pushing through pain, stretching her legs out for a first-place finish, again and again. Various studies indicate that imagery can give an athlete an extra boost.

Imagery is great for children too. For example, children who suffer from recurring tummy pain often miss school and other activities. A study in 2006 used guided imagery and progressive muscle relaxation for this problem and found that the children said they had less pain and also that they missed out on fewer activities.

Another way to use imagery is to face your fears in a less stressful way than meeting them for the first time in real life. You do this by repeatedly imagining yourself conquering your fears.

Chapter 6

Delving into Stress

. . . .

. . . .

S tress is what you experience when you believe you cannot cope effectively with a threatening situation.

What this means is that you experience stress whenever you're faced with an event or situation that you perceive as challenging to your ability to cope. If you see the event or situation as only *mildly* challenging, you'll probably feel only a little stress; however, if you perceive the situation or event as threatening or overwhelming your coping abilities, you'll probably feel a lot of stress. So, having to wait for a bus when you have all the time in the world triggers little stress. Waiting for that same bus when you're late for a plane that will take off without you triggers much more stress.

This difference between the demands of the situation and your perception of how well you can cope with that situation is what determines how much stress you will feel.

How this Whole Stress Thing got Started

Believe it or not, you have stress in your life for a good reason. To show you why stress can be a useful, adaptive response, you need to take a trip back in time.

Imagining you are a cave person

Picture this: You've regressed in time to a period millions of years ago when men and women lived in caves. You notice that you're roaming the jungle dressed in a loincloth and carrying a club in your hand. Your day, so far, has been routine. Nothing more than the usual cave politics and the ongoing problems with the in-laws. Nothing you can't handle. Suddenly, on your stroll, you spot a tiger. This is not your ordinary tiger; it's a sabre-toothed one. You experience something called the *fight-or-flight response*. This response is aptly named because, just then, you realise that you have to make a choice. You can stay and do battle (that's the fight part) or you can run like the wind (the flight part, and probably the smarter option here). Your body, armed with this automatic stress response, prepares you to do either. You're ready for anything.

Seeing how your body reacts

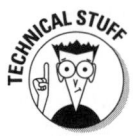

When you're in the fight-or-flight mode, your physiological system goes into high gear. The first thing you notice is that you're afraid, very afraid. You also notice that you're breathing much faster than you normally do, and your hands feel cool and more than a little moist. But that's just for starters. If you could see what's happening below the surface, you would also notice some other changes going on. Your sympathetic nervous system, one of the two branches of your autonomic nervous system, is producing changes in your body. Your *hypothalamus*, a part of your brain, is activating your *pituitary*, a small gland near the base of your brain, which releases a hormone into the bloodstream. This hormone (it's called ACTH or adrenocorticotropic hormone) reaches your adrenal glands, and they in turn produce more adrenaline (also known as epinephrine) along with other hormones called glucocorticoids (cortisol is one). This melange of biochemical changes is responsible for an array of other remarkable changes in your body. Some highlights include the following:

- ✔ Your heart rate speeds up, and your blood pressure rises (more blood is pumped to your muscles and lungs).

- ✔ You breathe more rapidly. Your nostrils flare, causing an increased supply of air.

- ✔ Your digestion slows. (Who's got time to eat?)

- ✔ Blood is directed away from your skin and internal organs and is shunted to your brain and skeletal muscles. Your muscles tense. You feel stronger. You're ready for action.

- ✔ Your blood clots faster, ready to repair any damage to your arteries.

- ✔ Your pupils dilate, so you see better.

- ✔ Your liver converts glycogen into glucose, which teams up with free fatty acids to supply you with fuel and some quick energy. (You'll probably need it.)

In short, when you're experiencing stress, your entire body undergoes a dramatic series of physiological changes that readies you for a life-threatening emergency. Clearly, stress has adaptive, survival potential. Stress, back then, was nature's way of keeping you alive.

Surviving the modern jungle

The reality is, in today's modern society, we are required to deal with very few life-threatening stresses on a normal day. Unfortunately, your body's fight-or-flight response is activated by a whole range of stressful events and situations that are *not* going to kill you. The physical dangers have been replaced by social or psychological stresses, not worthy of a full flight-or-fight stress response. Your body, however, does not know this and reacts the way it did when your ancestors were facing danger.

Panicking on the podium

In today's modern jungle, giving that presentation, being stuck in traffic, confronting a disgruntled client, facing an angry spouse, or trying to meet some unrealistic deadlines are what stresses you. These far less-threatening stresses now trigger that same intense stress response. It's overkill. Your body is now not just reacting; it is *overreacting*. And that is definitely not good.

Understanding stress is as simple as ABC

One of best ways of understanding stress is to look at a model of emotional distress elaborated by psychologist Albert Ellis. He calls his model the ABC model, and it's as simple as it sounds:

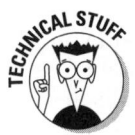

A→B→C where:

- ✔ A is the Activating event or potentially stressful situation.

- ✔ B is your Beliefs, thoughts or perceptions about A.

- ✔ C is the emotional Consequence or stress that results from holding these beliefs.

Managing stress: A three-pronged approach

This three-pronged model of dealing with stress provides you with a useful tool to help you understand the many ways you can manage and control your stress. You have three major choices, outlined in the following sections.

You can change your 'A'

Changing your 'A' means modifying your environment. Rats stress you out? Stay away from rats. Traffic stresses you? Leave home earlier. Hate deadlines? Finish the project earlier.

Many of the stress management tools in this book are designed to help you change those situations that are triggering your stress. But what if you can't? You can't avoid rats – you work in pest control. You can't leave home for work earlier. You can't finish the project before the deadline. You need to change you.

You can change your 'B'

Even if you cannot significantly change those situations and events that are triggering your stress, you can change the way you perceive them. An important subset of stress management skills focuses on ways of changing the way you view your world. You will see that much, if not most, of your stress is self-induced, and you can learn to see things differently.

You can change your 'C'

Even if you cannot change the situation, and cannot change the way you view that situation, you can still manage your stress by mastering other skills. You can learn how to relax your body and quieten your mind. You can learn the secrets of becoming calm and how to turn off your stress.

Tuning your strings: Finding the right balance

Stress is part of life. No one makes it through life totally stress free, and you wouldn't want to. You certainly want the good stress, and you even want some of the stress that comes with dealing with life's challenges and disappointments. What you don't want is too much stress in your life, or too little stress. Too much (or prolonged) stress can become a negative force, and can rob you of much of life's joy. Too little stress means you're missing out, taking too few risks, playing it too safe. Finding the right amount of stress in your life is like finding the right tension in a violin string. Too much tension and the string can break; too little tension and there is no music.

You want to hear the music, without breaking the strings.

Stressed-Out? Welcome to the Club!

Are you feeling more tired lately than you used to? Is your fuse a little shorter than normal? Are you worrying more? Enjoying life less? If you feel more stress in your life these days, you aren't alone. Count yourself among the ranks of the overstressed. Most people feel that they have too much stress in their lives. Your stress may come from your job, your personal life, or simply from not having enough time to do everything you have to do – or *want* to do. You could use some help. Thankfully, you can eliminate or certainly minimise much of the stress in your life and manage the stress that remains.

Understanding where all this stress is coming from

In his popular book, *Future Shock* (originally published in 1984), Alvin Toffler observed that people experience more stress whenever they are subjected to a lot of change in a short span of time. If anything characterises our lives these days, it is an excess of change. We are in a continual state of flux. We have less control over our lives, we live with more uncertainty, and we often feel threatened and, at times, overwhelmed. The following sections explain some of the more common sources of stress in our lives.

Getting frazzled at work

For most people, their jobs and careers are the biggest source of stress in their lives. Killer hours, a long commute, unrealistic deadlines, a boss from hell, office politics, toxic co-workers and testy clients are just a few of the many job-related stresses people experience. Workloads are heavier today than they were in the past, leaving less and less time for family and the rest of your life. A new lexicon of work-related stresses exists: downsizing, organisational redeployment, early retirement. Whatever the word, the effect is the same: insecurity, uncertainty and fear.

Feeling frazzled at home

After you leave work, you may start to realise that the rest of your life is not exactly stress-free. These days, life at home, our relationships, and the pressure of juggling everything else that has to be done only add to our stress level.

Life at home has become more pressured and demanding. True, we now have microwaves, hoovers and take-away menus, but the effort and stress involved seems to be growing rather than lessening. Meals have to be prepared, the house tidied, clothing cleaned, bills paid, chores completed, shopping done, the lawn and garden tended, the car maintained and repaired, phone calls returned, homework supervised, and the kids chauffeured. And that's for starters. Did we mention the dog?

A woman's work is never done

Add on the additional stress of being a mother with a family to manage at home, and you compound the level of stress. Women may find themselves in the not-so-unusual position of having to cope with the problems of ageing and ailing parents in addition to the problems of their own children. Caught in this generational divide, this 'stress sandwich' can be incredibly draining, both physically and emotionally. Although men give lip service to helping with the kids and the elderly (and they do, in fact, do more than their fathers or grandfathers), the woman is still the one who most often takes primary responsibility for these care-giving roles.

Managing the money malaise

Money may or may not be the root of all evil, but worrying about it certainly is a major source of stress in our lives. Actually, the *lack* of money is really the problem. Checking your bank statement at the end of the month (if you bother) reminds you that living is expensive. You remember that your parents bought their house for a pittance and now realise that you couldn't afford to buy that same house if you wanted to today. The mortgage, university tuition, medical expenses, travel, taxes, savings for retirement – it all adds up. And so does the stress. Money, however, can produce stress in other ways – especially for men. Many men tend to tie their self-worth to their financial worth. When their financial worth is down, they're down. And society doesn't help. Other people tend to equate success with their portfolios, and if they're not measuring up to what they think they should have, they may feel depressed, anxious or even angry.

Piling on new stresses (hint: Grandma never wore a personal alarm)

Our lives have become stressful in ways we never would have imagined even a decade ago. Whoever said there is nothing new under the sun probably never surfed the Web or carried a laptop. Changes in technology have brought with them new pressures and new demands; in short, new sources of stress.

The importance of hassle (or, the little things add up)

When we think of stress, we usually think of the major stresses we may face occasionally: death, divorce, financial ruin, a serious illness. And then of course there are those so-called moderate stresses: losing our wallets, denting the car, or catching a cold. Finally, we have the even smaller stresses: the mini-stresses and micro-stresses. These stresses are what we sometimes refer to as *hassles*.

Here is just a sample of the kinds of hassles we face every day (a complete list would be endless):

- Noisy traffic
- Loud neighbours

✔ Rude sales assistants

✔ Crowds

✔ Public telephones that don't work

✔ Cyclists from nowhere

✔ Deliveries made 'sometime between 9 and 5'

✔ Long queues

✔ No public toilets

✔ Mobile phones ringing in theatres

✔ People talking on mobile phones in restaurants and on public transport

Yes, we realise these things are relatively small. But the small things can add up. We can deal with one, maybe two, or even three of these at once. But when the number begins to rise, so does our stress level. When you reach a high enough level of stress, you notice that you overreact to the next hassle that comes along. And that results in even more stress. Alas, life is loaded with hassle. The funny part is, we usually deal fairly well with the bigger problems. Life's major stresses – deaths, illnesses, divorces or financial setbacks – somehow trigger hidden resources within us. We rise to each demand, summoning up some unrecognised inner strength, and we somehow manage to cope. What gets to us are the little things. It's the small stuff – the little annoyances, petty frustrations and minor irritations – that ultimately lead to a continuing sense of stress. Life's hassles are what becomes the real source of our stress.

Looking at the Signs and Symptoms of Stress

Here are some of the more benign, more commonly experienced stress signs and symptoms. Many will be all too familiar to you.

Physical signs of stress:

✔ Tiredness, fatigue, lethargy

✔ Heart palpitations, racing pulse, rapid, shallow breathing

✔ Muscle tension and aches

✔ Shakiness, tremors, tics, twitches

✔ Heartburn, indigestion, diarrhoea, constipation, nervousness

✔ Dry mouth and throat

✔ Excessive sweating, clammy hands, cold hands and/or feet

✔ Rashes, hives, itching

✔ Nail-biting, fidgeting, hair-twirling or hair-pulling

✔ Frequent urination

✔ Lowered libido

✔ Overeating, loss of appetite

✔ Sleep difficulties

✔ Increased use of alcohol and/or drugs and medications

Psychological signs of stress:

✔ Irritability, impatience, anger, hostility

✔ Worry, anxiety, panic

✔ Moodiness, sadness, feeling upset

✔ Intrusive and/or racing thoughts

✔ Memory lapses, difficulties in concentrating, indecision

✔ Frequent absences from work, lowered productivity

✔ Feeling overwhelmed

✔ Loss of sense of humour

That's just for starters. Prolonged and/or intense stress can have more serious effects.

Understanding how stress can make you ill

Researchers estimate that 75 to 90 per cent of all visits to GPs are for complaints and conditions that are, in some way, stress-related. Every week, 112 million people take some form of medication for stress-related symptoms. This statistic is not surprising given the wide-ranging physiological changes that accompany a stress response. Just about every bodily system or body part is affected by stress. Stress can play a role in exacerbating the symptoms of a wide variety of other disorders and illnesses as well. The following sections illustrate some of the more important ways stress can negatively impact your health and well-being.

How stress can be a pain in the neck (and other places)

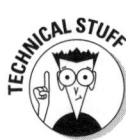

Your muscles are a prime target for stress. When you're under stress, your muscles contract and they become tense. This muscle tension can affect your nerves, blood vessels, organs, skin and bones. Chronically tense muscles can result in a variety of conditions and disorders, including muscle spasms, cramping, facial or jaw pain, bruxism (grinding your teeth), tremors and shakiness. Many forms of headache, chest pain and back pain are among the more common conditions that result from stress-induced muscle tension.

Taking stress to heart

Stress can play a role in circulatory diseases such as coronary heart disease, cardiac arrest and strokes. This fact is not surprising because stress can increase your blood pressure, constrict your blood vessels, raise your cholesterol level, trigger arrhythmias, and speed up the rate at which your blood clots. Stress is now considered a major risk factor in heart disease, right up there with smoking, being overweight and a lack of exercise. All of this becomes very important when you consider that heart disease kills more men over the age of 50 and more women over the age of 65 than any other disease.

Hitting below the belt

Ever notice how your stress seems to finds its way to your stomach? Your gastro-intestinal system can be a ready target for much of the stress in your life. Stress can affect the secretion of acid in your stomach and can speed up or slow down the process of peristalsis (the rhythmic contraction of the muscles in your intestines). Constipation, diarrhoea, gas, bloating and weight loss can all be stress-related. Stress can contribute to gastro-oesophageal reflux disease and can also play a role in exacerbating irritable bowel syndrome and colitis.

Stress can affect your immune system

In the last decade or so, growing evidence has supported the theory that stress affects your immune system. In fact, researchers have even coined a name for this new field of study. They call it *psychoneuroimmunology*. Quite a mouthful! Scientists who choose to go into this field study the relationships between moods, emotional states, hormonal levels, and changes in the nervous system and the immune system. Without drowning you in detail, stress – particularly chronic stress – can compromise your immune system, rendering it less effective in resisting bacteria and viruses. Research has shown that stress may play a role in exacerbating a variety of immune system disorders such as HIV and AIDS, herpes, cancer metastasis, viral infection, rheumatoid arthritis, and certain allergies, as well as other auto-immune conditions. Some recent studies appear to confirm this.

'Not tonight, dear. I have a (stress) headache.'

A headache is just one of the many ways stress can interfere with your sex life. Stress can affect sexual performance and rob you of your libido. When you're feeling stress, feeling sexy may not be at the top of your to-do list. Disturbed sexual performance may appear in the form of premature ejaculation, erectile dysfunction, and other forms of difficulty in reaching orgasm. The irony is, sex can be a way of *relieving* stress. In fact, for some people, sexual activity *increases* when they feel stressed.

Can stress be good?

Not all the news about stress is bad. As Hans Selye, the pioneer researcher in the field of stress said, 'Stress is the spice of life.' He termed the good kind of stress *eustress,* as opposed to *distress,* or the nasty kind of stress. (The *eu* part of *eustress* comes from the Greek, meaning 'good'.) Stress can be a positive force in your life. Watching a close play-off game, taking a ride at an amusement park, solving an interesting problem, falling in love – all can be stressful. Yet these are the kinds of stresses that add to the enjoyment and satisfaction of our lives. We want *more* of this kind of stress, not less.

And even many of the less pleasant uncertainties and surprises of life can be a source of challenge and even excitement and interest. Change and the pressures of modern life don't necessarily create the bad kind of stress. Rather, how you view the potential stresses in your life and how you cope with them makes all the difference. The good news is that, with a little help and the right direction, learning to manage your stress is easier than you think.

Chapter 7

Managing Stress Proactively

● ●

In This Chapter

▶ Understanding the effects of tension

▶ Slowing down your mind

▶ Controlling your anger

▶ Dealing with your worries

▶ Insulating yourself from stress

● ●

*W*hen you're under stress, your muscles contract and become tense. This muscle tension is nature's way of preparing you to cope with a potential threat – part of the fight-or-flight response described in Book V Chapter 6. Your body is now ready to fight that tiger. Unfortunately, this once adaptive response (and the accompanying muscle tension) can be triggered by less than life-threatening situations (such as the disagreeable taxi driver who doesn't seem to have a clue where he's going but is breaking speed records to get there). Muscle tension can result in a wide variety of stress-related conditions and disorders. Fortunately, you can catch your tension before it does its worst. All you need are the right stress-busting tools in your toolbox.

To help you manage stress proactively, this chapter describes strategies and techniques that can help you let go of tension, relax your body and quieten your mind. We also share some tips to control anger, learn how to worry less and generally have more fun.

Letting Go of Tension

Consider the following strategies and techniques to help you let go of tension and relax your body.

Breathing away your tension

Breathing properly is one of the simplest and best ways of draining your tension and relieving your stress. Simply by changing your breathing patterns, you can rapidly induce a state of greater relaxation. If you control the way you breathe, you have a powerful tool in reducing bodily tension. As important, you have a tool that helps prevent your body from becoming tense in the first place. This section shows you what you can do to incorporate a variety of stress-effective breathing techniques into your life.

Breathing 101: Breathing for starters

Here is one of the best and simplest ways of introducing yourself to stress-effective breathing.

1. **Either lying or sitting comfortably, put one hand on your tummy and your other hand on your chest.**

2. **Inhale through your nose making sure that the hand on your tummy rises, and the hand on your chest moves hardly at all.**

3. **As you inhale slowly, count to 3 silently, to yourself.**

4. **As you exhale, slowly count to 4, feeling the hand on your tummy falling gently.**

   Pause slightly before your next breath. Repeat for several minutes and whenever you get the chance.

Moving on to something more advanced: Taking a complete breath

Complete breaths (or *Zen breathing* as it is often called) helps you breathe more deeply, more efficiently, and maximise your lung capacity.

1. **Lie comfortably in bed, a reclining chair, or on a rug.**

   Keep your knees slightly apart and slightly bent. Close your eyes if you like.

2. **Put one hand on your abdomen near your tummy-button, and the other hand on your chest so that you follow the motion of your breathing.**

   Try to relax. Let go of any tension you may feel in your body.

3. **Begin by slowly inhaling through your nose, first filling the lower part of your lungs, then the middle part of your chest, and then the upper part of your chest.**

   As you inhale, feel your diaphragm pushing down, gently extending your abdomen, making room for the newly inhaled air. Notice the hand on your abdomen rise slightly. The hand on your chest should move very little, and when it does, it should follow your abdomen. Do not use your shoulders to help you breathe.

4. **Exhale slowly through your parted lips, emptying your lungs from top to bottom.**

   Make a whooshing sound as the air passes through your lips, and notice the hand on your abdomen fall.

5. **Pause slightly, and take in another breath repeating this cycle.**

   Continue breathing this way for ten minutes or so – certainly until you feel more relaxed and peaceful. Practise this technique daily if you can. Try this exercise while sitting and then while standing.

With a little practice, this form of breathing comes more naturally, and automatically. Over some time and some practice, you may begin to breathe this way much more of the time. Stick with it.

Emergency breathing: How to breathe in the trenches

Breathing properly is no big deal when you're lying on your bed or vegging out in front of the TV. But what's your breathing like when you're caught in gridlock, when you're approaching a deadline, or when the stock market drops 20 per cent? You're now in a crisis mode. You need another form of breathing. Here's what to do:

1. **Inhale slowly through your nostrils, taking in a very deep diaphragmatic breath, filling your lungs and filling your cheeks.**

2. **Hold that breath for about six seconds.**

3. **Exhale *slowly* through your slightly parted lips, releasing *all* the air in your lungs.**

   Pause at the end of this exhalation. Now take a few 'normal' breaths.

   Repeat Steps 1 to 3, two or three times, and then return to what you were doing. This form of deep breathing should put you in a more relaxed state.

The yawn that refreshes

Yawning is another way Mother Nature tells you that your body is under stress. In fact, yawning helps relieve stress. When you yawn, more air – and therefore more oxygen – enters your lungs, revitalising your blood stream. Releasing that plaintive sound that comes with yawning is also tension reducing. Unfortunately, people have become a little over-socialised, meaning they hold back with their yawns. You need to recapture this lost art.

The next time you feel a yawn coming on, go with it. Open your mouth widely and inhale more fully than you normally might. Take that breath all the way down to your abdomen. Exhale fully through your mouth, completely emptying your lungs. What a feeling! Enjoy it.

Quietening Your Mind

To be completely relaxed, you need to not only relax your body but also calm your mind. This chapter details how to quieten your mind. For many people, and you may be one of them, stress takes the form of psychological distress, and you find that your mind is filled with distressing thoughts that prevent you from feeling relaxed and at ease. It may be that your mind is racing a mile a minute. You may be worrying about your job, your relationships, your finances, or simply how you're going to juggle the hundred and one things that are on your plate. Whatever the source of your worry, you clearly are not going to relax until you stop – or at least slow – this mental mayhem.

Distract yourself

The simplest way to calm your mind is to distract yourself. This idea may sound obvious, but you'd be surprised how often people overlook this option. Psychologists know that concentrating on two things at the same time is very hard. Therefore, if your mind is flooded with distressing thoughts, change course. Find something else to think about. Here are some pleasant diversions you may want to consider:

- Watch some television
- Go to the cinema
- Read a book, newspaper or magazine
- Talk to a friend
- Work or play on your computer
- Play a sport
- Immerse yourself on some project or hobby
- Listen to some favourite music
- Think of something you're looking forward to

One of the best ways to distract yourself, calm your mind, and stop those unwanted, persistent worries is to use your imagination.

Imagine this

If you can replace that stress-producing thought or image with one that is relaxing, the chances are that you'll feel much better. Here's how:

1. **Find a place where you won't be disturbed for a few minutes and get comfortable, either sitting in a favourite chair or lying down.**

2. **Think of an image – a place, a scene or a memory – that relaxes you.**

   Use all your senses to bring that imagined scene to life. Ask yourself: What do I see? What can I hear? What can I smell? What can I feel?

3. **Let yourself become completely immersed in your image, allowing it to relax you completely.**

'Sounds good', you say, 'but what is my relaxing image?' Try taking one these mental flights (air fare included):

- **The Caribbean package:** Imagine that you're on the beach of a Caribbean isle. The weather is perfect. Lying on the cool sand, you feel the warm breeze caress your body. You hear the lapping of the ocean waves on the shore and the tropical birds chirping in the palms. You're slowly sipping a piña colada. You can smell your coconut-scented suntan lotion. You feel wonderful. You're relaxed. Your mind is totally at peace.

- **The pool package:** You're lying in a large inflatable raft, floating blissfully in an incredibly beautiful swimming pool. The day is perfect. The sky is a deep blue, the sun is warming your relaxed body. You feel the gentle rocking of the raft in the water. You can hear the soothing voice of the waiter announcing a buffet lunch in half an hour. You're very content. You could lie here forever.

- **The winter wonderland package:** Picture yourself in a small cabin in the Alps. You're snowed in, but that's fine because you don't have to be anywhere and no one needs to contact you. Also, you're not alone – a favourite person is with you and you're both lying in front of a crackling fire. Soft music is playing in the background. You're sipping hot toddies, mulled wine or champagne.

- **A pleasing memory:** Try to picture a memory, possibly when you were growing up, or one from more recent times that you find particularly happy and satisfying. It could be a holiday long ago, a birthday party you loved, or frolicking with a childhood pet.

None of these examples do it for you? Then come up with your own personal relaxation image. You might try one of these:

- Soaking in a hot, soapy bath . . . soft music . . . candle light . . .

- Walking in a quiet forest . . . birds chirping . . . leaves rustling . . .

- Lying under a tree in the park . . . warm breezes . . . more chirping . . .

- In your most comfortable chair . . . reading a great book . . . fire crackling . . .

Five signs that your mind is stressed

Below are some of the more common signs that indicate that your mind is working overtime. See how many of the following describe you.

1. Your mind seems to be racing.

2. You find controlling your thoughts difficult.

3. You're worried, irritable or upset.

4. You're preoccupied more often and find concentrating more difficult.

5. You find it difficult to fall asleep or to fall asleep again once awake.

What you see and hear usually dominates your imagination. But don't forget your senses of touch and smell. By adding these sensual dimensions you can enrich your images and make them more involving. Feel the sand between your toes; smell the freshly brewed coffee; taste the salt in the air.

Make things move

Your image need not be a static scene. It can change and move. You may, for example:

- ✔ Imagine a sports event that you enjoy. It could be a cricket match that you attended. Or make one up. Mentally follow the play as you work your way through the innings. Not a cricket fan? Try imagining a tennis match.

- ✔ Try replaying favourite films in your mind, visualising different scenes and filling in bits of dialogue. Scenic films work wonderfully.

- ✔ Remember the details of a trip you've taken in the past and retrace your journey from place to place.

This *Guided Imagery*, as it's called, can help keep you focused and interested in your image, and ensure that unwanted, intrusive thoughts stay out of the picture.

Stop your thoughts

Sometimes distracting yourself isn't enough to calm your mind. Sometimes you need stronger measures to eliminate, or at least slow, those unwanted and stress-producing worries and concerns. Perhaps you have an upsetting worry that continually intrudes into your thinking and keeps you from enjoying a pleasant evening with friends. Or maybe you're trying to fall asleep and the thoughts racing around in your head make sleeping impossible. You recognise that there is nothing you can do about your worry and that your worrying is only making things worse. You would be better off if you could somehow stop thinking about this. But how?

That's where a technique called *Thought Stopping* can be very useful. It is an effective way of not only keeping worries and upsets temporarily out of your mind, but also weakening those thoughts, making it less likely that they will return. Here are the steps you need to take to get this technique to work for you:

1. **Notice your thoughts.**

   When a worrisome thought runs through your mind, mentally step back and recognise that it is an unwanted thought. It may be a worry, a nagging concern, or a regret – anything that you feel is not worth the stress at this particular time.

2. **Find a Stop sign.**

   In your mind, picture a red and white Stop sign, you know, the kind you see on the street corner. Make your sign large and vivid.

3. **Yell 'Stop!'**

   In your head, silently shout the word STOP to yourself.

4. **Do it again.**

   Every time the worrisome or unwanted thought reappears, notice that thought, imagine your Stop sign, and yell STOP to yourself.

5. **Find a replacement thought.**

   Find a thought or image that you can substitute for the distressing thought or image. It may be something taken from the list of relaxing images above, or any other thought that is not the one you're trying to weaken.

The image of the sign and the verbal STOP disrupts your thought sequence and temporarily puts the unwanted thought out of mind. Be warned, however: It probably will return, and you may have to repeat this sequence again. If your stress-producing thought or image is very strong, it may take many repetitions of this technique to weaken or eliminate it. Stick with it.

Strike up the band (or better yet, a string quartet)

Music therapists know that listening to music can result in significant physiological changes in your body: Your heart rate drops, your breathing slows, and your blood pressure lowers. But not all music does the trick. Some music can upset you, making you more stressed. (Think of that Metallica fan living upstairs.) Other music may delight you, but still not have a calming effect.

Go for Baroque

Following is a short list of field-tested composers and compositions (Baroque and otherwise) that should slow your pulse.

- **Bach:** The slower second movements are particularly appropriate for relaxation. *The Air on a G-string* is a real calmer.
- **Handel:** *The Water Music.*
- **Chopin:** *Nocturnes.*
- **Schubert:** *Symphony No. 8 in B Minor.*
- **Pachelbel:** *Canon in D.*
- **Albinoni:** *Adagio in G.*
- **Mozart:** *Piano Concerto No. 21.*
- **Beethoven:** *Pastoral symphony.*
- **Elgar:** *Salut d'Amour.*

Not a fan of the classics?

Of course, relaxing music need not be all classical. Bach and Mozart probably aren't as effective as Miles Davis if you're a jazz fan. Other forms of music can be incredibly soothing. Many of the 'New Age' tapes and CDs work nicely.

No one piece of music works for everyone. Experiment. Find what relaxes you. Listen in your car while commuting, in bed before going to sleep, in your favourite chair in your favourite room. Headphones and a personal tape or CD allow you to take your music – and a state of relaxation – wherever you go.

Use some common scents

Your ears are not the only road to mental relaxation. Your nose can work as well. People have been using scents to relieve stress and tension for centuries. An aroma can elicit feelings of calm and serenity. In fact, a school of therapy called *aromatherapy* is devoted to using your sense of smell as a vehicle for emotional change.

Mix your own aroma cocktail

Some of the more common oils used to induce a relaxed, calming state include lavender, rose, jasmine, chamomile, orange blossom, vanilla, bergamot, geranium and sandalwood. Often, you can combine oils to produce a new, relaxing aroma.

Do nothing: Meditation is good for you

The sections that follow present meditation as an important stress-reducing tool that fits nicely in your stress toolbox.

The effects and benefits of meditation are wide and varied. Many of them you can notice immediately, while others are less obvious, affecting you in more subtle ways. Most importantly, meditation can help you relax your mind and body. It can help you turn off your inner thoughts. Meditating can help you feel less stressed; and your body will be less tense and your mind calmer. With some practice, after meditating you should feel rested, renewed and recharged. Meditation allows you to develop greater control over your thoughts, worries and anxieties. It is a skill, that once mastered, can serve you well throughout your life.

Preparing to meditate

Here is a step-by-step guide to preparing for meditation. Remember that there are many ways of meditating.

1. **Find a quiet place where you won't be disturbed for a while.**

   No telephones, mobiles, TV – nothing.

2. **Find a comfortable sitting position.**

   Contorting yourself in some yogi-like, snake-charmer squat (albeit impressive), may not be the best way to start meditating if you're a novice. Remember that you're going to remain in one position for 15 to 20 minutes.

3. **Focus on a sound, a word, a sensation, an image, an object or a thought.**

4. **Maintain your focus and adopt a passive, accepting attitude.**

   When you're focusing in meditation, intrusive thoughts or images may enter your mind and distract you. When those thoughts occur, notice them, accept the fact that they are there, and then let them go: no getting upset, no annoyance, no self-rebuke.

Try not to get hung up on the timing. Meditate for about 15 or 20 minutes. If you want to meditate longer, fine. If you find you're becoming uncomfortable, you can stop and try it again at another time. Remember, this is a non-pressured, non-ego-involved exercise.

Overcoming Your Anger

Are you angry because someone cut you up in traffic or kept you waiting for what seemed like an eternity? Are you angry because that clumsy guest spilled red wine on your sofa, or because your printer refuses to print? Everyone feels anger sometimes. Unfortunately, too many people – and you may be one of them – experience too much anger too much of the time. Anger is not only terribly stressful, it can be harmful to your physical well-being and destructive to your relationships with others. Fortunately, ways of reducing your levels of anger and limiting its consequences do exist. This section shows you how to control your anger – instead of letting your anger control you.

Examining the downside of anger

When you're angry, your body reacts much the same way it does when you're experiencing any other stress reaction. Your anger triggers your body to take a defensive stance, readying yourself for any danger that may come your way. When your anger is intense and frequent, the physiological effects can be harmful. Your health is at risk. And any or all of those nasty stress-related illnesses and disorders can become linked to excessive anger.

Tempering your temper

Anger is not an automatic reaction beyond our control, even though it may feel like that at times. Instead, anger is a response that can be managed.

Keeping an anger log

The first step in managing (and ultimately eliminating) much of your stressful anger is knowing what it looks like and where it comes from. A simple anger diary, or anger log, can help you identify those times when you're angry and give you the information you need to begin feeling less angry.

Simply enter in your log (a small notebook, a piece of paper, a file on your laptop – whatever works for you) the times when you became angry and what triggered your anger. Also, rate the level of your anger using a simple 10-point scale, where a rating of 10 means 'very, very angry', 5 means 'moderately angry' and 0 means 'not angry at all'.

Take a look at the example in Table 7-1:

Table 7-1	Rating Your Anger	
What Happened?	*Importance*	*My Anger Level*
My child spilled juice on the sofa.	3	6
I missed my train by one minute.	2	5
My boss blamed me for a mistake made by my co-worker.	4	7
My computer crashed, and I lost the last hour's work.	3	8

Checking your stress balance

You can find out if your anger is excessive and inappropriate by checking your stress balance. Just compare the level of your anger with the importance of the anger-producing situation. Use a 10-point scale, where 10 means 'incredibly important' and 0 means 'not at all important'. Insert that rating next to your description of the distressing situation as above. You're 'in balance' when the two numbers match; you're overreacting if your anger level is higher than the importance of the situation.

If you're in stress balance, chances are your level of anger is appropriate and functional. If not, you're overreacting. If your level of anger is way up there (8s, 9s or 10s), you may be experiencing rage and hostility and not just your typical common-or-garden anger.

Using the examples in Table 7-1, the juice spilled on the sofa is probably an importance level of 3; missing the train, a 2; being unfairly blamed, a 4, and the crashing of the computer, a 3. In each case, the person is overreacting and out of balance.

Modifying your mindset

Most often, your thinking and your perceptions of events are what make you angry.

Thoughts like, 'I was angry because that idiot cut me up in traffic' or 'Missing my train made me angry' suggest that an outside event or circumstance is what caused you to feel anger. But the reality is that these situations and events are only potential triggers that can cause your perceptions and interpretations to create your anger. Like your other stress emotions (anxiety, upset, frustration, and so on), your anger is largely self-created. It is your thinking – your perceptions and interpretations – that play a very important role in creating (and ultimately reducing) your stress.

Thinking about your thinking

See if you can identify your anger-producing thoughts. Ask yourself, 'What could I be saying to myself to make myself angry?' Take a look at Table 7-2 and try to complete it with your own experiences.

Table 7-2	Your Angry Thoughts and the Experiences That Triggered Them
Situation	*My Automatic Thoughts*
My son spilled juice on the sofa.	The sofa is ruined! He should have been more careful! How could he have been so careless? He knew he wasn't supposed to bring food into the living room!
I missed my train by one minute.	This is awful! This always happens! Now my whole day is ruined. I hate this!
My boss blamed me for a mistake made by my co-worker.	
My computer crashed, and I lost the last hour's work.	

Writing down these anger-producing thoughts helps you get a clearer picture of what you're saying to yourself to make yourself angry about a particular situation. By getting in touch with this thinking, you're now in a good position to begin changing that thinking, and thereby reducing the level of your anger.

Finding and fixing your Thinking Errors

Most likely, if your level of anger is excessive or prolonged, you're probably making at least one Thinking Error. Examine your automatic thoughts and see if there are any Thinking Errors to be found. Just about any of the Thinking Errors can result in some form of anger (for example, unrealistic demands).

Using your coping self-talk

When confronted with a potentially anger-provoking situation, you can either say things to yourself that make you angry, or you can say things to yourself that reduce or even eliminate any anger that may have been triggered. By consciously and explicitly talking to yourself, you have a powerful tool that can help you regulate your anger.

Here are some useful examples of anger-reducing self-talk that can help you reduce your level of anger. Choose the ones that best fit your situation, and try coming up with some of your own.

- Is this really worth getting so angry about?
- My getting angry is not going to help anything.
- People can look at things differently from how I do. They always have, and they always will.
- Don't take this personally.
- Let it go. It's not worth the emotional effort.
- I really do not have to feel angry about this if I choose not to.
- Relax. Take a deep breath. Hold it. And let it all out.
- Other people have different priorities.
- Just because someone says something, that doesn't make it true.
- How would Mr or Ms Mental Health handle this?
- Stay calm, stay cool.
- Don't rise to the bait.
- People have the right to be wrong. And often they are.
- Don't judge the person. Judge the behaviour.
- Is this really such a big deal?
- Will I remember this in three years? Three months? Three hours?

Rehearsing your anger

Often you may become angry because you're caught off guard, and your gut reacts before your head has had a chance to evaluate the situation a little more sensibly. One effective strategy for combating this irrational response is to begin to anticipate which situations and circumstances may trigger some of your anger and plan ahead accordingly. Before the situation occurs, rehearse what you will say and how you want to feel. You can always identify upcoming situations in which you know that your chances of becoming angry are pretty high. These situations may be just before you're about to discuss some point of disagreement or contention with someone, and you know that the person will be less than receptive or downright opposed to what you have to say. You may be dealing with a client, a fellow worker, a relative, or a sales assistant at the local shopping centre.

When you can anticipate the situation, imagine it occurring, and then imagine what you will say and how you will act. Your goal, of course, is not to go ballistic or become excessively angry. Choose the words you think will work best. Also, imagine that the other person is getting angry and is close to getting you very angry in turn. Use your coping self-talk. Imagine telling yourself to calm down, to not go for the bait, and keep your anger level low. Rehearse this situation several times in your head. Chances are, when the situation does materialise, you'll be much better prepared to handle it.

Breathing your anger away

When you're angry, your body is probably running in high gear. Your heart rate and blood pressure are up, and just about all the other measures of physiological distress are elevated as well. You can speed up the process of dissipating your anger by adding some physical strategies to your psychological bag of tricks. Relaxing your body is a good place to start. And because you can always find time to breathe, a deep breathing exercise can be an effective way of lowering your body's level of physiological arousal and can make reducing your anger an easier job.

The next time you find yourself getting angry, follow these steps:

1. **Take a deep breath, inhaling through your nostrils.**

   Hold that breath for three or four seconds.

2. **Slowly exhale through your slightly parted lips.**

   Let a wave of relaxation spread from the top of your head, down your body, to your toes.

3. **Wait a little bit, and then take another deep breath.**

   Repeat the process.

You'll feel more physically relaxed and less angry in a very brief period of time.

Seeing the funny side

Humour can be an excellent tool to help you defuse your anger. If you can find something about the anger-triggering situation to make you laugh or at least bring a smile to your face, you can be assured that your anger will be lessened and possibly even eliminated.

Worrying Less

Everybody worries at some time or another. In fact, worrying can be a *good* thing. You *should* worry about some things in your life. Worrying is healthy and appropriate when it motivates you and leads you to attempt to resolve a problem in a productive, adaptive manner. Some people, however, worry far more than they have to, and in turn they do very little to effectively resolve their worries. For these people, much of their stress takes the form of excessive worry. This inordinate and often useless worrying can rob people of much of life's joy and can interfere with their day-to-day functioning. And if a person's worrying becomes chronic, it can result in a wide variety of stress-related conditions and disorders. Controlling and managing your own worries becomes an essential part of managing your stress.

Get off your worry-cycle

Worrying is a process that starts when you perceive an event, situation or circumstance as potentially dangerous or threatening. You think about that situation – at times unconsciously and automatically – and depending on what you say to yourself about that situation, you create varying degrees of emotional stress. If your self-talk is positive and sensible, your stress level will be lower. On the other hand, if your self-talk is negative and irrational, you will cause yourself to feel excessive worry. This worry not only manifests itself emotionally, but also physically, producing all of the symptoms that characterise the fight-or-flight response. And the fight-or-flight response can result in even more worry.

> Situation/event → excessive worrying → physical/emotional stress → more worrying

Think straighter, worry less

If your worrying is excessive, chances are your self-talk and thinking are somewhat out of control, which means that you're probably making one or more Thinking Errors. The following sections outline the major Thinking Errors that can result in excessive worrying and tell you how to avoid those errors yourself. Each of these Thinking Errors can add to your anxiety level, make you worry more than you should, and make your worrying more stress-producing rather than stress-reducing.

Minimising the what-ifs

On the slowest day, some people can find a host of things to worry about. Chronic worriers can find worries in just about any situation. They dissect every potentially dangerous or threatening situation and ask themselves, 'What if. . . ?' Here are some examples of things chronic worriers worry about:

✔ What if that twinge in my shoulder means I'm having a heart attack?

✔ What if the plane crashes on my upcoming flight?

✔ What if my taxi driver is on drugs?

 ✔ What if this pimple turns out to be cancer?

 ✔ What if there's a hailstorm the day my daughter gets married?

You get the idea. One way of minimising your 'what-ifs' is by knowing just how likely it is that your what-if will actually happen.

Knowing the odds

Just about every nasty, scary, threatening event you could imagine has some chance of happening. However, for many, if not most, of these feared occurrences, the chances of them actually *happening* are really very slim. Most of us are not very good at estimating the odds that something will happen. Do you know the chances of your plane crashing or being hijacked, or the odds that you're developing a brain tumour or contracting some strange disease? Probably not. Too often, we worry about the wrong things. We worry about getting rare or unlikely diseases or worry about dying in horrible ways. The irony is, we worry less about not putting on our seat belts, going to our doctor for a regular check-up, or having an accident in the kitchen, all of which have a greater chance of causing us grief than the things we do worry about.

Getting more comfortable with not having control

A sense of not having control can easily trigger stress. We tend to feel uncertain when we feel out of control. In turn, feeling uncertain can create feelings of anxiety and upset. We would like to have control over the unpleasant and unsettling events in our lives, but frequently we can't. We cause ourselves to feel far more stressed than we have to. Becoming more comfortable with uncertainty and a lack of control is an essential part of your programme of stress management.

We can be incredibly limited when it comes to controlling our world and those who live in it. So, the next time you find yourself in a potentially stressful situation, ask yourself: 'How much control do I really have in this situation?' And, if your answer is 'not much', ask yourself a second question: 'Then why am I making myself so stressed?' Sometimes, just acknowledging that you have no control can reduce your level of worry. Because you can't change it, maybe you can accept it. Worrying won't help.

Asking yourself some good questions

People who worry too much tend to be somewhat limited in generating options, alternatives and solutions to potentially stressful problems. This is mainly because their anxiety limits their ability to think outside the box and come up with more creative ideas. They continue to worry in non-productive ways.

See if you can come up with some ideas and solutions that may resolve your worries or at least make your worries less troublesome. Some questions to ask yourself include the following:

✔ What am I afraid of?

✔ Is there another way, a more sensible way, of looking at this?

✔ Am I looking at worst-case scenarios?

✔ How likely is it that what I'm worrying about is really going to happen?

✔ How would someone else (a good friend or a role model, for example) look at this problem?

✔ How would someone who is more of an optimist look at this?

✔ What are some alternatives and solutions that I may have missed?

Using your coping self-talk

You probably have a pretty good idea of the importance we place on talking to yourself in a sensible, reasonable manner. This coping self-talk can help you change the way you feel. In short, it can help you reduce your stress. Using your coping self-talk to reduce (and at times eliminate) your feelings of anger is particularly useful. Here are some examples of coping self-statements that you can use whenever you find yourself over-worrying. See if you can come up with a few of your own.

✔ Don't assume the worst will happen.

✔ I can cope with this.

✔ Take a nice deep breath. Hold it. And let it all out slowly.

✔ Don't make this a bigger deal than it really is.

✔ I'm being a worrywart! Do I always want to be a worrywart?

✔ *Realistically*, what is the worst that can happen?

✔ Is this worrying helping me in any way?

✔ What can I do to distract myself from these worries?

✔ I will be able to figure out ways of coping with this.

✔ Stop 'what-if'-ing.

✔ On my 0–10 scale of importance, how important is this really?

Going for a walk

One of the frequently overlooked ways of coping with worry is to go for a walk. A brisk walk is even more effective. When you're walking, you're distracted, and you're releasing physical stress and tension – all terrific antidotes to stress.

Working up a sweat

Try worrying next time you're jogging, rowing, swimming, lifting, climbing, hitting a golf or tennis ball, or doing any other form of exercise or sport. It's not easy. After about ten minutes of working out on the exercise bike or on the treadmill at the gym, we find it very hard to concentrate on anything. Part of the positive effect comes from the physical relaxation that often follows physical exertion. With your body more relaxed, your mind slows. Also your body may be secreting *endorphins*, hormones that are known to have stress-reducing effects. The bonus: Not only can you control your unwanted worrying, you can stay in shape at the same time.

Talking about it

We feel better and worry less when we've had an opportunity to talk to someone about those things that are bothering us. When we can get our worries out on the table, it gives us some perspective, and with this perspective can come greater feelings of control and hope. Of course, you need someone to tell your worries to. This person could be a family member, a friend, or simply an understanding and sympathetic listener. Some of our best therapy sessions have resulted not from our brilliant insights, but from just letting our clients talk about their worries.

Maintaining a Stress-Resilient Lifestyle

Managing your stress is a little like managing your weight. In the beginning, you're enthusiastic and, with much gusto and determination, you start dropping those pounds. Weeks (or maybe only days) later, your enthusiasm has begun to wane. You're even gaining back any weight that you may have lost. Your attempts at stress reduction can easily fall victim to the same fate. Staying motivated and finding the time to practise your stress-management skills is not that easy.

You may also find that, even though you now have the right tools, you rarely use them. This common situation is much like belonging to a gym and never going. On most days, especially your busier ones, time flies by, and you don't even consider doing anything that even slightly resembles stress management.

Effective stress management means more than having the right stress-reducing tools and techniques. Stress management means knowing how to balance the pressures and demands in your life with positive satisfactions, personal pleasures and a lifestyle that insulates you from the negative impact of stress. This chapter shows you how to create that balance and how to use these positives to enhance your overall stress resilience.

Make an appointment with yourself

When you schedule something, you're more likely to follow through with it. You almost always show up for appointments with your doctor, your dentist, your lawyer, your accountant, your dinner-date, and the person who cuts your hair. So why not use that same principle for other things in your life, like managing your stress? Try some of the following suggestions:

✔ Schedule regular times during the week when you will do something to manage your stress. Make Thursdays 'Lunch-with-a-Friend Day'. Schedule Monday and Wednesday evenings as health club times.

✔ Make your coffee break a stress break. Set aside a few minutes mid-morning and mid-afternoon to drain some of that accumulating tension from your mind and body.

✔ Commit part of each lunch hour to some stress-reducing activity. Go to the gym or try meditating in a nearby park for 20 minutes.

✔ Designate specific chunks of time during your week as times when you do the kinds of activities you normally wouldn't. While these activities will be specific stress-management techniques, they can also be activities that are diverting and relaxing: listening to music, taking in a film, going for a swim, playing squash or tennis.

Finding your oasis (sand optional)

To effectively manage your stress, you need a place where you can escape the pressures and demands of everything going on around you. In fact, you need several such places. Ideally, these should be places that are quiet, peaceful and relaxing. These places become your oasis – your places of refuge in a stress-filled world. Places like this usually aren't that easy to come by. A wood-panelled study or a Zen garden may only be wishful figments of your imagination. The reality is, the place you use as an oasis may be your bathroom or your bedroom. But these can just as easily serve as places you retreat to when your soul needs a little peace and tranquillity. Continue to add to your list of peaceful places. Your oases don't need to be magnificent. All you need is a place where, for at least a small part of the day, you won't be disturbed. In the following sections, we start you off with some suggestions.

Create an inner sanctum

Try to create a space within your home that you really like to spend time in. Have at least one feel-good room or an area that is emotionally welcoming. Your private corner can be anywhere – maybe a window seat, a warm kitchen, an inviting bedroom or a cosy study – that you can close a door and feel hidden away from it all, where you feel unhurried and unhassled. This place is your inner sanctum, a space within a space to which you can retreat when the world outside feels less than hospitable, a place where you can sit, read, write, think, meditate or just daydream. Designate this space as somewhere that you don't worry, pay bills, answer the phone, or do anything else that could even remotely increase your level of stress. The rewards of having a quiet retreat are immense.

Take a bath

The bathroom may be the only room in your house where you feel like you can lock the door and be alone. One of the many things you can do in a bathroom is take a bath. A hot bath is a wonderful place to relax and totally let go. Stretched out and surrounded by warmth, in a bath you can give yourself permission to relax. Adding some soft lighting, gentle music and a soothing drink can make this place feel like heaven.

Park a while

Most towns and cities have wonderful parks where you can stroll aimlessly, taking in the activity around you, or becoming lost in your own thoughts and images. In the larger parks, you can often find yourself quite alone, one of the few places were there is no one else around. But the park doesn't have to be large. Some are no more than a small patch of grass, a few trees, and a bench or two. When we can, we find that walking through the park on our way to the office or coming home after work is a wonderful way of mellowing out and dissociating from a busy day.

Jogging and cycling in the park are great ways of combining exercise with a sense of solitude. You can bring headphones or, better still, simply enjoy being alone with your thoughts.

Seek sanctuary

We tend to think of houses of worship as religious sanctuaries, places for prayer. And, of course, they are. But churches and temples can also be visited for non-religious forms of expression. You can reflect, meditate or simply lose yourself in reverie. They are quiet and often softly lit – ideal settings in which to be alone. Many churches and temples are quite majestic and sweeping in their architecture, inspiring and revitalising even the most tired spirit. And, except for Midnight Mass and Yom Kippur, for example, your chances of finding an empty pew are excellent.

Become a lobbyist

Many hotels, especially some of the older ones, are wonderful buildings that can be a treat to spend time in. You won't be alone here, but chances are you won't be bothered. Although many people are coming and going, don't be surprised if you find a comfortable chair situated in a relatively quiet part of the lobby.

Got a life?

Respond to the following statements with 'very much', 'so-so' or 'not really'.

✔ I have family I can rely on when I need to.

✔ I have friends I can talk to when problems arise.

✔ I have friends I enjoy spending time with.

✔ I have hobbies and/or interests I enjoy.

✔ I look forward to certain activities during the week.

✔ I get satisfaction from the work I do.

✔ I find my life satisfying and involving.

✔ My spiritual beliefs give me support and comfort.

✔ I enjoy meeting new people.

✔ I like trying new things.

✔ I take a holiday regularly.

✔ I enjoy nature and the outdoors.

✔ I frequently do things that are fun.

✔ I have an adequate income.

✔ I do things for others less fortunate.

Lose yourself in the shelves

Bookshops, especially the larger ones, can be marvellous places to sit, write and escape the pressures all around you. You may consider your local bookstore as your personal library. It's a great place to escape to a quieter mode. The catch? It can be a madhouse at weekends. On good days, however, the unhurried, not crowded floors, lined with wonderful books, become an inviting setting to which you can retreat.

And don't forget the public libraries. Libraries, especially the larger ones, are great places to spend an hour or more in relative solitude. Large tables, vast spaces and enforced quiet all contribute to an ideal place to work, think and imagine.

Accentuate the positive (s)

When you think of reducing your stress, most often you think of ways of eliminating, or at least minimising the negatives in your life. Get rid of as many of those unpleasant pressures and demands, and your life will be much less stressful. However, creating a lifestyle that is truly stress-resilient means not only eliminating the negatives, it also means finding and building in positive sources of satisfaction and pleasure that compensate for those negatives that you haven't been able to eliminate. We call these your stress buffers. They include a wide range of activities, involvements and commitments that bring positive feelings to your life.

Get a life

One of the keys to creating a stress-resilient lifestyle is living more than a one-dimensional life. This means looking at your lifestyle and figuring out what's missing. Complete the checklist in the 'Got a life? box to determine whether your lifestyle is providing you with the stress buffers that are important in helping you resist the negative effects of stress.

Connecting with others

Having people in your life you can talk to, complain to, cry with and laugh with – not to mention go see a film with – represent important stress buffers in your life. Connecting with family members and with friends becomes one of the more important ways you can insulate yourself from stress and strengthen your ability to cope.

Family: The ties that bind

Although, at times, your family may seem like the source of much of your stress, for most people, family members can be an important source of caring and emotional support. After all, there are very few other people in your life who know you as well, and are by your side when the chips are down. Being with family, and sharing memories of times past can provide you with a sense of being part of something larger, something that feels warm and comforting. Family events such as birthdays, anniversaries, marriages, christenings and bar and bas mitzvahs all bring with them a sense of repeated experience and family reunion and provide you with a sense of emotional connectedness that can buffer you from stress.

However, as you well know, maintaining family ties and holding on to those good feelings takes some effort. Make the time to be with those you care about. Work at making these relationships positive and satisfying. It's worth it.

You need a Monica, a Rachel or a Chandler

When you ask people what they value most in life, near the top of that list, right under family, is friends. Most of us regret, or will come to regret, that we neglect our friendships at the expense of other, often less rewarding activities. We wish we had spent more time with friends, called them more often, and worked harder to maintain and nurture our friendships.

Your friendships are probably your most important stress buffers. Friends provide company for you, bring you pleasure, and help relieve feelings of loneliness. Good friends listen to your problems, give you guidance, and support you emotionally. They are your therapists.

People with a strong social support system report experiencing less stress and are better able to cope with the stress that they do feel. Studies show that friendships can insulate you from the effects of stress in your life.

Having friends can lower your blood pressure, improve your immune system, and even increase your life span. In one research study of some 7,000 women conducted over 17 years, the researchers found that those women who had few friendships had a higher risk of dying from all kinds of cancer. Having good friends, it appeared, was even more protective than being in a marriage. Another study found that among patients with coronary heart disease, those individuals who were neither married nor had close friends were more likely to die in a five-year period than were those who were married, had a close friend, or both. It seems that having friends and family can reduce the destructive effects of stress on your body.

Do something, anything, and have fun

Finding satisfaction in a hobby or interest is an important way of reducing your stress. Any hobby – whether it's collecting beer cans or stuffed animals, doing some bird-watching, or whatever else suits your fancy – can be absorbing and diverting. The fact is, it really doesn't matter that much what you do. It's a big mistake to reject or abandon a hobby because you think it's unworthy, or less esteemed by others. What counts is that you're doing something. Leave your ego out of it.

Join the group

Every city or town has groups and organisations that can put you together with other like-minded people: for example, a local church, school group, special interest group, and so on.

Learn a thing or two

You have numerous opportunities to attend classes or join a course on something you find interesting: for example, cookery classes, dancing or music lessons, and so on.

Get in the game

Or, consider getting involved in a sport or a game: for example, tennis, golf, swimming, and so on.

Get a pet

Having a pet is a marvellous way of combating your stress. Convincing data shows that pets can indeed reduce your stress, and serve as important sources of emotional comfort. The presence of a pet in the room can put you at ease, evoke feelings of caring and tenderness, and provide you with a companion. Pets can lower your blood pressure, make you feel more relaxed, and distract you from your own day-to-day worries and concerns.

Cultivate calm

Working in a garden can be satisfying. You can find something soothing and peaceful about potting a petunia or tending to a tomato. Why? Because you're in control. The pace is your own, with no one telling you what you're doing wrong or giving you a deadline. It's just you and nature. Your garden doesn't need to be extensive. It can be a small terrace, a shared plot of ground, an indoor herb garden in the winter months, or simply several house plants that you water and prune. A window-box works well, too – the effects are the same. A few square yards of paradise can bring a large measure of tranquillity to your life.

Cook, bake, grill, fry

Baking is especially comforting because of the wonderful aromas that emanate from the oven. Eating the end result is great fun too. Of course, this may not be the most exciting idea for you if you already spend hours in the kitchen supplying the rest of your family with sustenance. In that case, booking dinner out may be your idea of a good way to relieve stress.

Sometimes it's the little things

Here's a list of some simpler pleasures that can add to the quality of your life:

- The smell of newly cut grass
- Writing to a friend
- Spring rain
- New snow on a moonlit street
- The smell of the air after rain
- Someone's perfume
- The warmth of the sun
- Rustling leaves in the autumn
- The smell of burning wood
- The sound of children laughing
- The crackling of an open fire

- The smell of freshly baked cakes
- Birds chirping in the morning
- Sunrises and sunsets
- Completing a task

Get out of the house

When was the last time you did one of the following?

- Went out for dinner
- Went to the cinema
- Went dancing
- Saw a play
- Heard a concert
- People-watched
- Went to a nightclub
- Strolled in the park
- Went shopping just for fun
- Explored a new neighbourhood
- Saw a dance performance
- Went to a sports event
- Had lunch with friends
- Went to a museum
- Went to an art gallery

Take the time to find joy in the little things and to explore some new avenues – and reduce your stress while you're at it.

Taking a holiday

Holidays are a wonderful way of regrouping and regaining some perspective on your life. Try building in more frequent, shorter trips. These can take the form of half-days away, day trips, sleepovers, weekends, and long weekends. Think of your time away as a safety valve that needs to be opened from time to time. The trick is to evenly distribute these getaways throughout your year, before the pressure builds.

Taking your fun seriously

Ask yourself when was the last time you did something that was pure fun. When was the last time you just played? Or did nothing? Sometimes, doing nothing or having fun is just what the doctor ordered. It may seem sinful and decadent, and you may feel your guilt level rising just thinking about it, but taking time to do nothing really is an important part of your stress-management programme. Playing or taking time off can distract you from your problems. It can give you time to regroup and regain some equilibrium. You return to your world refreshed, and ready to jump back into the fray.

Index

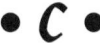

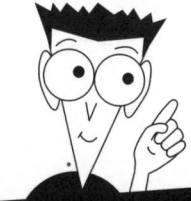

FOR DUMMIES®

Making Everything Easier! ™

UK editions

BUSINESS

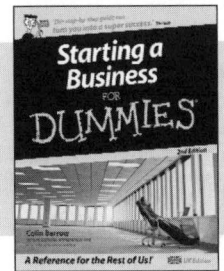

978-0-470-51806-9

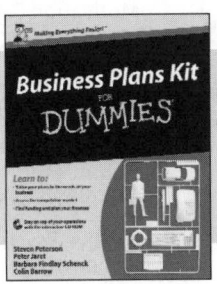

978-0-470-74381-2

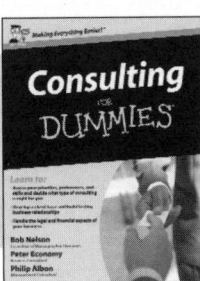

978-0-470-71382-2

FINANCE

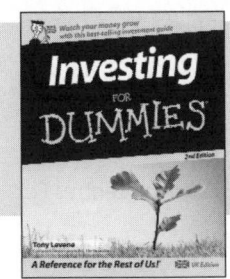

978-0-470-99280-7

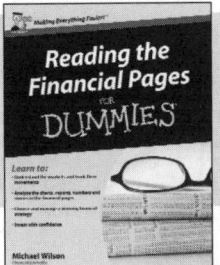

978-0-470-71432-4

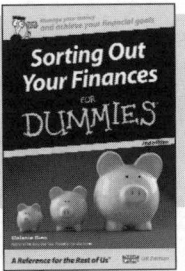

978-0-470-69515-9

HOBBIES

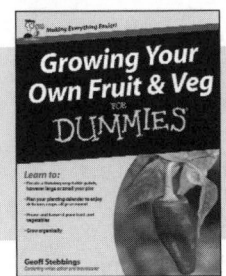

978-0-470-69960-7

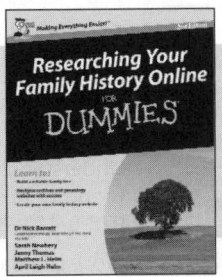

978-0-470-74535-9

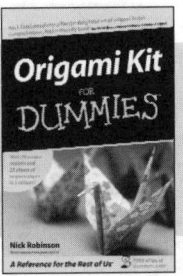

978-0-470-75857-1

British Sign Language
For Dummies
978-0-470-69477-0

Business NLP For Dummies
978-0-470-69757-3

Competitive Strategy For Dummies
978-0-470-77930-9

Cricket For Dummies
978-0-470-03454-5

CVs For Dummies, 2nd Edition
978-0-470-74491-8

Digital Marketing For Dummies
978-0-470-05793-3

Divorce For Dummies, 2nd Edition
978-0-470-74128-3

eBay.co.uk Business All-in-One
For Dummies
978-0-470-72125-4

Emotional Freedom Technique For
Dummies
978-0-470-75876-2

English Grammar For Dummies
978-0-470-05752-0

Flirting For Dummies
978-0-470-74259-4

Golf For Dummies
978-0-470-01811-8

Green Living For Dummies
978-0-470-06038-4

Hypnotherapy For Dummies
978-0-470-01930-6

IBS For Dummies
978-0-470-51737-6

Lean Six Sigma For Dummies
978-0-470-75626-3

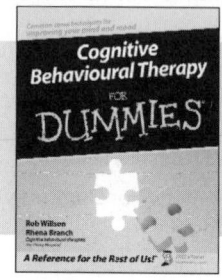
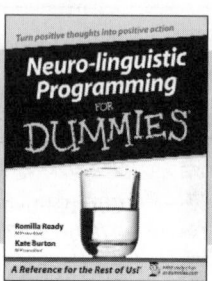
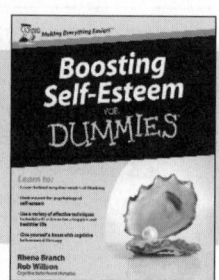
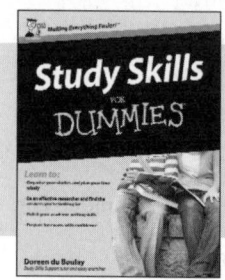
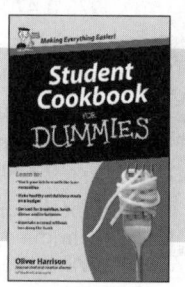
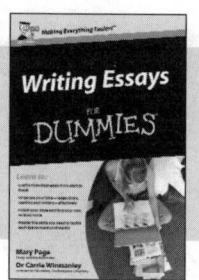
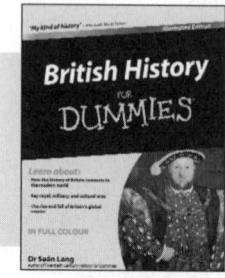
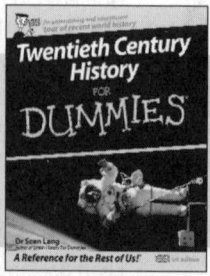
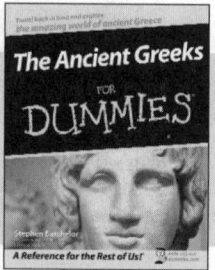

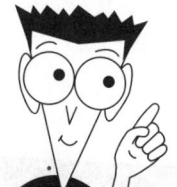

FOR DUMMIES®

The easy way to get more done and have more fun

LANGUAGES

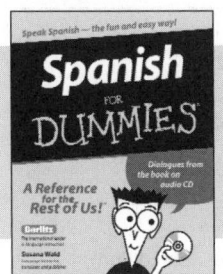

978-0-7645-5194-9

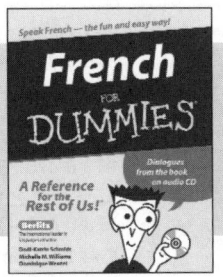

978-0-7645-5193-2

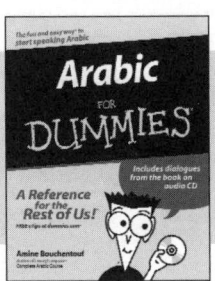

978-0-471-77270-5

MUSIC

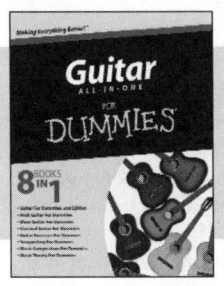

978-0-470-48133-2

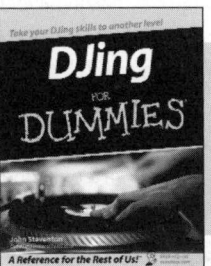

978-0-470-03275-6
UK Edition

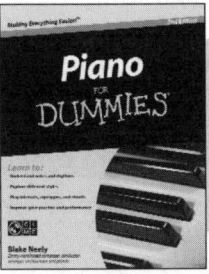

978-0-470-49644-2

SCIENCE & MATHS

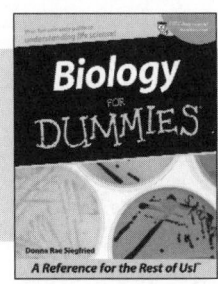

978-0-7645-5326-4

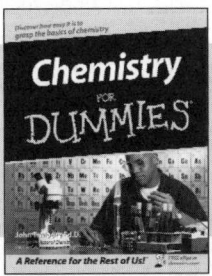

978-0-7645-5430-8

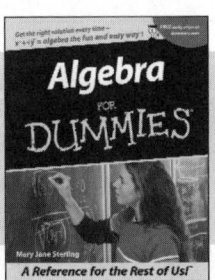

978-0-7645-5325-7

Art For Dummies
978-0-7645-5104-8

Bass Guitar For Dummies
978-0-7645-2487-5

Brain Games For Dummies
978-0-470-37378-1

Christianity For Dummies
978-0-7645-4482-8

Criminology For Dummies
978-0-470-39696-4

Forensics For Dummies
978-0-7645-5580-0

German For Dummies
978-0-7645-5195-6

Hobby Farming For Dummies
978-0-470-28172-7

Index Investing For Dummies
978-0-470-29406-2

Jewelry Making & Beading
For Dummies
978-0-7645-2571-1

Knitting For Dummies, 2nd Edition
978-0-470-28747-7

Music Composition For Dummies
978-0-470-22421-2

Physics For Dummies
978-0-7645-5433-9

Schizophrenia For Dummies
978-0-470-25927-6

Sex For Dummies, 3rd Edition
978-0-470-04523-7

Solar Power Your Home For Dummies
978-0-470-17569-9

Tennis For Dummies
978-0-7645-5087-4

The Koran For Dummies
978-0-7645-5581-7

Wine All-in-One For Dummies
978-0-470-47626-0

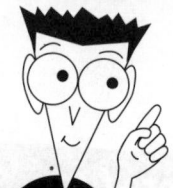

FOR DUMMIES®

Helping you expand your horizons and achieve your potential

COMPUTER BASICS

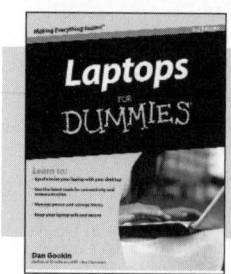

978-0-470-27759-1

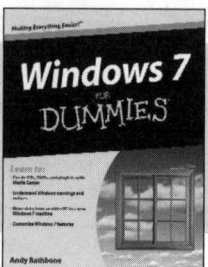

978-0-470-13728-4

978-0-470-49743-2

DIGITAL PHOTOGRAPHY

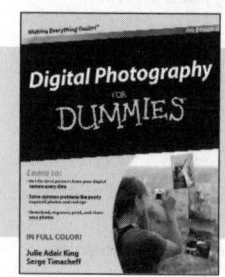

978-0-470-25074-7

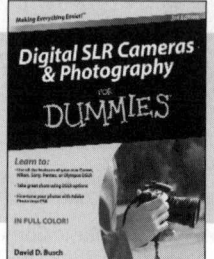

978-0-470-46606-3

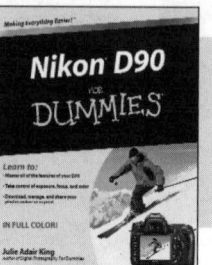

978-0-470-45772-6

MAC BASICS

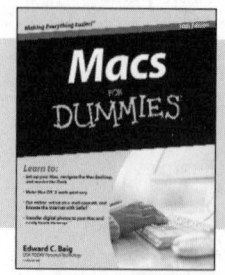

978-0-470-27817-8

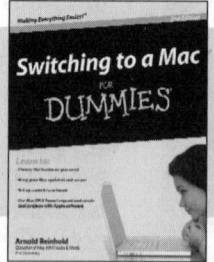

978-0-470-46661-2

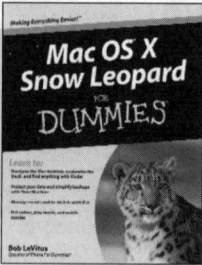

978-0-470-43543-4

Access 2007 For Dummies
978-0-470-04612-8

Adobe Creative Suite 4 Design
Premium All-in-One Desk Reference
For Dummies
978-0-470-33186-6

AutoCAD 2010 For Dummies
978-0-470-43345-4

C++ For Dummies, 6th Edition
978-0-470-31726-6

Computers For Seniors For Dummies ,
2nd Edition
978-0-470-53483-0

Dreamweaver CS4 For Dummies
978-0-470-34502-3

Excel 2007 All-In-One Desk Reference
For Dummies
978-0-470-03738-6

Green IT For Dummies
978-0-470-38688-0

Networking All-in-One Desk Reference
For Dummies, 3rd Edition
978-0-470-17915-4

Office 2007 All-in-One Desk Reference
For Dummies
978-0-471-78279-7

Photoshop CS4 For Dummies
978-0-470-32725-8

Photoshop Elements 7 For Dummies
978-0-470-39700-8

Search Engine Optimization
For Dummies, 3rd Edition
978-0-470-26270-2

The Internet For Dummies,
11th Edition
978-0-470-12174-0

Visual Studio 2008 All-In-One Desk
Reference For Dummies
978-0-470-19108-8

Web Analytics For Dummies
978-0-470-09824-0

Windows Vista For Dummies
978-0-471-75421-3